THE AIRWAY
EMERGENCY MANAGEMENT

The Airway Emergency Management

ROBERT H. DAILEY, M.D.
Clinical Professor of Medicine
University of California at San Francisco
San Francisco, California
Staff Emergency Physician
Summit Medical Center
Oakland, California

BARRY SIMON, M.D.
Assistant Clinical Professor of Medicine
University of California at San Francisco
San Francisco, California
Highland General Hospital
Oakland, California

GARY P. YOUNG, M.D.,
Associate Professor of Emergency Medicine
Assistant Professor of Internal Medicine
Oregon Health Sciences University
Chief, Emergency Medicine Service
Medical Director
Emergency Care Unit
Portland Veterans Affairs Medical Center
Portland, Oregon

RONALD D. STEWART, M.D., F.R.C.P.C.
Professor of Anesthesia (Emergency Medicine)
Dalhousie University
Attending Staff
Department of Emergency Medicine
Victoria General Hospital
Halifax, Nova Scotia, Canada

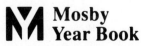 **Mosby Year Book**

St. Louis   Baltimore   Boston   Chicago   London   Philadelphia   Sydney   Toronto

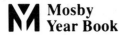
Mosby
Year Book

Dedicated to Publishing Excellence

Sponsoring Editor: James F. Shanahan
Assistant Editor: Joyce-Rachel John
Associate Managing Editor, Manuscript Services: Deborah Thorp
Senior Production Assistant: Maria Nevinger
Proofroom Manager: Barbara Kelly

Mosby–Year Book, Inc.
11830 Westline Industrial Drive
St. Louis, MO 63146

1 2 3 4 5 6 7 8 9 0 CL MV 96 95 94 93 92

Library of Congress Cataloging-in-Publication Data
The Airway : emergency management / [edited by] Robert H.
Dailey . . .
    [et al.].
        p.   cm.
    Includes bibliographical references and index.
    ISBN 0-8016-1270-5
    1. Respiratory intensive care.   2. Airway (Medicine)
  3. Respiratory organs—Obstructions.   4. Medical
emergencies.
    I. Dailey, Robert H., 1935–
    [DNLM: 1. Airway Obstruction—
therapy.   2. Emergencies.
    3. Intubation.   WF 140 A298]
    RC735.R48A47   1993   92-5948
    616.2'00425—dc20   CIP
    DNLM/DLC
    for Library of Congress

CONTRIBUTORS

DIANE M. BIRNBAUMER, M.D.
Assistant Clinical Professor of Medicine
UCLA
Associate Residency Director
Department of Emergency Medicine
Harbor-UCLA Medical Center
Torrance, California

STEPHEN V. CANTRILL, M.D.
Assistant Professor of Clinical Emergency Medicine
University of Colorado
Continuing Medical Education Coordinator
Denver General Hospital
Denver, Colorado

FREDERICK B. CARLTON, JR., M.D.
Associate Professor at Medicine
Director, Division of Emergency Medicine
University of Mississippi School of Medicine
Jackson, Mississippi

JONATHAN T. CLARKE, M.D.
Assistant Clinical Professor
Department of Anesthesia
University of California at San Francisco
San Francisco, California
Pediatric Anesthesiologist
Children's Hospital
Oakland, California

ROBERT H. DAILEY, M.D.
Clinical Professor of Medicine
University of California at San Francisco
San Francisco, California
Staff Emergency Physician
Samuel Merritt Hospital
Oakland, California

MOHAMUD DAYA, M.D., F.A.C.E.P.
Assistant Professor
Department of Medicine
University of Toronto
Emergency Department Physician
The Toronto Hospital
Toronto, Canada

DAVID K. ENGLISH, M.D.
Clinical Instructor in Medicine
University of California at San Francisco
San Francisco, California
Assistant Chief
Emergency Medicine

Highland General Hospital
Oakland, California

WILLIAM FEASTER, M.D.
Director, Department of Anesthesiology
Children's Hospital
Oakland, California

CHRISTOPHER FERNANDES, M.D., F.A.C.E.P.
Assistant Professor
Department of Medicine
University of Toronto
Staff Physician
The Toronto Hospital
Toronto, Canada

DAVID GOUGH, D.O.
Former Attending Faculty
Emergency Medicine Residency Program
Madigan Army Medical Center
Tacoma, Washington
Attending Physician
St. Luke's Regional Medical Center
Boise, Idaho

STEVEN HULSEY, M.D.
Emergency Physician
North Bay Medical Center
Fairfield, California

KEVIN HUTTON, M.D.
Assistant Clinical Professor of Medicine
Department of Emergency Medicine
University of California at San Diego Medical Center
San Diego, California

JAY A. JOHANNIGMAN, M.D.
Assistant Professor of Surgery
Uniformed Services University of Health Science
Medical Director
Surgical Intensive Care Service
Wilford Hall United States Air Force Medical Center
San Antonio, Texas

JON JUI, M.D.
Assistant Professor of Emergency Medicine
Oregon Health Sciences University
Portland, Oregon

ROY MAGNUSSON, M.D., F.A.C.E.P.
Assistant Professor
Director, Emergency Medicine Residency Program
Oregon Health Sciences University
Portland, Oregon

RONALD MARIANI, E.M.T.-P.
Clinical Instructor
Oregon Health Sciences University
Firefighter/Paramedic
Portland Fire Bureau
Flight Paramedic
Emanual Hospital Lifeflight
Portland, Oregon

CHERYL MELICK, M.D.
Chief Resident of Emergency Medicine
Denver General Hospital
Denver, Colorado

WILLIAM S. MEZZANOTTE, M.D.
Instructor of Medicine
Division of Pulmonary Sciences
University of Colorado Health Science Center
Denver, Colorado

MICHAEL F. MURPHY, M.D., F.R.C.P.C.
Assistant Professor of Anaesthesia
Dalhousie University
Director of Emergency Medicine
IWK Children's Hospital
Halifax, Nova Scotia, Canada

JAMES T. NIEMANN, M.D.
Associate Professor of Medicine
UCLA School of Medicine
Director of Research
Department of Emergency Medicine
Harbor-UCLA Medical Center
Los Angeles, California

STEVEN PACE, M.D., F.A.C.E.P.
Faculty Physician
Emergency Medicine Residency
Madigan Army Medical Center
Fort Lewis, Washington

JAMES E. POINTER, M.D., F.A.C.E.P.
Associate Clinical Professor
University of California at San Francisco
EMS Medical Director
City and County of San Francisco
San Francisco, California
Staff Emergency Physician
Providence Hospital
Oakland, California

CHARLES V. POLLOCK, M.D.
Associate Director of Emergency Medicine Research
Department of Emergency Medicine
Attending Physician
Maricopa Medical Center
Phoenix, Arizona

THOMAS PURCELL, M.D., F.A.C.E.P.
Adjunct Assistant Professor
Department of Medicine
UCLA
Los Angeles, California
Residency Director
Department of Emergency Medicine
Kern Medical Center
Bakersfield, California

DAVID M. RODMAN, M.D.
Assistant Professor of Medicine
University of Colorado Health Sciences Center
Director, Adult Cystic Fibrosis Center
University Hospital
Denver, Colorado

JEDD ROE, M.D.
Assistant Professor
Division of Emergency Medicine
Department of Surgery
University of Colorado Medical School
Assistant Director
Paramedic Division
Department of Health and Hospitals
Denver, Colorado

HERBERT ROGOVE, M.D.
Clinical Associate Professor of Medicine
Ohio State University
Director, Intensive Care Unit
Riverside Methodist Hospitals
Columbus, Ohio

PETER ROSEN, M.D.
Adjunct Professor of Medicine and Surgery
Director, Emergency Medicine Residency Program
Director of Education
Department of Emergency Medicine
University of California at San Diego Medical Center
San Diego, California

TERRI A. SCHMIDT, M.D.
Assistant Professor
Department of Emergency Medicine
Oregon Health Sciences University
Portland, Oregon

JAMES SCOTT, M.D.
Assistant Dean for Student Affairs
Associate Professor
Department of Emergency Medicine
The George Washington University Medical Center
Washington, D.C.

SARAH K. SCOTT, M.D.
Assistant Professor of Surgery
University of Colorado
Staff Physician
Emergency Medicine Services
Denver General Hospital
Denver, Colorado

BARRY SIMON, M.D.
Assistant Clinical Professor of Medicine
University of California at San Francisco
San Francisco, California
Highland General Hospital
Oakland, California

RONALD STEWART, M.D., F.R.C.P.C.
Professor of Anaesthesia (Emergency Medicine)
Dalhousie University
Attending Staff
Department of Emergency Medicine
Victoria General Hospital
Halifax, Nova Scotia, Canada

GLENN F. TOKARSKI, M.D.
Henry Ford Hospital
Henry Ford Health Systems
Detroit, Michigan

SUSAN W. TOLLE, M.D.
Associate Professor of Medicine
Oregon Health Sciences University
Director, Center for Ethics in Health Care
University Hospital
Portland, Oregon

RON M. WALLS, M.D., F.R.C.P.C.
Associate Professor and Head
Division of Emergency Medicine
Department of Surgery
University of British Columbia
Head, Department of Emergency Medicine
Vancouver General Hospital
Vancouver, British Columbia, Canada

RICHARD WOLFE, M.D.
Assistant Professor
University of Colorado Health Sciences Center
Associate Residency Director
Denver General Hospital
Denver, Colorado

GARY P. YOUNG, M.D.
Associate Professor of Emergency Medicine
Assistant Professor of Internal Medicine
Oregon Health Sciences University
Chief, Emergency Medicine Service
Medical Director
Emergency Care Unit
Portland Veterans Affairs Medical Center
Portland, Oregon

FOREWORD

The specialty of emergency medicine has now achieved an accepted presence within the corps of accepted medical specialties. While it may still require time and experience for all physicians to understand the field, the reality is that patients still present to the emergency department for the management of acute medical problems with greater frequency than with which they enter the medical delivery system through any other route.

It is true that most such emergency department visits do not represent life or limb threatening emergencies, but that does not relieve the burden of the emergency physician who must not only recognize the critical life threat in all its manifestations, subtle as well as obvious, but be prepared to intervene to achieve stabilization of that threat. This must often be done with a paucity of information, a scarcity of resources, and a lack of assistance from colleagues expert in other specialties.

The most critical of these problems is the expert management of the airway. Not only must the emergency physician be technically deft in ability, but it is almost always the case that those techniques must be performed on patients with the worst anatomy and preparation. For example, the anesthesiologist for elective intubations has the protection of working with a patient who has an empty stomach. The emergency physician almost always has a patient with a full stomach, altered consciousness, and a deteriorated physiology that leaves little room for anything but immediate success.

Given these difficulties, it is long since time that there is one place to which the practitioner, resident in training, and student can turn to assist with the knowledge that is requisite for these critical tasks.

It is this book that will play such a role, and for which I have been waiting impatiently for over 20 years. The question of who needs immediate intubation is one to which there is no easy answer. Even the patient in respiratory arrest, a condition that almost everyone thinks of to head the list of mandatory indications, may have this easily reversed in the right circumstances. There is little if any consensus on other mandatory indications. When there is a paucity of time to act, the emergency physician must possess the knowledge with which to respond rather than to try to solve the puzzle with the patient gasping his way into hypoxic arrest.

Not only is this knowledge not generally available, but there is also little consensus on what are the best techniques, what is the safest pharmacology, what are some of the most useful tricks derived from real encounters in busy emergency departments.

The authors of this text are all practicing emergency physicians. They come from a wide body of practice, and they have extensive experience with the clinical scenarios and the difficult problems with which the book is concerned.

There is no person involved with the care of the emergency patient who will not derive increased knowledge, as well as a sense of increased confidence, with which to approach the difficult airway problem. Sometimes the hardest part of any action is in its commencement. Having some clues as to when to initiate that action takes the physician a long way down the path to the desired success.

Even though it will be impossible not to present material that varies from your own experience and practice since as stated above there is no consensus upon these difficult matters, it will be profitable to challenge your own way of thinking and practice. Just trying to organize in your own mind the approach to these problems, and the suggested solutions, will help the next time you encounter the difficult patient.

In addition to the question of who needs the immediate intervention, there are the further difficult decisions: what route shall be most safely taken; when should the patient be paralyzed; when should surgical airway be utilized; what pharmacology is useful; what sedatives can be employed; what's different about the child?

Even if you have spent considerable time and effort in answering these questions for yourself, and feel comfortable with the answers, this text provides a wonderful opportunity to review the answers of many of the leaders in the field of emergency medicine.

Even after many years of facing these problems in busy emergency departments, I am still confounded by the variety of difficult airway problems that still present as new dilemmas.

I only wish that I had instant recall of everything in this book, had the combined experience of its authors, and could call upon their advice when I most needed it.

Without the ability to respond to the most critical life threats, there is no point in having a specialty of emergency medicine. It is therefore comforting to know that this excellent resource is available to provide the knowledge that leads to confident competency.

I am sure that our patients will be the recipients of improved management because of the wisdom of this book; and that, after all, is the main point of our specialty.

PETER ROSEN, M.D.
Adjunct Professor of Medicine and Surgery
Director, Emergency Medicine Residency Program
Director of Education
Department of Emergency Medicine
University of California at San Diego
San Diego, California

PREFACE

It may seem strange that this text has not already been written. The airway is the most critical aspect of acute care and has been one of the major components of anesthesia, critical care, trauma, cardiothoracic surgery, emergency medicine, and prehospital care. But, paradoxically, the fact that the emergency airway cuts across so many disciplines may be the very reason that none of them has taken it as its own. Furthermore, only in the past 25 years have the necessary knowledge and skills, experience, and consciousness developed to allow an in-depth examination of the subject. Looking back to the late 1950s and early 1960s when I began my medical career, I remember critically ill patients in dimly lit wards slipping into shock and then ventilatory failure, placed "close to the nurse's desk" for their imminent demise. The terminal "death rattle" of uncleared secretions often precipitated the final knell—a bloody bedside tracheostomy.

But look at what has happened: the ability to quantify ventilation and metabolic status by arterial blood gas (ABG) determinations, the establishment of intensive care units, and the development of instrumentation for measuring both cardiovascular and pulmonary physiology; the emergence of the endotracheal tube from the confines of the operating room; the development of mechanical ventilators and the initiation of BLS and ACLS courses that emphasize and codify airway support procedures; and, finally, the development of the specialty of emergency medicine, which has embraced the emergency airway as one of its most important components.

Yet as far as we have come, this text is largely an article of faith—much of what is presented is based solely on the experience and opinion of its authors; little has been subjected to the hard light of formal inquiry. For this we do not apologize; there is much clinical maturity here. However, further examination and research must be stimulated by the text and will make the following editions more informed, more advanced, and more authoritative. The con-

tent is meant first and foremost to be *practical and relevant to clinical practice*. Nevertheless, it must draw upon sound physiologic and anatomic principles. All sections have had computer literature searches to assure currency and completeness. Unfortunately, too often such searches have been relatively barren, underscoring the need for further experience and study.

At the outset, Section I provides an overall conceptual framework by examining in detail the three pillars upon which rest successful airway management. These three pillars are: (1) integrity of airflow, (2) protection from pulmonary aspiration, and (3) assurance of adequate ventilation/oxygenation (Figure). All clinical threats are to one or more of these "pillars," and all therapeutic interventions must take into consideration *all* of these factors. The design/evolution of the body is a series of compromises or tradeoffs between necessary functions; what is good design for some functions may be bad for others. Furthermore, more complex and interlocking func-

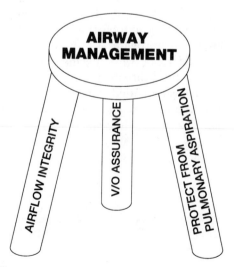

FIGURE.
Three pillars of successful airway management. V/O = ventilation-oxygenation.

tions demand numerous organs and complex physiologic interrelationships, making those functions more susceptible to disease and malfunction. Sometimes we may not be able to discern what advantages are conferred by a particular structuring. The airway is no exception. For example, ideally, respiration should be facilitated and protected so that the lungs are connected directly to their external oxygen source, without the interposition of other structures or functions. But air needs to be warmed, humidified, and filtered, demanding a nose and nasopharynx, entraining the possibility of obstruction, secretions, and bleeding. Speech demands a tongue and a larynx with airflow across it, introducing two critical sites for airflow obstruction. And the sharing of a common orifice for alimentation and respiration (conferring what advantage?) means that an organ of alimentation (stomach) can spill into and damage the organ of respiration (lung). Although the clever capping of the airway (epiglottis) usually serves with distinction to prevent such aspiration, critical illnesses sometimes cause fatal lapses. This functional "conflict of interest" further poses a therapeutic problem: the endotracheal tube needed to control airway or ventilation problems must be directed along an angled path into a narrow opening that is not visible externally.

Sections II and III progress from the anatomy and physiology of the three pillars to their practical clinical applications. Section II outlines the skills/techniques (maneuvers) for establishing and maintaining the airway, including pharmacological aids and ventilators. These maneuvers are described in detail, taking into account complicating factors, and emphasizing useful "tricks" if initial approaches fail, yet utilizing only those tools that might be mastered by a primary care provider.

Section III deals with specific common clinical situations that pose threats to the airway. Each clinical situation is subdivided into its various scenarios (variations on a theme), e.g., the clinical situation of grand mal seizures is subdivided into the scenarios

of (1) the postictal period, (2) the presumed isolated seizure, and (3) status epilepticus. In most clinical situations (e.g., COPD) variations are written according to a format of "stable" (ventilatory insufficiency), "crashing" (ventilatory failure), and "crashed" (ventilatory failure with decreased level of consciousness and/or circulatory consequences).

Algorithms are provided for each clinical situation and its scenarios. These are intended to simulate clinical thinking and a realistic flow of events. However, they should not be interpreted rigidly. No two real clinical situations are ever exactly alike, so clinical approaches must be adjusted accordingly. Overall, the authors have taken into account risks vs. benefits, advantages vs. disadvantages, cost-effectiveness, reality-testing, variability of knowledge and skills of the physician, and conflicting priorities (e.g., cervical spine vs. airway control). Sometimes, there may not be a *good* or "right" solution, but rather only a best bad one. Often we end in dilemmas, difficult/fuzzy choices, unfortunate options, and hastily improvised maneuvers. The unusual format of these chapters combined with the difficulties of real-world emergency airway management have translated into enormous difficulties for the authors. These difficulties have been compounded by the fact that true airway emergencies are uncommon in clinical practice, and little detailed literature is currently available that is relevant to the unstructured emergency situation.

We ask the readers' indulgence in the face of these problems. This is a first run. We hope that it will stimulate discussion, controversy, and, yes, even heated disagreement and debate. Out of this process will come resolution and new syntheses—the making of subsequent editions.

I wish especially to thank my fellow editors for their support, enthusiasm, ideas, and hard work, without all of which this book would not have been possible.

Robert H. Dailey, M.D.

CONTENTS

PART I

Airway and Breathing

Clinical Airway Anatomy

Gary P. Young, M.D.

As an introduction to emergency airway management, this chapter serves as a basic review (Fig 1–1). Clinical correlations are briefly outlined with regard to: (1) the sites of normal anatomic narrowing; (2) the sites of airway narrowing related to "normal" variants; and (3) clinical conditions known to cause acute airflow obstruction.[1–8] Knowledge of these correlations is essential to management of the threats to the three pillars of the airway, particularly airflow obstruction. A thorough understanding of anatomy is indispensable for performance of airway procedures, especially when structures are only partially visible. Finally, any clinician responsible for managing the emergency airway must be aware of the important anatomic differences in the infant, child, and adult airway.[9–15]

THE NOSE

As the anatomically superior part of the airway, the nose serves the following functions[4, 8, 16–18]: (1) it acts as a respiratory conduit for airflow; (2) the nasal mucosa warms and humidifies inspired air; and (3) the nasal hairs and the mucous film covering the nasal mucosa act as an initial barrier to aspiration of inhaled foreign matter. In the nasal passages, the points of normal airway narrowing and of common normal "variants" with potential to cause airflow obstruction include (Fig 1–2 and 1–3): (1) the openings of the anterior nares; (2) the inferior turbinates; (3) deviation of the septum; and (4) the acute posterior angle formed by the horizontal floor of the nose with the vertical nasopharynx. Table 1–1 lists ana-

tomic variants and pathologic conditions associated with nasal airflow obstruction.

THE MOUTH

The mouth provides a conduit not only for airflow (see Fig 1–2 and 1–3) but also for alimentation. The mouth includes the vestibule (between the lips and cheeks and the teeth and gums) and the oral cavity proper (encompassing the teeth, gums, alveolar arches, hard and soft palates, and tongue).[1, 4, 5, 8] The base of the tongue rises out of the hypopharynx to occupy the floor of the mouth. Utilizing the other passive structures of the oral cavity for support,[19, 20] the tongue and the oropharyngeal reflexes actively protect against threats to the airway. The extrinsic muscles of the tongue are innervated by the hypoglossal nerve (cranial nerve XII); this nerve is very superficial at the angle of the mandible. If these muscles are impaired by paralysis from nerve injury or (as examples) secondary to a cerebrovascular event, general anesthesia, or acute ethanol intoxication, the tongue falls posteriorly into the pharynx and airway occlusion occurs. Noisy respirations, or even stridor, is the clinical hallmark.[21, 22] Other common causes of oral airflow obstruction are listed in Table 1–2.

A brief dental examination is worthwhile before and after airway maneuvers.[1, 9, 11, 18, 23] Children aged 6 months to 6 years have only primary dentition. There are no roots and the teeth are easily dislodged. Older children aged 6 to 12 years have mixed dentition, both loose deciduous teeth and un-

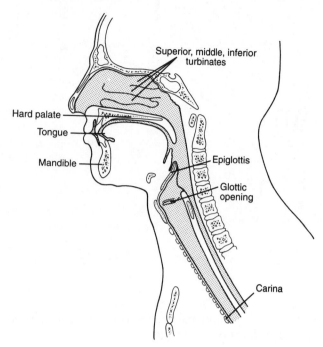

FIG 1−1.
The upper and lower airways meet at the glottic opening.

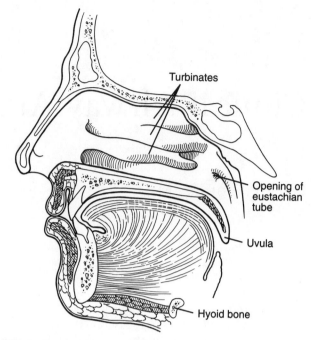

FIG 1−2.
Sagittal view of the nasal and oral airway anatomy.

derlying permanent teeth. Loose teeth in adults are usually caused by periodontal disease. Prostheses, particularly dentures, may become dislodged, causing upper airway or tracheal obstruction. Dentures also inhibit intraoral sensation of food and drink, putting their wearers at risk of inadvertent aspiration of inadequately chewed food.

THE NECK

Physicians are often concerned about aggravating or causing a neurologic deficit involving the cervical spinal cord.[24] The full range of motion of the neck is normally 90 to 165 degrees.[4] Limited neck motion may interfere with placing the patient in the "sniffing" position, the position most likely to relieve airflow obstruction (Fig 1−4). The reader is referred to the discussion in Chapter 3 of the alignment of the three airway axes. Factors associated with limited neck motion are listed in Table 1−3.

THE PHARYNX

The pharynx is a fibromuscular tube beginning at the base of the skull and ending at the lower bor-

der of the cricoid cartilage (Fig 1−5). [1, 4] It constitutes a common aerodigestive tract. With regard to airflow, it serves as a passive conduit of inspired air between the nasal and oral cavities above and the larynx below, which divide the pharynx into the naso-, oro-, and laryngopharynx, respectively.[8, 17] It is continuous from the esophagus through which re-

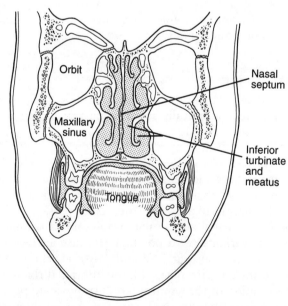

FIG 1−3.
Coronal view of the nasal and oral airway anatomy.

TABLE 1–1.

Causes of Nasal Airflow Obstruction*

Anatomic variants: narrow nares, hypertrophied turbinates, septal deviation, nasopharyngeal curvature
Traumatic: *nasal fracture, epistaxis, septal hematoma,* saddle nose deformity
Inflammatory: *nasopharyngitis, allergic and infectious rhinitis, coryza,* abscesses and furuncles, mucormycosis
Iatrogenic: postoperative epistaxis or septal edema, nasal packing
Neoplastic: *nasal polyps,* cysts, papilloma, fibroma, carcinoma, sinus tumors
Pediatric: foreign body, adenoidal tonsillar hypertrophy,* deviated septum, neonatal choanal atresia
Toxic: inhalational drug abuse

*Italic type indicates common cause.

gurgitated stomach contents may be aspirated. The junction of the pharynx with the esophagus constitutes the narrowest part of the alimentary canal; a foreign body trapped at this level places the patient at risk for airflow obstruction or aspiration.[14, 25, 26] Posteriorly, the pharynx is bounded by the fascia covering the prevertebral muscles and the cervical spine; here a potential space exists for the formation of abscesses. Pharyngeal causes of airway obstruction and difficult intubation are listed in Table 1–4.

THE LARYNX

The larynx is the boundary between the upper airway and the lower airway. The glottic opening (Figs 1–6 and 1–7) divides the larynx into two parts[6–8]: the upper compartment extends from the laryngeal outlet to the vocal cords; the lower compartment extends from the vocal cords to the lower border of the cricoid cartilage or the upper portion of the trachea.[1–5] The larynx functions as an open valve in respiration, as a partially closed valve which can modulate phonation, and as a closed valve protecting against aspiration during swallowing. *In the adult, the airway is narrowest at the vocal cords.*

In the adult, the larynx is at the level of the C–C5 vertebrae.[1–8] The larynx is a complex boxlike structure consisting of two suspensory systems and eight folds with fibroelastic membranes, and nine cartilages connected by ligaments and moved by nine muscles, all lined with mucous membrane. The three single cartilages (i.e., epiglottis, thyroid, and cricoid) and the three paired cartilages (i.e., arytenoids, corniculates, and cuneiforms) pivot and swing in relationship to one another; the connections between the cartilages are true joints with a built-in range of motion. The single cartilages form the basic structure of the larynx (particularly the thyroid and cricoid cartilages) and provide major internal (epiglottis) and external (thyroid and cricoid) landmarks. Three ligaments or folds of mucous membrane extend superiorly from the epiglottis to help form the laryngeal inlet. Paired fossae or small depressions on either side of the median ligament and between the lateral folds are known as the valleculae, or valleys.

The shieldlike thyroid cartilage is the largest laryngeal cartilage. Inferiorly, the thyroid cartilage articulates with the cricoid cartilage; it is further attached to the cricoid by the cricothyroid membrane which, on average, measures 1 by 3 cm. The cricothyroid membrane is relatively avascular, superficial, and removed from the major structures in the neck. The cricoid cartilage is shaped like a signet ring with

TABLE 1–2.

Causes of Oral Airflow Obstruction or Difficult Intubation*

Anatomic variants: macroglossia, short thick mandible, obtuse mandibular angle, reduced space between the angles of the mandibles, micrognathia, protruding upper incisor teeth, loose or absent teeth or the presence of dentures, deeply arched palate, elongated uvula, tori palatini
Traumatic: mandible or dental fractures and soft tissue injuries to the tongue or oral cavity
Neurologic: *tongue and oropharyngeal reflexes,* laxity of tongue muscles from hypoglossal paralysis secondary to cerebrovascular event, tetanus
Infectious: *oral and oropharyngeal infections with associated trismus,* parotid abscess, Vincent's angina (trench mouth), masticator space infection, mandibular osteomyelitis, sialoadenitis
Allergic: angioneurotic edema of the lips, tongue, oral cavity, oropharynx, uvula
Toxic: oral orifice scarring (caustic ingestion, electrical burns)
Neoplastic: tumors of the tongue, hard and soft palate, floor of mouth, sinuses, mandible
Pediatric: congenital defects (cleft palate)
Miscellaneous: temporomandibular joint dysfunction

*Italic type indicates common or potentially critical airway compromise.

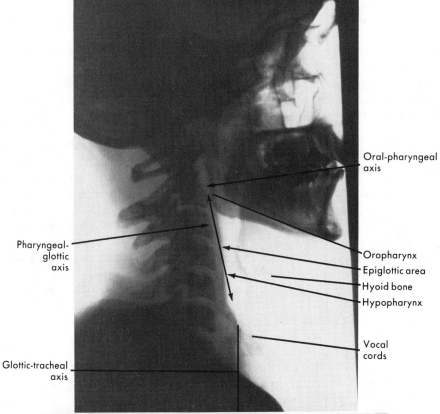

Oral-pharyngeal
axis

Pharyngeal-
glottic
axis

Oropharynx
Epiglottic area
Hyoid bone
Hypopharynx

Vocal
cords

Glottic-tracheal
axis

FIG 1−4.
Radiologic anatomy demonstrating closer
alignment of axes with occipital extension
and neck flexion. (From Kastendieck JG:
Airway management, in Rosen P, Baker FJ
II, Barkin RM, et al (eds): *Emergency
Medicine: Concepts and Clinical Practice*,
ed 2. St Louis, Mosby−Year Book, Inc,
1988, p 47. Used by permission.)

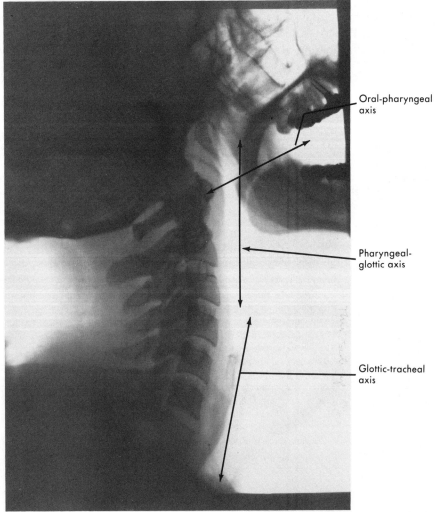

Oral-pharyngeal
axis

Pharyngeal-
glottic axis

Glottic-tracheal
axis

TABLE 1–3.

Factors Associated With Limited Neck Motion*

Anatomic variant: a short, muscular, or fat neck
Traumatic: cervical spine fractures/dislocations
Iatrogenic: cervical spine immobilization, postoperative neurologic or skeletal changes
Neurologic: cervical nerve root compression
Degenerative: arthritis or other musculoskeletal disorders
Muscular: neck muscle spasm
Inflammatory: meningismus
Pediatric: cervical hyperflexion secondary to prominent occiput

*Italic type indicates common or potentially critical airway compromise.

TABLE 1–4.

Causes of Pharyngeal Airway Obstruction and Difficult Intubation*

Traumatic: bleeding, hematoma, caustic or thermal burns
Infectious: pharyngitis or tonsillitis, oropharyngeal infections with associated trismus, peritonsillar abscess, prevertebral or retropharyngeal abscess, epiglottitis, diphtheria
Allergic: angioneurotic edema, anaphylaxis, oropharyngeal insect bite or bee sting
Neurologic: bulbar palsy
Neoplastic: tumors, polyps, *uvular or tonsillar hypertrophy*
Miscellaneous: emesis, posteriorly displaced tongue, foreign bodies

*Italic type indicates common or potentially critical airway compromise.

the broad bulky portion placed posteriorly. Because it is the only complete skeletal ring of the airway, pressure applied to its anterior surface is transmitted to the esophagus which lies directly posterior.[27] External pressure on either the thyroid or the cricoid cartilage will push the vocal cords, which are located inside the thyroid cartilage, posteriorly.[28–30] The oblique entrance, or aditus, of the larynx (defined by the epiglottis, the arytenoid cartilages, the aryepiglottic folds, and the posterior commissure) lies anteriorly

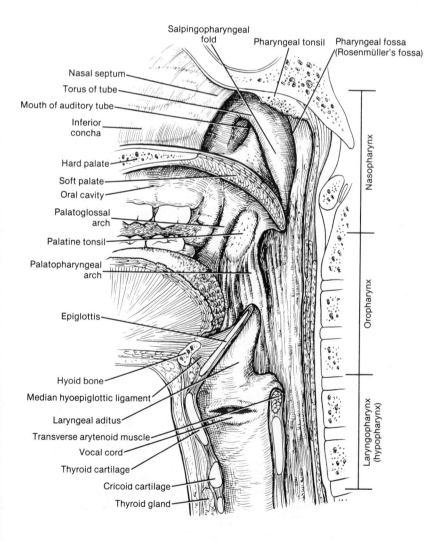

FIG 1–5.
Medial view of pharyngeal mucosa. (From Graney RO: Basic science: Anatomy, in Cummings CW, Fredrickson JW, Harker LA, et al (eds): *Otolaryngology—Head and Neck Surgery.* St Louis, Mosby–Year Book, Inc, 1986, p 1096. Used by permission.)

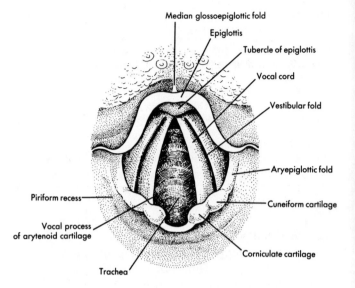

FIG 1–6.
Laryngoscopic view of the airway. (From Kastendieck JG: Airway management, in Rosen P, Baker FK II, Barkin RM, et al (eds): *Emergency Medicine: Concepts and Clinical Practice,* ed 2. St Louis, Mosby–Year Book, Inc, 1988, p 45. Used by permission.)

in the neck. Posteriorly, the larynx bulges into the laryngopharynx to leave deep recesses on either side of the laryngeal inlet, forming the piriform sinuses of the hypopharynx. The piriform fossae are a common site of perforation during instrumentation[31] and of lodging of swallowed foreign bodies such as fish bones.[25]

The paired arytenoid cartilages form the posterior attachment of the vocal folds; they are irregular pyramids mounted on top of the posterior aspect of the cricoid cartilage where they serve as important visual landmarks for intubation.[1, 21, 32] Functionally, the arytenoids are the dynamic structures of pronation and respiration; movement of the arytenoids

tenses, relaxes, and swings the vocal cords from side to side. This allows for phonation, breathing, coughing, and swallowing without aspiration. During swallowing, expiration, coughing, and straining, as the laryngeal muscles contract, the downward movement of the epiglottis and the closure and upward movement of the glottis prevent food from entering the larynx. Table 1–5 lists causes of laryngeal airflow obstruction.

The vocal cords are in nearly constant motion.[7, 8] At rest, they lie partially abducted. During quiet respiration, they move very little; but during forceful inspiration or hyperventilation, the cords open widely in order to minimize airflow resistance. By contrast, forceful cord closure and elevation of the larynx seal

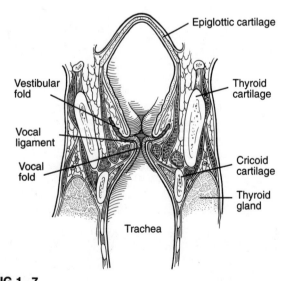

FIG 1–7.
Coronal view of the meeting of the upper and lower airway at the glottic opening.

TABLE 1–5.

Causes of Laryngeal Airway Obstruction and Difficult Intubation*

Infectious: epiglottitis, laryngotracheitis (croup), laryngitis
Traumatic: penetrating and blunt trauma
Toxic: thermal inhalation, caustic aspiration
Iatrogenic: intubation structural trauma, postintubation laryngospasm or edema or subglottic stenosis, postlaryngectomy scarring, contact ulcer
Allergic: anaphylaxis, angioneurotic edema, laryngospasm, laryngeal edema
Neurologic: vocal cord paralysis
Functional: hysterical aphonia, dysphonia plicae ventricularis
Degenerative: arthritis of arytenoid cartilages
Neoplastic: benign tumor (granuloma and nodule formation, polyp, papilloma, hyperkeratosis), carcinoma
Pediatric: laryngeal web
Miscellaneous: foreign bodies (cafe coronary), secretions

*Italic type indicates common or potentially critical airway compromise.

the airway. The larynx is one of the most powerful sphincters in the body; by effort closure, it assists in the development of intrathoracic pressure associated with coughing, micturition, defecation, and weightlifting. Laryngospasm, or spasmodic closure of the vocal cords, is the most marked form of airway closure.[6, 29, 30, 33–35] This reflexive, forceful contraction of all the laryngeal muscles commonly occurs when a foreign body lodges in the larynx. Laryngospasm produces the suffocating sensation and the loud, stridulous noises following accidental near-aspiration of liquids or solids. Although it normally serves a protective function, laryngospasm may exacerbate airway obstruction, totally prevent ventilation, and complicate or physically prevent the passage of an endotracheal tube. Forcing a tube through the cords with excessive pressure can dislocate an arytenoid and cause permanent hoarseness.[36]

The epiglottis is doubly innervated.[1, 2, 5–8] The superior portion is innervated by the glossopharyngeal nerve and the inferior portion is supplied by the vagus nerve. Theoretically, laryngospasm is less likely to occur with physical stimulation above the epiglottis as opposed to just below it. The larynx is innervated by two branches of the vagus nerve— the superior laryngeal and recurrent laryngeal nerves.[1, 2, 5–8] Damage to the superior laryngeal nerve causes hoarseness due to a loss of tension in the ipsilateral vocal cord. Usually the opposite cord compensates and the hoarseness is temporary. Injury to the recurrent laryngeal nerve is more common, producing vocal cord paralysis on the affected side. The left recurrent laryngeal nerve is paralyzed twice as often as the right; 25% of all recurrent nerve palsies are idiopathic. The remainder are caused by iatrogenic damage during thyroidectomy, trauma, and malignant infiltration.[18, 29, 30, 36–42]

Incomplete paralysis of the recurrent nerve tends to affect the abductors more than the adductors, because it is easier to damage the more superficial abducting fibers, in which case the cord adopts the midline adducted position. Complete paralysis of the recurrent nerve inactivates both the adductors and the abductors; however, the tensing action of the cricothyroid muscle innervated by the superior laryngeal nerve tends to maintain the affected cord in adduction. In the event of bilateral recurrent laryngeal nerve damage, complete adduction of the vocal cords results from the unopposed action of the superior laryngeal nerve; acute airway obstruction can result. Paralysis of both recurrent and superior laryngeal nerves, as with the use of muscle relaxants or with temporary or permanent iatrogenic damage

or malignant infiltration, produces a paralyzed cord in the cadaveric position of complete laryngeal relaxation, in which the cords are midway between abduction and adduction.[36–42] Muscular relaxation narrows the gap between the cords but does not alter air flow through the larynx; the resultant Bernoulli effect causes the cords to fall together and produces inspiratory stridor. Thus, the harder the patient tries to breath, the less air passes since the inrushing air forces the upper surface of the vocal cords together. Conversely, if the patient breathes more slowly, airflow obstruction diminishes.

THE TRACHEA

The trachea functions as a gas conduit.[2, 6–8] It consists of 16 to 22 **C**-shaped cartilaginous arches joined by fibroelastic tissue and closed posteriorly by the trachealis muscle to form a **D** shape on transverse section with the straight portion abutting against the esophagus and rigid cervical spine posteriorly (see Fig 1–1). The trachea extends 10 to 13 cm from the cricoid cartilage to the bronchial bifurcation at the carina (about the level of T5 at approximately the level of the angle of Louis, approximately 5 cm below the suprasternal notch).[1, 3–5] In

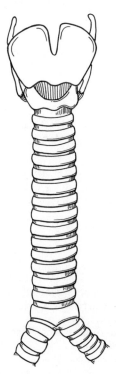

FIG 1–8.
External view of the larynx, trachea, and mainstem bronchi.

the adult, the outer diameter of the trachea is 2.5 cm and its inner diameter is 1.0 to 1.5 cm. In the elderly, its dimensions may be enlarged; during pregnancy, edema causes the internal diameter to diminish. The right mainstem bronchus is less angulated from the trachea than the left; in the adult it is at a 25-degree angle from the trachea and the left mainstem bronchus is at 45 degrees (Fig 1–8).[1–8] Thus, inadvertent endobronchial intubation of the right mainstem bronchus is a common complication in adults. The right upper lobe bronchus has its origin about 2 cm from the carina, whereas the left arises about 5 cm from the carina. As a result, aspirated material tends to gravitate into the right upper and lower lobes. Table 1–6 lists the causes of tracheal airway obstruction.

THE BRONCHI

When the bronchi are the site of lower airway obstruction (Table 1–7), alveolar gas exchange is significantly affected.[27–29, 43–45] Although the size of the individual airways decreases with each branching, the total amount of airway available for airflow (and the total area available for gas exchange) actually increases from the mainstem bronchi to the terminal bronchioles and the alveoli. However, because the individual airways become so small, there are many disease states that can interfere with airflow, and, secondarily, alveolar gas exchange (see Table 1–7).

PEDIATRIC PERSPECTIVE: COMPARATIVE AIRWAY ANATOMY

There are important anatomic differences in the upper and lower airways of the infant, child, and adult.[9–15, 46, 47] (An adult is considered here to be

TABLE 1–6.

Causes of Tracheal Airway Obstruction*

Traumatic: both blunt and penetrating trauma
Toxic: thermal or toxic gas inhalation, caustic liquid aspiration
Iatrogenic: tracheomalacia, stricture
Inflammatory: tracheitis, edema, secretions
Neoplastic: carcinoma, polyp
Pediatric: tracheal web, tracheomalacia
Miscellaneous: foreign object inhalation

*Italic type indicates common or potentially critical airway compromise.

TABLE 1–7.

Causes of Bronchial Airway Obstruction*

Bronchospastic: anaphylaxis, asthma, chronic obstructive lung disease, inflammatory tracheobronchitis, infectious bronchitis
Edema: congestive heart failure, noncardiogenic pulmonary edema
Toxic: thermal or toxic gas inhalation, caustic liquid aspiration, pesticide poisoning
Trauma: penetrating and blunt chest trauma
Neoplastic: *bronchogenic carcinoma,* adenoma, congenital cysts
Miscellaneous: foreign body aspiration

*Italic type indicates common or potentially critical airway compromise.

age 16 years or older; an older child or adolescent is 8 to 16 years old; a child is aged 1 to 8 years; and an infant is 1 year of age or less.) The older the child, the more the airway becomes like that of an adult; at age 8, the larynx of the child closely resembles that of the adult except in size. But size is all-important: airflow varies with the fourth power of the radius in idealized nonturbulent systems; in real terms it is sufficient to appreciate that there is a significant geometric, not linear, relationship between airflow and lumen size.

The differences between the adult and infant airway are not just in the diameter of the airway (Fig 1–9). The pharyngolaryngeal angle of the child is more acute and the hypopharyngeal space is more closed. The pediatric airway mucous membrane is softer, looser, and more fragile than in the adult, increasing the potential for obstructive edema and inflammation and for laceration and penetration leading to infectious and anatomic complications. The smaller air passage in infants and small children results in a decreased baseline airway reserve, increasing vulnerability to obstruction from edema and inflammation. The salient anatomic differences between the pediatric and adult airways are summarized below.[9–15, 46, 47]

Head

The infant's head is much larger in proportion to the rest of its body than is the adult's. In all children the occiput is pronounced so that in the supine position the neck is flexed as if in the sniffing position. Therefore, use of a pillow or a towel under the head to align the airway axes is not necessary in children below the age of 9 years, and it may actually result in airflow obstruction. Small infants sometimes have too much sniffing position, in which case placing a small towel under the back improves airflow.

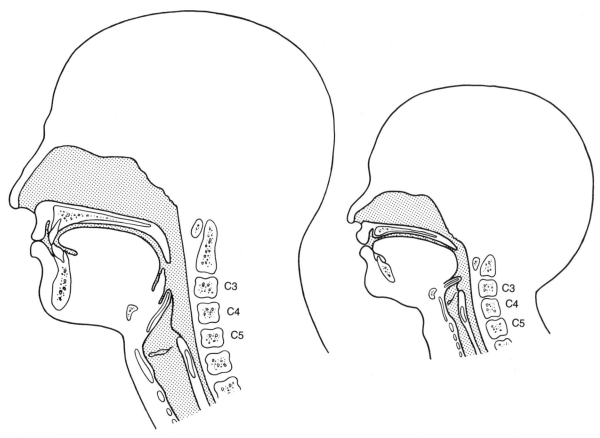

FIG 1–9.
Comparative sagittal view of the adult *(left)* and child *(right)* upper airway anatomy.

Nose

The infant is an obligate nose breather during most of the first year of life because of the more superior location of the epiglottis at C1 and the more anterior location of the larynx at C3–C4. The nose is easily obstructed by edema or secretions. The adenoid tissue in children is hypertrophied, increasing the potential for nasopharyngeal airflow obstruction. The nasopharyngeal passages are relatively narrow in the neonate, smaller in relation to the trachea than in adults.

Tongue

Posterior displacement of the tongue is the most common cause of airway obstruction in infants (as it is in adults). The infant's tongue is proportionately larger than that of the adult and respiratory efforts in the presence of diminished muscle tone tend to pull the tongue in a ball valve–like fashion over the airway, further contributing to obstruction. The tongue that is large relative to the size of the mouth also interferes with intubation. Finally, the smaller separation between the hyoid and the thyroid cartilage makes displacing the tongue and associated structures forward more difficult.

Larynx

The most significant difference between the adult and the infant larynx is that the overall diameter of the adult's airway is 8 mm or greater, whereas an infant's is typically 3 to 4 mm in diameter. In a neonate, a 1-mm reduction in this diameter, caused by either trauma or infection, will reduce the overall cross-sectional area of the airway by at least 50%. By comparison, in the adult airway, 1 mm of circumferential edema from intubation trauma leaves an airway with a diameter of at least 6 mm, at most a 25% reduction. Thus, in an infant, even minimal trauma can create life-threatening airway obstruction.

Cricoid Cartilage

The airway of the infant is narrowest at the level of the cricoid cartilage. Thus, an endotracheal tube that passes easily through an infant's cords may be too large at the cricoid ring. This precludes the use of cuffed tubes in children less than 9 to 12 years of age and increases complications of obstruction from subglottic stenosis, scarring, granuloma formation, and ulceration. The cartilage is very soft and pliable. Cricoid pressure or extremes of head position can cause obstruction of the airway. Cricoid pressure and overextension or overflexion of the head can make spontaneous or assisted ventilation difficult.

Trachea and Mainstem Bronchi

Compared with adults, the major conducting airways in infants are both narrower (3–4 mm in diameter in the newborn) and shorter (4–5 cm long in most infants, 7 cm by 18 months of age). The trachea of a premature infant may be as short as 2 cm. The epithelium of the trachea is loosely bound and susceptible to edema formation. The bifurcation of the trachea into right and left mainstem bronchi is also somewhat different in infants and children as compared with adults. The angulation of the infant carina at the right and left mainstem bronchi is symmetric at 55 degrees from the vertical. Even in older children, the bronchi are more symmetric and accidental endobronchial intubation and pulmonary aspiration in children are more evenly distributed between left and right mainstem bronchi.

The Increased Risk of Hypoxia in the Pediatric Patient

Finally, there are also a number of physiologic differences between the infant and adult that make the infant more susceptible to hypoxia. The most clinically obvious is that the infant's respiratory rate (35 breaths per minute) is more than double that of an adult. The neonate's oxygen consumption (>6 mL/kg/min) and carbon dioxide consumption (>6 mL/kg/min) rates are also almost double those of the adult. These clinically important anatomic and physiologic differences in the pediatric airway are discussed in Chapters 6, 7, and 8.

REFERENCES

1. Clemente CD (ed): *Gray's Anatomy of the Human Body,* ed 30. Philadelphia, Lea & Febiger, 1984.
2. Ellis H: *Clinical Anatomy—A Revision and Applied Anatomy for Clinical Students,* ed 6. Oxford, England, Blackwell Scientific Publishers, 1977.
3. Ellis H, Feldman S: *Anatomy for Anesthetists,* ed 4. Oxford, England, Blackwell Scientific Publishers, 1983.
4. Friedman SM: *Visual Anatomy.* vol 1: *Head and Neck.* New York, Harper & Row, 1970.
5. Graney DO: Basic science—Anatomy, in Cummings CW, Fredrickson JM, Harker LA, et al (eds): *Otolaryngology—Head and Neck Surgery.* St Louis, Mosby–Year Book, Inc, 1986, pp 217–226.
6. Kastendieck JG: Airway management. In Rosen P, Baker FJ II, Barkin RM, et al (eds): *Emergency Medicine: Concepts and Clinical Practice,* ed 2. St Louis, Mosby–Year Book, Inc, 1988, pp 41–68.
7. Meller SM: Functional anatomy of the larynx. *Otolaryngol Clin North Am* 1984; 17:1.
8. Morris IR: Functional anatomy of the upper airway. *Emerg Med Clin North Am* 1988; 6:639.
9. Brown TCK, Fisk GC: *Anesthesia for Children,* ed 1. Oxford, England, Blackwell Scientific Publishers, 1979.
10. Eckenhoff JE: Some anatomic considerations for the infant larynx influencing endotracheal anesthesia. *Anesthesiology* 1951; 12:407.
11. Godinez RI: Special problems in pediatric anesthesia. *Int Anesthesiol Clin* 1985; 23:88.
12. Kubota Y, et al: Tracheobronchial angles in infants and children. *Anesthesiology* 1986; 64:374.
13. Legvin RM: *Pediatric Anesthesia Handbook,* ed 2. Garden City, NY, Medical Examination Publications, 1980.
14. Majd NS, et al: Lower airway foreign body aspiration in children. *Clin Pediatr* 1977; 16:13.
15. Smith RE: *Anesthesiology for Infants and Children,* St Louis, ed 4. Mosby–Year Book, Inc, 1980.
16. Danzl D, Thomas D: Nasotracheal intubations in the emergency department. *Crit Care Med* 1980; 8:677.
17. Donlon JV: Anesthesia for eye, ear, nose and throat surgery, in Miller RD (ed): *Anesthesia.* New York, Churchill Livingstone Inc, 1981.
18. Hall IS, Coleman BH: *Disease of the Nose, Throat and Ear: A Handbook for Students and Practitioners,* ed 11. Edinburgh, Churchill Livingstone Ltd, 1975.
19. Block C, Vrechner V: Unusual problems in airway management. II—The influence of the temporomandibular joint, the mandible, and associated structures on endotracheal intubation. *Anesth Analg* 1971; 50:115.
20. Moukawa S, et al: Influence of the head-jaw position upon upper airway patency. *Anesthesiology* 1961; 11:165.
21. Cass N, James N, Lines V: Difficult direct laryngoscopy complicating intubation for anesthesia. *Br Med J* 1956; 1:488.
22. Kander P, White A: Anatomic factors in difficult direct laryngoscopy. *Br J Anaesth* 1975; 47:468.
23. Wright R, Manfield F: Damage to teeth during the administration of general anesthesia. *Anesth Analg* 1974; 54:405.
24. Collicott PE, et al (eds): *Advanced Trauma Life Support*

Course for Physicians. Chicago, Committee on Trauma, American College of Surgeons, 1984.

25. Danilidis J, et al: Foreign body in the airways. *Arch Otolaryngol* 1977; 103:570.

26. Kim IN, et al: Foreign body in the airway—A review of 202 cases. *Laryngoscope* 1973; 83:347.

27. Sellick BA: Cricoid pressure to control regurgitation of stomach contents during induction of anaesthesia. *Lancet* 1961; 2:404.

28. Atkinson RS, Rushman GB, Lee JA: *A Synopsis of Anaesthesia,* ed 8. Bristol, England, John Wright & Sons, 1977.

29. Collins VJ: *Principles of Anesthesiology.* Philadelphia, Lea & Febiger, 1966.

30. Dripps RD, Eckenhoff JE, Vandam LD (eds): *Introduction to Anesthesia: The Principles of Safe Practice,* ed 5. Philadelphia, WB Saunders, Co, 1982.

31. Lopez NR: Mechanical problems of the airway, *Clin Anesth* 1968; 3:8.

32. Morris IR: Techniques in endotracheal intubation and muscle relaxants, in Rosen P, Baker FJ II, Barkin RM, et al (eds): *Emergency Medicine: Concepts and Clinical Practice,* ed 2. St Louis, Mosby—Year Book, Inc, 1988, pp 69–82.

33. Gann DS: Emergency management of the obstructed airway. *JAMA* 1980; 243:1141.

34. Kryger M, et al: Diagnosis of obstruction of the upper and central airways. *Am J Med* 1976; 61:85.

35. Mcintyre J: The difficult tracheal intubation. *Can Anaesth Soc J* 1987; 34:204.

36. Holley HS, et al: Vocal cord paralysis after tracheal intubation. *JAMA* 1971; 215:281.

37. Walts LF, et al: Vocal cord function following short-term intubation. *Clin Otolaryngol* 1980; 5:103.

38. Arola MK, et al: Postmortem findings of tracheal injury after cuffed intubation and tracheostomy. *Acta Anaesthesiol Scand* 1979; 23:57.

39. Carroll R, et al: Intratracheal cuffs—performance characteristics. *Anesthesiology* 1969; 31:275.

40. Donnelly WH: Histopathology of endotracheal intubation. *Arch Pathol* 1969; 88:511.

41. Hedden M, et al: Laryngotracheal damage after prolonged use of orotracheal tubes in adults. *JAMA* 1969; 207:703.

42. Loeser EA, et al: Tracheal pathology following short-term intubation with low and high pressure endotracheal tube cuff. *Anesth Analg* 1978; 57:577.

43. West JB: *Respiratory Physiology.* Baltimore, Williams & Wilkins Co, 1979.

44. Wilson FR (ed): *Critical Care Manual—Principles and Techniques of Critical Care,* vol 1. Kalamazoo, Mich, Upjohn Co, 1977.

45. Dailey RH: Chronic obstructive pulmonary disease, In Rosen P, Baker FJ II, Barkin RM, et al (eds): *Emergency Medicine: Concepts and Clinical Practice,* ed 2, St Louis, Mosby—Year Book, Inc, 1988, pp 1141–1162.

46. Steward DJ: *Manual of Pediatric Anesthesia.* New York, Churchill Livingstone Inc, 1979.

47. Tucker JA: Obstruction of the major pediatric airway. *Symp Otolaryngol Head Neck Emerg* 1979; 12:329.

2

Aspiration

Richard Wolfe, M.D.

One of the main indications for active airway management is protection against aspiration. Patients at risk from altered mentation need airway protection, yet massive aspiration is the most feared complication of endotracheal intubation. Sir James Simpson, the Edinburgh obstetrician, reported the first anesthetic death from aspiration in 1861. However, a true understanding of the pathophysiology of aspiration only began in 1946 with Mendelson's landmark article alerting physicians to the dangers of abolishing protective airway reflexes.[1] Since that time, experimental data have clarified the pathophysiology, thus suggesting preventive measures. Aspiration frequently complicates emergency intubation and, when massive, carries a poor prognosis. Despite our understanding of the problem, the methodology of prevention of aspiration remains controversial and the methods variably applied. To be effective, airway management must involve more than tube placement. Intubator skill, judicious selection of route and technique of intubation, and the use of paralytic agents are the best means of protecting the tracheobronchial tree from gastric fluid.

EPIDEMIOLOGY

Lung damage and superinfection following aspiration are nonspecific and uncommon. Because of this, most studies have been of little help in defining the true incidence and risk of aspiration. The incidence of experimentally detected aspiration is vastly greater than clinically significant aspiration. A minimal degree of aspiration will occur in sleeping healthy subjects without complications 45% of the time.[2] Gastric aspirate can also be found in the tracheobronchial tree following intubation in 8% to 10% of anesthetized patients[3] and in 40% to 50% of patients undergoing emergency airway management.[4] This contrasts with the incidence of aspiration pneumonia, which is 4.7 per 10,000 patients in electively intubated patients.[5]

The morbidity of aspiration will vary considerably depending on the patient. Any condition that alters the laryngeal reflexes results in a higher risk (Table 2-1).

PATHOPHYSIOLOGY

For significant aspiration to occur, the tone of the lower esophageal sphincter and the laryngeal closure reflex must both be depressed.[5] The gastroesophageal sphincter is normally contracted during rest and exerts a pressure of 10 cm H_2O. This is higher than the average intragastric pressure and, under ordinary circumstances, prevents regurgitation.[6] An increase in intragastric pressure renders this barrier ineffective. Bag-mask ventilation inevitably exceeds sphincter pressure by insufflating air into the stomach and increasing intragastric pressure. High-risk conditions such as pregnancy and morbid obesity also favor aspiration by increasing abdominal pressure. Regurgitation also follows diaphragmatic relaxation due to paralyzing drugs and preexisting conditions such as hiatal hernia.[7] Nasogastric tubes increase the risk by depressing the laryngeal reflexes, as well as inducing hypersalivation, laryngopharyngeal trauma, and inhibition of sphincter function (Table 2-2).

Aspiration of gastric contents results in three separate syndromes: (1) chemical pneumonitis due to the direct toxic effect of gastric fluid; (2) mechanical obstruction due to food particles; and (3) infec-

TABLE 2–1.

Risk Factors of Spontaneous Aspiration

Depressed mentation
  Alcohol
  Drug overdose
    Narcotics
    Barbiturates
    Benzodiazepines
    Tricyclic antidepressants
  Closed head injury
  Coma
  Cerebrovascular accident
  Status epilepticus
  Seizure
Neurologic disease
  Myasthenia gravis
  Guillain-Barré syndrome
  Botulism
  Multiple sclerosis
  Polymyositis
Nasogastric tube placement

TABLE 2–2.

Patients at High Risk for Aspiration During Airway Management

Major trauma
  Delayed gastric emptying
  Decreased airway protection from head trauma and shock
Bowel obstruction
  Increased intragastric pressure
Pregnancy
  Increased intragastric pressure
  Increased gastrin production: increased gastric volume
  Decreased motilin production: delayed gastric emptying
Obesity
  Increased intragastric pressure

tion or superinfection due to aspiration of pyogenic material. Following aspiration, the gastric fluid can reach the alveolar space in 12 to 18 seconds. Direct toxic effects cause peribronchiolar hemorrhage, destruction of type I and type II alveolar cells, loss of surfactant, and increased compliance. There follows outpouring of fluid and blood into the alveoli and intrapulmonary shunting. This results in a clinical picture that is similar to left ventricular heart failure. There is often a drop in blood pressure and occasionally a shock state without reduction in cardiac indices.[8] Bronchospasm due to bronchial irritation may occur immediately and is often severe.

Clinical decompensation is related to the nature and volume of the aspirate, its distribution, and the patient's underlying condition. With increased hydrogen ion concentration, tissue damage reaches a plateau response at a pH of 1.5. The effect of a pH greater than 2.4 cannot be distinguished experimentally from water. Overall, if the pH is less than 2.5,

gastric acid aspiration carries a mortality of 40% to 90%.[9–12] Mortality reaches 100% if the pH is less than 1.8.[13] After gastric contents, blood is the next most common material aspirated. Unless a large enough volume is inhaled to cause asphyxia, blood is well tolerated in the tracheobronchial tree.

Most often, the aspirate is sterile. When infected material is aspirated a higher mortality is found. Pulmonary aspiration of pus is uncommon but may occur when intubating a patient with a peritonsillar or neck abscess or when a lung abscess spontaneously ruptures. In patients with bowel obstruction or ileus, enteric content aspiration carries a mortality of 100%.[14]

Aspirate volumes of greater than 0.4 mL/kg are necessary to induce clinically significant chemical pneumonitis.[12] Hypoxemia occurs with significant aspiration, regardless of the material aspirated. Aspiration of material with a nontoxic pH usually results in rapid recovery after a short period. The distribution of the aspirated material in the lungs also affects outcome. Fluid that is limited to one segment of the lung causes localized damage, whereas a large volume of acid spreading through all segments results in acute respiratory distress syndrome.

Aspiration can result from either active vomiting or passive regurgitation. Silent regurgitation of gastric contents has been reported in up to 25% of patients receiving general anesthesia and 10% to 75% of those had evidence of aspiration.[15] Unlike vomiting, the physician is unaware that the process is occurring. Regurgitation may be enhanced in Trendelenburg's position, in assisted ventilation in the unintubated patient, and by vigorous bouts of coughing.[16]

Vomiting requires that the breath be held, the diaphragm descend, the anterior abdominal wall contract, the pelvic diaphragm be raised, the pylorus be closed, and the esophageal sphincter be open. A pressure of over 40 cm H_2O is needed for the material to be ejected.[17] This implies that most patients who vomit have an intact brainstem and functioning striated muscle. Unless a preexisting condition has impaired protective airway reflexes (see Table 2–1), aspiration will not occur immediately. This underlines the importance of rapidly clearing the airway of vomitus.

CLINICAL FINDINGS

The onset of clinical signs occurs promptly after aspiration and tends to be similar in all patients, irrespective of their subsequent course or outcome. This includes tachypnea, diffuse rales, and serious hypoxemia. Chemical pneumonitis leads to an initial elevation in temperature that resolves spontaneously and is not a sign of infection. When superinfection occurs it is most often delayed until 3 days after aspiration. Cough, cyanosis, wheezing, and apnea are each seen in approximately one third of the cases. Apnea and early severe hypoxemia are particularly ominous events. Decreased intravascular volume from capillary leakage, vasovagal reaction, and decreased cardiac output result in low blood pressure, and in shock in 10% of patients.[18]

ANCILLARY STUDIES

Chest Films

Initial chest films are often normal. Within 6 to 12 hours, diffuse or localized alveolar infiltrates appear and progress during the next 24 to 36 hours.[17] The right lower lobe is the most common location, and the left upper lobe the least common. The extent of the infiltrates does not correlate with mortality.[10, 19, 20]

Arterial Blood Gases

Arterial blood gases demonstrate an acute decrease in arterial oxygen tension (PaO_2) with variable pH and arterial carbon dioxide tension ($PaCO_2$). Hypocapnia may occur initially secondary to tachypnea in response to the pulmonary changes; however, hypercapnia may ensue after frank respiratory failure. A respiratory alkalosis is common initially, followed by metabolic acidosis secondary to inadequate oxygen delivery to the tissues.[21-23]

PREVENTION OF ASPIRATION

Technique of Intubation

As noted earlier, endotracheal intubation carries a risk of aspiration that is markedly increased when managing the airway of a patient in the emergency department. Fortunately, most of the time the aspirate does not have a significant consequence, because of the small volume of fluid.[24-26] A number of measures play a key role in preventing aspiration. The route of intubation, use of paralyzing agents, and the intubator's skill and experience are all factors contributing to the risk of aspiration (Table 2–3). The selection of route and technique leads to

TABLE 2–3.

Iatrogenic Factors Increasing Risk of Aspiration

Impairment of airway protection
  Laryngeal trauma: multiple attempts, overaggressive technique
  Sedatives
Abolition of laryngeal closure reflex
  Succinylcholine
  Nondepolarizing agents
Delay in airway management
  Difficult airway
  Inadequate operator skill and experience
  Combative patient
Increase in intragastric pressure
  Bag-valve-mask ventilation
  Succinylcholine

a dilemma. Firstly, the procedure should be made as easy as possible to minimize the duration and the number of attempts. Secondly, maintaining natural airway protection prevents aspiration. The first consideration argues for the use of paralyzing agents; the latter argues against their use. A patient with intact airway protection requiring airway management rarely tolerates the procedure without sedation, and sedative drugs in turn impair the glottic reflex. When properly done, rapid-sequence induction (RSI) is probably the safest technique of intubation.[27] Intragastric pressure that is normally 7 cm H_2O[28] rises to 35 cm H_2O following administration of succinylcholine, perhaps because of fasciculations.[29] An antifasciculating dose of a nondepolarizing muscle relaxant can prevent this increase in intragastric pressure, reducing the incidence of silent regurgitation.[30] Although muscle relaxants do not affect reflux at the gastroesophageal sphincter, they do paralyze the cricopharyngeus and intrinsic muscles of the larynx, facilitating aspiration.

Close attention to technique will reduce the risk of aspiration. Cricoid pressure should be maintained until the endotracheal tube is placed and the cuff is inflated. When multiple attempts are required, and the patient requires active ventilation, the risk becomes substantially higher than with a patient who has intact airway reflexes. Bagging the patient after succinylcholine is contraindicated as this fills the stomach with air, increasing intragastric pressure and causing silent regurgitation. Thus failure to intubate promptly when using RSI may lead to a disaster. Worsening hypoxia necessitates bag-mask ventilation with its complications. Predicting a difficult airway is the true contraindication of RSI. The glottis may be exceedingly difficult to locate following blunt and penetrating neck trauma. Massive facial trauma, uncontrolled gastrointestinal bleeding, and severe epistaxis may dramatically impair visualization, even with adequate suctioning. The anatomy of the patient's mouth and neck, as well as a preexisting pathologic condition should be taken into consideration before opting for paralysis. Methods for predicting difficult airways are discussed in Chapter 6.

Oral intubation without paralyzing agents is often chosen to manage a difficult airway, in order to allow the patient to maintain airway protection and ventilation. Yet, with the exception of comatose patients, direct laryngoscopy under these conditions is poorly tolerated and technically difficult. Sedation of the patient and regional anesthesia of the upper airway favor aspiration, but if sedation is inadequate, vomiting may occur and subsequent passive aspiration.[31]

Blind nasotracheal intubation appears to offer an alternative in a breathing patient who is able to protect the airway.[32] Bone et al. reported a 10% incidence of aspiration while nasally intubating patients with drug overdose.[24] Repeated unsuccessful attempts may induce vomiting, and also result in pharyngolaryngeal trauma. Epistaxis also may produce aspiration of blood.[24]

Aspiration is unlikely with fiberoptic intubation and has been used with success in some high-risk patients.[33] However, fiberoptic intubation is often poorly suited for the management of the emergency airway because of bleeding or because the need to achieve intubation rapidly precludes the use of a slow technique.

Adjuncts

The endotracheal tube cuff is critical in preventing aspiration. Although the incidence of cuff-induced tracheal damage has been considerably reduced by the judicious use of tracheal tubes with large-volume, low-pressure cuffs, aspiration continues to be a problem. Aspiration can occur even with an inflated cuff: 40% of the time with low-volume, high-pressure cuffs, and 20% with high-volume, low-pressure cuffs. However, if the cuff is correctly inflated at 15 mm Hg, aspiration drops to 0%. It is recommended that the correct inflation pressure of cuffs be checked routinely.[34] In children, noncuffed tubes can wedge tightly at the cricothyroid membrane and are effective in preventing aspiration.[35]

In 1961, Sellick[36] described a maneuver to prevent silent regurgitation. By holding the cricoid cartilage firmly between finger and thumb and pressing it posteriorly, the esophagus can be compressed be-

tween the horizontal portions of the cartilage and the cervical spine. Firmly applied cricoid pressure is effective in sealing the esophagus against an intraesophageal pressure of up to 100 cm H_2O and can be used with a nasogastric tube in place.[37] It should not be used in a patient who is actively vomiting, as rupture of the esophagus could result. Positioning the patient in a 40-degree, head-up position will raise the pressure needed to allow gastric fluid to reach the glottis. In patients with reasonable hemodynamics, this anti-Trendelenburg's position should be used when depression of the lower esophagus is present or iatrogenically induced (e.g., during RSI).

Drug Prophylaxis

There are theoretical benefits to using histamine H_2 receptor antagonists prior to intubating patients. These benefits include an increase in gastric pH with a decrease in gastric volume. However, with the delay of onset of present H_2 blockers, little benefit is obtained if intubation is performed within 45 minutes to 1 hour after administration.[38-43] Newer agents under study with more rapid onset may solve this problem. Any patient with a surgical indication not needing immediate airway management should receive H_2 blockers as rapidly as possible to achieve the benefit. Antacid therapy has long been advocated for patients in labor to prevent gastric aspiration. No studies have documented a benefit from their use. Antacids will increase gastric volume and there is a direct toxic effect of the antacid leading to chronic pneumonitis.

Gastric emptying of the stomach with a nasogastric tube or wide-bore gastric tube will reduce gastric volume and intragastric pressure but also enhances regurgitation by decreasing protection at the upper and lower esophageal sphincters.[37, 44] Placement of these tubes is time-consuming and they do not guarantee complete emptying of gastric content.[44]

TREATMENT

Once a patient has aspirated, aggressively managing the airway takes first priority. If an oral intubation cannot be accomplished promptly, then strong consideration should be given to cricothyrotomy. The occurrence of vomiting during induction for airway management should be dealt with immediately. The patient should be placed head down in the right lateral position to drain vomit from the airway.[45] The pharynx should be cleared with suction, and with digital manipulations if the vomit is solid or particulate. Experimentally, corticosteroids have been shown to be of benefit only when given within 5 minutes after aspiration. Clinical studies have demonstrated no benefit from their use.[46–49] Bacteria rarely play a role in the initial event. Prophylactic antibiotics select out resistant strains and are of no benefit immediately following aspiration. Bronchodilators may be used when there is evidence of bronchospasm.

Most authors agree that when aspiration is observed, endotracheal suctioning should be performed. It stimulates coughing, removes aspirated material, and helps make the diagnosis. It is important to remember that aspirate will diffuse to the alveoli within 12 seconds and that only a small portion of the aspirate will be removed. Bronchial lavage has been performed with neutral or alkaline solutions. However, as the acid aspirate damage is almost immediate, this technique has resulted in either no benefit or increased damage. When severe right-to-left shunting develops, positive pressure ventilation with and without positive end-expiratory pressure (PEEP) has been shown to improve survival.[50]

Following aspiration pneumonia excessive intravenous fluid may worsen pulmonary edema because of the leaky alveolar-capillary membrane. Since it is difficult to estimate fluid loss, volume resuscitation should be guided by hemodynamic parameters and cardiac indices. While there is a theoretical advantage to the use of colloids to attempt to reduce fluid leak across damaged capillary membranes, there are no experimental data to confirm the benefit. Therefore, fluid demands can be met with crystalloid. Theoretically, by increasing serum osmolarity, colloids should decrease leakage of fluid across the pulmonary capillary membranes. Experimental studies have not supported this contention, and in view of the difference in cost, crystalloid is preferable.

SUMMARY

Despite extensive experimental work, further clinical studies are needed to assess which techniques of airway management are best suited to avoid significant aspiration. Prophylaxis geared toward decreasing gastric volume and increasing gastric pH are of little use at present, but newer agents with more rapid onset of action offer promise. Prevention by rapid and aggressive intubation, patient positioning, and Sellick's maneuver are key. Management of aspiration consists in positive pressure ventilation and supportive therapy with controlled volume resuscitation.

REFERENCES

1. Mendelson CL: The aspiration of stomach contents into the lungs during obstetric anesthesia. *Am J Obstet Gynecol* 1946; 52:191–204.
2. Huxley EJ, Viroslav J, Gray WR, et al: Pharyngeal aspiration in normal adults and patients with depressed consciousness. *Am J Med* 1978; 64:564–568.
3. Chokshi SK, Asper RF, Khandheria BK: Aspiration pneumonia: A review. *Am Fam Physician* 1986; 33:195–202.
4. Kinni ME, Stout MM: Aspiration pneumonitis: Predisposing conditions and prevention. *J Oral Maxillofac Surg* 1986; 44:378–384.
5. Olsson GL, Hallen B, Hambreus-Jonzos K: Aspiration during anesthesia: A computer-aided study of 185,358 anesthetics. *Acta Anaesthesiol Scand* 1986; 80:84–92.
6. Knoebel LK: Digestive Tract. B. Movements of the digestive tract, in Selkurtee (ed): ed 3. Boston, Little, Brown & Co, 1966, pp 579–598.
7. Jackson C: The diaphragmatic pinchcock in so-called cardiospasm. *Laryngoscope* 1922; 32:139–142.
8. Lewis RT, Burgess JH, Hampson LG: Cardiorespiratory studies in critical illness changes in aspiration pneumonitis. *Arch Surg* 1971; 103:335–340.
9. Cameron JL, Zuidema GD: Aspiration pneumonia: Magnitude and frequency of problem. *JAMA* 1972; 219:1194.
10. Cameron JL, Mitchell WH, Zuidema GD: Aspiration pneumonia: Clinical outcome following documented aspiration. *Arch Surg* 1973; 106:49–53.
11. Awe WB, Fletcher WS, Jacob SW: The pathophysiology of aspiration pneumonitis. *Surgery* 1966; 60:232–239.
12. Dines DE, Baker WG, Scantland WA: Aspiration pneumonitis. *Mayo Clin Proc* 1970; 45:347.
13. Tebeaut JR: Aspiration of gastric contents. An experimental study. *Am J Pathol* 1952; 28:51–67.
14. Hamelberg W, Bosomworth PP: Aspiration pneumonitis: Experimental and clinical observations. *Anesth Analg* 1964;43:669.
15. Manchikanti L, Colliver JA, Roush JR, et al: Evaluation of ranitidine as an oral antacid in outpatient anesthesia. *South Med J* 1985; 78:818–822.
16. Stark DC: Aspiration in the surgical patient. *Int Anesthesiol Clin* 1977; 15:13–48.
17. Brown HG: Anatomy of vomiting. *Br J Anaesth* 1963; 35:163.
18. Bynum LJ, Pierce AK: Pulmonary aspiration of gas-

tric contents. *Am Rev Respir Dis* 1976; 114:1129–1136.

19. Bynum L, Pierce AK: Pulmonary aspiration of gastric contents. *Am Rev Respir Dis* 1976; 114:1129.

20. Cameron JL, Anderson RP, Zuidema GD: Aspiration pneumonia. *J Sur Res* 1967; 7:44–53.

21. Brown M, Wynne JW: Aspiration pneumonitis: Which outcome for your patient? *J Respir Dis* 1982; 3:41–50.

22. James CF, Modell JH: Pulmonary aspiration. *Semin Anesthesiol* 1983; 2:177–182.

23. Schram JJ, Gibbs CP: Understanding aspiration pneumonitis. *Semin Anesthesiol* 1987; 11:180–187.

24. Bone DK, Davis JL, Zuidema GD, et al: Aspiration pneumonia: Prevention of aspiration in patients with tracheostomies. *Ann Thorac Surg* 1974; 18:30–37.

25. Spray SB, Zuidema GD, Cameron JL: Aspiration pneumonia: incidence of aspiration with endotracheal tubes. *Am J Surg* 1976; 131:701.

26. Elpern EH, Jacobs ER, Bones RC: Incidence of aspiration in tracheally intubated patients. *Heart Lung* 1987; 16:527–531.

27. Dronen SC, Merigian KS, Hedges JR, et al: A comparison of blind nasotracheal and succinylcholine-assisted intubation in the poisoned patient. *Ann Emerg Med* 1987; 16:650–652.

28. LaCour D: Rise in intragastric pressure caused by suxamethonium fasciculations. *Acta Anaesthesiol Scand* 1969; 13:255–261.

29. Roe RB: The effect of suxamethonium on intragastric pressure. *Anaesthesia* 1962; 17:179–181.

30. LaCour D: Prevention of the rise in intragastric pressure due to suxamethonium fasciculations by prior doses of D-tubo curarine. *Acta Anaesthesiol Scand* 1970; 14:5–15.

31. Walts LF: Anesthesia of the larynx in the patient with a full stomach. *JAMA* 1965; 192:121.

32. Hartung HJ, Osswald PM: Die nasotracheale Intubation am nicht-nüchternen, wachen Patienten. *Anaesthesist* 1980; 29:439–441.

33. Ovassapian A, Krejcie TC, Yelich SJ, Dykes MH: Awake fiberoptic intubation in the patient at high risk of aspiration. *Br J Anaesth* 1989; 62:13–6

34. McCleave DJ, Fisher M: Efficacy of high volume low pressure cuffs in preventing aspiration. *Anaesth Intensive Care* 1977; 5:167–168.

35. Goitein KJ, Rein AJ, Gornstein A: Incidence of aspiration in endotracheally intubated infants and children. *Crit Care Med* 1984; 12:19–21.

36. Sellick BA: Cricoid pressure to avoid regurgitation of stomach contents during induction of anesthesia. *Lancet* 1961; 2:404.

37. Salem MR, Joseph NJ, Heyman HJ, et al: Cricoid compression is effective in obliterating the esophageal lumen in the presence of a nasogastric tube. *Anesthesiology* 1985; 4:443–446.

38. Strain JD, Moore EE, Markovchick VJ, et al: Cimetidine for the prophylaxis of potential gastric acid aspiration pneumonitis in trauma patients. *J Trauma* 1981; 21:49–51.

39. Kowalsky SF: Cimetidine in anesthesia: Does it minimize the complications of acid aspiration? *Drug Intell Clin Pharmacol* 1984; 18:382–389.

40. Coombs DW, Hooper D, Pageau M: Emergency cimetidine prophylaxis against acid aspiration. *Ann Emerg Med* 1982; 11:252–254.

41. Coombs DW, Hooper D, Colton T: Pre-anesthetic cimetidine alteration of gastric fluid volume and pH. *Anesth Analg* 1979; 58:183–188.

42. Manchikanti L, Marrero TC, Roush JR: Preanesthetic cimetidine and metoclopramide for acid aspiration prophylaxis in elective surgery. *Anesthesiology* 1984; 61:48–54.

43. Cameron JL, Reynolds J, Zuidema GD: Aspiration pneumonia in patients with tracheostomies. *Surg Gynecol Obstet* 1973; 136:68–70.

44. Stone SB: Efficacy of cimetidine in decreasing the acidity and volume of gastric contents: Inadequacy of nasogastric suction and endotracheal intubation (letter). *J Trauma* 1981; 21:996–997.

45. McCormick PW: Immediate care after aspiration of vomit. *Anaesthesia* 1975; 30:658–665.

46. Stewardson RH, Nyhus LM: Pulmonary aspiration: An update. *Arch Surg* 1977; 112:1192.

47. Toung JK, et al: Aspiration pneumonia. Experimental evaluation of albumin and steroid therapy. *Ann Surg* 1976; 183:179.

48. Lawson DW, Defalco AJ, Phelps JA, et al: Corticosteroids as treatment for aspiration of gastric contents: An experimental study. *Surgery* 1966; 59:845–852.

49. Chapman RL, Downs JB, Modell JH: The ineffectiveness of steroid therapy in treating aspiration of hydrochloric acid. *Arch Surg* 1974; 108:858–861.

50. Weigelt JA, Mitchell RA, Snyder WH: Early positive end-expiratory pressure in adult respiratory distress syndrome. *Arch Surg* 1979; 114:497.

3

Ventilation and Oxygenation

William S. Mezzanotte, M.D.

David M. Rodman, M.D.

Proper oxygenation and ventilation is essential for fueling aerobic cellular activities and for helping to maintain acid-base balance. Ensuring adequate oxygenation and ventilation requires, firstly, that the other pillars of breathing—a patent, unobstructed airway and laminar airflow—are intact. However, the maintenance of proper oxygenation and ventilation also requires the coordinated functioning of neuromuscular, cardiovascular, and pulmonary physiology. Dysfunction of any of these components will hinder or even preclude the oxygenation and ventilation that the body requires. Two key goals are of utmost importance to the emergency physician: (1) to alertly recognize the existence of an aberration in ventilation or oxygenation, or both, and (2) to correctly identify the pathophysiologic break in the chain so that appropriate therapy may be instituted.

OVERVIEW OF PHYSIOLOGY

Normal Physiology

The prime function of the lung is gas exchange—moving ambient oxygen (O_2) into, and removing carbon dioxide (CO_2) from the bloodstream.[1] By acting as a CO_2 disposal system, the lung also serves as the body's most rapidly modulated buffering system. The concentration of CO_2 in the blood has a marked effect upon the resulting amount of hydrogen ion (H^+) in the blood. This can easily be seen from the following equation:

$$H_2O + CO_2 \leftrightarrow H_2O_3 \% H^+ + HCO_3^-$$

The lung (by regulating (CO_2) and the kidney [by regulating bicarbonate (HCO_3^-)] essentially work in concert to maintain the correct balance of H^+ ion in the body and therefore maintain the body's pH at an appropriate level. The relationship of the body's pH to HCO_3^- and CO_2 stores is expressed by the Henderson-Hasselbalch equation:

$$pH = 6.1 + \log\frac{(HCO_3^-)}{0.03\,(PCO_2)}$$

More clinically relevant, however, is the arterial blood gas (ABG) analysis which gives a rapid assessment of a patient's ability to maintain a normal pH, and the lung's influence (either positive or negative) on the pH, by the current level of CO_2 in the blood at the time of sampling. Because of the close association of ventilation to PCO_2 and pH, the ABG measurement is often thought of as a barometer of ventilation, and for the most part it is a reliable indicator of the net result of interaction of the individual components of breathing. These include the central nervous system with its peripheral chemoreceptors and mechanoreceptors; the musculature of the upper airway, which must function to maintain airway patency; and the chest wall musculature and diaphragm, which must function correctly to act as the bellows for the lungs. Obviously, the conduit airways are extremely important in maintaining normal gas exchange for the system. Obstruction of the airways for any reason, e.g., exuberant mucus production in asthma, foreign bodies, or tumors, will all negatively impact upon the body's normal ventilation. Similarly, an abnormality in other systems will also induce ventilatory dysfunction and therefore produce changes in the ABGs with rising PCO_2 and falling pH.

Along with being a functional assessment of ventilation, the ABG determination also gives a quantitative assessment of the arterial O_2 level. It is preferable to pulse oximetry as it provides information about a number of physiologic sequences that must be intact in order to produce a "normal" O_2 level.

First and foremost, the body must ventilate in order to oxygenate. This simple concept is extremely important to remember when evaluating patients. For without correct airflow in and out of the lungs, it is nearly impossible for the body to maintain normal oxygenation. There are many causes of hypoventilation which we have touched upon already, but will discuss at greater length later. However, the net result of all of these syndromes is the same: limited airflow producing decreased O_2 delivery to, and CO_2 removal from the body. The effect of hypoventilation on the ability to oxygenate is best described by the alveolar gas equation [2]*:

$$PAO_2 = [FiO_2 \times (PB - \text{water vapor pressure})] - \frac{PaCO_2}{RQ}$$

where PAO_2 = alveolar oxygen pressure
FiO_2 = fractional concentration of oxygen in inspired gas
PB = barometric pressure
$PaCO_2$ = arterial oxygen partial pressure
RQ = respiratory quotient

Assuming that FiO_2 and RQ are not changing and that PB and water vapor pressure are not changing minute to minute, *the single most important factor in the level of alveolar O_2 is the level of arterial CO_2*. And, as we have already discussed, the level of arterial CO_2 present is primarily dependent on the adequacy of ventilation.

Another important but subtle influence on the level of O_2 in the blood can be seen from the alveolar gas equation. The FiO_2 can be changed dramatically by both man-made and natural forces. Clearly, when a patient is given supplemental O_2, the FiO_2 changes to some extent and the PAO_2 should be expected to change as well. A more natural cause of changing arterial oxygenation is decreased inspired oxygen pressure (PiO_2) that results from falling

*At sea level, breathing room air, this formula can be approximated by $PAO_2 = 160 - (PCO_2/0.8)$.

barometric pressure as altitude increases.[1] Table 3–1 demonstrates the large differences in barometric pressure as altitude increases. Therefore, a "normal" PaO_2 at zero sea level can be almost 40 mm Hg higher than a "normal" PaO_2 in Mexico City (alt. 7,350 ft). Although this is rarely a problem for hospitalized patients, some North American clinics are located at elevations over 8,000 ft. In addition, many hospitals serve mountain populations and after discharge a patient may return to an altitude that is several thousand feet higher than the emergency room.

There are three other main ingredients required for adequate oxygenation in the body. They are: (1) proper matching of ventilation and perfusion in the lung ($\dot{V}/\dot{Q}$ matching), (2) adequate diffusion across the alveolar-capillary barrier, and (3) adequate O_2 transfer from the capillaries of the lung to the rest of the body. The last requires both adequate O_2-carrying capacity (i.e., hemoglobin) as well as an adequate cardiac output to ensure that the oxygen carried in the blood is circulated throughout the body.[1, 3]

Normally, most of the millions of alveolar capillary units in the lung receive an amount of blood flow proportional to the amount of their ventilation. This matching is not perfect, and some imbalance between ventilation and perfusion in various regions of the lung does occur. This is a result mainly of gravity- in the upright lung both ventilation and perfusion increase toward the bottom of the lung.[4] However, because perfusion increases more than ventilation, there is a spectrum of $\dot{V}/\dot{Q}$ matching throughout the lung, from $\dot{V}/\dot{Q} <1$ at the bottom of the lung, $\dot{V}/\dot{Q} = 1$ in the midlung, to $\dot{V}/\dot{Q} >3$ at the apex of the lung.[4] Obviously, the normal lung accommodates for this slight mismatch quite well. The normal gradient between alveolar and arterial blood gas (which we will discuss further) is mostly a function of normal $\dot{V}/\dot{Q}$ mismatching of the lung. However, as the $\dot{V}/\dot{Q}$ mismatch becomes greater, large disturbances in oxygenation occur. There are a large number of pathologic conditions that cause $\dot{V}/\dot{Q}$ mis-

TABLE 3–1.

Inspired (PiO_2) and Alveolar (PAO_2) Pressure at Various Altitudes

Location	Altitude (ft)	PB (mg)*	PiO_2 (mg)	PAO_2(mg)†
Sea level	0	760	160	102
Airplane cabin	6,000	608	128	70
Leadville, Colo.	10,200	517	110	51
Mexico City	7,347	580	120	64

*PB = barometric pressure.
†PAO_2 is calculated from the alveolar gas equation assuming $PCO_2 = 40$ mm Hg.

matches and these disturbances are discussed later in this chapter.

Oxygen and CO_2 transfer from the alveoli to the capillary and vice versa occur by the principle of diffusion. The physical law of gas diffusion states that the transfer of a gas through a membrane (in this case the alveolar-capillary barrier) is dependent on the difference in partial pressure of the gas on either side (the pressure gradient) as well as on the thickness of the membrane the gas has to pass through.[1] The pressure gradient of O_2 (60 mm Hg) and the area of the blood-gas barrier (50–100 m^2, the size of two tennis courts) in the normal lung are very large and the thickness of the barrier can be as small as 0.5 μm, making the lung ideal for efficient gas diffusion. Obviously, aberrations in the alveolar-capillary barrier will make gas exchange more difficult. There are a large number of pathologic conditions that cause diffusion abnormalities and these problems are also discussed below.

Lastly, once O_2 has successfully been transferred to an area of the lung where there is adequate ventilation and blood flow (a good $\dot{V}/\dot{Q}$ match) and once O_2 has successfully crossed the barrier into the bloodstream (good diffusion), it must still be carried to the various parts of the body to fuel cellular function. This job could not be done adequately by dissolving O_2 into the bloodstream alone because the amount of O_2 dissolved in blood is only equal to about 0.3 mL O_2/dL of blood.

Hemoglobin makes the O_2-carrying process much more efficient. One gram of hemoglobin can combine with 1.35 mL O_2 and, as normal blood has about 15 g of hemoglobin/dL, the O_2-carrying capacity of hemoglobin is about 20.8 mL O_2/dL of blood (a significant improvement over dissolved O_2 alone). Thus, it is obvious that all the effort of the lung would be wasted were there no hemoglobin or were hemoglobin unable to transport O_2 as efficiently as it can. However, a normal O_2 content in the blood from adequate hemoglobin does not ensure adequacy of O_2 transfer. Low or moderate cardiac output may impair O_2 delivery also. We can see this from the equation:

$$DO_2 = CO \times CaO_2$$

where DO_2 = tissue oxygen delivery
  CO = cardiac output
  CaO_2 = arterial oxygen content

Normal cardiac output is between 4 and 7 L/min; patients in shock can have a normal CaO_2, but because of low output have decreased DO_2. In such patients, merely knowing CaO_2 is not enough: assessment of cardiac output is also important. We discuss disorders that effect O_2 transfer later in this chapter.

Evaluating Physiologic Function

A number of diagnostic tools are normally available to the emergency room physician for evaluation of the adequacy or inadequacy of oxygenation and ventilation.[5] First and foremost, of course, is a good history and physical examination looking for signs or symptoms of cardiac, pulmonary, or neurologic dysfunction. Simple laboratory tests are invaluable and these include a chest film, electrocardiogram, and hemoglobin and hematocrit determinations. Abnormalities of any of these may help explain defects in ventilation or oxygenation. In the clinically appropriate setting drug screens may elucidate an unexplained hypoventilation.

Other ventilation disorders, especially asthma, are best assessed by some measurement of airflow. The ideal method of airflow assessment is spirometry, which plots volume vs. time. By knowing simple standards, the clinician can determine quickly whether a patient can expel an adequate volume of air (forced vital capacity, FVC) at an appropriate rate (the forced expiratory volume in 1 second, FEV_1). Often, a spirometer is not available to the emergency room physician, but a portable flowmeter is. Unlike the spirometer, which plots both volume and time, the flowmeter gives a single assessment of airflow (L/min). Despite its unsophisticated appearance, the flowmeter can be an extremely useful tool.[6] Firstly, peak flow measures the airflow that occurs in the first second and therefore correlates well with the FEV_1. Secondly, peak flow requires only an initial patient effort and not the prolonged effort that spirometry entails (7–10 seconds). This is especially helpful when performing repetitive measurements on ill patients in order to assess the efficacy of therapy. Thirdly, it is lightweight, portable, inexpensive, and easily used by the patient. In fact, in some instances, a compliant, intelligent patient can be sent home with a flowmeter and instructed to monitor peak flow with instructions to return if his or her disease worsens. As an adjunct to direct measurements of airflow, the PaO_2 is the best immediate indicator of the adequacy of both oxygenation and ventilation. In the present day and age it is far too common for medical personnel to replace the ABG with a percutaneous O_2 saturation (oximetry) reading. This is a mistake for two reasons. Firstly, there are occasions when a oximeter reading may be falsely low or high.[7] Secondly, the oximeter provides no information about the adequacy of ventilation. We believe that in the emergency room setting the ABG sample should be assessed first. Once ventilation is found to be adequate, then an oximeter can be used to monitor the response to interventions such as supplemental O_2. However, if on the initial ABG sample the patient's ventilation is found to be inadequate or inappropriate, then the efficacy of therapy should be assessed by repeated arterial sampling, in addition to oximetry.

Once the ABG sample is drawn, a number of assessments need to be made before conclusions are drawn.[8] Firstly, normal values are measured at 37°C and therefore any gross difference in the patient's body temperature should be noted so that corrections can be made for the ABG values. Hyperthermia raises in vivo PaO_2, but the blood sample is always measured in a water bath maintained at normal body temperature (37°C). For example, in a person whose body temperature is 39°C, the ABG measurement will be about 8 mm Hg lower than the actual partial pressure of oxygen (PO_2). Secondly, as a rule, the sum of PaO_2 and partial pressure of carbon dioxide (PCO_2) should be less than 140 mm Hg on room air; values higher than this suggest an error. A common cause of a falsely elevated PaO_2 is an air bubble in the sampling syringe. Thirdly, white blood cell counts in excess of $100,000/mm^3$ may consume enough O_2 that if there is a significant delay between the time the blood is drawn and the time the PaO_2 is measured, there may be a false lowering of the actual PO_2. Finally ABGs must be proved to be internally consistent, to assure that the pH measured and the PCO_2 measured are in fact accurate. Checking for internal consistency requires two pieces of information: the measured serum HCO_3^- and knowledge of the Henderson-Hasselbalch equation. It is important to remember that the HCO_3^- reported to the clinician on an ABG determination is calculated rather than measured. Therefore, in order to independently evaluate the validity of the blood gas numbers, we need to use the measured serum HCO_3^- (drawn in close proximity to the ABG).

A simple equation can be derived from the Henderson-Hasselbalch equation:

$$PCO_2 = \frac{[H^+] \times [HCO_3^-]}{24}$$

By rearranging the above equation, we can solve for $[HCO_3^-]$

$$\frac{PCO_2 \times 24}{[H^+]} = HCO_3^-$$

In order to use this equation, remember that in the range of pH 7.28 to 7.5 there is a fairly linear relation of pH to concentration of $[H^+]$:

pH	$[H^+]$
7.28	52
7.30	50
7.35	45
7.4	40
7.45	35
7.50	30

The ABG determination gives true measurements of pH (which can be converted to $[H^+]$) and PCO_2. The calculated HCO_3^- should be within 1 to 2 units of the measured serum HCO_3^-. Otherwise there is likely to be an error in measurement—usually with the pH or PCO_2, but possibly also with the serum HCO_3^-. A common error is a falsely low pH. This is generally the result of liquid heparin in the blood-gas syringe that was not fully expressed before drawing the blood sample.

Once the ABG sample has been validated, the results can be interpreted. The first step in interpreting ABGs is to note the pH. The normal pH range is about 7.37 to 7.43. A pH <7.37 indicates that the patient is acidemic; a pH >7.43 indicates alkalemia. Inspecting the PCO_2, then, often helps in interpreting whether alterations in the patient's PCO_2 are the cause or the result of the pH disturbance. For instance, if a patient's pH is 7.30 and the PCO_2 has risen to 50 mm Hg, then it is likely that the primary disturbance is reduced ventilation leading to a rising CO_2 level and therefore a fall in the pH. However, if the pH is 7.30, but the PCO_2 is 25 mm Hg, then it is likely that the primary disturbance is metabolic and that the change in PCO_2 is compensatory. The nature of pH and PCO_2 in various acid-base disturbances is shown in Figure 3–1.[9] In most clinical settings, interpretation of acid-base disorders is much simpler and can be done with the help of some simple equations.[10, 11]

The other major information from the ABG analysis is the PO_2. In determining whether the PO_2 is adequate, we must refer back to the alveolar gas equation and then determine the alveolar-arterial oxygen difference [P(A − a)O_2]. As stated earlier, to

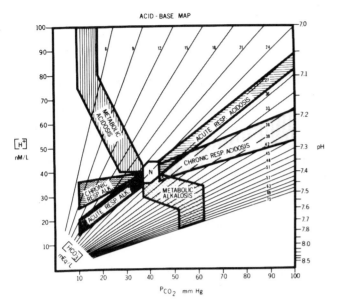

FIG 3–1.
An acid-base map helps to elucidate the type and duration of the acid-base disturbance. A point falling outside of the 95% confidence bands of the thick lines suggests that there is a mixed rather than a simple disturbance. (From McCurdy DK: *Chest* 1972;62(suppl):36S. Used by permission.)

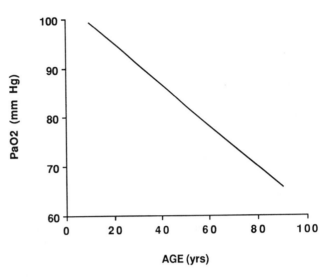

FIG 3–2.
Changes in PaO_2 with age. The line for PaO_2 is based on the regression equation: $PaO_2 = 103.5 - (0.42 \times age[yr])$. The equation is based on PaO_2 measurements in 152 normal subjects (aged 14–84 yr). The standard deviation of an estimate of PaO_2 from this equation is ±3.75 mm Hg. (From Sorbini C, Grassi V, Solinas V, et al: *Respiration* 1968;25:5. Used by permission.)

determine the O_2 level in the alveoli, we can use the alveolar gas equation:

$$PAO_2 = FiO_2 (PB - 47) - \frac{PaCO_2}{RQ}$$

The RQ is a simple approximation of the ratio of carbon dioxide production ($\dot{V}CO_2$) to oxygen uptake ($\dot{V}O_2$) by the lung, or $\dot{V}CO_2/\dot{V}O_2$. Normally more O_2 is taken up by the lung than CO_2 eliminated and therefore it is standard to insert the value 0.8 for RQ. However, at times RQ may be much closer to 1.0 as $\dot{V}CO_2$ production is increased out of proportion to increases in $\dot{V}O_2$ uptake (vigorous exercise, catabolic states, high carbohydrate intake). In most people, however, RQ = 0.8 is a fair assumption and is the most commonly used value to calculate PAO_2. Once PAO_2 is calculated, we can then determine the difference from the expected or calculated O_2 and the actual O_2 measured. This is the alveolar-arterial oxygen difference, or $P(A - a)O_2$. Normally, when breathing room air, the difference is less than 15 mm Hg. The difference that does exist is due to a small amount of intrinsic $\dot{V}/\dot{Q}$ mismatch in the lung.[4] The amount of intrinsic $\dot{V}/\dot{Q}$ mismatch normally increases with age and so the expected PaO_2 will decrease with age (Fig 3–2). Thus, at age 80 years a normal alveolar-arterial

gradient can be about 30 mm Hg.[12] The alveolar-arterial gradient can help distinguish some ventilation disorders from oxygenation disorders. Patients with a pure hypoventilation disorder or with decreased PO_2 due to high altitude (and decreased barometric pressure) will have a normal alveolar-arterial gradient. Ventilation-perfusion mismatching, diffusion problems, airway problems, and O_2 delivery problems all lead to widened alveolar-arterial gradients.

Tools for Physiologic Intervention

Interventions to improve oxygenation and ventilation are varied and depend on the disorder. Treatments can include bronchodilator therapy (inhaled or parenteral β agonists, parenteral methylxanthines, anticholinergic agents, and corticosteroids), narcotic antagonists (naloxone), antibiotics, blood transfusions, pressors (dopamine, dobutamine) or, at times, even intubation with mechanical ventilation. One of the most important interventional tools is supplemental O_2.

In the emergency room, O_2 is most commonly utilized to overcome the $\dot{V}/\dot{Q}$ mismatching that results from a variety of diseases including exacerbations of chronic obstructive pulmonary disease (COPD), diffuse pulmonary infiltrates, pulmonary embolism, and interstitial pneumonitis. In addition, O_2 is indicated for the treatment of low output states such as congestive heart failure and O_2-carrying disorders such as the anemias, hemoglobinopathies, and carbon monoxide poisoning. In disorders like pneumonia, pulmonary embolism, or cardiogenic pulmonary edema, patients are generally hypoxemic, but not hypercapnic (this can be determined with an ABG sample). In these patients, O_2 can be fairly safely administered, usually through a nasal cannula. On the other hand, patients with COPD that develop acute respiratory failure are often hypoventilating. In most cases, administration of controlled O_2 to hypoventilatory patients produces small but clinically insignificant increases in PCO_2. Since chronically hypoventilating patients develop renal compensation and elevation of the serum HCO_3^-, this small further increase in $PaCO_2$ generally does not give rise to significant worsening of the acidemia.[13, 14] Rapid administration of high-flow O_2 (100%) is also generally safe as long as the pH does not fall below 7.25.[15] Acute elevations of PCO_2 that produce a decrement in the pH below 7.25 have been associated with CO_2 narcosis and cardiopulmonary arrest. In such O_2-sensitive patients, O_2 should be administered in graded increments with repetitive arterial sampling to assess patient response. In these patients, O_2 may be delivered via a Venturi (Venti) mask (the preferred system) or nasal cannula. The advantages and disadvantages of each system are discussed in Chapter 18. The most reliable means of O_2 delivery is, of course, mechanical ventilation in which the amount of O_2 can be delivered accurately.

THE INTEGRATED SYSTEM FOR OXYGENATION AND VENTILATION-NORMAL AND ABNORMAL

Sensation and Regulation of Ventilation and Oxygenation

Sensation and regulation of ventilation and oxygen can be otherwise referred to as control of breathing. For the most part, respiratory control is the result of a negative feedback system. If the system is disrupted from its baseline state, the alteration is sensed by peripheral receptors (chemical and mechanical) that transmit signals via afferent receptors to the central respiratory controller—the central nervous system (CNS). The CNS consequently sends efferent signals out to the effectors of ventilation (the muscles and airways) producing the desired change in respiration.

Central Nervous System

The majority of the impulses emanating from the central controller come from the brainstem. The medulla houses the main portion of the respiratory center. There is likely both an inspiratory area (located on the dorsal side) and an expiratory area (located on the ventral side). The expiratory area is normally inactive since expiration is generally a result of passive relaxation of the chest wall back to its baseline position. However, this area can become active during more forceful breathing, as in exercise. The inspiratory area, on the other hand, is constantly active in maintaining normal respiration. The inspiratory area in the medulla can be either inhibited or excited by separate areas of the pons which seem to function to fine-tune the respiratory rhythm that is actually generated in the medulla. The cortex can voluntarily override the brainstem's function to a degree, especially when performing respiratory tasks not commonly encountered (i.e., breathing against a resistance). In general, hypoventilation due to CNS disorders are likely caused by insults to the brainstem.[16] These disorders include bulbar poliomyelitis, encephalitis, infarction, hemorrhage, trauma, neoplasms, multiple sclerosis, and sarcordosis, all of which either infiltrate, obliterate, or demyelinate the important neural cells in the medulla. Obviously, diffuse CNS depression can also be caused by narcotics, ethanol, and other sedatives which are often overlooked as a cause of respiratory depression, especially in the elderly. Diseases of the cerebral cortex, in general, do not affect involuntary respiratory control, but may produce loss of the ability to voluntarily hyperventilate. There are cases of massive hemorrhage and infarction of the cortex producing respiratory compromise, but generally this is secondary to increased intracranial pressure exerting unnatural force upon the medulla.

Peripheral Receptors

The main sensory input for ventilation emanates from chemoreceptors and mechanoreceptors. The chemoreceptors can be both central and peripheral. The central chemoreceptors are situated in the medulla, separate from the respiratory areas. These central chemoreceptors respond mainly to changes in H^+ or CO_2. They monitor these levels mainly in cerebrospinal fluid (CSF). CSF has, in general, much less buffering ability than blood and therefore the change in pH for a given change in PCO_2 is greater. Thus, small changes in $PaCO_2$ generally produce decreases in CSF pH which tend to stimulate ventilation. Chronically low CSF pH is avoided, however, by sustained influx of HCO_3^- which tends to reset the pH of the CSF to near normal. Therefore, in chronic CO_2 retention (COPD), PCO_2 in the blood may be high but CSF pH is also high and therefore the stimulus for reflex ventilation is not as great as expected. The result is chronic hypoventilation.

The peripheral chemoreceptors are located in the carotid bodies at the bifurcation of the common carotid arteries and the aortic bodies located above and below the aortic arch.[3] These receptors respond to decreases in PaO_2 and pH and to increases in PCO_2. The peripheral chemoreceptors are solely responsible for responding to arterial hypoxemia; loss of hypoxic ventilatory response has been shown in response to bilateral carotid body resection. While the role of the peripheral receptors in responding to changes in PCO_2 is much less than that of the central chemoreceptors, their response is more rapid and thus may play a role in quickly changing ventilation in response to abrupt changes in CO_2. The carotid bodies also respond to pH change, be it metabolic or respiratory, whereas the aortic bodies do not respond to pH changes.

There are a variety of other nonchemosensitive receptors that help to regulate ventilation.[1] Pulmonary stretch receptors lie in series with airway smooth muscle spindles and act mainly as a negative feedback system: the receptors sense inflation of the lung and decrease inspiratory activity. This reflex action is known as the Hering-Breuer reflex. Other receptors, called irritant receptors, lie among airway epithelial cells and respond to a variety of noxious stimuli (smoke, dust, cold air) and reflexly produce bronchoconstriction and hyperpnea. Juxtacapillary, or J receptors probably exist in alveolar walls close to capillaries and respond quickly to changes in pH in the pulmonary circulation by increasing ventilation. In addition, the J receptors may respond to the increased interstitial and pulmonary capillary pressure caused by left heart failure and the pulmonary leak of adult respiratory distress syndrome (ARDS), producing an increased sense of dyspnea and increased respiration. Dyspnea can also be produced by activation of other muscle stretch receptors present in the intercostal muscles and diaphragm. These receptors respond to elongation of muscle when large receptoral efforts are required as in asthmatic attacks. Their effect is to produce a sensation of dyspnea (sometimes out of proportion to the physiologic impairment) and also to strengthen contraction of accessory muscles in order to increase effective ventila-

tion. A variety of receptors that help to control ventilation exist in the upper airway. These include irritant receptors and stretch receptors similar to those mentioned above. In addition, there are receptors that reflexly respond to negative pressure, and which tend to produce airway collapse, helping to keep the upper airway patent and maintaining normal ventilation.

Disorders of the sensory aspect of ventilatory control include carotid body dysfunction or even congenital absence and trauma. This trauma may actually be iatrogenic; a form of subacute central alveolar hypoventilation has been described after various forms of cervical spine surgery that is presumably due to interruption of afferent fibers up through the spinal canal. In addition, surgical procedures of the chest may interrupt the vagus nerve which carries most of the afferent signals from the mechanoreceptors of the chest, although this interruption is rarely clinically relevant. Metabolic derangements can also cause the chemoreceptors to fire incorrectly. The most common derangement is a metabolic alkalosis (either acute or chronic) which by virtue of the increased serum pH produces an inhibitory effect upon the chemoreceptors and leads to hypoventilation. Rarely, over time, a chronic metabolic alkalosis may lead to depressed ventilation even with correction of the alkalosis. Prolonged hypoxia has also been shown to reduce the ability of the carotid bodies to respond to further hypoxia. This has been shown best with people living at very high altitudes who lose the ability to respond to low oxygen tensions and therefore develop chronic pulmonary hypertension and cor pulmonale. The best known defect in ventilatory control is primary (idiopathic) alveolar hypoventilation. This disorder, in which there is no other neurologic problem, represents either a failure of peripheral or central chemoreceptors or of the central regulator in the medulla to generate normal inspiratory activity. However, neuropathologic autopsy studies (albeit rare) have reported no abnormalities or lesions in medullary neurons, which suggests that this is more likely a peripheral receptor problem.[4]

The characteristics of primary alveolar hypoventilation and disorders affecting the peripheral or central control systems are similar. Often the only distinguishing feature is the clinical history. Signs likely to be present in these disorders include hypercapnia, chronic respiratory acidosis, and hypoxemia with a normal alveolar-arterial oxygen gradient. In general, dyspnea is not a complaint as these patients have abnormal reflex responses to exercise, hypercapnia, and hypoxemia. Generally, pulmonary function is normal as these patients maintain normal voluntary respiratory control (cortical override of the failing primary control center). This can be confirmed by asking the patient to voluntarily hyperventilate: these patients usually are able to normalize their blood gases, but will immediately revert to their baseline state when not hyperventilating. This is in contradistinction to patients with neuromuscular diseases (to be discussed next) which affect the underlying structural ability to ventilate.

Ventilatory control disorders generally produce the sequelae associated with blood chemistry abnormalities: cyanosis, polycythemia, pulmonary hypertension, and right ventricular failure. In addition, these patients often suffer the effects of chronic sleep deprivation—daytime somnolence, morning headaches, and lethargy. This likely occurs because as these patients go to sleep, they lose the cortical input that helped maintain what little respiratory activity they had and cessation of airflow (apnea) occurs. Apnea produces further derangement of blood chemistry which eventually becomes severe enough to stimulate even the most blunted control system. This chemical stimulation arouses patients from sleep, and cortical input resumes, with a return to the patient's baseline chemistry. The patient falls asleep again and the cycle is repeated.

Effectors of Ventilation and Oxygenation

The effectors of ventilation involve mainly the muscles of the upper airway and the thorax (both primary and accessory) as well as the underlying bony skeleton housing the respiratory system.

Upper Airway Musculature

The upper airway in man, unlike other animals, has no rigid bony support. This lack of rigidity makes phonation possible but also makes airway collapse a possibility. The airway is therefore dependent on the activity of pharyngeal dilator muscles for maintenance of patency. The pharyngeal muscles include the muscles of the soft palate, the main muscle controlling the tongue (genioglossus), and the hyoid muscle groups.

Failure of the upper airway muscles to function normally is the result of a variety of neuromuscular disorders affecting the brainstem, particularly bulbar poliomyelitis, the postpolio syndrome, myasthenia, and amyotrophic lateral sclerosis (ALS). The most common example of failed upper airway mus-

cle activity is the obstructive sleep apnea (OSA) syndrome, the pathogenesis of which is beyond the scope of this book. However, both OSA and neuromuscular disorders in general cause disturbances during sleep and produce sequelae similar to those mentioned above.

Primary and Accessory Muscles

The main muscles of inspiration are the diaphragm and the intercostals. More important is the diaphragm which, when it contracts, forces the abdominal contents downward and forward and so increases the vertical dimension of the chest cavity. In addition, the rib margins are lifted outward, which increases the transverse diameter of the thorax. Contraction of the intercostal muscles pulls the ribs upward and forward, increasing the lateral and anteroposterior diameter of the thorax.[17]

The accessory muscles of inspiration are inactive during normal, tidal breathing. However, during exercise or during other causes of respiratory distress, they can become quite active. These muscles include the scalene muscles, which elevate the first two ribs, and the sternomastoids, which raise the sternum. Also included are the alae nasi which dilate the nose (causing flaring) and reduce nasal airflow resistance during stressful periods, and the small muscles in the neck and head.

Dysfunction of primary or accessory muscles of the respiratory system are produced by poliomyelitis; motor neuron disease (ALS, myasthenia, muscular dystrophy); other myopathies, either primary or toxic (e.g., hypothyroidism); and peripheral neuropathies (Guillain-Barré syndrome). Disorders of respiratory muscles generally produce a syndrome of hypoventilation. However, unlike respiratory control disorders, there is often an increased alveolar-arterial gradient secondary to atelectasis at the bases of the lungs (causing increased $\dot{V}/\dot{Q}$ mismatch). This atelectasis is due to mechanical inability and therefore these patients, unlike those with respiratory control disorders, are unable to voluntarily hyperventilate. Dyspnea prevails because peripheral sensation is intact, and the supine position exacerbates the disorder. The chest film may also show diaphragmatic elevation suggesting paralysis. The history and physical examination should elucidate most muscular and chest wall disorders and explain the hypoventilation. The other major muscular disorder is diaphragmatic paralysis, which may be due to nerve trauma (occasionally iatrogenic), inflammation, or neoplastic infiltration, but is most commonly idiopathic. Unilateral diaphragmatic paralysis is often asymptomatic whereas bilateral diaphragm weakness or paralysis often leads to respiratory failure.

Thorax

Another important accessory structure is the bony thorax, which houses the lungs and allows for normal pulmonary mechanics. In normal states the thorax has no dynamic influence on ventilation. However, when abnormal, the thorax can cause major ventilatory compromise. The bony thorax can be affected by disorders such as kyphoscoliosis, chronic fibrothorax (secondary to chronic inflammatory disorders), ankylosing spondylitis, or old chest surgery (e.g., thoracoplasty). Chest trauma may also cause serious ventilatory limitation. Flail chest, a condition marked by rib separation in two places, is well known to cause hypoventilation because of pain and mechanical instability. Patients with disorders of the bony thorax often hypoventilate similarly to patients with primary muscular disorders. In addition, the restrictive effect of the abnormal bony skeleton may in itself inhibit the normal mechanical defense system (i.e., cough) and therefore predispose these patients to infectious complications.

Gas Exchange

The conduit airways of the respiratory system consist of 23 generations (or branchings) from the trachea. The first 16 generations make up the conducting airways. These airways start in the trachea and end in the terminal bronchioles, and they bring air to the gas exchange units while not taking part in gas exchange themselves. These airways thus are termed the anatomic dead space and their volume is about 150 mL. The last 7 generations of the airway, from the respiratory bronchioles to the alveolar spaces, are termed the respiratory zone, for it is here that gas exchange actually occurs. The respiratory zone is small (<5 mm), but it makes up most of the lung's volume (about 3 L).

The airways are mainly responsible for maintaining normal $\dot{V}/\dot{Q}$ matching in the lung. Obviously, diseases that affect the airways will alter normal $\dot{V}/\dot{Q}$ relationships.[18] Problems in the larger airways include foreign body obstruction, upper airway collapse, tumors, laryngospasm, and tracheal stenosis. The degree to which these disorders affect ventilation directly relates to the amount of airway lumen occluded (Fig 3–3,b). More diffuse disorders that affect the conducting airways include COPD and asthma. These disorders tend to have large effects upon $\dot{V}/\dot{Q}$ matching for two reasons. Firstly, their pathophysiology of exuberant mucus production and bronchoconstriction tends to affect the conducting airways diffusely. Secondly, these diseases also involve small airways and therefore produce effects at the gas exchange level (Fig 3–3,c). Therefore, these disorders tend to produce marked hypoxemia and abnormal ventilation. Parenchymal lung diseases tend to produce marked hypoxemia that is also due to effects similar to small airway problems. These disorders include pneumonias, pulmonary contusions, pulmonary edema, and inhalational injuries such as hypersensitivity pneumonitis.

In most of these patients, evaluation will reveal symptoms suggestive of airway problems: cough, wheezing, chest tightness. Exertional dyspnea may also be a problem. Signs include wheezing, stridor, or segmental loss of airway sounds. A chest film is generally helpful and an ABG determination is essential. Although O_2 helps most patients, therapy should be aimed at the underlying disorder—improving ventilation.

Diffusion and Perfusion: The Alveolar-Capillary Unit

Along with adequate ventilation, the other essential ingredients for adequate oxygenation are normal gas diffusion and appropriate perfusion. As stated earlier, the normal lung is ideal for gas diffusion because it consists of a very large (50–100 m^2), extremely thin (<1 μm) barrier for gas exchange. Oxygen and CO_2 are also fairly soluble gases (CO_2 much more so) and this aids in their ease of passage from lung to pulmonary circulation and vice versa. Under typical resting conditions and assuming normal hemoglobin avidity for oxygen, the PO_2 in a red blood cell in a capillary that is passing by an alveolus will become equal to PAO_2 about one third of the way along the capillary. This suggests that under these circumstances, the amount of O_2 that enters the blood is dependent primarily upon how many red blood cells are present to be oxygenated. However, this can change under conditions which make the barrier between the lung and the capillary thickened, increasing diffusion time to the point that equilibration between lung and capillary may be unable to be completed by the time the red blood cell passes the alveolus.[18]

The diseases which cause diffusion difficulties are varied, but all have in common an increased transit time for effective O_2 transfer.[19] These diseases include asbestosis, sarcoidosis, interstitial fibrosis, viral interstitial pneumonias, and collagen-vascu-

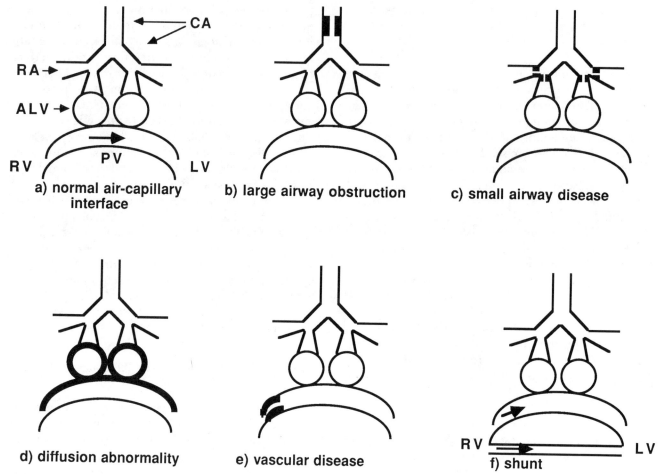

FIG 3–3.
Graphic demonstration of the pathophysiologic causes of hypoxemia. *(a)* represents the normal alveolar-capillary interface leading to nor-moxemia *(b–f)* demonstrate the various abnormalities leading to hypoxemia. *ALV* = alveoli; *CA* = conducting airways; *RA* = respiratory airways; *RV* = right ventricle; *LV* = left ventricle; *PV* = pulmonary vasculature. (Modified from West J: *Pulmonary Pathophysiology—the Essentials,* ed 3. Baltimore, Williams & Wilkins Co, 1985.)

lar diseases (especially scleroderma, Wegener's granulomatosis, Goodpasture's syndrome, and systemic lupus erythematosus), and lymphangitic carcinomatosis. Interstitial edema that develops due to a myriad of causes (high altitude, left ventricular failure, hypoproteinemia) may also cause some diffusion problems, but tends not to become clinically relevant until fluid moves from the interstitium to the alveoli.

In all of the above diseases, exercise clearly exaggerates the disorder. This is easily envisioned if you remember that normal O_2 equilibration takes about one third of total resting capillary transit time across an alveolus. In diffusion disorders, the resting equilibration time may increase to one half of the total capillary transit time (Fig 3–3,d). If a person then exercises, stroke volume increases, mainly by increased heart rate, and transit time is therefore re-

duced. If transit time is reduced to less than 50% of resting time, the person with a diffusion disorder will not have enough time to transfer O_2. The result is exercise-induced hypoxemia and severe dyspnea—the two hallmarks of diffusion disorders. Physical examination often demonstrates cyanosis of the skin and rales in the lung fields and the chest film often exhibits fibrosis. Patients are generally hyperventilating owing to stimulation of J receptors in the lung, stretch receptors on the chest wall, and carotid bodies. These patients rarely retain CO_2 because of its higher solubility and therefore more efficient transfer. Oxygen is particularly helpful to these patients because it increases the alveolar-arterial O_2 gradient making O_2 transfer more favorable.

The pulmonary circulation is a dense network of branching vessels and a large-mesh bed of capillaries that is surrounded by alveoli and gas. The pulmonary circulation is a low-pressure, low-resistance system, which under normal conditions perfuses all parts of the lung in a relatively uniform manner (except for the effects of gravity which causes more blood to flow to the lung bases than to the apices). The pulmonary circulation does, however, have the ability to change its orientation in response to the local milieu. The most notable example is vasoconstriction as a response to alveolar hypoxemia. This serves to redirect blood flow away from areas of poor ventilation and toward areas of normal ventilation to improve $\dot{V}/\dot{Q}$ matching.

A variety of disorders can cause an abnormality in the pulmonary circulation and therefore $\dot{V}/\dot{Q}$ mismatch. The most common and notable is pulmonary thromboembolism. This can be either acute or chronic, and is usually associated with chest pain, shortness of breath, tachycardia, tachypnea, and hypoxemia. The mechanism for hypoxemia is twofold, both of which involve $\dot{V}/\dot{Q}$ mismatching. Firstly, there is increase in dead space ventilation as areas of the lung are ventilated but inadequately perfused. This occurs because the airways have limited ability to redirect airflow to areas of better perfusion. Secondly, blood flow is diverted to other areas producing abnormally low $\dot{V}/\dot{Q}$ ratios which also adds to a reduced O_2 admixture. In massive embolism, pulmonary hypertension can also cause decreased blood flow to the lung and even right ventricular failure, which further decreases systemic oxygenation.[20]

Pulmonary hypertension is another cause of hypoxemia seen in the emergency room. Although the rise in pulmonary artery pressure may be acute, there is generally some degree of chronicity involved in the problem. The cause of hypoxemia in pulmonary hypertension is mainly $\dot{V}/\dot{Q}$ mismatching with areas of increased dead space ventilation. Exercise tends to exaggerate the hypoxemia in almost all of these cases. The causes of pulmonary hypertension are varied. Increased left arterial pressure due to mitral valve disease or left ventricular dysfunction can cause increases in pressure in the pulmonary arteries. Chronic hypoxemia (due to high altitude or chronic obstructive diseases) can cause chronic vasoconstriction with increases in pulmonary artery pressure. In addition, emphysema may cause additional pulmonary hypertension by actual destruction of part of the vascular bed along with the parenchymal destruction that occurs. Thromboembolism may cause increased pulmonary artery pressure either acutely (with massive emboli) or chronically (with multiple small emboli). Rare diseases like vasculitis (affecting the small arteries) and veno-occlusive dis-

ease (affecting the small veins) may obliterate the vascular bed causing increases in pulmonary artery pressure. Finally, pulmonary hypertension may be idiopathic, a disease characterized by smooth muscle hypertrophy of small pulmonary arteries. Pulmonary hypertension is generally found in young people (20–40 years old) with a female predominance. Like the above diseases, people with primary pulmonary hypertension have dyspnea, often at rest but definitely with exercise. Chest pain, hemoptysis, hyperventilation, and hypoxemia are other common manifestations of these diseases.

The most extreme form of $\dot{V}/\dot{Q}$ mismatch is a shunt—a mixing of totally unventilated, unoxygenated blood with ventilated, oxygenated blood.[18] There are two main types of shunts. Anatomic shunt occurs where an anatomic defect exists allowing blood to bypass the lungs and go directly from the right side to the left-sided circulation (Fig 3–3,f). Examples of anatomic shunts include atrial or ventricular septal defects, patent ductus arterosus, and pulmonary arteriovenous fistula. A second type of shunt occurs when a portion of the cardiac output circulates normally through the pulmonary vasculature but, because of parenchymal problems, does not come into contact with any alveolar air. The best example of this is complete lobar atelectasis, especially in the lower lobes (where $\dot{V}/\dot{Q}$ ratios tend to be low already). In both anatomic and physiologic shunts, oxygenation is low. However, the hypoxemia of anatomic shunts cannot be corrected by increasing the FiO_2. In contrast, increasing FiO_2 in physiologic shunts does improve oxygenation because even in lobar collapse there is some collateral ventilation to alveoli occurring via the pores of Kohn and canals of Lambert rather than via normal conduit airways.

Oxygen-Carrying Capacity

We have discussed at length disorders that may cause hypoxemia (low CaO_2). *Hypoxia* is a more general term and signifies a lack of O_2 in the body's tissues. Hypoxia is usually caused by hypoxemia, but may also result when the CaO_2 is normal, but the body cannot deliver the O_2 efficiently (e.g., in low cardiac output) or the tissues cannot adequately remove or use the available circulating O_2 (e.g., in distorted hemoglobin function or cyanide toxicity).

Oxygen Transfer (Hemoglobin)

The total CaO_2 is the sum of the amount of O_2 bound to hemoglobin and the amount of O_2 dissolved in plasma. As discussed earlier, the amount of dissolved O_2 (0.1% of total O_2 available) is negligible compared to the amount of O_2 bound to hemoglobin (99.9% of total O_2 available).[1]

Figure 3–4 demonstrates the hemoglobin dissociation curve which relates PaO_2 to saturation of arterial blood with oxygen (SaO_2).[21] A number of important remarks need to be made about this curve. Firstly, the PaO_2 is not affected by either changes in hemoglobin or percent saturation. Secondly, changes in hemoglobin concentration do not affect the SaO_2. Changes in hemoglobin concentration affect the total amount of bound O_2 and therefore play a major role in determining total CaO_2. The right side of Figure 3–4 shows CaO_2 with a normal hemoglobin (15 g/dL [or gm%]) and with anemia (10 g/dL [or gm%]). Clearly, PaO_2 content falls with anemia, making less O_2 available to vital tissues like the brain and myocardium. Considerable debate exists as to the critical juncture at which anemia produces its deleterious effects on tissue oxygenation and the patient's underlying condition becomes predominant. However, hemoglobin levels of less than 7.5 to 8.0 g/dL (especially acutely) are generally considered the point at which cardiovascular complications arise.[22, 23] The shape and position of the curve shows the relationship between PaO_2 and SaO_2 when the pH, PCO_2, body temperature, and other factors are normal. Alteration of any of these factors will shift the dissociation curve from its normal position.

The P_{50} represents the PaO_2 at which 50% of the hemoglobin is saturated with O_2; normally this is about 27 mm Hg. A P_{50} >27 mm Hg is a rightward shift of the O_2 dissociation curve: blood picks up less O_2 at the pulmonary capillary level but delivers more O_2 to the tissues. Acidemia, hypercapnia, and hyperthermia will shift the curve to the right; this shift is considered a helpful, protective adaptation.[1] A P_{50} <27 represents a leftward shift of the curve, meaning that blood picks up O_2 more avidly at the pulmonary level, but is less apt to deliver this O_2 to the tissues when PO_2 is low. This is a less favorable adaptation. A shift to the left is caused by alkalemia which produces a higher SaO_2 for any given PaO_2. This can be clinically important when using an oximeter (which measures SaO_2) on a patient who is hyperventilating (causing alkalemia). The SaO_2 recorded will not truly reflect PaO_2. This reinforces the value of ABG determinations.

There can be many derangements of this system. Firstly, as we have mentioned, although anemia does not adversely affect either PaO_2 or SaO_2, it does affect total CaO_2. It is total CaO_2 that affects the tissues and so reduced CaO_2 can aggravate angina, pulmonary impairment, or even claudication despite seemingly normal O_2 measurements. Secondly, a relatively common problem is carbon monoxide toxicity. Carbon monoxide combines more avidly with hemoglobin than with O_2 to form carboxyhemoglobin. As carboxyhemoglobin is increased, oxyhemoglobin and CaO_2 are decreased. In addition, CO, by changing the nature of hemoglobin binding, shifts the O_2 dissociation curve to the left, making it more difficult for tissues to receive the O_2 present in red blood cells. The additive effect of decreased CaO_2 and ineffective delivery of O_2 to the tissues can produce profound tissue hypoxia.

The diagnosis of CO toxicity includes an inappropriately low *measured* SaO_2 (ABGs report *calculated* SaO_2) despite a normal PaO_2. Thus, an elevated carboxyhemoglobin (% HbCO) level[24] can be best detected by a direct CO measurement. Less than 2% HbCO is considered normal, whereas smokers can have HbCO levels of 5% to 10%. Higher levels than these suggest a pathologic condition. Automobile exhaust and fires are the commonest causes of acute CO poisoning. Other causative agents are wood stoves, malfunctioning fireplaces, and space heaters. Symptoms include headache, lethargy, dyspnea, confusion, and angina. Dilation of cutaneous vessels

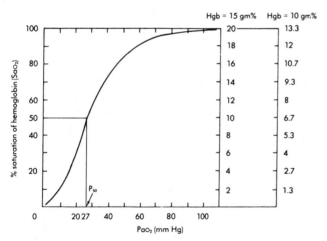

FIG 3–4.
PaO_2 vs. SaO_2 and oxygen content. The oxygen dissociation curve relates only PaO_2 to SaO_2 and is the same regardless of hemoglobin content. P_{50} = the PaO_2 at which hemoglobin is 50% saturated with oxygen, and is normally about 27 mm Hg. On the right is arterial oxygen content (CaO_2) which is a function of both PaO_2 and hemoglobin concentration. CaO_2 is given in a healthy *(Hgb=15 gm%)* and an anemic subject *(Hgb=10 gm%)*. (From Martin L: *Pulmonary Physiology in Clinical Practice.* St Louis, Mosby–Year Book, Inc, 1987, p 116. Used by permission.)

(cherry-red color) can occur, as well as ventricular arrhythmias.

Another major cause of reduced O_2 content is methemoglobin. Methemoglobin occurs when the ferrous (Fe^{2+}) moiety of hemoglobin is oxidized to the ferric state (Fe^{3+}). This oxidized hemoglobin is unable to bind O_2. Like carboxyhemoglobin, methemoglobin has two effects: (1) it decreases the amount of hemoglobin available for O_2 binding and (2) it increases the avidity of hemoglobin for O_2, shifting the dissociation curve to the left.[25]

The most common cause of methemoglobinemia are drugs, including nitrites (e.g., metabolites of nitro-vasodilators) and sulfonamides (Table 3–2). Normally, about 1.5% of hemoglobin is in the oxidized (methemoglobin) state. A value greater than this suggests methemoglobinemia. Diagnosis is suggested by history and by profound cyanosis despite a seemingly normal PaO_2. Once again, *measured* SaO_2 will be low and an increased methemoglobin level can also be measured. Another situation in which SaO_2 and PaO_2 may truly be normal but in which tissue hypoxia still persists is cyanide toxicity. Cyanide inhibits the function of mitochondria and therefore causes cellular hypoxia. Anaerobic metabolism and cell death ensue producing (predominantly) CNS and respiratory toxicity followed quickly by death.

Abnormal hemoglobin may also adversely affect the body's ability to oxygenate. As shown in Figure 3–4, anemia causes decreased total CaO_2. In addition, a variety of abnormal hemoglobins[26] exist that may shift the oxygen dissociation curve to the left or right. Their clinical impact rests largely upon the direction in which they shift the curve.

Cardiac Output

As stated earlier, adequate O_2 delivery to the tissues requires adequate CaO_2, normal hemoglobin to deliver this O_2, and a normal cardiac output. Patients in cardiogenic shock can have a normal CaO_2, but still have severe tissue hypoxia due to inadequate O_2 delivery. Obviously, such patients require further evaluation to determine their hemodynamic state.

Reduction in either cardiac output or CaO_2 threatens O_2 delivery. In either case, tissue death ensues if tissue VO_2 is not maintained. Assessing whether VO_2 is maintained can be a difficult task. In practice, this is done by pulmonary artery (Swan-Ganz) catheterization.[27] This can impart two important pieces of information: (1) cardiac output and

TABLE 3–2.

Drugs and Environmental Agents Reported to Cause Methemoglobinemia

Drugs
  Phenazopyridine
  Benzocaine
  Prilocaine
  Nitroglycerin
  Amyl nitrite
  Metaclopramide
  Dapsone
  Primaquine
  Trimethoprim
Environment agents
  Aniline derivatives (varnishes, dyes, inks, crayons, paints)
  Nitrate salts (fertilizers, contaminated water, spinach)
  Sodium nitrite (food preservatives)

(2) mixed venous oxygen saturation ($S\bar{v}O_2$). The blood in the pulmonary artery represents the mixed venous blood from various parts of the body. $S\bar{v}O_2$[28] represents the *net* result of the initial CaO_2 after O_2 has been extracted by the tissues ($\dot{V}O_2$). The $S\bar{v}O_2$ is normally 75% while normal mixed venous partial pressure of oxygen ($P\bar{v}O_2$) is about 40 mm Hg.

When cardiac output or CaO_2 are reduced, the tissues generally respond by extracting a higher percentage of the available O_2. This leads to a decreased $P\bar{v}O_2$ or $S\bar{v}O_2$. A low $S\bar{v}O_2$ indicates inadequate O_2 delivery to the tissues. This is true whether the problem be low cardiac output due to left ventricular failure or septic shock (producing increased $\dot{V}O_2$). The differentiation of cardiogenic from noncardiogenic shock is obviously aided by the pulmonary artery measurements, including cardiac output and pulmonary capillary wedge pressure.

There are certain conditions in which a normal $S\bar{v}O_2$ does not adequately assess the body's oxygenation. Firstly, regional hypoperfusion to one or several organs may be masked by normal perfusion to other areas, resulting in a net normal $S\bar{v}O_2$. Secondly, in both septic and cardiogenic shock, left-to-right shunts may develop peripherally. These shunts send blood directly from arteries to veins, bypassing the capillaries of the tissues. This results in a "normal" $S\bar{v}O_2$ despite tissue hypoxia. Thirdly, in the case of cyanide toxicity, cells are unable to utilize O_2, resulting in anaerobic metabolism and lactic acid accumulation. In this case $\dot{V}O_2$ by the tissues is reduced and $S\bar{v}O_2$ is falsely normal. However, keeping these exceptions in mind, the $S\bar{v}O_2$ can be a powerful tool in assessing proper oxygen delivery.

SUMMARY

The act of ventilation and oxygenation is a complicated and coordinated process involving most of the human body. Derangements in the process can occur at every step along the pathway. The clinical armentarium for assessing and correcting these defects is vast, and requires that the clinician have a working knowledge of the various segments of this integrated process if he or she is to make correct therapeutic decisions.

REFERENCES

1. West JB: *Respiratory Physiology—the Essentials,* ed 3. Baltimore, Williams & Wilkins Co, 1990.
2. Gilbert R, Keighley J: The arterial/alveolar oxygen tension ratio: An index of gas exchange applicable to varying inspired oxygen concentrations. *Am Rev Respir Dis* 1974; 109:142.
3. Murray J: *The Normal Lung.* Philadelphia, WB Saunders Co, 1986.
4. Murray J, Nadel J: *Textbook of Respiratory Medicine.* Philadelphia, WB Saunders Co, 1988.
5. Braman S: Pulmonary signs and symptoms. *Clin Chest Med* 1987; 8:177–188.
6. Hetzel MR, Clark TJ: Comparison of normal and asthmatic circadian rhythms in peak expiratory flow rate. *Thorax* 1980; 35:732.
7. Alexander CM, Teller LE, Gross JB: Principles of pulse oximetry: Theoretical and practical considerations. *Anesth Analg* 1989; 68:368.
8. Dowd J, Jenkins LC: Some problems associated with measurement of physiologic blood gases. *Can Anaesth Soc J* 1973; 20:132.
9. McCurdy D: Mixed metabolic and respiratory acid-base disturbances: Diagnosis and treatment. *Chest* 1972; 62(suppl):35.
10. Narins R, Gardner L: Simple acid-base disturbances. *Med Clin North Am* 1981; 65:321.
11. Winters RW: Terminology of acid-base disorders. *Ann Intern Med* 1965; 63:837.
12. Sorbini C, Grassi V, Solinas V, et al: Arterial oxygen tension in relation to age in healthy subjects. *Respiration* 1968; 25:3.
13. Shoemaker W: *Textbook of Critical Care.* Philadelphia, WB Saunders Co, 1989.
14. Bone RC: Acute respiratory failure and chronic obstructive lung disease: Recent advances. *Med Clin North Am* 1981; 65:563.
15. Aubier MD, Murciano Milic-Emili J, et al: Effects of the administration of O_2 on ventilation and blood gases in patients with chronic obstructive pulmonary disease during acute respiratory failure. *Am Rev Respir Dis* 1980; 122:747.
16. Williams MH: Disturbances of respiratory control. *Clin Chest Med,* 1980, vol 1.
17. Belman MJ: Respiratory muscles in health and disease. *Clin Chest Med,* 1988, vol 9.
18. West JB: *Pulmonary Pathophysiology—the essentials,* ed 3. Baltimore, Williams & Wilkins, 1987.
19. Schwarz M, King T: *Interstitial Lung Disease.* Toronto, BC Decker, Inc, 1988.
20. Moser K: Venous thromboembolism. *Am Rev Respir Dis* 1990; 141:235.
21. Martin L: *Pulmonary Physiology in Clinical Practice.* St. Louis, Mosby–Year Book, Inc, 1987.
22. Shoemaker WC, Reinhard JM: Tissue perfusion defects in shock and trauma states. *Surg Gynecol Obstet* 1973; 137:1980.
23. Varat MA, Adolph RJ, Fowler NO: Cardiovascular effects of anemia. *Am Heart J* 1972; 83:415.
24. Myers RA, Linberg SE, Crowley RA: Carbon monoxide poisoning: The injury and its treatment. *JACEP* 1979; 8:479.
25. Mansouri A: Methemoglobinemia. *Am J Med Sci* 1985; 289:200.
26. Edwards J, Mathay K: Hematologic disorders affecting the lungs. *Clin Chest Med* 1989; 10:723–746.
27. Wiedman H, Mathay M, Mathay R: Cardiovascular-pulmonary monitoring in the intensive care unit. *Chest* 1984; 85:537.
28. Kandel G, Aberman A: Mixed venous oxygen saturation: Its role in the assessment of the critically ill patient. *Arch Intern Med* 1983; 143:1400.

ADDITIONAL READINGS

Belman MJ: Respiratory muscles in health and disease. *Clin Chest Med* 1988; 9:

Bordow R, Moser K: *Manual of Clinical Problems in Pulmonary Medicine.* Boston, Little, Brown Co, 1985.

Fick RB: Inflammatory disorders of the airways. *Clin Chest Med* 1988; 9:

Gilbert R, Keighley J: The arterial/alveolar oxygen tension ratio: An index of gas exchange applicable to varying inspired oxygen concentrations. *Am Rev Respir Dis* 1974; 109:142.

Hyers T: Pulmonary emobllism and hypertension. *Clin Chest Med* 1984; 5:

Ingram R, Miller R, Tate L: Acid-base response to acute carbon dioxide changes in chronic obstructive pulmonary disease. *Am Rev Respir Dis* 1973; 108:225.

Murray J, Nadel J: *Textbook of Respiratory Medicine.* Philadelphia, WB Saunders Co, 1988.

Murray J: *The Normal Lung* WB Saunders Co, 1986.

Narins R, Gardner L: Simple acid-base disturbances. *Med Clin North Am* 1981; 65:321.

Moser K: Venous thromboembolism. *Am Rev Respir Dis* 1990; 141:235.

Shaver JA: Hemodynamic monitoring in the critically ill patient. *N Engl J Med* 1983;308:277.

Shoemaker W: *Textbook of Critical Care*. WB Saunders Co, 1989.

Smith J, Stone R, Muschenheim C: Acute respiratory failure in chronic lung disease. Observations on controlled oxygen therapy. *Am Rev Respir Dis* 1968; 97:791.

PART II

Airway Maneuvers

4

Basic Life Support

Mohamud Daya, M.D.

Ronald Mariani, E.M.T.–P.

Christopher Fernandes, M.D.

Basic life support (BLS) is an essential component of resuscitation and of fundamental importance in the practice of emergency medicine. Victims of cardiorespiratory arrest must have breathing and circulation restored within 4 minutes if irreversible neurologic injury is to be prevented. The goal of BLS is to provide adequate oxygenation to all vital tissues, in particular the brain and heart, until spontaneous circulation can be restored through the use of advanced life support (ALS) measures. The success of ALS is critically dependent upon prompt and effective BLS. BLS can be performed anywhere and by anyone (trained lay public, health care providers, and so forth) since little or no equipment is needed. The sequence of steps performed during BLS can be summarized as follows:

1. Establish unresponsiveness; beware of cervical spine injury.
2. Call for help.
3. Properly position the victim—supine on a hard surface.
4. Airway: open and maintain the airway.
5. Breathing: assess and ensure adequate ventilation.
6. Circulation: assess and ensure adequate perfusion and oxygenation of tissues.

The American Heart Association (AHA) defines BLS as those aspects of cardiopulmonary resuscitation (CPR) which can be performed without the use of mechanical adjuncts.[1] The World Federation of Societies of Anaesthesiologists (WFSA) uses BLS to describe all methods used to achieve emergency oxygenation in CPR, irrespective of the use of ancillary equipment.[1] This chapter approaches BLS using a combination of these two definitions. Although simple mechanical adjuncts are covered, esophageal airways and tracheal intubation are not discussed.

HISTORY

The earliest record of a successful resuscitation using mouth-to-mouth ventilation is in the Bible.[1] In II Kings 4:34, the story of how the prophet Elijah breathed life into the son of a Shunammite woman in 850 B.C. is described as follows: "And he went up, and lay upon the child, and put his mouth upon his mouth . . . and the flesh of the child waxed warm." Despite this auspicious beginning, mouth-to-mouth ventilation was not accepted into the practice of resuscitation medicine until the middle part of this century.

Early methods of resuscitation were based on the principles of restoring warmth to the body and physically stimulating the victim back to life.[2] Hot water, warm ashes, or burning excrement were often placed on the body in an attempt to revive the victim.[2] Physical stimulation involved the use of loud noises, slapping, whipping, or tongue stretching to "awaken" the victim.[2] The use of warmth and physical stimulation remained a part of resuscitation medicine well into the 19th century.

Other methods of resuscitation included the use of rhythmic chest compressions to achieve ventilation and revive victims of drowning.[2] Victims were placed on the back of a trotting horse or rolled over barrels in the hope that this would restore spontaneous breathing.[2] The procedure of blowing air or tobacco into a victim's mouth or rectum (fumigation) was a popular method of resuscitation in the 18th century.[2] Concerns over the potential toxicity of tobacco led to the discontinuation of fumigation in 1811.[2] The use of fireside bellows to blow air into the victim's mouth was first described by Paracelsus in the 16th century.[2] The bellows figured prominently in resuscitation until 1829 when d'Etiolles showed that overdistention of the lungs could kill an animal.[2]

In the same paper, d'Etiolles also advanced the concept of manual ventilation through the use of chest and abdominal pressure.[2] This concept was subsequently expanded on by a number of investigators including Dalrymple, Hall, Silvester, Schafer, Eve, and Nielsen.[2] The various methods of manual ventilation described by these authors were eventually integrated into resuscitation practices. In 1951, Gordon used intubated volunteers to study six methods of manual ventilation and found that the push-pull or active inspiration and expiration methods produced superior tidal volumes.[2,3] Gordon favored the Nielsen method of back pressure–arm lift and this method was subsequently adopted and taught by the American Red Cross.[2]

In the 1950s Elam, Safar, Gordon, and their colleagues and others began some of the basic research on the fundamentals of modern resuscitation medicine. Earlier studies demonstrating the effectiveness of manual ventilation in intubated curarized patients were criticized because they did not take into account the behavior of the upper airway in the unconscious patient.[4-6] It was noted that upper airway obstruction due to posterior relaxation of the tongue and epiglottis in the unconscious patient limited the efficacy of all methods of artificial respiration.[3,4,7] This obstruction could be corrected by backward tilt of the head and forward displacement of the mandible.[4,7] The importance of head tilt and mandible support to prevent pharyngeal obstruction by the relaxed tongue during anesthesia had actually been described in the 1870s by Esmarch and Heiberg.[1]

The first successful application of mouth-to-mouth ventilation in an adult was reported by Tossach in 1743.[8] Although the use of mouth-to-mouth ventilation had been recommended by many authors, the method was used infrequently by rescue personnel. Reluctance to come into contact with the lips of a moribund patient and the low oxygen content of expired air were frequently cited as the major objections to mouth-to-mouth ventilation.[8] The first objective evaluation of mouth-to-mouth ventilation was reported by Elam et al. in 1954.[8] They showed that apneic patients could be ventilated effectively with exhaled air to keep the arterial oxygen saturation above normal and the alveolar carbon dioxide tension below normal.[8] In 1958, Safar et al.[5] demonstrated that mouth-to-mouth resuscitation was superior to the chest pressure–arm lift (Silvester) or back pressure–arm-lift (Nielsen) methods of manual ventilation. Expired air ventilation produced larger tidal volumes and left both hands of the operator free to support the head and mandible.[3,5] Similar findings were subsequently reported in children by Gordon.[1] The use of simple adjuncts such as a face mask or an artificial airway also made mouth-to-mouth ventilation more acceptable and less unpleasant for the operator.[5,8]

In 1960 Kouwenhoven, an electrical engineer at Johns Hopkins Hospital in Baltimore, serendipitously discovered that external chest compressions could maintain circulation in arrested animals.[9] In 1961, Safar combined artificial ventilation and external cardiac compression and the concept of CPR was born.[10]

In the 1960s, the feasibility of teaching CPR to the public was demonstrated, followed by the creation of innovative teaching aids.[11] During the same time, national and international meetings established standards and guidelines for CPR.[1]

The last two decades have been characterized as periods of rediscovery and refinement.[10] Kouwenhoven's theory that blood flow during CPR occurred as a result of cardiac compression between the sternum and the vertebral bodies was challenged. Criley et al. reported that vigorous coughing produced effective systemic blood flow during cardiac arrest in the absence of direct cardiac compression.[2,12,13] The importance of intrathoracic pressure increases (thoracic pump theory) was recognized and the heart was now seen as simply a conduit for blood flow during CPR.[12] Methods to improve the effectiveness of CPR by further increasing the intrathoracic pressure are currently under investigation.[12,13]

At this time, CPR has emerged as a valid concept, delivered in a continuum from the field to the hospital. Revision of standards has continued, based on ongoing studies.[13] New methods and adjuncts are on the horizon, awaiting the test of time, and comparison with the advances of the last 40 years.

THE AIRWAY

General Considerations

Upper airway obstruction can result from either central or peripheral causes.[14] Any condition that depresses the central nervous system (CNS) and reduces muscle tone will allow the tongue to fall posteriorly against the pharynx resulting in airway obstruction. The tongue is the most common (and most important) cause of upper airway obstruction. Causes of CNS depression include cardiac arrest, shock, head trauma, drug overdose, general anesthesia, metabolic derangements, and cerebrovascular events.[14] Peripheral causes of airway obstruction include all conditions that directly encroach upon the upper airway. Included in this category are congenital anomalies, infections (epiglottitis, croup), trauma, burns, anaphylaxis, and tumors.[14]

Airway obstruction resulting from prolapse of the tongue is best understood by reviewing the anatomy of the upper airway. The oropharynx has a rigid posterior wall consisting of the cervical vertebrae and a collapsible anterior wall formed by the tongue and epiglottis. The tongue is firmly attached to the mandible, hyoid bone, and epiglottis through a number of muscles and ligaments.[14] The epiglottis is attached inferiorly to the thyroid cartilage and superiorly to the tongue and hyoid bone. In the conscious patient, tone within the oropharyngeal muscles keeps the tongue and epiglottis away from the pharynx and larynx, respectively. In the unconscious patient, these muscles relax, allowing the tongue to relax posteriorly and occlude the hypopharynx. Recession of the tongue and hyoid bone also allows the epiglottis to fall posteriorly against the laryngeal opening.

Other factors also contribute to airway obstruction in the unconscious person. The loss of tone in the neck muscles and the effect of gravity allow the neck to flex on the cervical vertebral column, resulting in acute angulation and narrowing of the hypopharynx.[15] In addition, the relaxed tongue may act as a valve and increase airway obstruction during inspiratory efforts.[14, 16] Airway obstruction in the unconscious patient is therefore dependent upon the position of the jaw and neck. This obstruction will occur regardless of whether the patient is in the supine, prone, or lateral position.[1] Gravity alone is ineffective in correcting hypopharyngeal soft tissue obstruction.[1]

Upper airway obstruction compromises gas exchange resulting in hypercarbia and hypoxia. If un-

corrected, this can rapidly lead to irreversible neurologic injury or death. Thus, the first step in any resuscitation attempt is to open the airway. This can be accomplished using a variety of manual methods outlined below.

Airway Opening Techniques

Head Tilt

The head tilt is the easiest and most effective method for opening the airway.[4, 7, 17] One hand is placed on the forehead and firm pressure is applied to tilt the head backward at the atlanto-occipital joint. This maneuver stretches the anterior soft tissue structures between the chin and larynx, thereby lifting the tongue and epiglottis away from the posterior pharyngeal wall.[17] By reestablishing the normal cervical curve, the maneuver also corrects the acute angulation and narrowing of the hypopharynx.[16] The head tilt is especially useful for securing the airway in the seated victim. In the presence of residual oropharyngeal muscle tone, the head tilt alone may be adequate to open and maintain the airway. More often, the head tilt is combined with other manual maneuvers to establish an open airway.

Head Tilt–Chin Lift

The head tilt–chin lift (Fig 4–1) was described by Elam et al.[18] in 1960 and is recommended by the AHA as the preferred method of opening the airway in the unconscious victim.[19] One hand is placed on the victim's forehead and firm pressure is applied to tilt the head backward. The maneuver is completed by placing the fingers of the other hand un-

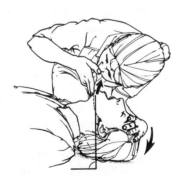

FIG 4–1.
The head tilt–chin lift maneuver. The perpendicular lines reflect proper neck extension, i.e., a line along the edge of the jaw bone should be perpendicular to the surface on which the victim is lying. (From *Heartsaver Manual.* Dallas, American Heart Association, 1987, p. 34. Used by permission.)

der the bony part of the lower jaw and lifting the chin forward. The addition of the chin lift leads to further stretching of the anterior soft tissue structures between the chin and larynx. This is important since the degree of stretch determines the degree of separation of the base of the tongue from the posterior pharyngeal wall.[17] The fingers must not press on the soft tissue structures of the neck since this can worsen airway obstruction.[18, 19]

The AHA adoption of the head tilt–chin lift was based on the results of a comparison study by Guildner[19] in 1976 on the efficacy of various airway opening techniques in anesthetized patients. Guildner found that the head tilt–chin lift method was the most consistent in facilitating untroubled and adequate ventilation.[16] This method was also less fatiguing and allowed for better control of loose dentures during mouth-to-mouth ventilation.[16]

Head Tilt–Neck Lift

The neck lift was originally described by Elam et al. in 1960.[18] The head tilt–neck lift method is accomplished by placing one hand on the forehead and the other hand under the neck. The neck is then lifted and extended while the forehead is tilted backward. The neck lift adds additional stretch to the anterior soft tissue structures between the chin and larynx. Guildner found the head tilt–neck lift to be less effective and more fatiguing than the head tilt–chin lift method.[16] He also found that the head tilt–neck lift worsened airway obstruction in persons with loose dentures.[16]

Jaw Thrust (Triple Airway Maneuver)

The jaw thrust was introduced by Safar in the late 1950s.[4, 17] The jaw thrust combines backward tilt of the head with displacement of the mandible and opening of the mouth.[1] The jaw thrust is very useful when other manual maneuvers have failed to open the airway. The studies of Safer and colleagues showed that backward head tilt and anterior neck stretch failed to open the airway in 20% of unconscious patients.[4, 17] In these cases, additional forward displacement of the mandible (jaw thrust) was required to establish a patent airway.[4, 17] Mandibular displacement further stretches the anterior soft tissue structures of the neck, helping to lift the tongue away from the posterior pharyngeal wall. Furthermore, it was noted that expiratory nasopharyngeal obstruction occurred in 30% of unconscious patients.[4, 11] This was attributed to a valve-like behavior of the soft palate during expiration.[1, 4] It was

corrected by holding the mouth slightly open during expiration.

To open the airway using this technique, the head should be tilted back in extension (Fig 4–2). The fingers of both hands are then used to grasp the ascending rami of the mandible. The mandible is displaced forward and upward to open the airway. The mouth is opened by retracting the lower lips with both thumbs. The jaw thrust is very useful when a face mask is to be used for rescue breathing. The nose is closed with the operator's cheek during mouth-to-mask ventilation. In his comparison studies, Guildner found that the jaw thrust was difficult to perform, tiring to execute, and poor at controlling loose dentures.[16]

Modified Jaw Thrust

This method of airway opening is identical to the jaw thrust maneuver with the exception that the victim's head is not tilted back. The AHA recommends the modified jaw thrust as the safest first approach to opening the airway of a patient with a suspected cervical injury.[19] Flexion, extension, and rotational movements must be avoided at all costs in patients with suspected neck injuries. The modified jaw thrust produces minimal neck movement and is the procedure of choice in this setting. If the modified jaw thrust alone does not open the airway, slight backward tilt of the head is recommended. Guildner found that the modified jaw thrust with no or minimal backward head tilt satisfactorily opened the airway in all instances.[16]

Thumb–Jaw Lift (Older Method)

In the very relaxed patient, the thumb–jaw lift can also be used to open the airway.[1] With this maneuver, the thumb is inserted into the victim's

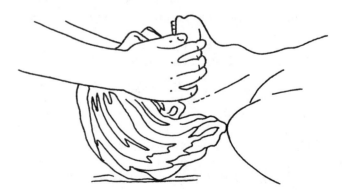

FIG 4–2.
The jaw thrust or triple airway maneuver. (From Finucane BT, Santora AH: *Principles of Airway Management.* Philadelphia, FA Davis Co, 1988. Used by permission.)

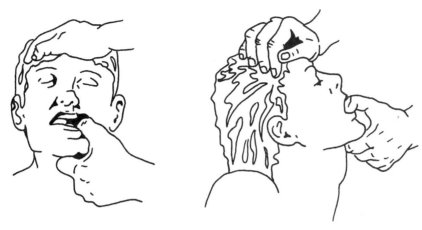

FIG 4–3.
The tongue–jaw lift or mandibular thrust. (From Safar P, Bircher NG: *Cardiopulmonary Cerebral Resuscitation,* ed 3. Philadelphia, WB Saunders Co, 1988. Used by permission.)

mouth while the other fingers are used to grasp the mandible at the chin (Fig 4–3). The mandible is then lifted anteriorly to open the airway. Unfortunately, the presence of the thumb will interfere with the seal during mouth-to-mouth ventilation.[18] In addition, the use of this maneuver carries with it the risk of being bitten by the partially obtunded victim.[1]

Summary

Training, performance, and efficacy issues must be considered prior to the selection of a particular airway opening maneuver. The 1985 national conference on standards and guidelines for CPR and emergency cardiac care (ECC) recommended the head tilt–chin lift maneuver as the preferred method for opening the airway because it is safe, simple, and effective.[20] Since all of the methods, with the exception of the modified jaw thrust cause movement of the neck, the latter was recommended as the method of choice for opening the airway in patients with suspected cervical spine injuries.[20]

BREATHING

Once the airway has been established, the adequacy of ventilation is assessed using the look-listen-and-feel technique. The rescuer *looks* to see if the victim's chest rises and falls, while he or she *listens* and *feels* for air movement through the mouth and nose. This step in the BLS sequence should take only 3 to 5 seconds.[19]

In the event of spontaneous respirations, the rescuer must simply ensure that an open airway is maintained at all times. The unattended victim should be placed onto the side (coma position) to allow secretions to drain out of the mouth and reduce the risk of aspiration (Fig 4–4). Trauma victims should have spinal alignment maintained prior to being logrolled onto the side.[21]

Should the victim have agonal or no spontaneous respirations, positive pressure ventilation must be provided immediately using either an exhaled air or forced air method. Current AHA recommendations call for two slow breaths to be delivered initially in all cases of respiratory or cardiac arrest. Rescue breathing in the presence of cardiac activity is then performed using slow (1.5–2.0 seconds) breaths at a rate of 12 times per minute. In the absence of cardiac activity, two slow breaths (1.0–1.5 seconds) should be delivered after every 15 chest compressions during one-rescuer CPR and one slow breath every 5 chest compressions with two-rescuer CPR.[22] The volume of air delivered with each breath should be large enough to make the victim's chest rise. For adults, the AHA recommends a tidal volume of 800 mL per breath.[19] The use of slow breaths allows for a longer inspiratory time and lower peak inspiratory pressures, thereby reducing the risk of gastric insufflation. Breath stacking and rapid ventilations were rejected at the 1985 conference on CPR and ECC because they produce higher peak airway pressures resulting in gastric insufflation.[22]

Exhaled Air Techniques

Mouth-to-Mouth Ventilation
In the absence of ancillary equipment, this ancient method is extremely effective at delivering air

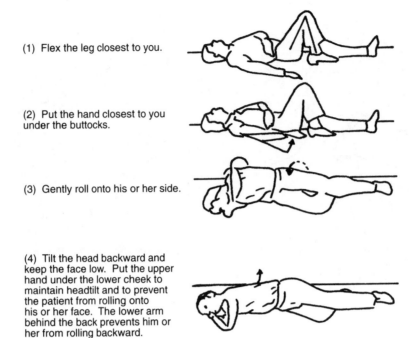

(1) Flex the leg closest to you.

(2) Put the hand closest to you under the buttocks.

(3) Gently roll onto his or her side.

(4) Tilt the head backward and keep the face low. Put the upper hand under the lower cheek to maintain headtilt and to prevent the patient from rolling onto his or her face. The lower arm behind the back prevents him or her from rolling backward.

FIG 4–4.
The stable side (coma) position for the spontaneously breathing conscious patient. (From Safar P, Bircher NG: *Cardiopulmonary Cerebral Resuscitation,* ed 3. Philadelphia, WB Saunders Co, 1988. Used by permission.)

to a victim of respiratory arrest. Having opened the airway, the rescuer's mouth is placed directly over the victim's mouth. The nose is pinched shut using the thumb and index finger of the hand which maintains backward tilt of the head. Alternatively, the rescuer's cheek may be placed against the nose to seal it during ventilation. Exhaled air is blown into the victim's lung while the chest is watched to ensure expansion. The nose is released and the mouth opened to allow for passive exhalation. During exhalation, the rescuer's head should be turned away from the victim to protect against contact with vomitus and other oral secretions.

Mouth-to-Nose Ventilation

The mouth-to-nose technique should be used when the victim cannot be ventilated using the standard mouth-to-mouth method. Mouth-to-nose ventilation is useful in the presence of trismus and other disease processes (trauma, arthritis, infections) that interfere with opening of the mouth. Positioning of the victim is the same as with the mouth-to-mouth method. The mouth is held shut using one hand while head tilt is maintained with the other hand. The rescuer then exhales into the nose of the victim, ensuring that the chest rises with each delivered breath. A nasopharyngeal airway (see Pharyngeal

Intubation below) is a useful adjunct with this method of ventilation.

Mouth-to-Stoma or Mouth-to-Tracheostomy Ventilation

Health professionals are frequently called upon to resuscitate victims that have tracheostomy tubes in place. These patients may be ventilated using the standard mouth-to-mouth method while the tracheostomy site is occluded with one finger.[23] Unfortunately, this can be difficult to perform if both hands are required to maintain a patent airway. Alternatively, the rescuer can provide direct mouth-to-stoma ventilation. Esthetic considerations, however, may limit the desirability of this method.[23] Safar and Park have recommended the following method for ventilation of the tracheotomized patient.[23] The inner cannula of the tracheotomy tube should be withdrawn partially so as to leave only its tip in the outer cannula. The inner cannula serves as the operator mouthpiece and is turned to the side to allow for easier patient accessibility. The victim's head should be tilted backward, preferably by elevating the shoulders with a rolled sheet. The efficacy of this method can be assessed by observing for chest movement during positive pressure ventilation. Air leaks can be minimized by closing the victim's mouth and nose with one hand during ventilation. Mucous plugs, if present, should be suctioned or removed manually.

Mouth-to-Mask Ventilation

Adjuncts were introduced in the 1950s and 1960s to overcome public objection toward mouth-to-mouth ventilation.[24] Many types of masks are available for use during exhaled air positive pressure ventilation. These range from simple face shields (Microshield) to elaborate masks (Laerdahl pocket mask, SealEasy) with one-way valves and oxygen ports. Shields are small, lightweight, and inexpensive. They can be carried for use as an immediate tool until more elaborate equipment is available. Masks are the most commonly used adjuncts during resuscitation. They may be used alone or in conjunction with a self-inflating resuscitator bag. Masks must be large enough to fit over the mouth and nose of a patient and be sealed tightly against the cheeks.[25] They should have pliable borders to enhance the seal and be clear to allow visualization of cyanosis, vomiting, and clouding with exhalation.[24, 25] Although the exact operation of a shield or mask will vary depending on style, the basic steps are very similar. When using face shields, the head should be positioned in the same manner as described for mouth-to-mouth ventilation. The shield should be placed on the face and the victim ventilated in the normal fashion. During mouth-to-mask ventilation (Fig 4–5), the mask is placed on the victim's face to completely cover the mouth and nose. The jaw thrust (triple airway) maneuver is used to hold the mask firmly in place and exhaled air is blown through a port on top of the mask.

Tube-Valve-Mask Ventilation

The tube-valve-mask ventilator uses a long corrugated tube between the operator and the mask that acts as an oxygen reservoir.[26] This design allows adequate tidal volumes to be delivered while increasing the percent of oxygen delivered (FDO_2) to the patient.[26]

Advantages and Disadvantages

The major advantage of the exhaled air ventilation methods is that they require no or only a minimal amount of ancillary equipment. This allows the rescuer to deliver lifesaving ventilation to a victim of respiratory arrest in a rapid and effective manner. In addition, all of the methods described are simple to use and can be taught to relatively inexperienced personnel in a short period of time. This simplicity improves the retention of skills and allows a single rescuer to perform both ventilation and external cardiac compression during CPR. Exhaled air techniques are also able to deliver larger tidal volumes when compared with one-operator bag-valve-mask ventilation.[26–28] In a manikin study, Harrison et al.[27] found that mouth-to-mask ventilation delivered tidal volumes equivalent to those achieved with endotracheal intubation. Hess and Baran,[28] using a similar model, found that both mouth-to-mouth and mouth-to-mask ventilation delivered larger tidal volumes than one-person bag-valve-mask ventilation. Finally, the use of exhaled air ventilation allows for better assessment of airway resistance and lung compliance.

One major disadvantage is that expired air has a low oxygen and high carbon dioxide content. The FDO_2 with exhaled air ventilation ranges from 16% to 18%.[24, 26, 29] This can be increased from 16% to 27% by having the rescuer breathe oxygen by nasal cannula at 10 L/min.[29] The FDO_2 can be improved to 40% to 50% through the use of face masks with oxygen ports during mouth-to-mask ventilation.[24, 26] The large oxygen reservoir with the tube-valve-mask method further improves the FDO_2 to 91%.[26] The high carbon dioxide content is only a theoretical concern, since moderate hypocarbia in the operator can maintain the victim's partial pressure of arterial carbon dioxide ($PaCO_2$) at nearly normal levels.[8, 24]

Mouth-to-mouth ventilation can be distasteful to

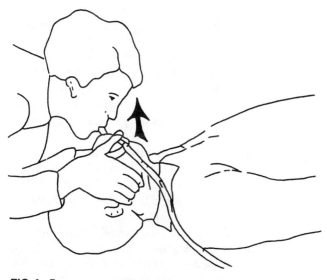

FIG 4–5.
Technique for mouth-to-mask ventilation. (From Elling R, Politis J: *Ann Emerg Med* 1983; 12:765. Used by permission.)

perform in the victim who is regurgitating or who has massive facial trauma.[26] Concerns over the transmission of infectious pathogens such as the human immunodeficiency (HIV) and hepatitis viruses (see Infection Issues) may further limit the use of this method. The use of one-way valves with the mouth-to-mask and tube-valve-mask methods allows expelled air to be diverted away, protecting the rescuer from contact with breath-borne infectious microorganisms.[26] The principal disadvantage of expired air mask ventilation is the presence of air leaks due to a poor face-to-mask seal. The face-to-mask seal must constantly be checked to assure delivery of adequate tidal volumes.

Cricoid Pressure

The delivery of large tidal volumes or generation of high pressures during ventilation increases the risk of gastric insufflation with resultant regurgitation and aspiration. Gastric insufflation may also interfere with ventilation efforts by elevating the diaphragm.[30] Therefore, the Panel on Ventilation at the 1985 conference on CPR and ECC recommended that the Sellick maneuver (cricoid pressure) be taught to all rescue personnel to reduce the possibility of gastric insufflation and passive regurgitation during artificial ventilation with an unprotected airway.[22] Cricoid pressure, by compressing the esophagus, reduces gastric insufflation during positive pressure ventilation. The cricoid cartilage is located one fingerbreadth below the thyroid cartilage prominence. Cricoid pressure (Fig 4−6) is applied by placing the thumb and middle finger of one hand on either side of the cartilage. The index finger is then used to exert firm pressure toward the spine. Since the cricoid is a complete cartilage, compression will not result in airway obstruction.[31] Pressure should not be applied over the thyroid or tracheal cartilages. In addition, cricoid pressure *must* not be used during active vomiting to avoid esophageal injury or rupture.[31] Ruben et al.[30] reported that the lower esophageal sphincter consistently opened at airway pressures between 15 and 25 cm H_2O in the anesthetized patient. The use of cricoid pressure, however, prevented gastric insufflation despite airway pressures that exceeded 50 cm H_2O.[30]

Forced Air Techniques

The most common type of forced air technique used for ventilation of the apneic patient is the self-inflating bag-valve-mask (BVM) resuscitator (Fig

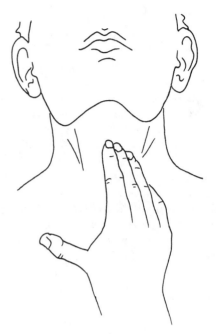

FIG 4−6.
Cricoid pressure (Sellick maneuver). (Adapted from Sellick BA: *Lancet* 1961; 2:404. Used by permission.)

4−7). Self-inflating bag-valve resuscitators can also be used with a wide variety of adjuncts such as endotracheal tubes, esophageal obturator airways (EOAs), pharyngeal-tracheal lumen (PTL) airways, and tracheostomy tubes. BVM resuscitators come in a variety of sizes and types to fit neonatal, pediatric, and adult populations. These devices should consist of a self-refilling bag with an one-way inlet valve which can be attached to a reservoir bag or tube.[1] These devices should also have side ports for supplemental oxygen, standard 15- or 22-mm fittings, and a nonsticking non-rebreathing valve at the mask end. Some devices may be equipped with a pop-off valve to minimize excessive airway pressures during ventilation. BVM devices must be easy to clean and maintain and be capable of functioning under a variety of environmental conditions.

Although considered an essential skill, many studies have demonstrated that BVM ventilation requires extensive experience and special training.[24, 26, 28] Ideally, BVM ventilation should be performed by two rescuers. One rescuer maintains a tight mask seal using the jaw thrust (triple airway maneuver) while the other compresses the bag. When the bag is compressed, air is expelled through a one-way valve into the victim's lungs. Between compressions, the bag refills with air drawn in through the one-way demand valve. During one-rescuer BVM ventilation, one hand

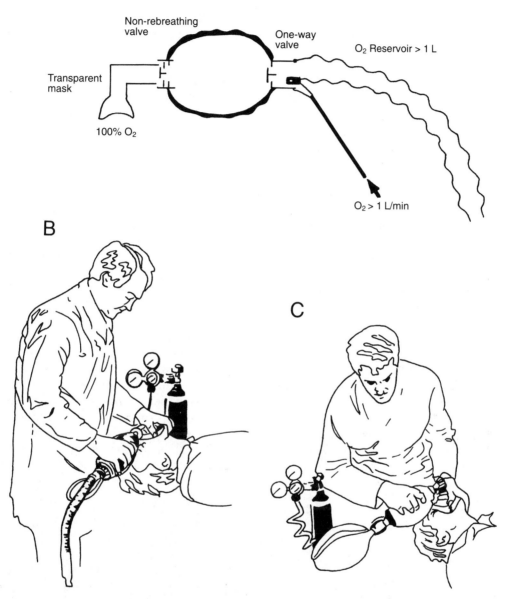

A

Non-rebreathing
valve

One-way
valve

O_2 Reservoir > 1 L

Transparent
mask

100% O_2

O_2 > 1 L/min

B

C

FIG 4-7.
A, bag-valve-mask (BVM) design. **B,** BVM ventilation with tube oxygen reservoir. **C,** BVM ventilation with bag oxygen reservoir. (From Safar P, Bircher NG: *Cardiopulmonary Cerebral Resuscitation.* Philadelphia, WB Saunders Co, 1988. Used by permission.)

is used to open the airway and maintain a tight mask seal while the other hand squeezes the bag. The rescuer should be positioned at the top of the patient's head. The head is tilted backward and the thumb and index fingers of one hand are used to hold the mask firmly against the face. The remaining fingers of the hand are used to hook and lift the chin upward to further open the airway. The free hand then compresses the bag at the appropriate ventilation rate.

Advantages and Disadvantages

In the presence of a good face mask seal, these devices are able to deliver very acceptable tidal volumes. Disease transmission is minimized and the devices also allow the experienced operator to assess lung compliance during ventilation. The use of room air will result in an FDO_2 of 21%. This can be increased by adding an oxygen source to the bag, so that the bag fills with both air and oxygen.[32] The

FdO_2 can be increased even more by manually controlling the refill time of the bag to allow for greater entrainment of oxygen.[32]

Very high FdO_2 values can be achieved through the use of a reservoir tube, a reservoir bag, or demand valve.[33] Reservoir tubes must have a volume of at least 1 L while reservoir bags must be able to hold at least 2.5 L. The inlet port is used to supply oxygen to both the bag and the reservoir. A constant supply of oxygen should be maintained to keep the reservoir full at all times. This requires flow rates greater than 15 L/min in most instances. Campbell et al.[33] found that a 2.5-L bag reservoir or a demand valve with an oxygen flow rate of 15 L/min consistently produced FdO_2 values of 0.95 to 1.00. Reservoir bags should be watched carefully to ensure an adequate flow of oxygen at all times. A deflated bag may indicate a disconnected line, a leak in the system, or an empty oxygen cylinder.[33] Similarly, demand valves provide a level of protection in that a hissing sound is heard when oxygen is being supplied to the resuscitator bag device.[33] In this closed system, valve malfunction will prevent the bag from refilling. Corrugated reservoir tubes do not provide these warning systems.

The training process for BVM ventilation is usually longer and technically more difficult. The most common problem encountered with this technique is an inadequate face mask seal resulting in large air leaks. Large air leaks lead to reduced tidal volumes and a lower FdO_2. Several studies have shown one-rescuer BVM ventilation to be inferior to mouth-to-mouth and mouth-to-mask ventilation with respect to tidal volumes.[26–28, 34] Experience has not been shown to improve the efficacy of one-rescuer BVM ventilation.[34] Better mask designs, however, have been shown to improve the efficacy of one-person BVM ventilation.[35] Efficacy is also improved in the presence of two-rescuer BVM ventilation.[28] In the event of excessive airway pressures, BVM ventilation can result in pulmonary barotrauma and gastric insufflation with regurgitation. The latter may be minimized by the concurrent application of cricoid pressure.

CIRCULATION

The maintenance of artificial circulation until spontaneous circulation can be restored is the next step in the BLS sequence. This ensures that vital organ perfusion is maintained until ALS measures are available or effective. Artificial circulation is accomplished through the use of external chest compressions (Fig 4–8). Current AHA recommendations call for compression rates of 80 to 100/minute.[13, 22] Chest compressions must be synchronized with ventilation to ensure maximum oxygen availability. Current standards call for two ventilations per 15 compressions during one-rescuer CPR and a single ventilation per 5 compressions during two-rescuer CPR. Compressions should be stopped for the delivery of ventilation in both one- and two-rescuer CPR.

The ability of chest compressions to maintain adequate vital organ perfusion has been questioned in recent years, prompting a search for additional

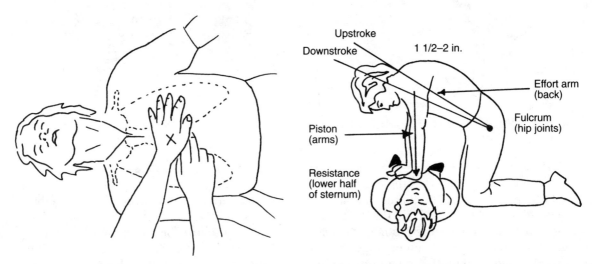

FIG 4–8.
External chest compression. *Left,* locating the correct hand position on the lower half of the body. *Right,* proper position of the rescuer, with shoulders directly over the victim's sternum and elbows locked. (Adapted from American Heart Association: *JAMA* 1986; 255(suppl):2841. Used by permission.)

methods to improve blood flow during CPR. Data now exist that carotid blood flow can be augmented by techniques that increase intrathoracic pressure (thoracic pump theory) during external cardiac compression. This includes techniques such as simultaneous ventilation and compression (SVC), interposed abdominal compression (IAC), simultaneous chest and abdominal compression (SCAC), and longer compression duration.[13, 36, 37] Unfortunately, these techniques have not improved neurologic outcome in animal or human studies to date.[13] To be useful, these techniques must also be easy to apply and not cause undue fatigue in the single rescuer.[13]

PHARYNGEAL INTUBATION

Airway obstruction resulting from posterior displacement of the tongue and epiglottis can usually be relieved by manual maneuvers. When manual maneuvers fail (e.g., in obese or short-necked patients), it may be necessary to use artificial adjuncts to secure and maintain a patent airway. An artificial airway inserted nasally or orally provides a route through and around which ventilation can be maintained.[14] These artificial adjuncts can also be used to reduce the fatigue associated with prolonged and continuous application of manual maneuvers. In addition, the efficacy of bag-valve-mask ventilation may be improved by the use of these airway adjuncts.

The oropharyngeal (OPA) and nasopharyngeal (NPA) airways (Fig 4–9) hold the base of the tongue forward and away from the posterior pharyngeal wall and counter obstruction by the teeth and lips. In effect, these devices substitute for the jaw thrust

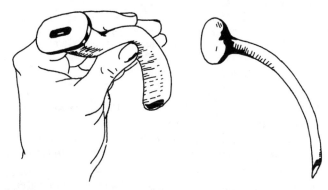

FIG 4–9.
Simple artificial airways: oropharyngeal *(left)* and nasopharyngeal *(right)*. (From Clinton JE, Ruiz E: Emergency airway management procedures, in Roberts JR, Hedges JR (eds): *Clinical Procedures in Emergency Medicine*, ed 1. Philadelphia, WB Saunders Co, 1985. Used by permission.)

and mouth-opening components of the triple airway maneuver.[1] Despite the use of these airways, backward tilt of the head is still required since flexion of the neck leads to partial withdrawal of the adjunct, allowing the tongue to relax against the posterior pharyngeal wall. Some patients may also require forward displacement of the mandible (chin lift or jaw thrust) to maintain an open airway. These points were well illustrated in an early study by Safar and colleagues using anesthetized volunteers.[4] They found that flexion of the neck resulted in complete airway obstruction in 98% and partial obstruction in 2% of patients despite the presence of an OPA. With the head extended, 88% of patients had an open airway in the presence of the OPA and the addition of forward mandibular displacement improved this figure to 98%.[4]

These adjuncts should only be used in unconscious patients with absent upper airway reflexes. Their use in patients with intact protective reflexes can precipitate laryngospasm and vomiting.

Oropharyngeal Airways

The OPA is a plastic semicircular device manufactured in various lengths, sizes, and designs. The OPA is constructed such that there is a flange outside the lips, a straight portion between the lips, and a curved portion that extends upward and backward corresponding to the shape of the palate and tongue. The standard Guedel type is tubular whereas the Berman type has the air channels along the side. The Berman variety is easier to clean and less likely to be obstructed by oral secretions, vomitus, or blood.[38] The Williams Airway Intubator is a modified Guedel-type OPA with an enlarged circular opening for the subsequent insertion of an endotracheal or an orogastric tube.[21] Some OPAs have modified proximal ends that protrude through the lips, allowing for a better seal during bag-valve-mask ventilation.[21]

An appropriate size (Table 4–1) should be selected and the oropharynx cleared of vomitus, blood, and other secretions prior to insertion. With the mouth open, the OPA is inserted backward with the distal tip pointing up toward the hard palate (Fig 4–10,A). As the posterior pharyngeal wall is approached, the OPA is rotated 180 degrees so that it lies along the tongue with its distal end immediately posterior to the epiglottis.[21] Alternatively, the mouth can be opened and the tongue depressed anteriorly using a finger or a wooden tongue depressor (Fig 4–10,B). The OPA can then be inserted and moved

TABLE 4–1.

Recommended Sizes of Oropharyngeal and Nasopharyngeal
Airways for Use in Adults*†

Size	Oropharyngeal Airway (OPA)	Nasopharyngeal Airway (NPA)
Large	100 mm (Guedel 5)	8–9mm
Medium	90 mm (Guedel 4)	7–8mm
Small	80 mm (Guedel 3)	6–7mm

*Adapted from *Advanced Life Support Manual.* Dallas, American Heart Association, 1987.
†OPA size is based on the distance from flange to distal tip. NPA size is based on internal diameter.

posteriorly following the normal curvature of the tongue.[14] With either method of insertion, it is important to ensure that the lips and tongue are not caught between the teeth and the OPA.[1] Proper position should be confirmed by assessment of airflow and efficacy of ventilation. As mentioned, head tilt must be maintained despite the presence of the OPA.

In general, it is difficult to insert an OPA in patients whose jaws are tightly clamped due to muscle spasticity. Under no circumstances should the OPA be used as an adjunct to open the mouth since this can result in severe dental and oral trauma.[21] If manual maneuvers fail to open the mouth (see Foreign Body Upper Airway Obstruction), a nasopharyngeal airway should be considered.

The OPA should only be used in patients with relaxed jaws and absent upper airway reflexes. Its use in the semiconscious patient can provoke vomiting and laryngospasm. However, shortened OPAs can be used as a bite-block in the semiconscious patient, to prevent obstruction or kinking of endotracheal and orogastric tubes.[39] Incorrect insertion of the OPA may actually worsen airway obstruction (Fig 4–10,C) by pushing the tongue posteriorly against the pharyngeal wall.[39] Selection of an airway of improper size can also worsen airway obstruction by either pushing the tongue posteriorly (too short) or pushing the epiglottis against the laryngeal opening (too long).[39] Improper or forceful placement can cause trauma to the teeth, lips, tongue, and pharynx.

Nasopharyngeal Airways

The NPA is an uncuffed tube made of soft rubber or plastic that comes in various lengths and diameters. The NPA is beveled laterally at its pharyngeal end and has a funnel-shaped slip joint at its nasal end. The latter, often reinforced by a safety

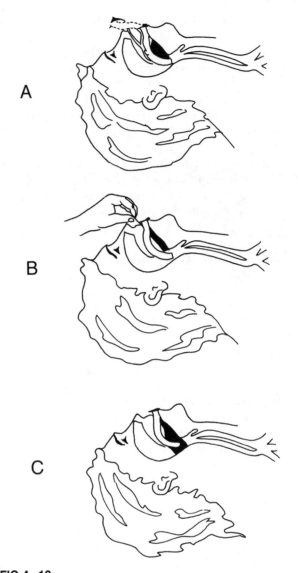

FIG 4–10.
Insertion of an oropharyngeal airway. **A,** airway is inserted backward and rotated into position. **B,** tongue depressor airway. **C,** airway obstruction from incorrect insertion. (Adapted from Stewart RD: Field airway control for the trauma patient, in Campbell JE (ed): *Basic Trauma Life Support,* ed 2. Englewood Cliffs, NJ, Prentice-Hall, Inc, 1985, p 59. Used by permission.)

pin, helps to guard against accidental slippage of the airway into the esophagus or trachea.[14]

Indications for its use include inability to insert an OPA (trismus, maxillomandibular wiring) and relative contraindications to the use of an OPA (severe oral trauma).[39] The NPA is also better tolerated by patients with marginal stupor or coma who require an artificial airway. In addition, the NPA is sometimes used to facilitate the passage of nasogastric and nasotracheal suction catheters. The NPA is contraindicated in patients with severe maxillofacial trauma and possible injury to the cribriform plate.

The largest airway that fits through the external nares should be selected.[21] Size options are summarized in Table 4–1. The airway should be well lubricated, preferably with an anesthetic containing a water-soluble agent.[1] The airway is inserted into the nasal passage parallel to the hard palate with the bevel turned toward the floor or the septum to avoid trauma to the lateral nasal turbinates. If excessive resistance is encountered, the operator should stop and attempt insertion into the opposite nostril. Alternatively, a smaller size can be selected and the procedure repeated in the same nostril. At no point should excessive force be used. The majority of NPAs are designed to be inserted into the right nostril. In 10% to 15% of the population, a deviated septum will prevent insertion into the right side.[40] To insert the airway into the left side, the NPA is turned upside-down with the bevel toward the septum. It is then inserted in the usual fashion until it hits the nasopharynx, at which point it is turned 180 degrees and advanced further into the pharynx.[40] Slight rotation can help overcome the occasional resistance encountered when the airway reaches the angle between the nasal passages and the nasopharynx. Once in place, the NPA extends from the external nares to the base of the tongue and rests posterior to the epiglottis (Fig 4–11). Proper placement should be confirmed by assessment of airflow and efficacy of ventilation. Despite the presence of the NPA, head tilt and occasionally chin lift must be con-

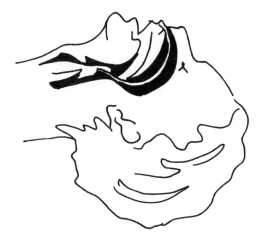

FIG 4–11.
Nasopharyngeal airway in place. Note head tilted back for proper insertion. (Adapted from *Advanced Cardiac Life Support Manual.* Dallas, American Heart Association, 1987, p 28. Used by permission.)

tinued to maintain an open airway (see Fig 4–11).

The most common complication associated with the NPA is trauma to the fragile and vascular nasal mucosa resulting in epistaxis and tracheal aspiration of blood. This can be minimized by using the correct insertion technique in conjunction with a soft, well-lubricated tube. Use of the NPA in patients with intact upper airway reflexes can precipitate laryngospasm and vomiting. Elevated local pressure in conjunction with prolonged use may predispose the patient to sinusitis or tissue necrosis.[14] Deep insertion of an excessively long NPA can lead to esophageal intubation, resulting in gastric insufflation and inadequate ventilation.[1,14]

SUCTIONING

Airway patency achieved through the use of manual maneuvers and artificial adjuncts can be compromised by the presence of blood, vomitus, and other secretions in the oropharynx. The availability of appropriate and functioning suction equipment is therefore essential for optimal airway management. Wall-mounted or portable suction pumps should be powerful enough to clear particulate matter, blood, and other thick secretions from the oropharynx. Most wall-mounted suction pumps can generate negative pressures ranging from 0 to 750 mm Hg.[41] The maximal negative pressure generated can be determined by briefly occluding the suction tubing and monitoring the gauge reading. To adequately suction the oropharynx, the suction apparatus should generate a negative pressure of at least 300 mm Hg and airflow of at least 30 L/min.[1] While the maximum negative pressure generated is a property unique to each particular suction device, the airflow rate achieved is primarily dependent on the size of the suction catheter.[42] Increasing the internal diameter of the suction catheter is the most effective way to improve airflow. Passage of aspirated material into the working part of the suction pump is prevented by the use of reservoir bottles.

There are basically three types of suction tips (Fig 4–12) available to the emergency physician, each suited for a different type of airway obstruction problem.[43]

1. The dental tip or rigid pharyngeal suction catheter is very useful for removing vomitus from the oropharynx. These suction tips are preferred

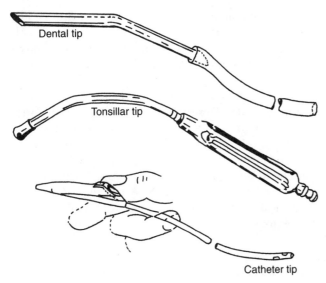

FIG 4–12.
Three types of suction tips: dental, tonsillar, and catheter tips. (From Clinton JE, Ruiz E: Emergency airway management procedures, in Roberts JR, Hedges JR (eds): *Clinical Procedures in Emergency Medicine,* ed 1. Philadelphia, WB Saunders Co, 1985. Used by permission.)

during critical resuscitation, since they are less likely to be obstructed by particulate matter.[43]

2. Metal or plastic rigid tonsillar suction tips are very effective in removing blood and other secretions from the upper airway. The distal end of the tonsillar tip is round with multiple holes.[1] This design reduces local trauma and also prevents the tonsillar tip from being occluded by blood or tissue.[43]

3. Flexible soft suction catheters are primarily used to suction the nasopharynx and the endotracheal tube. Unfortunately, the small negative pressures and the low airflow rates achieved with these devices are limiting factors with regard to oropharyngeal suctioning.[43]

Ideally, all three types of suction tips should be available for optimal airway management. Interchangeability may be facilitated by the use of latex suction tubing.[43] A suction trap added to the base of the suction tip can help prevent clogging of the latex tubing.[43]

All patients should be hyperventilated with 100% oxygen for at least 2 minutes prior to suctioning. Suctioning should be limited to 10 seconds per attempt and the patient must be hyperventilated and hyperoxygenated between attempts.[14, 39, 44, 45] The mouth is opened manually and the dental or tonsillar tip suction is applied in a sweeping fashion (Fig 4–13) across the oropharynx.[1] Ideally, this should be performed under direct visualization (laryngoscopy), since blind attempts at suctioning can actually worsen airway obstruction.

Endotracheal tube suctioning is performed using sterile technique. Use of a catheter that is approximately half the size of the endotracheal tube allows air to enter the lung during suctioning and reduces the risk of pulmonary deflation.[1] To minimize tracheobronchial mucosal injury, the suction pump negative pressure must not exceed 100 to 120 mm Hg.[41] The soft, well-lubricated catheter is advanced through the endotracheal tube to an appropriate depth (see Fig 4–13). Intermittent suction is then

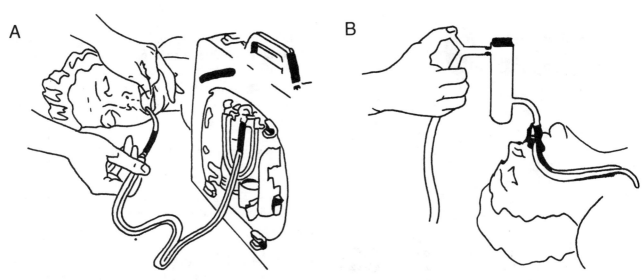

FIG 4–13.
Technique for **(A)** pharyngeal and **(B)** tracheal suctioning. (From Safar P, Bircher MD: *Cardiopulmonary Cerebral Resuscitation,* ed 3. Philadelphia, WB Saunders Co, 1988. Used by permission.)

applied (proximal side port opening) and the catheter withdrawn with a rotating motion.[39] The presence of a flexible catheter tip allows for suctioning of both the right and left main bronchi.[1] Left main bronchus insertion can be facilitated by turning the patient's head to the right.

Although there are no specific contraindications to suctioning, overzealous or incorrect use of the suction device can result in a number of complications. All types of suction devices that are available can induce laryngospasm or cause vagal stimulation resulting in bradycardia and hypotension.[39] Tracheobronchial suctioning can also precipitate cough and reflex bronchospasm. Rigid tonsillar suction tips can damage teeth and other oral structures.[14] Vigorous suction of the nasal passages and nasopharynx can lead to mucosal injury and epistaxis.[43] Prolonged suctioning of tracheobronchial secretions can cause significant hypoxemia, resulting in cardiac arrhythmias or respiratory arrest.[44, 45] This can be minimized by limiting suctioning attempts to 10 seconds and ensuring that patients are hyperventilated and hyperoxygenated prior to and between attempts.[14, 41, 44, 45] The use of large catheters and excessively high negative pressures during endotracheal tube suctioning can produce mucosal injury and cause dangerous reductions in lung volumes (functional residual capacity).[44] The latter, if severe, may lead to lung collapse and cardiac arrest.[39]

INFECTION ISSUES

Although mouth-to-mouth and mouth-to-nose expired air ventilation are extremely effective methods of artificial respiration, concerns over the possibility of acquiring infectious diseases may delay or limit their widespread use. In recent years, these concerns have prompted a thorough evaluation of the risks of acquiring infectious diseases through participation in CPR training or by performing CPR on victims of circulatory or respiratory arrest.[19] This evaluation has been directed primarily to health care workers and public safety personnel who frequently perform mouth-to-mouth ventilation on victims about whom they have little or no prior medical knowledge.[19]

The risk of disease transmission during CPR training appears to be negligible. Over the last 25 years, there have been no reported cases of bacterial, fungal, or viral disease transmission through a CPR training manikin.[19] Strict adherence to the current AHA guidelines for the cleaning and maintaining of manikins provides an extremely high safety level for CPR training participants.[19] The AHA also recommends simulation of finger sweeps and respirations during two-rescuer CPR to further reduce the risk of disease transmission.[19]

Health care workers are often exposed to blood and other body fluids during resuscitation and rescue efforts. Although both the hepatitis B virus (HBV) and HIV are present in salivary secretions, there is no evidence that either virus can be transmitted by mouth-to-mouth ventilation.[46] There have been several instances of persons providing mouth-to-mouth ventilation to HIV-positive patients but no reports of transmission.[46] Attempts to infect animals by direct exposure of oral mucosa to high concentrations of HIV have also been unsuccessful.[46] Although the risk of acquiring HIV infection through occupational exposure appears to be extremely low, the consequences of becoming infected are obviously grave, and every precaution should be taken to protect the rescuer from infectious particles present in blood, saliva, and other body secretions. Protective devices should be simple and must provide a good seal as well as adequate airflow to ensure effective ventilation.

The risk of infectious disease transmission may be reduced by the use of clear face masks with one-way valves (Laerdahl Pocket-Mask or SealEasy) or filters that divert the victim's exhaled air away from the rescuer.[19, 47, 48] Unfortunately, the effectiveness of these devices in reducing the potential for disease transmission has not been well defined.[19] If they are used, it is extremely important that the rescuer has been properly trained in the technique of mouth-to-mask ventilation, especially with respect to maintaining an adequate face-to-mask seal. Rescuers should also wear latex gloves to prevent the inadvertent transfer of blood and other body secretions onto the hands.[19]

In the absence of such adjuncts, some authors recommend the use of a clean handkerchief for protection against disease transmission.[1] Recently, the Resusci Face Shield (Laerdahl Medical Co.) has been recommended as an adjunct for expired air ventilation.[49] The face shield is a one-time-use foil-wrapped sheath measuring 32.5 by 19.5 cm with a hydrophobic circular filter with a diameter of 3.5 cm in its center. In one study, the face shield was able to retain up to 80% of aerosolized bacterial particles measuring 0.5 to 5.0 µm.[49] In contrast, cotton handkerchiefs showed no evidence of particle trapping. When used on manikins, the face shield achieved effective tidal volumes and did not increase ventilation resistance.[49] Although the face shield appears to be an effective device for the trapping of bacteria, its value in trapping the smaller viral particles remains unclear. This device, however, does offer the potential for protection against transmission of respiratory droplets and body fluids during resuscitation and may help prevent delays in initiating mouth-to-mouth ventilation.[49]

FOREIGN BODY UPPER AIRWAY OBSTRUCTION

History

The correct treatment of foreign body upper airway obstruction (FBUAO) has generated much controversy and debate over the last two decades. Existing recommendations are based largely on anecdotal reports and airflow studies using models, animals, and human volunteers. There are no (nor are there likely to be any) well-constructed clinical trials on this issue.

The first written description in English of a foreign body in the air passages appeared in the form of a letter read before The Royal Society of London in 1677.[50] The letter described a patient who had accidentally aspirated a musket ball into a bronchus while attempting to cure "colic." The letter outlined the failure of downward suspension, fume inhalation, and concussions of the body to expel the projectile. The patient ultimately succumbed to recurrent pulmonary infections. This presentation led to the account of another case in which inversion, shaking, and coughing were effective in expelling a bullet from the lungs. Thus, the 17th century approach to FBUAO relied primarily on inversion and back pounding.[50]

Almost 200 years later, in 1854, Samuel D. Gross published a book entitled *A Practical Treatise on Foreign Bodies in the Air Passages*.[50, 51] In this oft-quoted treatise, Gross outlined in detail the diagnostic, pathologic, therapeutic, and operative aspects of FBUAO. With regard to therapy, he warned that inversion and backslapping were potentially dangerous since they could cause the foreign body to impact on the underside of the larynx, leading to asphyxiation.[50] He also warned of the dangers of finger probing.[50] Gross concluded that tracheotomy was the most effective way to relieve FBUAO.[50] Unfortunately, his work has generated much confusion with respect to the treatment of supraglottic vs. subglottic airway obstruction.

In 1963 the classic work by Haugen described the "cafe coronary."[52] This paper showed that the typical middle-aged or elderly person who collapsed suddenly in a restaurant was often stricken by FBUAO, and not coronary artery disease. In autopsied subjects, Haugen found food obstructing the airway from the hypopharynx to the major bronchi.[52] Like Gross, Haugen also felt that immediate tracheotomy was the treatment of choice. This, however, proved to be impractical in most situations.

From 1917 to 1973, the Chevalier Jackson Clinic in Philadelphia recorded observations on nearly 6,000 victims of choking. The clinic recommended that finger probing, inversion, and back blows be used only as a last resort.[50] Subsequently, the American Red Cross, which had been teaching the use of back blows for choking victims from 1933 to 1969, changed its recommendations. In 1973, the Red Cross began to recommend back blows only as "a last desperate effort."[50, 51]

In 1974, Henry Heimlich introduced the abdominal thrust, or Heimlich maneuver, to relieve FBUAO.[53] His preliminary studies on beagles suggested that this should be the method of choice for relieving FBUAO.[53, 54] Without further clinical study, the maneuver received widespread media coverage and was quickly adopted by the general public as a first-aid measure to treat the choking victim.[53, 54] Subsequently, anecdotal case reports were submitted which seemed to confirm the efficacy of the technique.[50, 54]

In 1976, the Red Cross, under its new adviser, Dr. Archer Gordon, changed its recommendations and began advocating back blows in the initial management of these victims.[51] This sparked a debate which continued in the literature until the 1985 conference on CPR and ECC. At this conference, the panel on FBUAO recommended that the Heimlich maneuver be adopted as the treatment of choice for FBUAO in adults and children over 1 year of age.[55] Concerns over abdominal trauma, as well as the declining death rate from FBUAO in infants treated with existing techniques, prompted the panel to recommend the continued use of back blows and chest thrusts to relieve FBUAO in children less than 1 year of age.[55] Unfortunately, the latter recommendations have continued to spark debate in the recent literature.[56–61]

Epidemiology

There are over 3,000 deaths per year in the United States from foreign body asphyxiation.[62, 63] This figure is probably an underestimation, since many additional deaths may be attributed to cardiac or other causes. Victims of FBUAO are either very old or very young. Risk factors that contribute to FBUAO include the use of dentures, poor mastication of food, talking while eating, hurried swallowing, and elevated blood alcohol levels.[20, 52, 63]

Clinical Presentation

Early recognition and management is essential since anoxia of 4 to 6 minutes can result in irreversible brain damage. In the typical scenario, a middle-aged person will be in a restaurant, dining, say on lobster or filet mignon, with perhaps wine accompanying the meal. In the middle of conversation, the subject becomes pale, then cyanotic, and finally collapses.[52, 54, 63] Prior to collapse, the victim may demonstrate the universal distress signal for choking (Fig 4–14) by grasping the neck between the thumb and index finger of one hand. FBUAO should also be considered if one cannot ventilate an unconscious and apneic person after manual opening of the airway. FBUAO must be differentiated from other causes of collapse and respiratory distress such as cardiac arrest, a cerebrovascular event, and drug overdose. The prognosis is influenced by the level of obstruction (supraglottic vs. subglottic), type of foreign body (meat can be difficult to expel), and the degree of obstruction (partially obstructing foreign bodies are easier to expel).[51, 62]

Approach

At the present time management is dictated primarily by the type of airway obstruction (partial or complete) and the degree of air exchange (good or poor).[19] Partial airway obstruction is characterized by supraclavicular and intercostal muscle retractions, snoring, crowing, gurgling, or wheezing, depending on the level of obstruction.[1, 19] The patient with par-

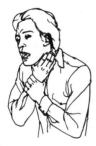

FIG 4–14.
Universal distress signal. (From *Heartsaver Manual*. Dallas, American Heart Association, 1987, p 42. Used by permission.)

tial airway obstruction may have either good or poor air exchange. Patients with partial obstruction and good air exchange are usually conscious and able to cough forcefully. As long as good air exchange persists, these patients should be encouraged to cough and manual attempts to expel the foreign body avoided. This is supported by the studies of Gordon et al.[64] which showed that none of the artificial maneuvers produced air pressures, volumes, or flows comparable to those generated by a normal cough. Ruben and MacNaughton[65] have also shown that a normal cough can generate sufficient intratracheal pressures to expel a foreign body.

Patients with partial airway obstruction and poor exchange usually have a weak cough, high-pitched inspiratory noises, respiratory distress, and cyanosis. These patients and those whose good air exchange progresses to poor air exchange are treated the same as patients with complete upper airway obstruction. Complete airway obstruction is characterized by the inability to speak or breathe. The patient is unable to cough and there is no airflow. These patients must be rapidly treated with the Heimlich maneuver (subdiaphragmatic abdominal thrust).

The Heimlich maneuver is based on the principle that elevation of the diaphragm compresses the lungs, producing increased airway pressures. The pressures generated are enhanced by the fact that FBUAO usually occurs during inspiration. The increased pressure forces air out through the trachea, thereby ejecting the foreign body. The maneuver can be thought of as an artificial cough, although the air pressure, volume, and flow generated are considerably less.

Technique

In the standing or sitting conscious victim, the rescuer stands behind the victim and wraps his or her arms around the victim's waist. Making a fist with one hand the rescuer places the thumb side against the victim's abdomen between the navel and the xiphoid process. Grasping the fist with the other hand, the rescuer presses into the victim's abdomen with a quick upward movement (Fig 4–15).

The unconscious victim should be placed supine. The rescuer kneels astride the victim's thighs and places the heel of one hand on the victim's abdomen between the navel and the xiphoid process (Fig 4–16). The other hand is placed on top of the first. The rescuer then presses into the abdomen with a quick upward thrust.[1, 20, 54]

The Heimlich maneuver can also be used for

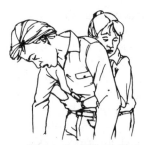

Abdominal Thrust

FIG 4–15.
Subdiaphragmatic abdominal thrust (the Heimlich maneuver) administered to a conscious (standing) victim of foreign body airway obstruction. (From *Heartsaver Manual*. Dallas, American Heart Association, 1987, p 42. Used by permission.)

self-treatment. If the fist technique fails, the upper abdomen can be pressed quickly over a firm surface such as the edge of a table or back of a chair.

For the pregnant or markedly obese patient in whom abdominal thrusts are difficult to apply, the AHA recommends the use of chest thrusts.[19] In the conscious victim, sitting or standing, the rescuer stands behind the victim and wraps his or her arms around the victim's chest (Fig 4–17). The rescuer places one fist on the middle of the sternum, thumb side down, then grabs the fist with the other hand and performs backward thrusts. In the supine unconscious patient, the rescuer kneels beside the body, positions the hands as for external chest compression, and thrusts slowly.

Management Sequence

Patients with FBUAO should be managed using the sequence of steps outlined in Table 4–2. Finger sweeps should only be performed on the unconscious patient. The mouth can be opened using either the crossed-fingers, finger-behind-teeth, or the tongue–jaw lift maneuvers (Fig 4–18).[1]

1. The crossed-fingers maneuver for the relaxed jaw consists of a scissors movement in the far corner of the mouth exerted by placing the index finger against the upper teeth and the thumb against the lower teeth.
2. The finger-behind-teeth maneuver for the tight jaw consists of wedging the tip of the index finger behind the patient's last molar teeth.
3. The tongue–jaw lift maneuver for the fully relaxed jaw consists of grasping the tongue with the thumb and the mandible with the other fingers and lifting anteriorly.

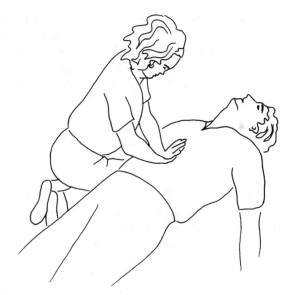

FIG 4–16.
Chest thrust administered to an unconscious victim (supine) of foreign body upper airway obstruction. (Adapted from *Heartsaver Manual*. Dallas, American Heart Association, 1987, p 46. Used by permission.)

After the mouth has been opened, the finger sweep is carried out using a wrapped finger to decrease friction and prevent salivary slippage (Fig 4–19). The foreign body should be removed using a hooking technique. Finger sweeps should not be performed in children unless the foreign body is visualized when the mouth is opened. The sequence outlined in Table 4–2 must be repeated until the airway has been cleared.

TABLE 4–2.
Recommended Sequence for Management of Foreign Body Upper Airway Obstruction*

1. Conscious victim or victim who becomes unconscious
   a. Identify airway obstruction
   b. Apply Heimlich maneuver—foreign body expelled
      or
   c. Victim becomes unconscious: open the mouth and perform finger sweep
   d. Open the airway—attempt rescue breathing
   e. If unable to ventilate, perform six to ten abdominal thrusts
   f. Repeat sequence c–e if unsuccessful in expelling foreign body
2. Unconscious victim
   a. Attempt to ventilate
   b. If unsuccessful, reposition head and reattempt ventilation
   c. Abdominal thrust
   d. Finger sweep
   e. Repeat sequence if unsuccessful

*Adapted from *Basic Life Support Manual*. Dallas, American Heart Association, 1988.

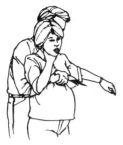

Chest Thrust

FIG 4–17.
The chest thrust administered to a pregnant woman with foreign body airway obstruction. (From *Heartsaver Manual*. Dallas, American Heart Association, 1987, p 42. Used by permission.)

If manual methods fail and a laryngoscope is available, direct visualization should be performed. A Kelly clamp or Magill forceps can be used to remove the foreign body. If unsuccessful, a surgical airway must be considered.

The Controversy

The Heimlich maneuver has become the accepted standard of care for FBUAO after much controversy. Heimlich's initial studies on anesthetized beagles demonstrated the effectiveness of the abdominal thrust in relieving FBUAO.[53, 54] He also found that manual rib compressions (chest thrusts) were unsuccessful in expelling the foreign body.[54] In 1975, Heimlich reported on 162 personal communications that demonstrated the apparent success of the technique.[54] He also performed physiologic studies on ten healthy volunteers using a closed pressure gauge system. In these studies, the abdominal thrust generated an average air pressure of 31 mm Hg and expiratory airflow of 205 L/min.[54]

In 1976, Guildner et al.[66] studied six anesthetized volunteers and found that back blows were ineffective in increasing air pressures or flow. The authors also found that chest thrusts generated higher air pressures, flow, and volumes than the abdominal thrust.[66]

Gordon et al.,[64] using anesthetized baboons, found that back blows generated higher airway pressures over a shorter time period then either the abdominal or chest thrust. They found that this brief but rapid rise in airway pressure was often necessary to dislodge the foreign body.[64] The back blows, however, produced considerably less air volume than the

A   B   C

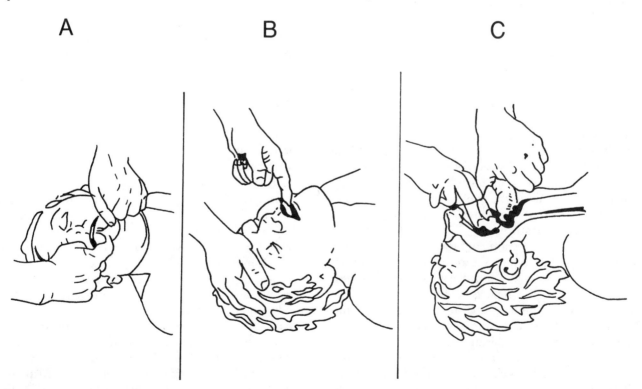

FIG 4–18.
Three methods to open the mouth: **A,** the crossed-fingers maneuver. **B,** the finger-behind-the-teeth maneuver. **C,** the tongue–jaw lift maneuver. (From Safar P, Bircher NG: *Cardiopulmonary Cerebral Resuscitation*, ed 3. Philadelphia, WB Saunders Co, 1988. Used by permission.)

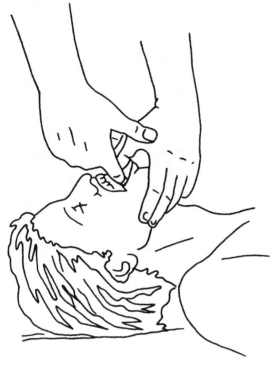

FIG 4–19.
The finger sweep. (From Finucane BT, Santora AH: *Principles of Airway Management.* Philadelphia, FA Davis Co, 1988. Used by permission.)

abdominal or chest thrust. These findings led the authors to recommend the use of a combination of methods, i.e., back blows (to dislodge the foreign body) followed by abdominal thrust or chest thrust (to move the foreign body out of the air passage).[64]

Ruben and MacNaughton, in 1978,[65] confirmed the observations of Gordon et al., that back blows produced higher airway pressures, and that the Heimlich maneuver displaced larger volumes of air. These authors also emphasized the use of gravity (head down) to aid in the management of FBUAO.[65] Heimlich criticized these studies and characterized back blows as "death blows."[50, 67] He cited observations from Gross's treatise and the Chevalier Jackson Clinic experience, which showed that back blows actually increased airway obstruction. Heimlich also used anecdotal case reports to further support the use of the abdominal thrust.[50, 67] He also condemned the use of chest thrusts because of their potential for serious complications.[67]

Redding addressed the issue in 1979 by analyzing 225 cases of food choking treated by various artificial maneuvers.[68] He found that no single technique was effective in all situations and often a combination of techniques was required to relieve the FBUAO.[68] Statistical analysis of the data, how-

ever, showed the abdominal thrust to be four times as effective as the back blow in relieving the choking episode.[69]

In 1982, Day and co-workers[70] used an accelerator model to show that back blows could actually push a supraglottic foreign body further into the airway. This reasoning was based on Newton's third law of motion which states that "for every action there is an equal and opposite reaction."[70] In volunteer studies, the authors found that the abdominal thrust produced peak airway pressures of 32 mm Hg compared with 13 mm Hg with back blows.[70] They felt that the differences between their findings and those of previous studies could be explained by design (anesthetized vs. nonanesthetized patients) and body position.[55, 69, 70] As a result, back blows were discontinued because "as a single method, back blows may not be as effective as the Heimlich maneuver in adults" and "in an effort to simplify training, the Heimlich maneuver is the only method recommended at this time."[20] This statement from the FBUAO panel at the 1985 conference on CPR and ECC ended much of the previous controversy.[20, 55]

Complications

The most common complication following application of the Heimlich maneuver is vomiting.[71] If this occurs, the head should be turned to one side and the mouth cleared of vomitus prior to resuming efforts to relieve the FBUAO. Other reported complications include fractured ribs,[50] pneumomediastinum,[72, 73] ruptured stomach,[74] splenic laceration,[74] ruptured bioprosthetic aortic valve,[75] retinal detachment,[62] ruptured jejunum,[76] and abdominal aortic thrombosis.[77]

Although Heimlich maintains that the majority of complications are related to improper technique, complications have arisen following correct application of the maneuver. As a result, it is recommended that all patients subjected to the Heimlich maneuver be examined by a physician.[19, 63]

Improperly performed finger sweeps can worsen airway obstruction by pushing a foreign body distally. Finger sweeps can also cause pharyngeal trauma and have the potential for infectious disease transmission. If possible, fingers should be protected with gloves prior to sweeping.

Although complications from chest thrusts have not been reported, Heimlich has suggested that chest thrusts have the potential to cause complications similar to those reported with external cardiac compressions.[67] These include fractures of the ribs and sternum, liver and splenic lacerations, myocardial contusion, and pneumothorax.

PEDIATRIC CONSIDERATIONS

Airway

The AHA also recommends the use of the head tilt–chin lift maneuver to open the pediatric airway.[19] Hyperextension should be avoided in the very young child since this can increase airway obstruction as a result of tracheal collapse (immature cartilage support).

Breathing

Mouth-to-nose ventilation may be easier to perform in the young child. Tidal volumes must be carefully monitored to avoid gastric insufflation and pulmonary barotrauma. The increased resistance during mouth-to-nose ventilation is beneficial in reducing peak airway pressures.[22] Cricoid pressure can also help reduce gastric insufflation and regurgitation.

Circulation

Hand position and compression rates vary according to age. Current guidelines of the AHA should be adhered to during CPR.[19]

Pharyngeal Intubation

The 180-degree method of inserting an OPA is contraindicated in children since this can lead to significant soft tissue trauma. Only the tongue depressor method should be used to insert the OPA. Size selections will vary with age. The NPA can cause adenoidal trauma and may actually increase airway resistance during positive pressure ventilation.[14]

Suction

The presence of oral secretions, vomitus, and blood can also compromise the pediatric airway. The availability of effective suctioning devices is paramount for adequate airway management. The use of nasal suctioning is of particular value in young infants who are obligatory nose breathers. This can be done using bulb syringes or soft nasopharyngeal catheters. Negative pressure during either oral or

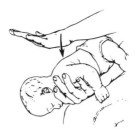

FIG 4–20.
Back blows in an infant. (From *Heartsaver Manual*. Dallas, American Heart Association, 1987, p 59. Used by permission.)

nasal suctioning should not exceed 30 cm H_2O to avoid mucosal injury and prevent lung collapse.

Foreign Body Upper Airway Obstruction

The Heimlich maneuver is also recommended as the method of choice for relieving FBUAO in the child.[19] The conscious child with partial airway obstruction and good air exchange must not be placed in the head-down position. The sequence of steps followed is similar to that described for adults (see Table 4–2) with the exception that blind finger sweeps are not permitted in the pediatric patient. Finger sweeps are recommended only if the foreign body is visible after the mouth has been opened. In the infant, the AHA continues to recommend the use of back blows and chest thrusts.[19] The declining death rate from FBUAO in infants and concerns over the possible abdominal visceral injury with the abdominal thrust were the basis behind this recommendation at the 1985 conference.[55] Unfortunately, this too has become a controversial issue and awaits further clarification.[56–61] Back blows (Fig 4–20) are applied by straddling the infant over the rescuer's arm with the head lower then the trunk and delivering four forceful strikes between the shoulder blades with the heel of the hand. To perform chest thrusts (Fig 4–21), the infant is placed face up on the rescuer's thigh and forearm with the infant's head lower than the trunk. Using two fingers, four chest

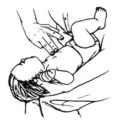

FIG 4–21.
Chest thrusts in an infant. (From *Heartsaver Manual*. Dallas, American Heart Association, 1987, p 59. Used by permission.)

thrusts are performed in the same location used for external cardiac compression but at a slower rate.

REFERENCES

1. Safar P, Bircher NG: *Cardiopulmonary Cerebral Resuscitation,* ed 3. Philadelphia, WB Saunders Co, 1988.
2. Liss HP: A history of resuscitation. *Ann Emerg Med* 1986; 15:65.
3. Safar P: Failure of manual respiration. *J Appl Physiol* 1959; 14:84.
4. Safar P, Escarraga LA, Chang F: Upper airway obstruction in the unconscious patient. *J Appl Physiol* 1959; 14:760.
5. Safar P, Escarraga LA, Elam JO: A comparison of the mouth-to-mouth and mouth-to-airway methods of artificial respiration with the chest-pressure arm-lift methods. *N Engl J Med* 1958; 258:671.
6. Safar P: Ventilatory efficacy of mouth-to-mouth artificial respiration. *JAMA* 1958; 167:335.
7. Asmussen E, Hahn-Petersen A, Rosendal T: Air passage through the hypopharynx in unconscious patients in the prone position. *Acta Anaesthesiol Scand* 1958; 3:123.
8. Elam JO, Brown ES, Elder JD: Artificial respiration by mouth-to-mask method. *N Engl J Med* 1954; 250:659.
9. Kouwenhoven WB, Jude JR, Knickerbocker GG: Closed-chest cardiac massage. *JAMA* 1960; 173:1064.
10. Criley JM, Niemann JT, Rosborough JP: Cardiopulmonary resuscitation research 1960–1984: Discoveries and advances. *Ann Emerg Med* 1984; 13:756.
11. Lind B: Teaching mouth-to-mouth resuscitation in primary schools. *Acta Anaesthesiol Scand Suppl* 1961; 9:63.
12. Criley JM, Niemann JT, Rosborough JP, et al: Modifications of cardiopulmonary resuscitation based on the cough. *Circulation* 1986; 74(suppl 4):42.
13. Paraskos JA: External compression without adjuncts. *Circulation* 1986; 74(suppl 4):33.
14. Finucane BT, Santora AH: *Principles of Airway Management.* Philadelphia, FA Davis Co, 1988.
15. White RD: CPR: Basic life support. *Clin Symp* 1983; 35:1.
16. Guildner CW: Resuscitation—opening the airway. *JACEP* 1976; 5:588.
17. Morikawa S, Safar P, DeCarlo J: Influence of head-jaw position upon upper airway patency. *Anesthesiology* 1961; 22:265.
18. Elam JO, Greene DG, Schneider MA, et al: Head-tilt method of oral resuscitation. *JAMA* 1960; 172:812.
19. American Heart Association: *Basic Life Support Manual.* Dallas, American Heart Association, 1988.
20. American Heart Association: Standards and guidelines for cardiopulmonary resuscitation (CPR) and emergency cardiac care (ECC). *JAMA* 1986; 255(suppl):2841.
21. Stewart RD: Field airway control for the trauma patient, in Campbell JE (ed): *Basic Trauma Life Support,* ed 2. Englewood Cliffs, NJ, Prentice-Hall Inc, 1988, pp 42–90.
22. Melker RJ: Alternative method of ventilation during respiratory and cardiac arrest. *Circulation* 1986; 74(suppl 4):63.
23. Safar P, Park CJ: Mouth-to-tracheotomy tube breathing. *Anesthesiology* 1958; 19:802.
24. Safar P: Pocket mask for emergency artificial ventilation and oxygen inhalation. *Crit Care Med* 1974; 2:273.
25. Jorden RC: Airway management. *Emerg Med Clin* 1988; 6:671.
26. Giffen PR, Hope CE: Evaluation of a prototype tube-valve-mask ventilator for emergency artificial ventilation (abstract). *Ann Emerg Med* 1990; 19:478.
27. Harrison RR, Maull KI, Keenan RL, et al: Mouth-to-mask ventilation: A superior method of rescue breathing. *Ann Emerg Med* 1982; 11:74.
28. Hess D, Baran C: Ventilatory volumes using mouth-to-mouth, mouth-to-mask and bag-valve-mask techniques. *Am J Emerg Med* 1985; 3:292.
29. Hess D, Kapp A, Kurtek W: The effect on delivered oxygen concentration of the rescuer's breathing supplemental oxygen during exhaled-gas ventilation. *Respir Care* 1985; 30:691.
30. Ruben H, Knudsen EJ, Caraguti G: Gastric inflation related to airway pressure. *Acta Anaesthesiol Scand* 1961; 5:107.
31. Sellick BA: Cricoid pressure to control regurgitation of stomach contents during induction of anaesthesia. *Lancet* 1961; 2:404.
32. Priano LL, Ham J: A simple method to increase the F_DO_2 of resuscitators bags. *Crit Care Med* 1978; 6:48.
33. Campbell PP, Stewart RD, Kaplan RM, et al: Oxygen enrichment of bag-valve units during positive pressure ventilation: A comparison of various techniques. *Ann Emerg Med* 1988; 17:232.
34. Elling R, Politis J: An evaluation of emergency medical technicians' ability to use manual ventilation devices. *Ann Emerg Med* 1983; 12:765.
35. Stewart RD, Kaplan R, Pennock B, et al: Influence of mask design on bag-mask ventilation. *Ann Emerg Med* 1985; 14:403.
36. Barranco F, Lesmes A, Irles JA, et al: Cardiopulmonary resuscitation with simultaneous chest and abdominal compression: Comparative study in humans. *Resuscitation* 1990; 20:67.
37. Babbs CF, Tacker WA: Cardiopulmonary resuscitation with interposed abdominal compression. *Circulation* 1986; 74(suppl 4):37.
38. Berman RA, Lilienfeld SM: Correspondence. *Anesthesiology* 1950; 11:136.
39. American Heart Association: *Advanced Cardiac Life Support Manual,* Dallas, American Heart Association, 1987.

40. Campbell JE: *Basic Trauma Life Support,* ed 1. Bowie, Md, Brady Communications Co, Inc, 1985.

41. Hoffman LA, Maszkiewicz RC: Airway management for the critically ill patient. *Am J Nurs* 1987; 87:39.

42. Rosen M, Hillard EK: The use of suction in clinical medicine. *Br J Anaesth* 1960; 32:486.

43. Clinton JE, Ruiz E: Emergency airway management procedures, in Roberts JR, Hedges JR (eds): *Clinical Procedures in Emergency Medicine,* ed 1. Philadelphia, WB Saunders Co, 1985, pp 2–29.

44. Shim C, Fine N, Fernandez R, et al: Cardiac arrhythmias resulting from tracheal suctioning. *Ann Intern Med* 1969; 71:1149.

45. Marx GF, Steen SN, Arkins RE, et al: Endotracheal suction and death. *NY State J Med* 1968; 68:565.

46. Baker JL: What is the occupational risk to emergency care providers from the human immunodeficiency virus? *Ann Emerg Med* 1988; 17:700.

47. Hildebrand RM: Mouth-to-mask ventilation in the dental office. *J Indiana Dent Assoc* 1986; 65:19.

48. Caccomo A: A simple device for filtering mouth-to-mouth resuscitation. *Anesthesiology* 1984; 61:638.

49. Blenkharn JI, Buckingham SE, Zideman DA: Prevention of transmission of infection during mouth-to-mouth resuscitation. *Resuscitation* 1990; 19:151.

50. Heimlich HJ, Uhley MH: The Heimlich maneuver. *Clin Symp* 1979; 31:1.

51. Montoya D: Management of the choking victim. *Can Med Assoc J* 1986; 135:305.

52. Haugen RK: The cafe coronary. *JAMA* 1963; 186:142.

53. Heimlich HJ: Pop goes the cafe coronary. *Emerg Med* 1974; 6:154.

54. Heimlich HJ: A life-saving maneuver to prevent food-choking. *JAMA* 1975; 234:398.

55. White RD: Foreign body obstruction: Considerations in 1985. *Circulation* 1986; 74(suppl 4):60.

56. Greensher J, Montgomery WH: Treatment for choking infants: Some controversy lingers (letter). *Public Health Rep* 1986; 101:454.

57. Heimlich HJ: Back blows and chest thrusts for choking victims? Dr. Heimlich answers (letter). *Public Health Rep* 1986; 101:454.

58. Schwartz B: More on the choking controversy (letter). *Public Health Rep* 1987; 102:115.

59. Montgomery WH, Greensher J: Doctors Montgomery and Greensher reply (letter). *Public Health Rep* 1987; 102:115.

60. Heimlich HJ: Choking victims: Back blows and chest thrusts are hazardous, even lethal (letter). *Public Health Rep* 1987; 102:561.

61. Greensher J, Montgomery WH: Abdominal thrusts: Overzealous application may be hazardous to small children (letter). *Public Health Rep* 1987; 102:562.

62. Hoffman JR: Treatment of foreign body obstruction of the upper airway. *West J Med* 1982; 136:11.

63. Kitay G, Shafer N: Cafe coronary: Recognition, treatment and prevention. *Nurse Pract* 1989; 14:35.

64. Gordon AS, Belton MK, Ridolpho PF: Emergency management of foreign body obstruction, in Safar P, Elam JO (eds): *Advances in Cardiopulmonary Resuscitation,* New York, Springer-Verlag, 1977.

65. Ruben H, MacNaughton FI: The treatment of food-choking. *Practitioner* 1978; 221:725.

66. Guildner CW, Williams D, Subitch T: Airway obstructed by foreign material: The Heimlich maneuver. *JACEP* 1976; 5:675.

67. Heimlich HJ: First aid for choking children: Back blows and chest thrusts cause complications and death. *Pediatrics* 1982; 70:120.

68. Redding JS: The choking controversy: Critique of evidence on the Heimlich maneuver. *Crit Care Med* 1979; 7:475.

69. Day RL: Differing opinions on the emergency treatment of choking (commentary). *Pediatrics* 1983; 71:976.

70. Day RL, Crelin ES, DuBois AB: Choking: The Heimlich abdominal thrust vs back blows: An approach to measurement of inertial and aerodynamic forces. *Pediatrics* 1982; 70:113.

71. Orlowski JP: Vomiting as a complication of the Heimlich maneuver. *JAMA* 1987; 258:512.

72. Agia GA, Hurst DJ: Pneumomediastinum following the Heimlich maneuver. *JACEP* 1979; 8:473.

73. Fink JA, Klein RL: Complications of the Heimlich maneuver. *J Pediatr Surg* 1989; 24:486.

74. Visintine RE, Choong HB: Ruptured stomach after Heimlich maneuver. *JAMA* 1975; 234:115.

75. Passik CS, Ackermann DM, Piehler JM, et al: Traumatic rupture of Ionescu-Shiley aortic valve after the Heimlich maneuver. *Arch Pathol Lab Med* 1987; 111:469.

76. Razaboni RA, Brathwaite CEN, Dwyer WA: Ruptured jejunum following Heimlich maneuver. *J Emerg Med* 1986; 4:95.

77. Roehm EF, Twiest MW, Williams RC: Abdominal aortic thrombosis in association with an attempted Heimlich maneuver. *JAMA* 1983; 249:1186.

5

Esophageal Airways

Diane M. Birnbaumer, M.D.

James T. Niemann, M.D.

Ventilating a patient using an esophageal airway device is a concept that was introduced in 1968.[1] In the years following the introduction of this "mouth-to-lung airway" the esophageal obturator airway (EOA) was developed. The use of this airway became widely accepted in the early 1970s and in 1974 it was endorsed by the American Heart Association CPR Committee on Standards.[2] Since that time the EOA has been used over 3 million times in the prehospital setting.[3] Criticisms of the EOA led to the development of other types of esophageal airways, including the esophageal gastric tube airway (EGTA),[4] the pharyngotracheal lumen airway (PTLA),[5] the esophageal tracheal Combitube (ETC),[6] and the tracheo-esophageal airway (TEA).[7] For information on ordering these esophageal airways, see the Appendix.

With the nationwide trend toward training prehospital personnel in laryngoscopy and endotracheal intubation techniques, the use of esophageal airways has declined. Despite this shift from the use of esophageal airways to endotracheal intubation in the field, there are still some settings in which the use of the esophageal airway may be preferable.

INDICATIONS AND CONTRAINDICATIONS

The primary indication for use of an esophageal airway is when conventional endotracheal airway management cannot be performed (i.e., when medical personnel are not trained in endotracheal intubation techniques, when endotracheal intubation equipment is unavailable, or when attempts at endotracheal intubation are unsuccessful). The contrain-

dications to the use of the esophageal airway are (1) age less than 16 years, (2) presence of a gag reflex, (3) a conscious or semiconscious patient, (4) known or suspected esophageal disease or injury, and (5) known or suspected caustic ingestion. The presence of maxillofacial injuries is considered to be a relative contraindication to the use of esophageal airways.

EQUIPMENT

Esophageal Obturator Airway

The EOA consists of a plastic tube 34 cm long and 13 mm in diameter (Fig 5–1). The proximal end of the tube has an adaptor which attaches to a face mask with an inflatable cushion to seal it against the patient's face. The distal end of the tube is closed and rounded. A 35-mL balloon lies at the distal end of the tube and is inflated from the proximal end through a small tube with a one-way valve and a pilot bulb. Sixteen 3-mm perforations are present about one third of the way along the tube, designed to rest at the level of the pharynx when the EOA is fully inserted. The EOA is intended to be used no more than five times, with sterilization between uses.

Esophageal Gastric Tube Airway

The EGTA is a modification of the EOA described above. Instead of the distal end being closed, this tube has the distal end of the tube open to allow for passage of a 16F nasogastric tube for decompression of the stomach (Fig 5–2). The EGTA is to be used no more than five times, with sterilization between uses.

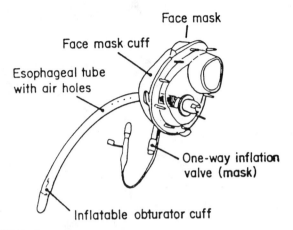

FIG 5–1.
The esophageal obturator airway. (From Brown CG: *Emerg Med Surv*, 1984, p 282. Used by permission.)

Pharyngotracheal Lumen Airway

The PTLA is a two-tube, two-cuff system with two tubes of unequal length running in parallel (Fig 5–3). Each tube has a proximal adaptor for use with a ventilation system. Both tubes are attached proximally to a teeth plate or bite-block, which, when inserted, sits at the level of the patient's incisors. This bite-block has a strap attached to secure the device around the patient's head. The first tube is 31 cm in length with an internal diameter of 8 mm. This tube contains a semirigid, cushioned, occluding stylet for maintaining proper shape during insertion and for occluding the tube if it passes into the esophagus. A large, low-pressure cuff is attached to the distal end of this tube. The second tube is 21 cm in length. A larger, low-pressure cuff is attached to this tube near its end and at the halfway point along the longer tube. When this cuff is inflated, it seals off the oro-

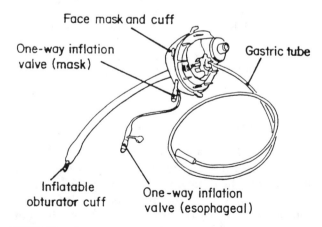

FIG 5–2.
The esophageal gastric tube airway. (From Brown CG: *Emerg Med Surv*, 1984, p 282. Used by permission.)

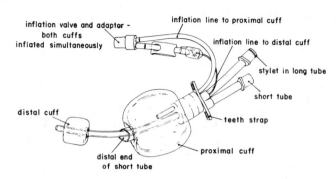

FIG 5–3.
The pharyngotracheal lumen airway. (From Niemann JT, Rosborough JP, Myers R, et al: *Ann Emerg Med* 1984;13:593. Used by permission.)

pharynx. The cuffs are inflated simultaneously through an in-series valve system located at the proximal end of the airway. The PTLA is intended for one-time use only.

Esophageal Tracheal Combitube

The ETC is a double-lumen airway that does not use a stylet (Fig 5–4). It has two balloons. The distal balloon holds 15 to 20 mL of air and is inflated through a proximal pilot balloon with a one-way valve adaptor. The proximal balloon, designed to be positioned between the root of the tongue and the soft palate to seal off the mouth and nasopharynx, holds 100 to 140 mL of air and is also inflated through a proximal pilot bulb system. One lumen is open to the distal end of the airway; the other lumen is blocked distally and is perforated along the mid-

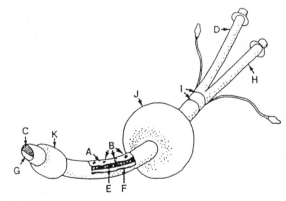

FIG 5–4.
Esophageal-tracheal Combitube (ETC): *A*="esophageal" lumen; *B*=perforations of lumen *A*; *C*=distal closed end of lumen *A*; *D*=longer connector for lumen *A*; *E*=partition wall; *F*="tracheal" lumen; *G*=distal open end of lumen *F*; *H*=shorter connector for lumen *F*; *I*=printed ring marks indicating depth of insertion; *J*=pharyngeal balloon; *K*=distal cuff. (From Frass M: *Crit Care Med*, Spring 1991, p. 610. Used by permission.)

portion of the tube. The ETC is to be used one time and discarded.

Tracheoesophageal Airway

The TEA consists of a mask with an adaptor attached with holes for passage of an endotracheal tube and for attaching an Ambu bag (Fig 5–5). Adaptors are available for use with various endotracheal tube sizes. The endotracheal tube is to be discarded after use; the mask can be sterilized and reused.

PROCEDURE

Several procedural points are applicable to the use of esophageal airways. When using these airways in the emergency patient, a 100% oxygen source should be used. In addition, airway alignment is important not only in aiding the placement of the airways. It is also critical that this alignment be maintained during the entire course of using these airways if they are to be effective.

Esophageal Obturator Airway and Esophageal Gastric Tube Airway

1. Place the patient in the supine position with the neck in the neutral position or slightly flexed.
2. Place the thumb deep into the back of the patient's mouth; grasp the tongue and lower jaw between the thumb and index finger, and open the mouth fully (Fig 5–6,A).

3. Insert the tube blindly, attached to the mask, through the mouth and into the esophagus (Fig 5–6,B).
4. Seal the mask against the patient's face (this may take two hands) (Fig 5–6,C).
5. Ventilate; listen over the lungs and stomach; watch for the chest to rise to confirm the position (Fig 5–6,D). If no chest rise is noted or breath sounds heard, remove the EOA or EGTA and reinsert it, repeating the above steps.
6. Inflate the balloon with 30 to 35 mL of air (palpate the pilot bulb to determine the correct amount to be used).
7. When endotracheally intubating a patient with an EOA or EGTA in place, leave the device in place until successful endotracheal intubation has been performed.
8. Have suction ready and consider positioning the patient in the lateral decubitus position when removing the airway.

Theory of Use

After the tube is inserted into the esophagus and the balloon is inflated to occlude the esophagus, the mask is sealed tightly against the face and air is forced through the perforations and into the lungs.

Pharyngotracheal Lumen Airway

1. Place the patient in the supine position with the neck in the neutral position.
2. Place the thumb deep in the back of the mouth; grasp the tongue and lower jaw between the thumb and index finger, and open the mouth fully.

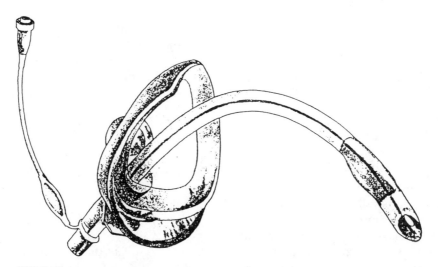

FIG 5–5.
The tracheoesophageal airway. (From Eisenberg RS: *Ann Emerg Med* 1980;9:272. Used by permission.)

A

B

C

D

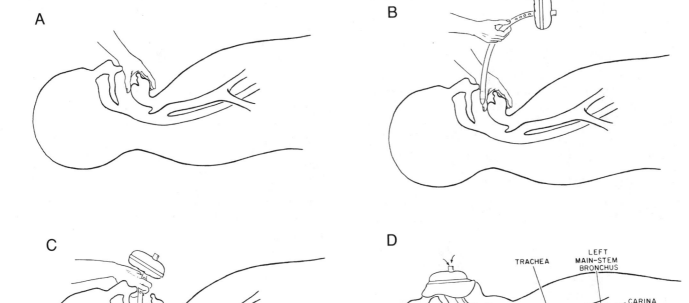

FIG 5–6.
A–D, insertion and use of the esophageal obturator airway or the esophageal gastric tube airway. See text for details.

3. Insert the airway blindly until the teeth touch the bite-block or teeth plate.

4. Inflate both cuffs through the in-series system until the pilot bulb is firm.

5. Ventilate through the short tube; if the chest rises and breath sounds are heard, ventilation is continued through this tube, i.e., the long tube is in the esophagus (Fig 5–7,A).

6. If the chest does not rise or breath sounds are not heard, remove the stylet from the long tube and ventilate through this tube. If chest rises and breath sounds are heard, continue ventilation through this tube (Fig 5–7,B).

7. Attach a strap around the patient's head to secure the airway in place.

Theory of Use

The tube is inserted blindly and the balloons are inflated. If the tube passes into the esophagus, ventilation can be performed through the shorter tube with the longer tube (stylet in place) occluding the esophagus. If the longer tube passes into the tra-

chea, the stylet is removed and the patient is ventilated through this tube.

Esophageal Tracheal Combitube

1. Place the patient in the supine position with the neck in the neutral position.

2. Place the thumb deep in the patient's mouth; grasp the tongue and lower jaw between the thumb and index finger and open the mouth fully (Fig 5–8,A).

3. Insert the Combitube blindly until the printed ring is aligned with the teeth.

4. Inflate line 1 (the pharyngeal balloon, with the blue pilot balloon) with 100 mL of air (Fig 5–8,B).

5. Inflate line 2 (the distal balloon, with the white pilot balloon) with 15 mL of air (see Fig 5–8,B).

6. Ventilate the patient through the longer blue tube (Fig 5–8,C). Listen for breath sounds and

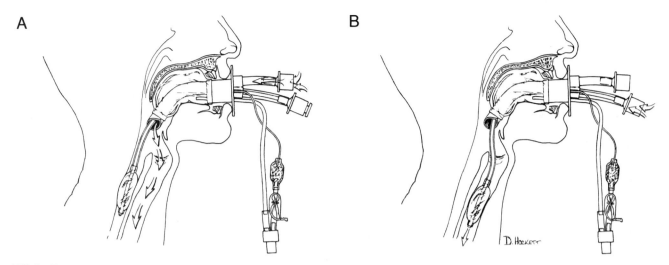

FIG 5–7.
The pharyngotracheal lumen airway. **A,** inserted in the esophageal position. **B,** inserted in the tracheal position. See text for details.

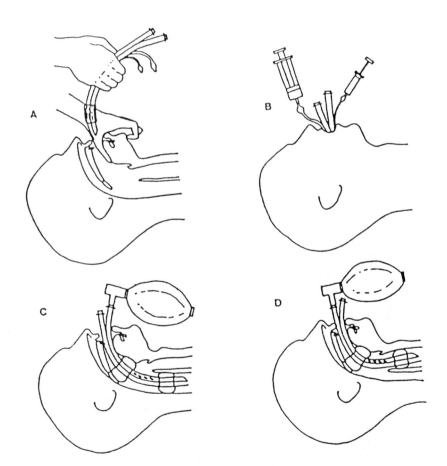

FIG 5–8.
A, blind insertion of the esophageal-tracheal Combitube (ETC). **B,** inflation of the pharyngeal balloon and then the distal cuff. **C,** ventilation in the esophageal position of the ETC. **D,** ventilation in the tracheal position of the ETC. See text for details. (From Fras M: *Crit Care Med,* Spring 1991, p. 610. Used by permission.)

watch for the chest to rise. If present, continue ventilating the patient through this tube.

7. If no breath sounds are heard or chest rise seen ventilate the patient through the shorter clear tube (Fig 5–8,D). Again listen for breath sounds and watch for the chest to rise. If present, continue ventilating patient through this tube.

Theory of Use

If the tube passes into the esophagus, the patient can be ventilated through the side holes of the tube and the stomach aspirated through the other tube, as needed. If the tube passes into the trachea, the patient can be ventilated through the hole at the end of the tube.

Tracheoesophageal Airway

1. Place the patient in the supine position with the neck in the neutral position.
2. Insert the endotracheal tube with the mask attached, either blindly or with the aid of a laryngoscope.
3. Inflate the endotracheal tube balloon with 10 mL of air.
4. Ventilate the patient through the endotracheal tube (Fig 5–9,A). Listen for breath sounds and watch for chest rise. If present, continue ventilation through the endotracheal tube.
5. If breath sounds are not heard and the chest is not seen to rise, attach an Ambu bag to the other mask port and ventilate the patient through the mask (Fig 5–9,B). Listen for breath sounds and watch for the chest to rise.

Theory of Use

If the endotracheal tube is inserted into the trachea, the patient can be ventilated through this tube as with a conventional endotracheally intubated patient. If the endotracheal tube passes into the esophagus, the tube acts as an oropharyngeal airway, keeping the airway open, and the gastric contents can be aspirated through this tube. The patient can then be ventilated via the mask as in bag-valve-mask ventilation.

EFFICACY AND COMPLICATIONS

Esophageal Obturator Airway and Esophageal Gastric Tube Airway

Table 5–1 lists the complications associated with the use of the EOA or EGTA. The two most dire

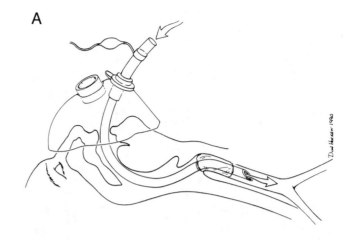

A

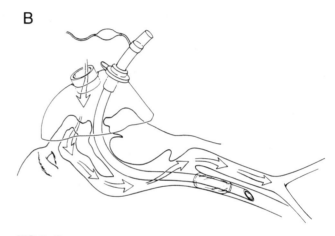

B

FIG 5–9.
A, the tracheoesophageal airway. A, in the tracheal position. B, in the esophageal position. See text for details.

complications are tracheal intubation and esophageal perforation. The incidence of these complications is not known and the cases reported probably represent an underreporting as autopsies are not done on all cases with fatal outcomes when these airways are used.

Since the EOA is a blind-ended tube, if it is passed into the trachea it acts to occlude the airway

TABLE 5–1.
Complications of the Esophageal Obturator Airway and Esophageal Gastric Tube Airway

Tracheal intubation
Esophageal rupture
Inadequate ventilation/oxygenation
Aspiration of contents of hypopharynx
Bleeding
Gastric rupture
Aspiration of gastric contents on removal

and the patient cannot be ventilated. The EGTA, although vented at the end of the tube, is not adapted for ventilation through this port in the event of tracheal intubation. The outcome of unrecognized tracheal intubation with the EOA is almost always fatal.[8-10] Several measures have been suggested to minimize the likelihood of inadvertent tracheal intubation with the EOA.[11] Positioning the patient's head in the neutral or flexed position aids in passing the tube into the esophagus; hyperextension of the head tends to favor passage into the trachea. Improper storage of a previously used EOA may cause excessive curvature of the device and lead to tracheal intubation; the manufacturer's recommended storage techniques should be followed. Careful auscultation of the lung fields for breath sounds and observation of the chest for rise are the most effective ways to prevent deaths from use of these airways.

Cases of esophageal perforation associated with the EOA have been reported widely in the literature.[12-22] The incidence of esophageal perforation is reported to be 0% to 2%[14]; the true incidence of this complication, however, is unclear because it is not known in nonsurvivors. The mortality rate of esophageal perforation is reported in the literature as 15% to 30%,[23, 24] and it has been suggested that this rate may be as high as 50% in patients with esophageal perforation as a complication of EOA use.[18]

Several mechanisms have been proposed as causes of esophageal perforation when using the EOA.[11, 21] Of these, the most readily remediable are overinflation of the balloon and removal of the EOA with the balloon still partially inflated. Proper inflation of the balloon can be gauged by palpating the pilot bulb when inflating the balloon; it should be firm to palpation and backpressure on the syringe will be felt when inflating the balloon. Under no circumstances should more than 35 mL of air be used to inflate the balloon. The balloon should always be completely deflated when removing the EOA.

Whether or not the use of the EOA can provide the patient with adequate oxygenation and ventilation is a topic of intense debate. While some studies comparing endotracheal intubation with esophageal intubation show no significant difference in oxygenation [25-27] and others show that the endotracheally intubated patients have a significantly higher arterial oxygen partial pressure (PaO_2),[28, 29] most studies show that arterial oxygen levels are adequate with both airways. On the other hand, several studies show that the $PaCO_2$ is significantly higher in patients being ventilated with the EOA[28-30] and the

blood pH of these patients is significantly lower. The effect of this acidosis and hypercarbia is unclear. Studies addressing survival data that compare patients in whom the EOA was used with those who were endotracheally intubated have generally shown no difference in outcome in the two groups.[22, 29, 31] These data suggest that the EOA or EGTA is a reasonable alternative to endotracheal intubation in the prehospital setting when used in cardiac arrest patients.

Several technical problems encountered by prehospital personnel may contribute to the difficulty in adequately ventilating the patient in whom the EOA is used. Although one study showed an 88% success rate in inserting the EOA in the field, it also showed only a 73% success rate in both inserting the tube and ventilating the patient.[32] The main complaint among prehospital personnel is difficulty in maintaining a mask seal, particularly in edentulous patients and during transport. This may account for the hypercarbia seen in some patients in whom the EOA is used. Other complications reported with the use of the EOA are bleeding,[10, 13] gastric rupture from balloon malfunction,[33, 34] and loss of the EOA into the hypopharynx when attempting to use the EOA with a conventional mask rather than the mask adapted for it.[35]

Pharyngotracheal Lumen Airway

Only two studies in the literature address the use of the PTLA in humans in the prehospital setting.[5, 36] One study[5] evaluated oxygenation, ventilation, and pH in six patients initially endotracheally intubated, then reintubated with the PTLA and ventilated. No significant difference was found between the two airways when PaO_2, arterial carbon dioxide partial pressure ($PaCO_2$), and pH were compared, and these data parallel the findings in the canine model in the same study. The other study[36] evaluated the successful intubation rates of the PTLA airway as compared to the endotracheal airway in the prehospital setting and found the rates to be equivalent for both airways. This study did not address the adequacy of oxygenation and ventilation with the PTLA. No complications have been reported with the use of this airway, but clinical data are limited.

Esophageal Tracheal Combitube

To date, all published studies of the ETC have been done by the same group[37-42] and its use has been confined to the hospital setting. All of the studies have shown adequate oxygenation when patients are ventilated with the ETC, and several show significantly higher PaO_2 levels in patients in whom the ETC was used compared with those who were endotracheally intubated.[37-39] One study showed no difference in outcome between patients endotracheally intubated compared with those in whom the ETC was used.[39] No complications have been reported with the use of this airway, but, as with the PTLA, use has been limited.

Tracheoesophageal Airway

One study of the TEA is reported in the literature.[7] The study reports 400 cases in which the TEA was used with "considerable success," but does not give success or complication rates nor does it address efficacy.

CONCLUSIONS

Although the esophageal airway is an airway management alternative in the prehospital setting, endotracheal intubation offers several advantages over esophageal airway management techniques (Table 5–2). In addition to the obvious direct airway control and protection from aspiration, endotracheal intubation provides a route for administration of

most resuscitative drugs and a route for tracheal suctioning. Moreover, direct laryngoscopy during intubation may visualize foreign bodies in patients who aspirate them and allow for their removal prior to intubation. These advantages are significant, and, as a result, endotracheal intubation is considered the method of choice in patients requiring airway management.

Training prehospital personnel in endotracheal intubation techniques has become prevalent across the country and endotracheal intubation is becoming the recommended standard of care.[43] Studies have shown that properly trained emergency personnel have endotracheal intubation success rates comparable with those of physicians.[22, 29, 31, 44, 45] Training, however, can be costly and time-consuming. Training a paramedical worker in endotracheal intubation can cost 12.5 times more than training him or her to use the EOA.[22] Although the didactic training time involved with these airways is comparable,[31] hands-on practice in endotracheal intubation took as much as 7 months longer to complete.[31] In small communities with limited resources, these factors may preclude training prehospital personnel in endotracheal intubation. In this situation, esophageal airway training and use is a reasonable alternative.

Despite the advantages of endotracheal intubation described above, studies showing no significant difference in outcome between the two airways[22, 29, 31] suggest that the esophageal airway is an adequate al-

TABLE 5–2.

Comparison of Endotracheal Intubation and Esophageal Airway Techniques*

	Placement Success	Overcoming Obstruction	Prevention of Aspiration	Oxygenation	Ventilation	Complications	Reusablity	Comments
ETT	88%–97%[22, 30, 31, 44, 45]	0 to +1	+2	+2	+2	Up to 50%[48]	No	Becoming prehospital standard of care
EOA	88%–95%[10, 22, 30, 31]	0 to–1	+1†	0 to +1[25-29]	0[28-30]	See text	×5	Viable alternative airwayif ETT cannot be done
EGTA	88%–95%[10, 22, 30, 31]	0 to–1	+1†	0 to +1[25-29]	0[28-30]	See text	×5	Viable alternative airwayif ETT cannot be done
PTLA	82%–83%[36, 46, 47]	0 to–1	+2†[47]	+1 to +2[5]	+1[5]	None reported‡	No	Limited prehospital data
ETC	100%[6]	0 to–1	+1†	+1 to +2[37-42]	+1 to +2[38-42]	None reported‡	No	No prehospital data in literature; may have potential
TEA	Not reported	Not reported	+1†	Not reported	Not reported	None reported‡	No	Very limited data available

*ETT = endotracheal intubation; EOA = esophageal obturator airway; EGTA = esophageal gastric tube airway; PTLA = pharyngeal-tracheal lumen airway; ETC = esophageal tracheal Combitube; TEA = tracheal-esophageal airway.
†Patient may aspirate any contents present in mouth and pharynx.
‡Reported uses are limited, and data may not reflect accurate complication rate.

ternative when endotracheal intubation cannot be successfully performed. In settings where training of pre-hospital personnel in endotracheal intubation is economically or technically impossible, the esophageal airway should be considered in emergency management of the unconscious patient.

REFERENCES

1. Don Michael TA: "Mouth-to-lung airway" for cardiac resuscitation. *Lancet* 1968; 2:1329.
2. American Heart Association CPR Committee on Standards: Standards for cardiopulmonary resuscitation (CPR) and emergency cardiac care (ECC). *JAMA* 1974; 227(suppl):833–868.
3. Don Michael TA: The role of the esophageal obturator airway in cardiopulmonary resuscitation. *Circulation* 1986; 74(suppl 4):134–137.
4. Gordon AS: Improved esophageal obturator airway (EOA) and new esophageal gastric tube airway (EGTA), in Safar P, Elam JO (eds): *Advances in Cardiopulmonary Resuscitation.* New York, Springer-Verlag, 1977, pp 58–64.
5. Niemann JT, Rosborough JP, Myers R, et al: The pharyngeo-tracheal lumen airway: Preliminary investigation of a new adjunct. *Ann Emerg Med* 1984; 13:591–596.
6. Frass M, Frenzer R, Rauscha F, et al: Evaluation of esophageal tracheal combitube in cardiopulmonary resuscitation. *Crit Care Med* 1986; 15:609–611.
7. Eisenberg RS: A new airway for tracheal or esophageal insertion: Description and field experience. *Ann Emerg Med* 1980; 9:270–272.
8. Gertler JP, Carmeron DE, Shea K, et al: The esophageal obturator airway: Obturator or obtundator? *J Trauma* 1985; 25:424–426.
9. Yancy W, Wears R, Kamajian G, et al: Unrecognized tracheal intubation: A complication of the esophageal obturator airway. *Ann Emerg Med* 1980; 9:18–20.
10. Donen N, Tweed WA, Dashfsky S, et al: The esophageal obturator airway: An appraisal. *Can Anaesth Soc J* 1983; 30:194.
11. Aguilar RC: Prevention of EOA complications. *Ann Emerg Med* 1980; 9:444–445.
12. Scholl DG, Tsai SH: Esophageal perforation following the use of the esophageal obturator airway. *Radiology* 1977; 122:315–316.
13. Johnson KR Jr, Genovesi MG, Lassar KH: Esophageal obturator airway: Use and complications. *JACEP* 1976; 5:36–37.
14. Strate RG, Fischer RP: Midesophageal perforations by esophageal obturator airways. *J Trauma* 1976; 16:503–509.
15. Carlson WJ, Hunter SW, Bonnabeau RC Jr: Esophageal perforation with obturator airway. *JAMA* 1979; 241:1154–1155.
16. Walloch Y, Zer M, Dintsman M, et al: Iatrogenic perforations of the esophagus. *Arch Surg* 1974; 16:503–509.
17. Pilcher DB, DeMueles JE: Esophageal perforation following use of esophageal airway. *Chest* 1976; 69:377–380.
18. Harrison EE, Nord HJ, Beeman RW: Esophageal perforation following use of the esophageal obturator airway. *Ann Emerg Med* 1980; 9:21–25.
19. McElroy CR: The esophageal obturator airway. *J Emerg Nurs* 1978; 4:232–233.
20. Kassels FJ, Robinson WA, O'Barak J: Esophageal perforation associated with the esophageal obturator airway. *Crit Care Med* 1980; 8:386–389.
21. Hoffman JR, Pietrafesa CA, Orban DJ: Esophageal perforation following use of esophageal obturator airway (EOA). *Am J Emerg Med* 1983; 3:282–287.
22. Goldenberg IF, Campion BC, Siebold CM, et al: Esophageal gastric tube airway vs. endotracheal tube in prehospital cardiopulmonary arrest. *Chest* 1986; 1:10–96.
23. Rosoff LR, White EJ: Perforations of the esophagus. *Am J Surg* 1974; 128:207.
24. Loop FD, Groves LK: Esophageal perforations. *Ann Thorac Surg* 1970; 10:571.
25. Hammargren Y, Clinton JE, Ruiz E: A standard comparison of esophageal obturator airway and endotracheal tube ventilation in cardiac arrest. *Ann Emerg Med* 1985; 14:953–958.
26. Meislin HW: The esophageal obturator airway: A study of respiratory effectiveness. *Ann Emerg Med* 1980; 9:54–59.
27. Schofferman J, Oill P, Lewis AJ: The esophageal obturator airway: A clinical evaluation. *Chest* 1976; 69:67–71.
28. Auerbach PS, Geehr EC: Inadequate oxygenation and ventilation using the esophageal gastric tube airway in the prehospital setting. *JAMA* 1983; 250:3067–3071.
29. Geehr EC, Bogetz MS, Auerbach PS: Pre-hospital tracheal intubation versus esophageal gastric tube airway use: A prospective study. *Am J Emerg Med* 1985; 3:381–385.
30. Smith JP, Bodai BI, Aubourg R: A field evaluation of the esophageal obturator airway. *J Trauma* 1983; 23:317–321.
31. Shea SR, MacDonald JR, Gruzinski G: Prehospital endotracheal tube airway of esophageal gastric tube airway: A critical comparison. *Ann Emerg Med* 1985; 14:102–112.
32. Bass RR, Allison EJ, Hunt RC: The esophageal obturator airway: A reassessment of use by paramedics. *Ann Emerg Med* 1982; 11:358–360.
33. Adler J, Dykan M: Gastric rupture: An unusual complication of the esophageal obturator airway. *Ann Emerg Med* 1983; 12:224–225.
34. Crippen D, Olvey S, Graffis R: Gastric rupture: An

esophageal obturator airway complication. *Ann Emerg Med* 1981; 10:370–373.

35. Berkebile PE, Narla R: An unusual complication of esophageal obturator airway (EOA). *Anesthesiology* 1982; 57:414–415.

36. McMahon S, Ornato J, Racht E, et al: Prehospital multiagency comparison of the pharyngeo-tracheal lumen airway tube (abstract). *Ann Emerg Med* 1990; 19:478.

37. Frass M, Frenzer R, Popovic R, et al: Esophageal tracheal Combitube (ETC) compared to endotracheal airway during mechanical ventilation after emergency intubation (abstract). *Ann Emerg Med* 1987; 16:1103.

38. Frass M, Frenzer R, Zdrahal F, et al: The esophageal tracheal Combitube: Preliminary results with a new airway for CPR. *Ann Emerg Med* 1987; 16:768–772.

39. Frass M, Frenzer R, Rauscha F, et al: Ventilation with the esophageal tracheal Combitube in cardiopulmonary resuscitation: Promptness and effectiveness. *Chest* 1988; 93:781–784.

40. Frass M, Frenzer R, Traindl O, et al: Evaluation of esophageal tracheal Combitube during cardiopulmonary resuscitation (abstract). *Ann Emerg Med* 1988; 17:411.

41. Frass M, Frenzer R, Mayer G, et al: Mechanical ventilation with the esophageal tracheal Combitube (ETC) in the intensive care unit. *Arch Emerg Med* 1987; 4:219–225.

42. Frass M, Rodler S, Frenzer R, et al: Esophageal tracheal Combitube, endotracheal airway, and mask: Comparison of ventilatory pressure curves. *J Trauma* 1989; 29:1476–1479.

43. Pepe PE, Copass MK, Joyce TH: Prehospital endotracheal intubation: Rationale for training emergency medical personnel. *Ann Emerg Med* 1985; 14:1085–1092.

44. Jacobs LM, Berrizbeitia LD, Bennett B, et al: Endotracheal intubation in the prehospital phase of emergency medical care. *JAMA* 1983; 250:2175–2177.

45. Stewart RD, Paris PM, Winter PM, et al: Field endotracheal intubation by paramedical personnel: Success rates and complications. *Chest* 1984; 85:341–345.

46. Hunt RC, Sheets CA, Whitley TW: Pharyngeal tracheal lumen airway training: Failure to discriminate between esophageal and endotracheal modes and failure to confirm ventilation. *Ann Emerg Med* 1989; 18:947–952.

47. Bartlett RL, Martin SD, Perina D, et al: The pharyngeo-tracheal lumen airway: An assessment of airway control in the setting of upper airway hemorrhage. *Ann Emerg Med* 1987; 16:343–346.

48. Taryle DA, Chandler JG, Good JT, et al: Emergency room intubations: Complications and survival. *Chest* 1979; 75:541.

APPENDIX

Ordering Information

Esophageal Obturator Airway (EOA)
Esophageal Gastric Tube Airway (EGTA)
Brunswick Biomedical Technologies, Inc.
6 Thatcher Lane
Wareham, MA 02571
Telephone: (508) 291-1830
FAX: (508) 295-6615

Pharyngotracheal Lumen Airway (PTLA)
Respironics, Inc.
1001 Murray Ridge
Murraysville, PA 15668-8550
Telephone: (412) 733-0200

Esophageal Tracheal Combitube (ETC)
Sheridan Catheter Corp.
Route 40
Argyle, NY 12809-9684
Telephone: (518) 638-6101
FAX: (518) 638-8493

Tracheoesophageal Airway (TEA)
Contact:
Robert Eisenberg, M.D.
Department of Respiratory Services
Huntington Memorial Hospital
100 Congress St.
Pasadena, CA 91105

6

Oral Endotracheal Intubation

James Scott, M.D.

HISTORY

The use of oral endotracheal intubation begins at least a thousand years ago. The Arab Avicenna (c. 980–1037) recorded the oral endotracheal intubation of a pig using a "golden or silver. . . tubus" inserted into the neck.[1,2] In 1796 Herholdt and Rafn described a resuscitation protocol for drowning victims that included digital oral intubation, and in 1878 Sir William Macewen popularized this method of intubation as an adjunct to surgical anesthesia.[3] It was not until the early 20th century when Kuhn introduced flexible metal tubing, and Jackson endorsed laryngoscopy and endotracheal intubation, that these became the definitive means of airway management.[4] Over the next 50 years oral intubation was standardized as an anesthesia procedure, but it was not until the 1960s that its usefulness in the areas of emergency medicine and resuscitation became recognized. With the advent of advanced cardiac life support (ACLS), the mechanics of this technique were disseminated to physicians practicing outside the operating suite. The use of intubation as a prehospital procedure has an even shorter history, as only in the last 15 years has this become an accepted procedure for prehospital care providers.

INDICATIONS

The general indications for oral endotracheal intubation are the same as the indications for management of an airway. These have been discussed previously. Specifically, endotracheal intubation is used to establish, maintain, or protect an airway that is compromised or has the potential for compromise. In addition, it is used to improve pulmonary toilet and to enhance the physiologic aspects of breathing: improved oxygenation and ventilation (Table 6–1).

In general, oral endotracheal intubation is the first choice for invasive airway management if simple positioning or bag-valve-mask ventilation is inadequate. The indications for other options, such as a surgical airway or nasotracheal intubation, are discussed elsewhere. If nasotracheal intubation is preferred but unsuccessful, oral endotracheal intubation may be the second choice for management of that airway. There is debate concerning the desirability of oral vs. nasotracheal intubation for patients in whom a prolonged intubation is expected. Although a nasal airway is generally better tolerated by the patient and is clearly more easily stabilized for prolonged ventilation, it carries the risk of turbinate necrosis and sinusitis with prolonged use.[5] Oral endotracheal intubation should always be chosen if a large tube is necessary. If the patient should require subsequent bronchoscopy, a large-diameter tube is needed and this is often not acceptable or possible via the nasal route. Also, for patients that have a contraindication to nasotracheal intubation, such as anatomic or pathologic conditions that would make this difficult, oral endotracheal intubation should be the choice.

CONTRAINDICATIONS

In addition to the controversy surrounding nasal vs. oral intubation for prolonged ventilation, an-

TABLE 6–1.

Indications and Contraindications for Oral Intubation

Indications
    Establishment, maintenance, or protection of the airway
    Improvement of pulmonary toilet
    Enhancement of the physiologic aspects of breathing;
      oxygenation and ventilation
    After unsuccessful nasotracheal intubation
    Intubation requiring a large tube
Contraindications
    Anticipated surgical access through the mouth
    Major maxillofacial trauma
    Significant bleeding in the supraglottic area
    Potential unstable cervical spine injuries (relative)
    Epiglottitis (relative)
    Miscellaneous (rheumatoid arthritis, ankylosing
      spondylitis)(relative)

other contraindication to oral intubation is the need for anticipated surgical access. If oral or facial surgery is expected, a nasal or surgical airway may be preferred for that patient. The major contraindications to oral endotracheal intubation are anatomic (see Table 6–1). The patient with major facial trauma that prevents recognition of landmarks, or isolated mandibular trauma where the temporomandibular joint (TMJ) may be immobile, will be difficult to intubate orally. Isolated maxillary trauma is usually not a contraindication to oral endotracheal intubation, unless a significant distortion of the hard palate is present.[6] In addition to mandibular trauma, other causes of trismus, such as arthritis, status epilepticus, or tetanus, may limit oral intubation. Significant bleeding in the oral pharynx or supraglottic area may inhibit visualization of necessary anatomy. The epiglottitis may require a surgical airway if landmarks are obscured or passage of a tube is made impossible.[7] The final anatomic considerations concern the neck and cervical spine. A patient with a suspected unstable cervical spine injury should have a lateral cervical spine radiograph prior to oral intubation, if possible. If this preintubation film is unobtainable, oral intubation may be acceptable if strict in-line immobilization is maintained, but a surgical airway may be necessary.[8] Cervical arthritis, degenerative joint disease, and ankylosing spondylitis may make oral intubation more difficult, but are not absolute contraindications. Rheumatoid arthritis, however, with degeneration of the odontoid process and transverse ligament of the first cervical vertebra may produce an unstable cervical spine and the technique of oral intubation may need to be modified or a substitute technique employed.[9]

EQUIPMENT AND EQUIPMENT PREPARATION

In the emergency setting there is often little notice of the immediate need for intubation, as patients present without warning or develop complications which need immediate or unanticipated intervention. Nonetheless, the physician usually has a few minutes to prepare for the procedure, and if these moments are well spent the overall procedure proceeds much more smoothly. Regardless of the acuteness of the situation, there is no need for hastily proceeding to laryngoscopy and endotracheal intubation without preparing the other necessary materials, medications, and personnel. A few minutes of preparation while the patient is ventilated with a bag-mask apparatus are moments well spent.

The first requirement is an adequate and immediately available oxygen source. Whether from a portable tank or wall source, it is imperative that at least 50 psi of O_2 be available after the regulator. It is best to use high-flow O_2 initially, then decrease the fractional concentration of oxygen in inspired gas (FiO_2) as the patient's requirements are more clearly delineated. All fittings should be examined to ensure that they are secure and that the tubing is not kinked. The O_2 source is turned on fully and the ball should move freely in the regulator or the humidifier should bubble vigorously. When a hand occludes the mask or the connection to the ET tube, the reservoir bag should fill rapidly. If any of these do not occur, the fittings must be rechecked or an alternative O_2 source located.

Simultaneous with establishing an O_2 source is documenting the presence of adequate suction. The time to do this is prior to attempting intubation and not at the moment that the posterior pharynx is found to be filled with stomach contents or blood. Suction may be wall-mounted or portable but should provide a minimum of 30 L/min at 30 mm Hg pressure.[10] The tubing should be 14F or larger to maximize the evacuation of larger particles. The rigid tonsillar tip suction catheter is preferred at the time of intubation as it is more suitable for large volumes of suction in the oropharynx. The flexible catheter tip is substituted after intubation to clear material from the lower trachea and bronchi. It may also be used prior to intubation to clear the deep posterior pharynx or esophagus. It must be kept in mind that when a patient is suctioned there is a period of time when the patient is not receiving O_2, is at a very high risk for coughing or vomiting, and is experiencing an increase in intracranial pressure if this reflex has not been pharmacologically blunted. Each period of suctioning should be limited to 10 seconds and repeated only after a period of oxygen-rich ventilation.

Although the end point of this preparation is an endotracheally intubated patient, it is important to have a bag and well-fitting mask immediately available. This is necessary for preoxygenation and ventilation of the patient who is not spontaneously breathing, and for ventilation once the intubation is complete. The proper equipment and technique for bag-mask ventilation are discussed elsewhere. Which bag is used for ventilation after intubation is a matter of individual preference.

The next decision is of the proper endotracheal (ET) tube. All currently available ET tubes are made of polyvinylchloride (PVC) and tested to be free of irritants. Although there are unique situations where specifically modified tubes are indicated, the single decision in the vast majority of instances is what size tube should be used. The size noted on the outside is the internal diameter of the ET tube and 2 to 3 mm should be added to estimate the external diameter. The adult airway ranges from 9 to 15 mm in diameter. In general, a 7.0- or 7.5-mm tube is appropriate for women and 8.0- to 8.5-tube for men. When there is uncertainty, it is prudent to choose a slightly smaller tube if immediate airway access is needed. The choice of pediatric tubes is discussed in Chapter 7.

The ET tube cuff is a high-volume, low-pressure cuff designed to prevent mucosal necrosis. Prior to intubation it is necessary to check that the cuff is patent. The cuff should be filled and the amount of air required to fully inflate the cuff should be mentally recorded. The pilot balloon that remains outside the patient's mouth is helpful in determining if the cuff has become deflated (Fig 6–1). However, it is not helpful in estimating cuff pressure; this must be assessed prior to intubation or by use of a manometer. If the cuff leaks or there is a question about its ability to remain inflated, it should be discarded and replaced. The problem of cuff leakage after intubation is discussed later.

In addition to the hole at the end of the ET tube, there is usually a second hole in the barrel and above the bevel, called Murphy's eye. This hole enables airflow even if the end is occluded by the tracheal wall, blood, or secretions (see Fig 6–1).

An alternative ET tube that is particularly useful

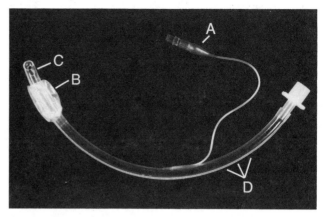

FIG 6–1.
Endotracheal tube. Note pilot balloon *(A)*, cuff *(B)*, Murphy's eye *(C)*, and centimeter markings of tube length from tip *(D)*.

is the Endotrol tube. This has a flexible stylet and circular trigger built into the side wall of the tube. This trigger is pulled and the stylet redirects the angle of the distal end of the tube. For patients with a distinctly anterior larynx this can be used to get

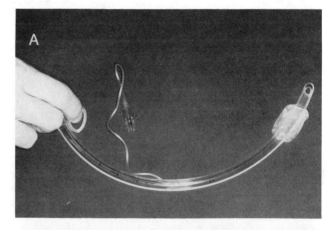
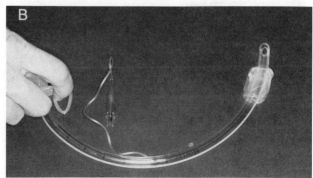

FIG 6–2.
Endotrol tube. **A,** relaxed position. **B,** trigger pulled. Note increased angulation to direct tip of tube anteriorly.

around the sharp angle, even when direct visualization is impossible (Fig 6–2). Another alternative, a double-lumen tube, is sometimes used for selective right or left bronchial intubation, but has little usefulness in the emergency setting. After selecting the correct ET tube and checking the cuff, a second tube, 0.5 mm smaller, and a 10-mL syringe should be placed within easy reach.

The next piece of required equipment is a stylet. A stylet is a malleable metal or plastic wand that is placed through the lumen of the ET tube and used to change the curvature of the tube (Fig 6–3). Use of the stylet is not absolutely necessary but is desirable in all emergency intubations. It is important that when the stylet is placed in the tube, that it does not project beyond the end of the tube as this may be a source of pharyngeal or laryngeal trauma when an attempt is made to pass the tube. It is also imperative that the stylet be put in and pulled out of the tube at least once prior to intubation. There are many instances where an attempt is made to remove the stylet after intubation only to have it stick in the

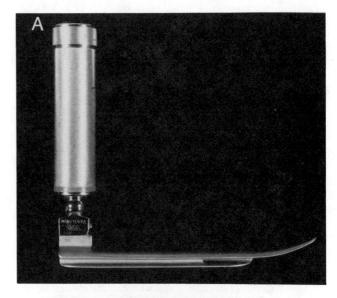

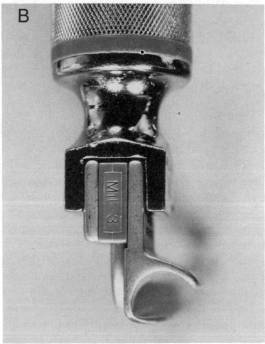

FIG 6–4.
Miller blade. **A,** side view **B,** intubator's view down the blade.

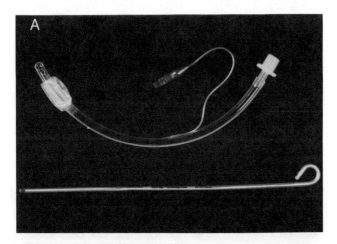

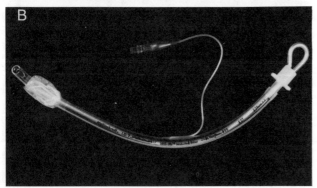

FIG 6–3.
A, endotracheal tube and malleable stylet. **B,** stylet in the ET tube. Note that the tip of the stylet does not extend past the tip of the tube.

lumen and remove the entire tube from the trachea. If the stylet does not withdraw easily, it should be lubricated and checked again to ensure that it passes easily in and out of the tube.

The next piece of equipment is the laryngoscope. It is important that laryngoscopes are checked daily to make sure that there are fresh batteries and that the light source is adequate. There are several manufacturers of laryngoscope handles and blades, so the compatibility of a particular blade and handle must be assured. If the bulb is dim or out, the blade is confirmed as securely attached to the handle, and the bulb is screwed tightly. If this does not provide a strong light source, the handle and blade should be changed until a properly functioning light is assured. The choice of which blade to use is almost exclusively a matter of personal preference. Straight (Miller) blades are narrow blades with a curved central channel (Fig 6–4). These may be better in patients with thick necks that are difficult to maneuver, but this is a source of considerable disagreement.[11]

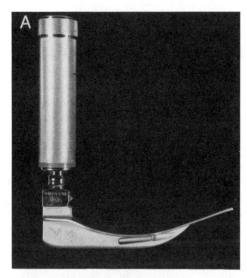

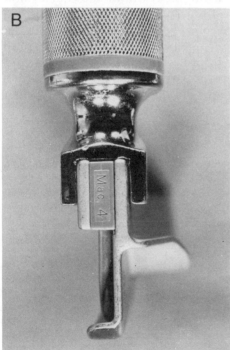

FIG 6–5.
MacIntosh blade. **A,** side view **B,** intubator's view down the blade.

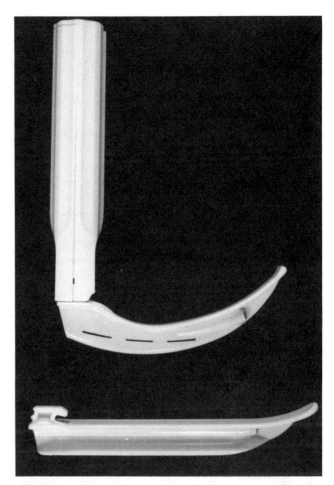

FIG 6–6.
Plastic disposable laryngoscope.

The curved (MacIntosh) blade has a broad flat surface and a tall flange to enhance movement of the tongue (Fig 6–5). There are special blades with different curves, mirrors, and prisms to further enhance visualization of the vocal cords and these are discussed later. Rarely are these available in the emergency department. At least two handles and several blades should be available at all times. Even after a particular blade is chosen, an alternative type and size should be immediately accessible in anticipation of any difficulty. For adults, a MacIntosh no. 3 or no. 4 or a Miller no. 2 blade is most useful. Occasionally a patient with a thick neck will require a Miller no. 3. The new disposable laryngoscopes are available with straight or curved blades. They are especially popular in prehospital situations because they are light and do not require cleaning (Fig 6–6). In addition to the aforementioned equipment it is desirable to have Magill forceps available. These are used to redirect tubes into the cords if proper angulation cannot be assured with simple manipulation of the tube. Unfortunately, Magill forceps are exclusively right-handed.

Lidocaine spray should be available and may be helpful to anesthetize the posterior pharynx and larynx. It is inconsistently effective at producing anesthesia at the level of the vocal cords, however. By spraying lidocaine or cocaine through a nasopharyngeal airway, more anesthesia will be delivered to the supraglottic structures.[12] Another effective means of achieving local anesthesia is nebulized lidocaine or aerosolized epinephrine and lidocaine mixtures administered prior to intubation, if time allows.[13]

Lubricating jelly should be available and used in almost all situations. Any available lubricating jelly is adequate. Lidocaine jelly may be used as a lubricant but has little local anesthetic effect because it is not applied uniformly to the mucosa and is in place for only a short period of time. It should not be used as a substitute for topical, aerosolized anesthetics.

Several miscellaneous pieces of equipment are also necessary. If the patient is not paralyzed and has any amount of voluntary motor activity, a bite-block may be helpful to prevent occlusion while intubating and to prevent damage to the tube after intubation. A highly adhesive and strong tape should be at the bedside for stabilization of the tube after intubation. Properly fitting gloves must be worn during intubation for protection against communicable diseases. As this procedures takes place through the mouth, it is not a sterile technique. Sterile gloves, therefore, are not necessary. Several folded towels should be available. These can be invaluable in assuring proper positioning of the head prior to intubation or in an attempt to facilitate a difficult visualization. Arrangements should be made for a ventilator. This serves as the initial recruitment of the respiratory therapy department, and eliminates the need for prolonged bagging of the patient. Finally, a stethoscope should be immediately available in its best position: around the neck of the physician. It is very common for the physician to be scrambling for a stethoscope when the time comes for documenting correct tube position. It is important that sedating and paralyzing agents be prepared ahead of time. These medications should be drawn up in syringes as should any antidotes or reversing agents that may be necessary. These syringes should be properly identified by the nurse. It is important that the nurse also fully understand the timing and order of administration of these agents. Other adjunctive equipment, such as a lighted stylet or fiberoptic intubating laryngoscope, should be made available at this time.

A last consideration is where to place this equipment. Often the equipment is placed haphazardly around the area or even behind the physician. This only further complicates what is often a very hectic moment. The ET tube, laryngoscope handle and blades, syringe, bag, mask, and suction apparatus should all be placed to the right side of the patient. This makes it easily accessible to the free right hand of the intubator without necessitating turning or moving away from the patient (Fig 6–7).

The equipment needed for oral endotracheal intubation is summarized in Table 6–2.

EVALUATING THE PATIENT

Although time often precludes an opportunity for a full evaluation of a patient prior to intubation, a few seconds or minutes are usually available. This time is best spent attempting to predict the patient who may be a difficult to intubate. This may allow the preparation of adjunctive means of intubation or surgical equipment in anticipation of an alternative airway.

Historical data are invaluable in assessing the ease or difficulty of intubation. A history of previous surgery with successful intubation or difficult airway management is often known by the patient or family and is highly predictive of subsequent difficulty. A history of previous oral or neck surgery, TMJ problems, rheumatoid arthritis, degenerative joint disease, or upper airway burns or angioedema is equally helpful. A discussion of other medical problems, particularly pulmonary and cardiovascular conditions, will help predict those patients least

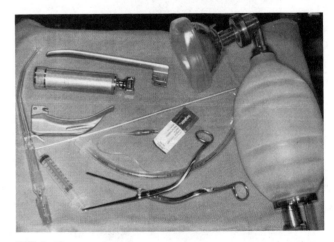

FIG 6–7.
Necessary intubating equipment, placed to the patient's and intubator's right.

TABLE 6–2.

Equipment for Oral Intubation

1. Immediately available oxygen source
2. Adequate suction
3. Bag and well-fitting mask
4. Endotracheal (ET) tube (7.0–7.5 mm for women, 8.0–8.5 mm for men)
5. A replacement ET tube
6. Two laryngoscope handles with batteries
7. Two Miller blades
8. Two MacIntosh blades
9. Magill forceps
10. Malleable stylet
11. Lidocaine spray and lubricating jelly
12. Gloves
13. Folded towels for head of patient
14. Stethoscope
15. Sedating and paralyzing agents

equipped to weather a difficult or prolonged intubation attempt. It is also important to ascertain the time of the patient's last meal. A meal within the previous 6 hours has predictive value for subsequent aspiration.[14]

In the general physical examination of the patient it is important to assess the patient's general state of health. As part of this, vital signs are important as documentation of the patient's current status and as estimations of both respiratory and cardiovascular reserve. The patient with reactive airway disease, profound tachypnea, and tachycardia is equally as tenuous as the victim of a drug overdose with significant bradycardia and bradypnea. At times simply listening to the patient will give indications of potential intubation difficulties. A stridorous or muffled voice is an indicator of upper airway obstruction that needs to be anticipated.

Inspection of the mouth may also predict the difficult passage of an oral ET tube. The TMJ should be assessed by opening the mouth and measuring the distance between the central incisors. A normal opening is 50 to 60 mm or approximately three adult fingerbreadths. If the joint allows less than 20 mm, or one fingerbreadth, problems for passage of the laryngoscope blade into the mouth and visualization of the vocal cords should be expected.[15] A standard Macintosh no. 3 blade has a flange height of 20 mm and will not pass between the teeth if the opening is less than this distance.

In assessing the oropharynx it is also important to determine the distance from the mandibular symphysis to the hyoid bone. If this distance is less than three fingerbreadths, or 60 mm, this predicts a difficult, short, anteriorly placed larynx.[6] This is the pa-

tient for whom many experts would consider a straight blade rather than a curved Macintosh. It is important to look at the teeth for dentures, loose teeth, plates, or caps which may become dislodged and seated in the posterior pharynx or larynx. The tongue should be examined for both size and mobility. Large tongues, which are relatively immobile, are more difficult to intubate around. If the uvula and tonsils cannot be visualized without the assistance of a tongue blade, expect some problem in passage between the posterior tongue and the soft palate.

When looking at the neck it is important to look for evidence of previous surgery or radiation which would distort the anatomy or narrow the underlying airway. In addition, tracheal deviation may be apparent and this will direct the intubator to the correct placement of the tube when intubation is attempted. In general, a thick or muscular neck will have limited mobility. This mobility should be assessed relative to the neck on the shoulders and the head on the neck. For a patient who cannot flex the neck on the shoulders more than 30 degrees or extend the head on the neck more than 45 degrees, it will be difficult to establish a line of sight from the opening of the mouth to the vocal cords. The distance from the inferior edge of the mandible to the thyroid notch should be greater than 6.5 cm. If it is less than 6.0 cm, establishing a line of sight to the larynx will be problematic.[16]

A general pulmonary and cardiovascular examination should follow. Other studies may be helpful, although they are usually not necessary. A chest radiograph may note tracheal, bronchial, or lung abnormalities and is helpful is to identify or rule out a pneumothorax prior to instituting positive pressure ventilation. For appropriate patients, the necessity of a cervical spine radiograph through the body of T1 has been previously stated. Arterial blood gas determinations may be helpful to identify the need for oxygenation or ventilation and are useful as a baseline. An electrocardiogram (ECG) may reveal evidence of ischemia which will increase the immediacy of airway concern.

PREPARING THE PATIENT

The initial preparation is to discuss the procedure with the patient in as much detail as the circumstances allow. This is standard practice in routine preanesthesia care, but is often overlooked in emergency intubation. If the patient is awake and aware of his or her surroundings, it is important to explain the risks and benefits of the procedure, and if possible, obtain informed consent. Even in patients who appear unresponsive, no harm can be done by talking to the patient and telling him or her what you are doing as you proceed. Commonly, patients who appear to be unaware will have recollections of the procedure which can be improved by a caring discussion with the physician.

In the general preparation of the patient an intravenous line should be established. If the patient is going to be paralyzed and sedated, it is desirable that two lines be available in the event that reversal is necessary and the first line is inadequate. An ECG monitor should be applied to detect dysrhythmias or bradycardia. A pulse oximeter is helpful to warn of desaturation prior to the bradycardia of hypoxia. Although this device is of little usefulness in determining initial oxygenation status, it is very useful for following trends in saturation. It is also important at this time to completely expose the face, neck, and chest of the patient to enhance intubation and subsequent auscultation.

At the same time that the patient is exposed, the oral pharynx should be examined for foreign bodies, food, or teeth, and these should be removed. The mouth and posterior pharynx should be gently suctioned to remove any secretions or blood. An absolute prerequisite to intubation is preventilating the patient with 100% O_2. This serves to increase the O_2 reserve which will be needed during the apneic period of intubation. If the patient is not capable of self-ventilating, he or she should be gently hyper-ventilated to decrease the carbon dioxide partial pressure (PCO_2). If the patient is breathing spontaneously, simple oxygenation is all that is necessary. The importance of preoxygenation to prevent hypoxia during intubation cannot be overstated. A difficult or prolonged intubation will be well tolerated if the patient is physiologically prepared, but even short episodes of hypoxia may result in immediate and extended complications.

The preparatory measures are summarized in Table 6–3.

PROCEDURE

At the time of intubation it is important to again verify that all the necessary equipment is readily available. All necessary medications should be drawn up in syringes by the nurse or assistant. All personnel needed for the intubation or for any postintubation tasks should be in position and should clearly understand their roles. The physician or intubator should assume a position at the head of the bed with all of the equipment immediately to his or her right. The patient should be adequately preventilated and should be informed and aware of what is going to take place.

It is most important to establish the position of the patient to enhance visualization of the vocal cords. To establish this line of sight there are three axes that must be maintained (Fig 6–8). The first is the axis of the mouth to the posterior pharynx. The second is a line running parallel to the posterior

FIG 6–8.
Resting position of three critical axes: mouth, posterior pharynx, larynx.

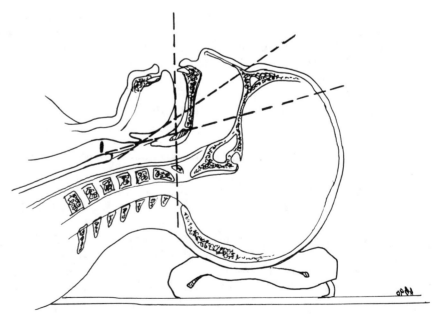

TABLE 6–3.

Preparation of the Patient: Prerequisites to Oral Intubation

1. Discussion of the procedure fully with the patient
2. Intravenous access
3. ECG monitor
4. Pulse oximeter
5. Complete exposure of head, neck, and chest
6. Removal of foreign bodies, food, or teeth in the mouth or posterior pharynx
7. Preoxygenation with 100% O_2

pharynx. The third is the line of the larynx as it traverses into the trachea. At rest none of these axes are completely aligned. In order to establish a clear line of sight it is important to first flex the neck on the shoulders to align the posterior pharynx and the larynx. Approximately 30 degrees of flexion is necessary to achieve this alignment. It is very useful to place towels or folded sheets under the occiput of the patient to assist in holding the patient in this position. It is next important to extend the head on the neck to approximate the line of sight of the mouth with the line of the pharynx and with the now aligned larynx. This requires approximately 20 degrees of extension although more may be necessary depending on the soft tissues of the posterior pharynx. This extension occurs at the atlanto-occipital joint and is thus the cause of difficulty if there is arthritis or cervical spine abnormality. This final align-

ment is conducive to a direct visualization of the vocal cords and is called the intubating or "sniffing" position (Fig 6–9).

It is next important to get the mouth open as widely as possible. Although several techniques exist, the scissors technique is most effective (Fig 6–10). The thumb of the intubator's right hand is placed on the right lower central incisor of the patient and the middle finger on the right upper central incisor. The thumb and middle finger are then scissored to force the mouth open. If this still does not achieve adequate visualization it may be necessary for an assistant to help in opening the mouth or in lifting the angle of the mandible to disengage the TMJ. Once the mouth is open as wide as possible, it is important that adequate suction is performed to remove any apparent secretions or foreign bodies.

At this point the laryngoscope is placed into the mouth and an attempt is made to visualize the cords. With a MacIntosh blade the blade is inserted with the left hand into the side of the tongue. From here the intubator should be able to identify the uvula and tonsillar pillars. It is important that no part of the tongue is trapped between the blade of the laryngoscope and the teeth as this will cause injury to the tongue. The blade is then gently moved to the left, sweeping the tongue out of the line of sight (Fig 6–11). The blade should be gently advanced to the base of the epiglottis until the epiglottis is clearly visualized, falling from the superior aspect of the view

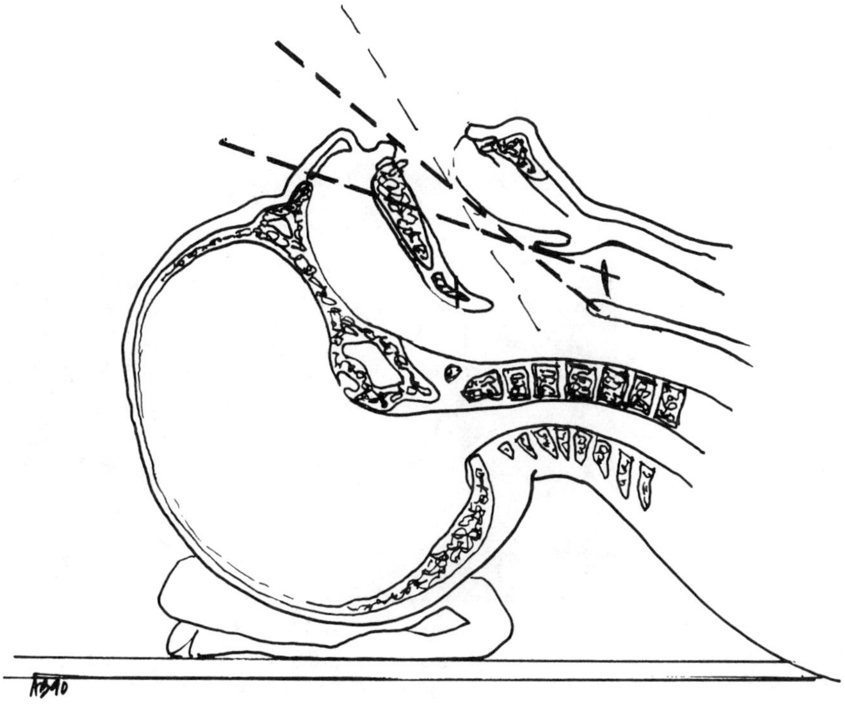

FIG 6–9.

Intubating or "sniffing" position. Note approximation of three critical axes.

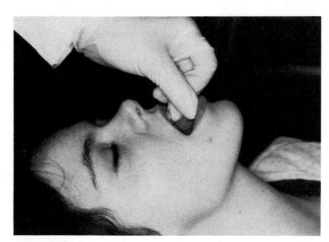

FIG 6–10.
Scissors technique to open mouth.

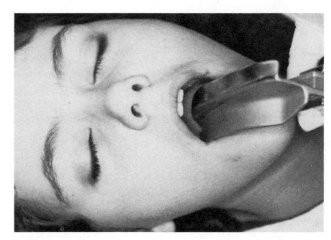

FIG 6–11.
MacIntosh blade sweeping the tongue to the left.

and into the line of sight. The laryngoscope handle is then gently but firmly pulled at a 45-degree angle to the patient until the epiglottis is lifted and the cords are clearly visualized (Figs 6–12 and 6–13). It is important that the intubator does not twist the wrist in an attempt to enhance visualization. This has the potential for causing damage to the upper incisors as the blade is rocked against the superior aspect of the mouth. Moreover, it does not enhance the line of sight of the cords as it actually disengages the tip of the blade from its firmly seated place in the vallecula (Fig 6–14). At the time of visualization the epiglottis should be clearly visualized superiorly and just below it the vocal cords should become apparent (see Fig 6–13). The true vocal cords are white linear structures which are angled outward from the center. The aryepiglottic folds are the cartilaginous folds to either side and they should be equally apparent.

If a Miller blade is used instead of the MacIntosh, the technique for inserting the blade into the mouth is similar. Because the blade has no flange an attempt to sweep the tongue is often unsuccessful. However, even if the tongue is not completely removed to the left it will be compressed against the floor of the mouth allowing visualization. The Miller blade is advanced past the epiglottis toward the vocal cords (Fig 6–15). It is not placed in the vallecula like the MacIntosh blade. Once the blade has been advanced the handle is lifted identically to the MacIntosh blade, and the same warnings are given to any attempt to twist the wrist while attempting visualization. It should be noted that since the Miller blade causes compression and lifting of the soft tissues, less lifting is usually needed to obtain visualization. This

is important to remember for patients with a suspected cervical spine injury, since less movement of the neck will be required. The view at the time of intubation will be somewhat different since the epiglottis will not be apparent. The intubator should be able to follow down the line of sight of the Miller blade to the level of the true vocal cords.

For intubators who are left-handed these techniques may be somewhat cumbersome. Handling the laryngoscope blade is not difficult for a left-handed intubator but placing the tube with the right hand is often awkward. The best option is to practice this in a right-handed fashion until it becomes manageable. For physicians who are intubating on a regular basis there are left-handed blades available and the technique is the same from the opposite side. Alternatively, the technique can be done with the blade in

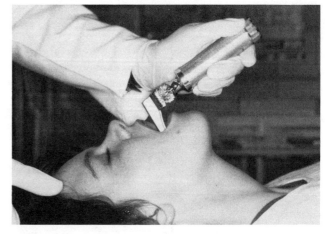

FIG 6–12.
MacIntosh blade inserted and the handle pulled at a 45-degree angle from the body. Note that the handle is not twisted.

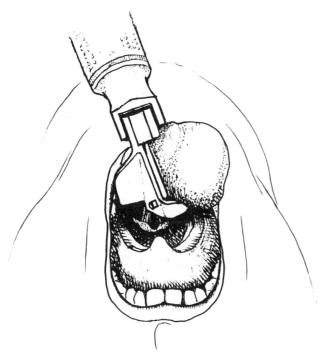

FIG 6–13.
View of vocal cords with the MacIntosh blade.

the right hand sweeping to the left and inserting the tube directly from above. The difference here is that the tube will not be inserted from the right side and there will have to be a crossing of the hands at the time of intubation. Although somewhat cumbersome, this technique has been mastered by some physicians who intubate regularly.

It is important, prior to placing the ET tube through the vocal cords, to apply cricoid pressure. This moves the trachea posteriorly and may enhance the line of sight down the larynx. More important, this occludes the esophagus and decreases the risk of aspiration in the unconscious or paralyzed patient. It must be kept in mind that if the patient is actively vomiting this pressure must be released and measures taken to clear the vomitus. This Sellick maneuver of occluding the esophagus with cricoid pressure has been shown to prevent aspiration in patients for periods up to 30 minutes while patients are being bagged prior to intubation.[16] Occasionally this technique will narrow the trachea and make intubation more difficult at the time that the tube is being placed. In this instance, the pressure should be released prior to another attempt.

The ET tube, equipped with a stylet, is placed into the mouth from the right side. The tube should be gently curved at the end toward the ceiling. Once the tube is just above the level of the cords the intu-

bator should wait for inspiration, if the patient is still breathing, or pass the tube when the cords appear relaxed. It is imperative that the tube is not forced through the cords as this can result in significant and often irreversible damage. The tube should pass through the cords easily without force. The tube should be advanced approximately 3 cm past the cords or until the cuff disappears just below the level of the cords. In an adult, placing the tube so that the teeth are approximately at the 21-cm mark on the tube will usually ensure that the tip is above the carina.[15]

A

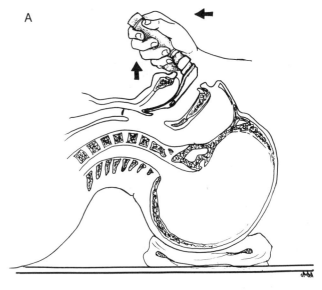

B

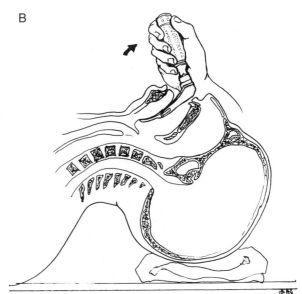

FIG 6–14.
A and **B,** with twisting of the wrist, the tip of the MacIntosh blade is unseated from the base of the epiglottis. Note the epiglottis falling back into the line of sight.

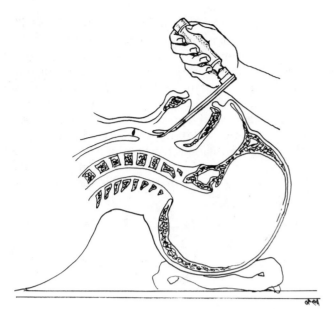

FIG 6–15.
Positioning of the Miller blade. Note placement past the epiglottis and compression of soft tissues.

The position of the tube should then be verified to rule out esophageal intubation or inadvertent right mainstem bronchus intubation. The absolute best way to verify tube position is to have observed the tube actually passing between the cords. This is undoubtedly the single best insurance against esophageal intubation. If there is doubt after the intubation has taken place, repeat laryngoscopy can be performed to verify the tube's position through the cords. Once the patient is ventilated condensation in the tube will suggest that the tube is in the trachea rather than the esophagus. This is not totally reliable but is a very reassuring sign that the tube is properly placed in the trachea. The lungs should be auscultated in both axillae and in the anterior lung fields for equal breath sounds. Auscultating the left axilla is especially important as this may identify an inadvertent right mainstem bronchus intubation. The epigastrium should also be auscultated for gurgling sounds, which suggest esophageal intubation. Normal breath sounds are often transmitted to this area and should not be interpreted as esophageal intubation. The chest wall should be observed for symmetric motion with inspiration. This provides reassurance that the intubation is in the trachea although it is not completely sensitive for either esophageal or right mainstem intubation. Some abdominal wall motion should be expected even with proper intubation and thus cannot be used as a suggestion of inadvertent esophageal intubation. In patients who are awake and making sounds, phonation should stop as the tube is passed through the cords. The patient

who has been intubated and is still able to talk has an esophageal intubation. End-tidal CO_2 monitoring has been shown to be very helpful in verifying correct tube placement.[17] End-tidal CO_2 should be close to 0 on inspiration and should rise to at least 6% on aspiration.[6] If there is no variation with respiration this is highly suggestive of esophageal intubation. End-tidal CO_2 monitoring has not been found to be effective in ruling out right mainstem bronchus intubation.

A portable chest film is helpful in discovering a right mainstem bronchial intubation, but without a lateral film, which is rarely available in the emergency setting, it is of little help in identifying esophageal intubation because the trachea directly overlies the esophagus. There should never be a time where a patient has an esophageal intubation suggested or documented by the chest film. Clearly, this should be a clinical diagnosis made far before a chest film is obtained. Pulse oximetry can be helpful in documenting correct intubation. If it is placed before intubation and the hemoglobin saturation is normal, any evidence of desaturation suggests esophageal intubation. However, inadvertent esophageal intubation will usually be diagnosed prior to O_2 desaturation. Lastly, difficulty in bagging a patient may suggest right mainstem or esophageal intubation. This is nonspecific as there are other sources of airway obstruction. However, with a patient who is initially easy to ventilate and in whom bagging then becomes more difficult, intubation in the right mainstem bronchus or esophagus should be suspected.

The cuff should be inflated to the predetermined volume established prior to intubation. This reinforces the importance of checking the volume needed to inflate the cuff prior to intubation. It is important to inflate the cuff until no air leak is noted around the cuff. If an airway pressure gauge is in place, the airway pressure should be elevated to 20 cm H_2O and the cuff inflated until there is no leak at that pressure. This has been found to be the most advantageous pressure to prevent necrosis of the tracheal mucosa.[16] If there is a persistent air leak it is most often caused by a faulty valve at the pilot balloon. A simple technique is to attach a stopcock to that balloon, reinflate it, and close the stopcock (Fig 6–16). This very often will eliminate the need to extubate and reintubate the patient. It is also important to recheck tube placement. A persistent air leak suggests that the ET tube is actually in the esophagus or in the larynx but above the vocal cords. Cuffs can of course become damaged during the procedure of intubation. If rechecking the placement of

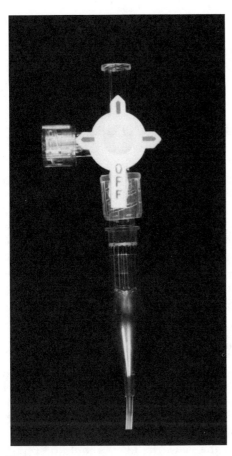

FIG 6–16.
Stopcock on pilot balloon.

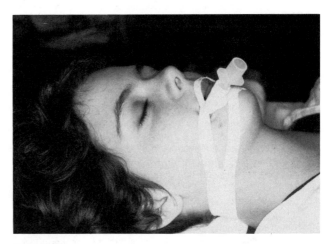

FIG 6–17.
Properly secured ET tube. Note tape on mandible and maxilla and sparing of lips.

the tube and attempting to stop a leak with a stopcock does not result in elimination of the air leak, the cuff must be assumed to be damaged and the tube will need to be replaced.

An often overlooked but uniquely important step is to secure the tube. The tube should be moved to the corner of the mouth to make it more comfortable for the patient and to prevent tonguing of the tube, which can dislodge it from the trachea. A bite-block may be essential if the patient is awake or may awake and become uncooperative. Benzoin should be liberally applied to the upper cheek and lips and allowed to dry completely prior to application of any tape. Although there are many techniques for securing the tube, it is important that whatever method is used, the intubator and the nurse who will be caring for the patient are equally assured that the tube is secure. One method is to place 1-in. tape along the face and as the tape approaches the tube, split the tape and wrap it around the tube. There is no advantage to this over multiple pieces of tape but it allows securing the tube with less tape. It is important that the tape be attached to the maxilla and the man-

dible since the mandible is mobile if the patient is awake. No tape should be placed on the lips or the vermilion border as this may be damaged at the time of removal. The tape should be securely attached to the upper lip and around the tube (Fig 6–17). If the patient has a beard the tape should go completely around the head. On the back of the head and beard, two pieces of tape may be placed together to prevent the tape from sticking to the hair and beard. Although some intubators believe that this technique is desirable on all patients, it is not absolutely necessary.

The intubation procedure is summarized in Table 6–4.

POSTINTUBATION TASKS

The most important task to be performed immediately after intubation is proper ventilation of the patient. Bagging of the patient should be done in a regular rhythmic fashion at a rate that is dictated by the clinical situation. A patient with cardiac arrest, sepsis, diabetic ketoacidosis, or with other reason to be acidotic should have a rate that will ensure hypocapnia in the first 2 to 3 minutes. The rate of ventilation will not usually effect oxygenation to a great degree, as this is more dependent on the FiO_2. It is equally important to use a more physiologic rate, e.g., 10 to 15 breaths per minute, for a patient in whom normal oxygenation and ventilation was assumed prior to intubation. The volume of ventilation must be determined by patient size and chest movement. A pressure valve can be placed between the bag and the ET tube to assess end points of ventilation. Ventilator settings are discussed in each of

TABLE 6–4.

Procedure for Oral Intubation

1. Gather all necessary equipment, medication, and personnel
2. Place the patient in the intubating or "sniffing" position
3. Carefully place the laryngoscope blade into the right side of the mouth
4. Gently sweep the tongue to the left
5. Advance the blade into the vallecula to the base of the epiglottis
6. Pull the laryngoscope blade at a 45-degree angle; avoid twisting the laryngoscope handle
7. Visualize the epiglottis and vocal cords
8. Apply cricoid pressure
9. Pass the tube through the cords until the balloon has completely disappeared
10. Remove the stylet
11. Bag the patient and auscultate the axillae and anterior chest for breath sounds
12. Inflate the cuff
13. Secure the tube

the clinical situation chapters in Part III. It is important that the patient be attended closely when initially placed on the ventilator. Most complications arise in the first few minutes and can be corrected at that time. The patient should not be placed on the ventilator until easily and comfortably bagged without significant resistance.

A nasogastric (NG) tube should be placed to decompress the stomach of any air that may have been introduced during preintubation or mask ventilation of the patient. If there are evident secretions or difficulty ventilating the patient with the bag, the ET tube should be suctioned with a flexible-tip catheter. This should be done only when the patient is well oxygenated, should never take longer than 10 seconds, and precautions should be taken against increasing intracranial pressure (ICP) if this is a concern.

A postintubation chest film should be performed to verify tube placement in or above the carina and to rule out complications such as a pneumothorax. An arterial blood gas sample should be obtained several minutes after intubation to assess the adequacy of ventilation and to help gauge the amount of continuous O_2 that will be required.

It is essential that the patient who initially underwent sedation and muscle relaxation for the purpose of intubation have these measures continued. This is often overlooked and the patient awakes only to self-extubate. Even cooperative patients benefit from mild sedation after intubation. If there is concern about increased ICP with intubation, this concern must continue after intubation. It must be remembered that the ET tube remains through the vocal cords, providing a very strong stimulus for increased ICP, and continued sedation and relaxation are absolutely necessary to blunt this reflex.

Postincubation tasks are summarized in Table 6–5.

UNSUCCESSFUL INTUBATION

Three percent to 4% of intubations will be unsuccessful even in the hands of experienced intubators.[11] Many of these failures can be predicted from anatomic abnormalities identified previously. A large tongue, a thick or short neck, evidence of previous surgery, or distorted anatomy are often predictive. Another large percentage of unsuccessful intubations results from flaws in the technique of the intubator. Others are due to anatomic complications which may require creative intubation measures.

Inadequate Oral Access

Inadequate access to the oropharynx may result from not opening the mouth adequately. It is important that the mouth be opened as far as possible and that the blade be used to firmly lift and maintain the mandible upward. If the tongue seems to be obstructing the view, the blade should be repositioned to the right and the tongue moved again to the left without allowing any of the tongue to slide back under the blade.

Anatomic complications may make access to the posterior pharynx difficult, even with proper technique. If the mouth cannot be opened two finger-breadths, even after muscle relaxation, this is evidence of an immobile TMJ and an alternative approach may be necessary (e.g., nasal or fiberoptic). As stated previously, one fingerbreadth of opening is the minimum necessary for passage of a MacIntosh blade into the mouth. If the patient has very large teeth or a severe overbite, there may be difficulty in making the turn of the blade into the poste-

TABLE 6–5.

Postintubation Tasks

1. Verify that the ET tube is secure and in its proper location
2. Bag the patient to document ease of ventilation
3. Place the patient on the ventilator if appropriate
4. Place the nasogastric tube to decompress the stomach
5. Obtain a postintubation chest film and arterial blood gas sample
6. Continue initial sedation and muscle relaxation if indicated for agitation or suspected increased intracranial pressure

rior pharynx without hitting the teeth. In this case it is important to open the mouth wider and try to lift the mandible higher in order to gain further posterior access. Another option is to try a smaller blade, especially a Miller blade, where it may be possible to place the entire blade and the top of the handle inside of the mouth. To achieve this it may be necessary to place the blade sideways and then rotate the blade after it is in the mouth.

A large or overly mobile tongue may obscure the view. The use of a larger MacIntosh blade with a taller flange may help to move and maintain the tongue out of the way. Another technique is to put gauze between the blade and the tongue in order to hold the tongue as one unit and sweep it out of the way. A final option is to have an assistant grasp the tongue with gauze and move the tongue to the left at the time of intubation.

Another anatomic complication which may limit oral access is a very high barrel chest. This enlarged chest will impinge on the handle of the laryngoscope as the blade is inserted into the mouth. If this happens it may be necessary to use a smaller blade and insert it from the side, or a straight blade which has a less acute angle of insertion into the mouth. Sometimes overextending the neck will allow introduction of the blade into the mouth and then the head and neck can be placed back into the proper intubating position. If all this fails there is a polio blade which has an obtuse takeoff from the handle and thus does not have the problem of impacting the chest when inserted.

Inadequate Visualization of the Cords

The most common cause of unsuccessful intubations is inability to properly visualize the cords. This often results from improper positioning of the patient during the intubation. Extension of the head on the neck may be inadequate but it is more likely that the flexion of the neck on the shoulders is poor. Thus, visualization of the posterior pharynx is obtained but actual alignment of the axes of the pharynx and the larynx is prevented. When this happens the patient should be repositioned and towels or other support should be placed under the patient's head to achieve the proper flexion of the neck. An alternative is to have an assistant lift the head from the base of the skull. This will flex the neck but allow the head to extend.

A second common cause of failure to visualize the cords is haste in the intubation process. Often the intubator is so anxious to place the tube that the landmarks are not fully identified. If the cords are not visualized on the first look, it is important to identify any visible landmarks to determine what procedures are needed to improve the location. If lateral landmarks are appreciated (aryepiglottic folds, tonsilar pillars) then it should be obvious in which direction to move to gain a midline position. If the epiglottis is in view but the cords are still obscured, the head has not been lifted vigorously enough. A more forceful lifting at a 45-degree angle to the bed will bring the cords into the line of sight. It is important that there be no twisting of the wrist which will give a better view of the epiglottis or vallecula but usually will not pull the epiglottis out of the way and enhance visualization of the cords.

A common problem is insertion of the blade too far into the pharynx. A MacIntosh blade placed on the epiglottis is usually not long enough to lift all of the epiglottic tissue. The base of the epiglottis will continue to obscure the view of the cords even when lifted. It is necessary in this situation, in which part of the epiglottis can be identified but the cords are still not seen, to pull the MacIntosh blade back until the epiglottis falls into view. The blade is then reseated in the vallecula and a repeat attempt at lifting and intubation is attempted. With a Miller blade it is not uncommon to place the blade too distal so that the end is down the esophagus. With this view no clear landmarks are seen other than generalized mucosal tissue. It is necessary to gently withdraw the blade while maintaining upward pull on the laryngoscope until the point where the cords come into view.

A final technical mistake is not inserting the blade far enough. The epiglottis cannot be lifted with the MacIntosh blade if the blade is not firmly seated in the vallecula. To reposition the blade, it must be advanced gently while maintaining a slight amount of lift on the handle. With the Miller blade, the epiglottis will fall into the line of sight, thus indicating that the blade is not inserted far enough. To correct this, the blade must be pulled back and then redirected downward to get past the epiglottis and to the level of the cords.

Anatomic complications that may inhibit visualization of the cords include a very anteriorly displaced larynx. The patient who has less than three fingerbreadths from the symphysis of the mandible to the hyoid is at high risk for this possibility. If it occurs it is important to reposition the neck so that there is more neck flexion and less head extension. Cricoid pressure may also force the larynx posteriorly, although this maneuver is rarely successful by itself. Often the larynx will be off center and this can usually be predicted. If it has not been anticipated but it appears that the larynx is to the right or left, the blade should be redirected. Another option is to use the tube itself to pull or push the tissues laterally as the tube approaches the cords. A final option is to angle the stylet in the tube to direct it more toward the side of the cords. A very generous or floppy epiglottis often obscures an adequate view of the vocal cords. When this occurs the MacIntosh blade should be seated more deeply into the vallecula to the base of the epiglottis, and the procedure repeated. Often this is a situation where a Miller blade, which flattens the epiglottis in addition to lifting it, will often be successful.

Despite these efforts, in a small number of patients the cords cannot be identified. A significant number of these patients may nonetheless be intubated. This may be interpreted as simply a fortuitous event, but there are maneuvers to improve the chances of a successful intubation. One is to make a sharp angle or "hockey stick" deformity in the ET tube with the stylet. This will enable a more anterior angulation of the tube and often will direct it through the cords even if they cannot be clearly seen. It is important to identify any landmarks that are visible, such as the esophagus or epiglottis, in order to direct this blind placement of the tube. Often the person applying cricoid pressure will feel the tube passing through the cords and this can be used as a sign of correct intubation. This is not completely specific, however, as a cord passing through a narrowed esophagus will also transmit pressure through the tracheal rings. Another technique to increase the likelihood of a successful blind intubation of a patient breathing spontaneously is to look for bubbles in the larynx during expiration. Although the cords cannot be seen, intubating in the direction of the bubbles will often be effective. Another option is to use the Endotrol tube to angulate the tube at the moment it is passed through the cords. The stylet must be withdrawn from the last 5 to 6 cm of the ET tube to permit this maneuver. Similar to the Endotral is the Flexiguide, a flexible stylet that passes through the tube and has a trigger to change its angulation. Hooks are available to pass through Murphy's eye and direct the end of the tube, but they have little advantage over a normal stylet. A final adjunct is Magill forceps. These are used to move the tube as far anteriorly as possible when it is felt to be at the level of the cords, but care must be taken to avoid laceration of the cuff. None of these efforts is foolproof, but each can enhance the success of a semiblind intubation.

Inability to Pass the Tube Through the Vocal Cords

Technical problems that can inhibit the passage of the tube through the vocal cords are usually related to the tube being too large or too flexible. A stylet to maintain some rigidity and the use of a smaller tube is often all that is necessary. Another technical problem occurs when an attempt is made to pass the tube when the cords are closed or in spasm. If this occurs the intubator should wait for the patient to breath or cough and then attempt to pass the tube. If this does not occur, attempts at intubation should be stopped, the patient should be ventilated with a mask, and muscle relaxation should be achieved prior to reattempting intubation. Under no circumstances should the tube be forced through cords that are closed.

A small opening in the cords or below the cords can also limit passage of the tube. Abnormal anatomy, scarring, a goiter, a fixed vocal cord, or glottic or subglottic edema may be the cause of this complication. A smaller tube is necessary in this situation. The intubator should not be reluctant to use even a very small tube. Especially if edema is present, this small tube may be lifesaving and the edema will provide an adequate seal. If the opening is still too small, a flexible stylet, such as an NG tube, can be advanced through the tube and past the tip in a Seldinger technique. Once the NG tube is placed below the cords the tube can be gently advanced over it and the NG tube removed. Another option is to use topical epinephrine to diminish any glottic or supraglottic edema that may be present in an attempt to enlarge the size of the opening. Another technique is moving the tube off the midline so that the tip of the bevel of the tube is on the midline. By placing the bevel on the midline, it can be used as a wedge, enhancing passage of the remainder of the tube through the cords. Finally, if the airway is displaced or angled, it is sometimes possible to remove the stylet after the tube is through the cords and then to continue to pass the tube. This will allow the tube to accommodate any changes in angulation below the level of the cords.

Alternatives After Unsuccessful Intubation

An unsuccessful intubation is defined as three or more attempts that are unsuccessful. In this case alternatives, such as fiberoptic intubation, digital intubation, intubation with a lighted stylet, or a surgical airway may be indicated. Except in cases where there is inadequate oral access, nasotracheal intubation rarely succeeds after attempted oral endotracheal intubation has failed. It must be emphasized that failed intubation is not the time to allow one's ego to interfere with necessary clinical care. If there is another, more experienced intubator available, that person should attempt intubation.

COMPLICATIONS OF ORAL ENDOTRACHEAL INTUBATION

Complications associated with endotracheal intubation can be divided into those which occurred during the intubation procedure, those which are a complication of being intubated, and those which occur during extubation (Table 6–6).

The most significant complication during the process of intubation is an unsuccessful intubation. The reasons for this have been discussed. The most dire end point of this complication is prolonged hypoxia. If the patient cannot be intubated, other means of oxygenation and ventilation must be substituted. It is not uncommon for a patient to desaturate while multiple attempts are made at oral endotracheal intubation. This is to be avoided at all costs and the availability of pulse oximetry should completely prevent this outcome. A second common complication during the intubation procedure is inadvertent esophageal intubation. This is especially a problem if the airway is assumed to be secure and the esophageal intubation goes unrecognized until there is evidence of clinical deterioration. This must be evaluated by direct visualization of the tube through the cords or by ausculation that clearly identifies the tube in the trachea. Right mainstem bronchus intubation is also a complication and may

lead to inadequate ventilation and left lung atelectasis. This is less of a problem in the emergency department, where ventilation and oxygenation can usually be maintained with single lung ventilation. However, it must be corrected prior to prolonged ventilation in the intensive care unit.

Trauma may occur to the eyes, lips, teeth, or tongue during the intubation procedure. This usually results from a hurried approach to the intubation or a difficult intubation in which many hands are around or on the face. Specifically, twisting the handle of the laryngoscope can cause injuries to the teeth. Injuries to the epiglottis or larynx may occur. Mucosal or submucosal injuries and vocal cord damage are rare but avoidable complications. Minor mucosal bleeding is very common, however. These can all be avoided by careful and controlled tube passage with no attempts at forcing the tube.

Aspiration is a common occurrence during the procedure of intubation. Unlike an intubation being performed in the operative suite, patients in the emergency department have not had their stomachs emptied prior to the attempt at establishing an airway. Aspiration usually occurs at the time the blade is placed in the posterior pharynx which causes a strong reflex for retching. It is important that suction be immediately available, that the patient's head be turned to the side if there is no suspicion of a neck injury, and that the patient is not ventilated with a bag until a reasonable attempt is made to clear vomit from the pharynx. Positive pressure ventilation via a bag-mask apparatus will only force vomitus in the posterior pharynx down into the trachea if it is not cleared beforehand.

In order to avoid hypoxia and hypercapnia it is important that the patient receive adequate preoxygenation and ventilation, and that prolonged intubation attempts not be made. Time limits should be set for how long an attempt at intubation will proceed before the patient is ventilated by an alternative method. If cardiopulmonary resuscitation (CPR) is being performed it should not be interrupted for more than 15 seconds for any single intubation attempt. It is often the case when an intubation is most hurried that the longest period of time goes by without adequate airway control and ventilation.

A serious complication from intubation is spinal cord injury from movement of an unstable cervical spine. If possible, cervical spine radiographs should be obtained prior to intubation to rule out any obvious fracture or ligamentous instability. If this is impossible, strict immobilization without distraction should be maintained or nasotracheal surgical alter-

TABLE 6–6.

Complications of Endotracheal Intubation

Unsuccessful intubation with prolonged hypoxia
Inadvertent esophageal intubation
Inadvertent right mainstem bronchus intubation
Trauma to eyes, lips, teeth, or tongue
Mucosal or submucosal injuries of the pharynx or vocal cords
Aspiration
Spinal cord injury from hyperextension of unstable cervical spine
Increased intracranial pressure
Precipitated dysrhythmias
Laryngospasm, bronchospasm
Tube obstruction
Cuff leak
Pneumothorax, pneumomediastinum

natives sought. Although the exact incidence of spinal cord injury resulting from intubation is unknown, there are many case reports and pathologic specimens showing the amount of movement of a cervical spine with oral intubation.[10] Passing a tube through the larynx may be the single most potent stimulus for increasing ICP. This response must be suspected in any patient with head injury or suspected intracranial hemorrhage and must be prevented by preventilation and the use of paralyzing or sedating agents.

Dysrhythmias may occur unrelated to hypoxia. The act of passing a tube through the vocal cords is stimulus enough to generate both supraventricular and ventricular dysrhythmias. These are especially common in patients that are hypothermic or are experiencing an acute myocardial infarction. Preparations should be made for the most gentle intubation possible. Intubation may also exacerbate bronchiolar reactivity in patients with asthma, and irritation of the carina can cause airway reaction even in patients without asthma. This generally quickly resolves once the tube is in place, but β-agonist inhalation therapy is sometimes necessary to reverse this reaction.

While the patient is intubated, several complications may occur which will cause further injury or inadequate oxygenation and ventilation. Tube obstruction from a kink or biting, or a tube clogged with blood or sputum can cause inadequate ventilation. It is important that tube placement and patency be checked initially and rechecked if there is any change in the patient's condition. Adequate suctioning and securing of the tube will minimize kinks and obstruction. Sedation, paralyzing agents, or a bite-block may be necessary to prevent the patient from occluding the tube. Accidental extubation should be expected if the patient is not cooperative during transfer from one location to another. The tube must be firmly secured and manually held in place during any seizure, bed transfer, or combative behavior. Adequate sedation and relaxation should be provided to minimize the chance of this adverse experience.

The problem of cuff leak has been discussed but it must be kept in mind that it may not be evident until some time after the patient is intubated. The same procedures should be used to check the cuff at this time as are used at the time of initial intubation. Mucosal erosion can occur from cuff pressures greater than 25 cm H_2O. Although this is not a major concern in the emergency department, the pressure should be checked if a patient is going to be intubated for more than a few hours, in order to maintain an adequately inflated, but not overly pressurized cuff.

Pneumothoraces may be caused or exacerbated by positive pressure ventilation. A small emphysematous bleb or pleural injury may be rapidly transformed into a large, even tension pneumothorax. Even if the preintubation radiograph is normal, postintubation films should be evaluated for any evidence of even the smallest pneumothorax. In addition, any change in the patient's clinical status must be reassessed while simultaneously documenting tube placement and patency. Laryngospasm is usually a problem after extubation but may occur while the patient is intubated, especially in children. Positive pressure ventilation, epinephrine, or inhaled β-agonist may be helpful in reversing this.

One of the most common problems encountered while caring for an intubated patient is difficultly in ventilating. This may be manifested as increased pressure required to maintain lung volumes or by an alteration in blood gases or vital signs. This is most commonly from tube obstruction, bronchus obstruction, bronchospasm, mainstem intubation, esophageal intubation, or a severe pulmonary pathologic condition. The physician must see to it the tube is properly placed and patent and that suction is attempted to clear any obstruction before making a diagnosis of bronchospasm or stiff lung.

At the time of extubation aspiration is very common. It is important to empty the stomach by NG tube and place the patient on the left side prior to extubation. Laryngospasm may occur after extubation. This is more frequent if the patient is half-awake, so it is important that the patient be fully awake and cooperative. It is also more common with prolonged intubation where tracheal stenosis may be present in addition to the smooth muscle irritation caused by removing the tube. Intravenous lidocaine prior to extubation and racemic epinephrine are useful in this situation. If laryngeal spasm becomes pronounced, it may be advisable to reintubate the patient and pretreat with steroids prior to another attempt at extubation. Mucosal irritation, hoarsness, and minor edema are common after even short-term intubations. These are usually not serious but may manifest as extubation croup in children. Saline mist or racemic epinephrine may be helpful in reducing this problem. Vocal cord avulsion is very rare and usually secondary to a traumatic intubation or extubation with the cuff inflated. In most situations, even removing the tube with the cuff inflated will not cause serious vocal cord injury. Nonetheless, this should be avoided at all cost. Recurrent laryngeal, lingual, or hypoglossal nerve injuries are also reported, but again are very rare and usually secondary to traumatic intubation.

REFERENCES

1. Frostad AB: Tracheostomy in acute obstructive laryngitis. *J Laryngol Otol* 1973; 87:1101.
2. Mihic D: The first endotracheal intubation (letter). *Anesthesiology* 1980; 52:523.
3. Atkinson RS, Rushman GB, Lee JA: *A Synopsis of Anaesthesthia*, ed 8. Bristol, England, John Wright & Sons Ltd, 1977.
4. Jackson C: The technique of insertion of intratracheal insufflation tubes. *Surg Gynecol Obstet* 1913; 17:507.
5. Danzl DF, Thomas DM: Nasotracheal intubation in the emergency department. *Crit Care Med* 1980; 8:677.
6. Finucane BT, Santora AH: *Principles of Airway Management*. Philadelphia, FA Davis Co, 1988.
7. Handler SD: Stridor, in Fleisher G, Ludwig S (eds): *Textbook of Pediatric Emergency Medicine* ed 2. Baltimore, Williams & Wilkins Co, 1988, p 300.
8. Rhee KJ, Grenn W et al: Oral intubation in the multiply injured patient: The risk of exacerbating Spinal Cord Damage. *Ann Emerg Med* 1990; 19:511.
9. Hess, EV: in Schumacher RH (ed): *Primer on the Rheumatic Diseases*, ed 9. Atlanta, Arthritis Foundation, 1988, pp
10. McIntyre KM, Lewis AJ (eds): *Textbook of Advanced Cardiac Life Support*. Dallas American Heart Association, 1983.
11. Whitten CE: *Anyone Can Intubate*. San Diego, Medical Arts Publications, 1990.
12. Barash PG, Cullen BF, Stoelting RK (eds): *Clinical Anesthesia*. Philadelphia, JB Lippincott Co, 1989.
13. Block C, Brechner VL: Unusual problems in airway management and the influence of TMJ, mandible and associated structures and endotracheal intubation. *Anesth Analg* 1971; 50:114.
14. Patic V, Stheling L, Zauder H: *Fiberoptic Endoscopy in Anesthesia*, ed 1. St Louis, Mosby–Year Book, Inc, 1983.
15. Dronen S, Chadwick O, Nowak R: Endotracheal tip position in the arrested patient (letter). *Ann Emerg Med* 1982; 11:116.
16. Sellick BA: Cricoid pressure to control regurgitation of stomach contents during induction of anesthesia. *Lancet*, 1961; 2:404.
17. Sanders AB: Capnometry in emergency medicine. *Ann Emerg Med* 1989; 18:1287.

7

Oral Endotracheal Intubation: Pediatric Perspective

William W. Feaster, M.D.

In its broadest definition, the pediatric age group extends from late adolescence down to the smallest premature infant. Differences in anatomy, equipment, and technique encountered when intubating the pediatric patient are greatest at the younger ages.

ORAL VS. NASAL INTUBATION

In children, the orotracheal route for emergency intubation is used almost exclusively. The anterior and superior position and anterior angulation of the larynx, coupled with relatively large turbinates, creates a difficult passage for a nasal tube in a younger child. In the preschool and school-age child, adenoidal hypertrophy makes tube passage difficult. Damage to the adenoids may result in copious bleeding or the dislodgment of adenoidal tissue and subsequent aspiration into the trachea as a foreign body. A medical condition leading to a clenched jaw, as in status epilepticus, is not a contraindication to oral intubation when a muscle relaxant is used.

EQUIPMENT

The equipment used during intubation of the pediatric patient varies primarily in size, with the exception of suction catheters for oral suctioning, as small suction catheters are unable to quickly clear tenacious secretions. Small catheters of appropriate size must be used for endotracheal tube suctioning. A smaller bag on a self-inflating bag or bag-valve-mask setup is desirable, but essential in only the smallest infant. Masks of all sizes must be available so that a good seal around the mouth and nose can be obtained.

Oral airways of several sizes should be available and will often be needed in the severely obtunded or comatose child with large adenoids. To determine the correct size of the oral airway, the airway should be laid along the side of the face in its position of use. The tip should extend to the angle of the mandible. A shorter airway may push the tongue back and obstruct the airway. A longer one may traumatize the supraglottic structures.

Endotracheal tubes used in children younger than 8 years of age are usually uncuffed. Since the narrowest part of the airway in this age group is the circular cricoid cartilage, an adequate seal around the tube can be obtained without inflation of a cuff. The submucosal tissues in this area are quite loose and swell easily in response to trauma or inflammation, so care must be given to place the correct-size tube atraumatically (Table 7–1). In preparation for intubation, tubes that are 0.5 mm internal diameter (ID) larger and smaller than the tube intended for use should be available. Since small tubes tend to be quite flexible, a stylet should be used during emergency intubations. Placement of the tube in the child's anterior larynx may require a "hockey stick" angulation of the end of the tube. Lubrication of the stylet is advised, as some tubes stick to the larger-size stylet.

Laryngoscope handles and blades are functionally the same, but again, differ in size. Difference in handle size is related to operator preference. Straight Miller blades are most often used for pediatric intubation, as the straight blade is believed to

TABLE 7–1.

Endotracheal Tube Sizes

Age*	Size (mm ID)
Premature	
<1,000 g	2.5
1,000–2,500 g	3.0
Neonate–6 mo	3.0–3.5
6 mo–1 yr	3.5–4.0
1–2 yr	4.0–4.5
2–4 yr	4.5–5.0
4–6 yr	5.5
6–8 yr	6.0
>8 yr	6.0 cuffed

*Formula for >2 yr: (age + 16)/4.

more easily expose the anterior and superior larynx by lifting up the epiglottis. Figure 7–1 is a graphic representation of these anatomic diferences. The Miller 0 blade is used for the premature and smallest newborns, and the Miller 1 blade is used for the group ranging from the larger newborn to the child 2 years of age. A Miller 2 blade can be used on any child over 2 years of age; however, the Wis-Hippel 1.5 blade is very useful in children 2 to 6 years of age. As with the adult, other blades should be available for difficult visualizations, and the MacIntosh 2 blade is often helpful in children over 2 years of age. For children older than 12 years of age, the MacIntosh 3 is frequently the blade of choice.

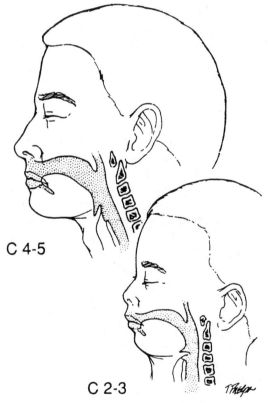

FIG 7–1.
Comparative anatomy of the adult and infant airway. (From Yaster M: Airway management, in Nichols DG, Yaster M, Lappe D, et al (eds): *Golden Hour—The Handbook of Advanced Pediatric Life Support*. St Louis, Mosby–Year Book, Inc, 1991; p 10. Used by permission.)

EVALUATING THE PEDIATRIC PATIENT

In an emergency setting, little time is available for patient evaluation. If the patient presents with airway obstruction, consideration must be given to foreign bodies, croup, epiglottitis, and so forth (see Chapter 34). A head-injured child requires special consideration during intubation in order to avoid increases in intracranial pressure (ICP), through the use of barbiturates, muscle relaxants, and hyperventilation. Certain congenital syndromes make intubation more difficult. Patients with Down's syndrome have small mouths and large tongues. Patients with the Pierre Robin anomaly have a hypoplastic mandible, posteriorly placed tongue, and cleft palate, and are extremely difficult to intubate.

PREPARATION FOR INTUBATION

If time permits, informed consent for intubation should be obtained from the parents. An intravenous (IV) line is essential for administration of medications and volume as required. An interosseous line may substitute for an IV line. Monitoring should include an electrocardiogram (ECG), frequent blood pressure readings (particularly if the patient is sedated and paralyzed for the intubation), and pulse oximetry. Smaller pulse oximeter probes should be available for younger patients.

PHARMACOLOGIC AGENTS

Pharmacologic agents are administered prior to intubation, to blunt consciousness, produce amnesia, relax muscles, and reduce unwanted side effects. As a minimum, a benzodiazepine should be given prior to intubating a conscious patient. Sodium pentothal in the appropriate dose produces anesthesia, but caution should be exercised with the hypovolemic patient. Patients at risk for a serious head injury and increased ICP should have a controlled intubation after sodium pentothal, a muscle relaxant (high-dose vecuronium or succinylcholine), and lidocaine are given to blunt tracheal reflexes. The seizing patient with a clenched jaw requires a muscle relaxant as a minimum, but a benzodiazepine or sodium pentothal may stop the seizures as well as blunt the stimulation of intubation.

Atropine should be administered to all children receiving succinylcholine and to young infants to block vagal stimulation. In early infancy the cardiac output is very rate-dependent and bradycardia is universally associated with hypotension.

PROCEDURE FOR INTUBATION

The patient should be placed in the "sniffing" position, with anterior displacement of the cervical spine and mild extension of the head on the neck. Newborns, with their large occiputs, do not require a towel under their heads for this maneuver. The laryngoscope is used in the same fashion as in the adult, except for the occasional use of the Miller 0 or 1 blade as a "curved" blade. Cricoid pressure is often required for visualization of the anteriorly placed larynx. Of course, cricoid pressure will automatically be applied during emergency intubations of children as well as adults, because of the concern about passive regurgitation of stomach contents and pulmonary aspiration.

The selected endotracheal tube should be passed through the cords, ideally to a position midway down the trachea. A newborn's trachea is only 5 cm long. An 18-month-old infant has a trachea 7 cm long. Therefore, in these younger patients, 2 to 3 cm below the cords is the appropriate depth. Some tubes have lines marking the distance to the end of the tube. The double line at the cords is usually the proper depth.

As soon as the tube is placed, attention should be given to the depth of the tube at an external landmark, such as the teeth or lips. A general rule is that the depth of the tube in centimeters is three times the ID numeral of the tube size. For example, a 1-year-old would take a 4.0-mm tube that most often will be taped at 12 cm at the lips. This rule of thumb applies to premature infants as well as adults when the appropriate-size tube for the patient's age is in place.

Auscultation of the chest to confirm bilateral breath sounds is the next essential step. Esophageal intubation may yield bilateral "breath sounds" in the chest, owing to the easy transmission of sounds from the stomach. End-tidal carbon dioxide monitoring remains the best check to confirm tracheal intubation. Oxygen saturation should stay high or increase after correct tube placement. A chest film to confirm proper placement should always be performed when time permits.

If positive pressure is applied to the endotracheal tube, a leak of air around the tube may be heard. This represents the snugness of the fit of the tube within the cricoid ring. Ideally the leak should occur between 20 and 30 cm H_2O pressure. If a tube passes through the cricoid ring with minimal effort, the absence of a leak does not mandate an immediate change to a smaller tube. This change can be made later, after the patient has fully stabilized. If the leak is prominent even at low inflating pressures, the tube should be changed to a larger size to better protect the airway and provide adequate ventilation.

Securing the tube in the child is even more important. If the child awakens, his or her first effort will be to remove the endotracheal tube, then the IV line, and anything else that is attached to the body. Placement of appropriate restraints, or continuing sedation, with or without paralysis, will prevent this. The stomach should be emptied of air or fluid by nasal or oral gastric tube.

VENTILATION

Ventilation for children of all ages should begin with 100% oxygen. In the child of less than 44 weeks' gestation, the fractional concentration of oxygen in inspired gas (FiO_2) should be decreased to 0.30 or below as soon as is practical, to avoid oxygen toxicity to the immature retina. Hand ventilation should provide an adequate chest expansion at whatever peak inflating pressure is required to achieve the expansion. In the premature infant, ventilating pressures will be quite low, usually less than 20 cm H_2O.

Initial respiratory rates used for controlled ventilation should approximate normal spontaneous respiratory rates based on age (Table 7–2). Adjust-

TABLE 7–2.
Normal Respiratory Rates in Children

Age	Breaths per Minute
Newborn	30–40
Infant	20–30
Child	16–24
Adolescent	12–18

ments are then made after blood gas determinations are made.

Adult ventilators can be used in either a volume- or pressure-cycled mode. With small tidal volumes (12–15 mL/kg), the volume lost into the compliance of the ventilator tubing will become significant. Also, with large leaks around the endotracheal tube, a large percentage of the tidal volume may be lost. In all cases, the volumes and pressures should be adjusted to ensure good chest expansion.

SPECIAL TECHNIQUES FOR DIFFICULT INTUBATIONS

The techniques of fiberoptic, digital, lighted stylet, and guide wire–assisted intubations apply for children as well as adults, but all are very rarely used. Fiberoptic intubation is limited in the youngest children. The smallest fiberoptic bronchoscope with direction controls and a suction channel is 3.1 mm outside diameter (OD). Tubes 4.0 mm ID or larger will fit over this scope if the 15-mm airway adaptor is removed and the scope is lubricated. Bleeding from adenoid trauma may obscure visualization of the larynx.

COMPLICATIONS OF INTUBATION

The most common cause of an unsuccessful pediatric intubation is operator inexperience. Anatomic landmarks are different in children than in adults, the emergent situation is highly stressful, and the wrong equipment may have been pre-selected. The patient's position may be improper, with a hyperextended neck, leaving the larynx too far ante-

rior to visualize. The child's relatively large tongue may be difficult to sweep aside during laryngoscopy or may occlude the light on the Miller blade.

Other complications include right mainstem bronchus intubation accompanied by airway obstruction, atelectasis, difficult ventilation, and hypoxemia. Esophageal intubation, if unrecognized, more quickly leads to hypoxemia, bradycardia, and cardiopulmonary arrest in the child. Trauma to the lips, teeth, or airway is common. A dislodged loose deciduous tooth may be aspirated.

Ventilation after correct tube placement may be difficult, particularly in patients with a history of asthma, bronchopulmonary dysplasia, or foreign body aspiration. Wheezing, without a history of asthma, may be caused by tracheal stimulation.

EXTUBATION

Extubation usually occurs outside of the emergency room. The usual precautions prior to extubation apply to both adults and children. The patient should receive nothing by mouth and be preoxygenated, and should have the oropharynx suctioned. Equipment and supplies for reintubation should be at hand. Postextubation croup is common in children. It is treated with cool mist, and, if severe, with racemic epinephrine aerosols.

SUGGESTED READING

Cote CJ, Todres ID: The pediatric airway, in *A Practice of Anesthesia for Infants and Children,* Orlando, Fla, Grune & Stratton, 1986, pp 35–56.

8

Oral Endotracheal Intubation: Prehospital Perspective

Jedd Roe, M.D.

Airway management in the prehospital setting has been a controversial topic and under investigation for many years. Endotracheal intubation (ETI) has long been recognized as the preferred method of airway control, and in the last two decades there has been increasing utilization of this technique by emergency medical systems (EMS) personnel. Yet, there remain wide disparities throughout the United States in the selection of techniques for airway management.[1] In those states that do not permit the performance of ETI by EMS personnel, generally an esophageal obturator airway (EOA) or one of its variants, usually the esophageal gastric tube airway (EGTA), is used. The controversy regarding ETI vs. EOA has been fueled by perceived differences in the expertise required to perform the techniques, training requirements, and their efficacy in providing ventilatory support.

Critical patients, particularly those in shock, have an increased survival rate with aggressive, early management of the pulmonary and cardiovascular systems.[2, 3] Endotracheal intubation provides maximum ventilatory support to the patient in the form of appropriate tidal volume (10–15 mL/kg) and delivery of the highest possible fraction of inspired oxygen (FiO$_2$). From a pulmonary standpoint, this results in a reduction of hypoxemia, dead space, and intrapulmonary shunting caused by inadequate ventilation.[4] Unconscious patients or those with an altered mental status are at high risk for aspiration of gastric contents owing to an absent or diminished gag reflex, and this risk increases with the use of cardiopulmonary resuscitation (CPR) or a bag-valve-

mask (BVM) device.[5] A marked decrease in gastric aspiration has been reported where paramedical personnel achieved successful ETI in the field.[6] Prehospital ETI is also advantageous in that it offers an alternative method of drug delivery in the field. During CPR, epinephrine, atropine, and lidocaine can be administered via the endotracheal route while intravenous (IV) access is being obtained.[7]

When the EOA was introduced by Don Michael in 1968, its arrival was heralded with a great deal of enthusiasm.[8] The advantages of using an EOA were said to include: (1) less skill and dexterity required by EMS personnel; (2) the possibility of blind insertion; (3) a more rapid performance than ETI; (4) less training required; and (5) the necessity for less movement of the head and neck.[9] Although the technique of EOA insertion is described in Chapter 5, it is important to review here those studies evaluating the use of EOA vs. ETI in the field.

The literature reveals a wide range of success rates for ETI and EOA or a EGTA, ranging from 88% to 95% for both techniques.[9] A number of studies have attempted to define the ability of these two techniques to achieve adequate ventilation and oxygenation. Auerbach and Geehr reported statistically significant higher arterial oxygen partial pressures (PaO$_2$) and lower arterial carbon dioxide (PaCO$_2$) values with ETI when compared with EGTA.[10] Merrifield and King performed a cadaver study involving the use of ETI, EOA, and the EGTA, and noted acceptable ventilation and tidal volumes with all of the devices.[11] Don Michael[12] reviewed the findings of five separate studies and concluded that statistically better levels of pH, PaO_2, and $PaCO_2$ were seen with ETI. However, no difference in survival or neurologic outcome was seen. He concluded that ETI was the preferred method of airway management yet was impractical in some settings.[12] A major criticism of these studies is that they were performed in a controlled setting by physicians, and thus bear little resemblance to the prehospital environment.

Several studies have been performed in the field. Bass et al.[13] found a 73% success rate for EGTA placement (mean 1.4 attempts), but noted that in 15% of patients successfully ventilated that paramedical workers experienced difficulty in maintaining an adequate airway secondary to inadequate mask fit, difficulty with oropharyngeal secretions, or unrecognized balloon leak.[13] Other studies have documented inadequate oxygenation in the field in 69% of cases with EOA use, and lower tidal volume with EOA than either mask, oropharyngeal airway, or ETI.[14] In a study of 171 cases, Smith et al.[15] showed that the EOA required 4 minutes or longer to be placed in 47% of patients. In a prospective, randomized study comparing EGTA and ETI, Goldenberg et al.[16] noted a similar success rate between the two groups: 92.2% and 90.2% respectively. However, of those successfully intubated, 23.9% of the EGTA group were inadequately ventilated as compared to 0.8% of the ETI group.[16] Shea et al.[5] compared EGTA to ETI in the field and found a statistically significant difference in the incidence of aspiration: 4.1% in the EGTA group compared to 0.7% in the ETI group.

A purported advantage of EOA and EGTA is that less training time is required. Yet this time varies from 4 to 16 hours of clinical and didactic time.[9] In one of the largest studies of ETI in the field to date, Stewart et al.[17] evaluated the components of an ETI training program that consisted of didactic instruction, manikin and animal laboratory training, and supervised operating room (OR) experience. An initial overall success rate of 90% was reported, which improved to 95% toward the end of the study. Initially, those that received more training (e.g., OR training) showed a slightly higher success rate: 92.1% vs. 86.2%. After field experience had been obtained, there was no difference between the two groups. Of interest, only 14 of 779 patients in this study were found to have esophageal intubation, and in the 3 patients in whom this was not detected the standard technique of auscultation of lung fields *and* the epigastrium was not followed.[17] Other studies confirm that the optimal ETI training program

should consist of didactic, manikin, and OR training.[18, 19]

Initial ETI training is clearly important, but as others[5, 18, 20] have noted, maintenance of this skill requires equal attention. If field personnel do not perform ETI with sufficient frequency, then continuing education will be required, preferably utilizing OR patients under supervision. Quality assurance programs and close physician supervision will help determine the need for continuing education to raise ETI skills to the appropriate level.

Prehospital intubation of traumatized patients has also been studied. In Denver, the airway management of consecutive *blunt* trauma victims was evaluated.[21] In this study, 35 patients underwent ETI which was accomplished nasotracheally in 22 cases (77% success rate) and orotracheally in 14 cases with in-line cervical stabilization (100% success rate). The protocol specified that the nasotracheal route was preferred where cervical spine injury was suspected. Other than failure to achieve nasotracheal intubation, no complications of ETI were observed. As well, 1.3 IV lines per patient were initiated which resulted in a mean on-scene time of 13.9 minutes.[21]

With the same EMS system, a similar study involving 203 consecutive *penetrating* trauma patients was performed by Pons et al.[22] Twenty-one patients underwent oral ETI with a 100% success rate. The average patient in this study had 1.8 IV lines started and the mean on-scene time was 9.5 minutes.[22] In a study of 131 trauma patients, Copass et al. found that successful ETI had the highest correlation with survival. The conclusion was made that paramedical personnel can have a positive effect on survival rates by airway management with ETI and transport to the nearest trauma center.[3] Clearly, ETI can be accomplished expeditiously and proficiently in the prehospital setting of multiple trauma, and is a key component in its management.

In prehospital management of children, successful ETI has correlated with survival.[23, 24] Losek et al.[24] showed an ETI success rate of between 83% and 86% in 101 patients aged 18 months to 18 years. In the 13 patients less than 18 months of age the success rate dropped to 58%.[24] In 36 patients under 14 years of age, Pointer found a 93.3% ETI success rate in patients over 18 months of age, and 85.7% in infants below that age. It is of interest that there was no difference in success rates with straight or curved blades.[25] Losek and colleagues[26] found several problems associated with ETI failure in the pediatric age group, including inability to visualize the vocal cords owing to secretions, the use of inappropriately small endotracheal tubes or large laryngoscope blades, seizure activity and patient resistance, and lastly, accidental extubation during transport.

Endotracheal intubation in the prehospital setting can be particularly challenging given the extraordinarily diverse environments field personnel must adapt to. Paramedical personnel at Denver General Hospital were surveyed in this regard. As in other medical environments, the majority of those responding emphasized the need for familiarity with, and the checking of, intubation equipment prior to each attempt, as well as the need for appropriate positioning of the patient before undertaking ETI. In many cases these workers preferred a straight laryngoscope blade for patients in whom the larynx was anticipated to be or was found to be anterior. In some nontrauma patients, ETI was facilitated by having an assistant grasp the patient by the hands and lift him or her slightly off the ground. This afforded greater ease in aligning the axes of the mouth, posterior pharynx, and trachea. The most common problem encountered by this group was failing to anticipate the need for suction or having inadequate suction capability.[27]

Adaptability is the trait most required of those who deal with airway problems in prehospital settings. With a patient in acute respiratory distress, performing ETI in the sitting position has been suggested as an alternative.[28] There is at least one report of this technique achieving successful ETI in a patient who was buried up to his shoulders in gravel and who needed airway control.[27]

Tactile (digital) intubation shows promise in prehospital situations where laryngoscopic ETI is impossible. Specific indications include obese or short-necked patients, in whom bleeding or secretions obscure direct visualization of the vocal cords, and selected trauma patients.[29] Hardwick and Bluhm reported a success rate of 89% in 66 patients in whom tactile intubation was attempted. It was believed that 41% of these patients would have incurred substantial delay in the management of their airway had this technique not been attempted.[30]

Discussion of the more controversial areas in prehospital airway management, such as the use of succinylcholine, the role of ETI in patients with potential cervical spine injury, and the possible superiority of nasotracheal intubation in certain situations, awaits further study.

Requisites for field performance of ETI are: (1) an adequate training program, (2) continuing medical education, and (3) strict physician guidance and control. These requirements are similar to those required for any paramedical procedures, and their effectiveness has been demonstrated. Airway management in the emergency department mandates ETI; patients deserve a similar standard of treatment in the prehospital setting.

REFERENCES

1. Smith JP, Bodai BI: The urban paramedic's scope of practice. *JAMA* 1985; 253:544–548.
2. Siegel JH, Farrell EJ, Miller M, et al: Cardiorespiratory interactions as determinants of survival and the need for respiratory support in human shock states. *J Trauma* 1973; 23:976–981.
3. Copass MK, Oreskovich MR, Bladergroen MR, et al: Prehospital cardiopulmonary resuscitation of the critically injured patient. *Am J Surg* 1984; 148:20–26.
4. Pepe PE, Copass MK, Joyce TH: Prehospital endotracheal intubation: Rationale for training emergency medical personnel. *Ann Emerg Med* 1985; 14:1085–1092.
5. Shea SR, MacDonald JR, Gruzinski G: Prehospital endotracheal tube airway or esophageal gastric tube airway: A comparison. *Ann Emerg Med* 1985; 14:102–112.
6. DeLeo BC: Endotracheal intubation by rescue squad personnel. *Heart Lung* 1977; 6:851–854.
7. Greenberg MI: The use of endotracheal medication in cardiac emergencies. *Resuscitation* 1984; 12:155–165.
8. Don Michael TA, Lambert EH, Mehran A: "Mouth-to-lung airway" for cardiac resuscitation. *Lancet* 1968; 2:1329.
9. Pons PT: Esophageal obturator airway. *Emerg Med Clin North Am* 1988; 6:693–698.
10. Auerbach PS, Geehr EC: Inadequate oxygenation and ventilation using the esophageal gastric tube airway in the prehospital setting. *JAMA* 1983; 250:3067–3071.
11. Merrifield AJ, King SJ: The oesophageal obturator airway: A study of cadaver lung ventilation through obturator airways and tracheal tubes. *Anesthesia* 1981; 36:672–676.
12. Don Michael TA: Comparison of the esophageal obturator airway and endotracheal intubation in prehospital ventilation during CPR. *Chest* 1985; 87:814–819.
13. Bass RR, Allison EJ Jr, Hunt RC: The esophageal obturator airway: A reassessment of use by paramedics. *Ann Emerg Med* 1982; 11:358–360.
14. Smith JP, Bodai BI, Seifkin A, et al: The esophageal obturator airway: A review. *JAMA* 1983; 250:1081–1084.

15. Smith JP, Bodai BI, Aubourg R, et al: A field evaluation of the esophageal obturator airway. *J Trauma* 1983; 23:317–321.

16. Goldenberg IF, Campion BC, Siebold CM, et al: Esophageal gastric tube airway vs. endotracheal tube in prehospital cardiopulmonary arrest. *Chest* 1986; 90:90–96.

17. Stewart RD, Paris PM, Winter PM, et al: Field endotracheal intubation by paramedical personnel: Success rates and complications. *Chest* 1984; 85:341–345.

18. Guss DA, Posluszny M: Paramedic orotracheal intubation: A feasibility study. *Am J Emerg Med* 1984; 2:399–401.

19. Stewart RD, Paris PM, Pelton GH, et al: Effect of varied training techniques on field endotracheal intubation success rates. *Ann Emerg Med* 1984; 13:1032–1036.

20. Paris PM: Airway interventions in the field (letter). *Am J Emerg Med* 1984; 2:459–461.

21. Cwinn AA, Pons PT, Moore EE, et al: Prehospital advanced trauma life support for critical blunt trauma victims. *Ann Emerg Med* 1987; 16:399–403.

22. Pons PT, Honigman B, Moore EE, et al: Prehospital advanced life support for critical penetrating wounds to the thorax and abdomen. *J Trauma* 1985; 25:828–832.

23. Torphy D, Minter M, Thompson B: Cardiorespiratory arrest and resuscitation of children. *Am J Dis Child* 1984; 138:1099–1102.

24. Losek JD, Hennes H, Glaeser P, et al: Prehospital care of the pulseless, nonbreathing pediatric patient. *Am J Emerg Med* 1987; 5:370–374.

25. Pointer JE: Clinical characteristics of paramedics' performance of pediatric endotracheal intubation. *Am J Emerg Med* 1989; 7:364–366.

26. Losek JD, Bonadio WA, Walsh-Kelly C, et al: Prehospital pediatric endotracheal intubation performance review. *Pediatr Emerg Care* 1989; 5:1–4.

27. Roe EJ: Survey of Denver General Hospital paramedics. Unpublished data.

28. Fontanarosa PB, Goldman GE, Polsky SS, et al: Sitting oral-tracheal intubation. *Ann Emerg Med* 1988; 17:336–338.

29. Stewart RD: Tactile orotracheal intubation. *Ann Emerg Med* 1984; 13:175–178.

30. Hardwick WC, Bluhm D: Digital intubation. *J Emerg Med* 1984; 1:317–320.

9

Nasotracheal Intubation

James E. Pointer, M.D.

Nasotracheal intubation is performed routinely in the operating room and emergency department, and now sometimes even in prehospital care. There is considerable controversy concerning the indications for nasotracheal intubation and its use as the advanced airway method of choice over available alternatives.[1] In the last 10 years, there have been more than 120 English-language references alone that discuss nasotracheal intubation. The majority discuss either the use of endoscopy in the operating room as an adjunct to the technique, or the indications for blind nasotracheal intubation in the emergency department. Recently, there has been considerable interest in nasotracheal intubation performed under digital and lighted stylet techniques.[2, 3]

Franz Kuhn, in 1902, first reported nasotracheal intubation.[4] In 1920, Rowbotham recorded accounts of intratracheal anesthesia administered by the blind passage of nasal catheters for oral surgery.[5] However, it was not until World War I that both orotracheal and nasotracheal intubation were developed as standard airway management techniques.[6]

Magill popularized nasotracheal intubation in the 1930s. His 1930 paper describing the use of this technique in anesthesia is a classic.[7] Since that time, the procedure has enjoyed both acceptance and controversy. Canuyt, in 1922, reported the injection of anesthetic agents through the cricoid membrane.[8] The use of translaryngeal anesthesia as an adjunct to the performance of endotracheal intubation first appeared in the literature in 1949.[9] The linking of anesthetic techniques with endotracheal intubation brought nasotracheal intubation from obscurity. The instillation of translaryngeal anesthetic agents expanded the application of nasotracheal intubation to the fully alert (and apprehensive) patient. Yet, the use of translaryngeal anesthesia has never been widely accepted,[1] probably owing to the necessity of puncturing the cricoid membrane.

INDICATIONS AND CONTRAINDICATIONS

Oral endotracheal intubation has been discussed in Chapter 6. Endotracheal intubation, either orotracheal or nasotracheal, is the advanced airway method of choice for hospital and prehospital care.[10]

Nasotracheal intubation is materially different from orotracheal intubation. One of the most important distinctions is that, generally, the awake blind nasotracheal intubation procedure requires a breathing patient. However, as will be discussed shortly, there are modifications of the nasotracheal technique which allow its use in the apneic patient. The nasal procedure is somewhat more difficult, and studies have shown that the success rates are slightly higher for the orotracheal route than for the nasotracheal route.[1, 11] In general, the nasotracheal technique requires more time than the orotracheal. One study showed that the time required for nasotracheal tube placement is 2.5 times longer than that for orotracheal intubation (26 ±30 seconds vs. 62 ±41 seconds).[12] On the other hand, there are many advantages to nasotracheal intubation compared with the orotracheal technique (Table 9–1).

Indications

Indications for nasotracheal intubation can be divided into five broad categories. Table 9–2 provides the specific patient categories that should be considered for the technique. The first broad cate-

TABLE 9–1.

Advantages of Nasotracheal Intubation vs. the Orotracheal Technique

1. The tube is more easily secured, hence less easily dislodged
2. More comfort in the awake intubation situation and upon patient awakening
3. Easier insertion in a patient with impaired neck or jaw motion
4. No danger of the patient biting the tube
5. Facilitates surgery to the oral cavity
6. Favored in patients in whom laryngoscopy is difficult or contraindicated[13, 14]
7. Useful in patients in whom neuromuscular blockade is hazardous[15]

TABLE 9–2.

Indications for Nasotracheal Intubation

1. Dsypneic patients who would worsen or who cannot cooperate with supine positions (e.g., COPD, asthma, pulmonary edema)
2. Oral cavity not sufficiently accessible to permit orotracheal intubation
   a. Wired jaws
   b. Anatomic problems (e.g., small mouth, temporomandibular joint ankylosis)
   c. Trismus (e.g., tetanus, intraoral infections)
   d. Active seizing
   e. Obstructing lesions of the anterior oropharynx (e.g., tumors, Ludwig's angina, lingual swelling/hematoma, dental abscesses)
3. Inability to attain proper sniffing position
   a. Suspected/proven unstable cervical spine injury
   b. Decerebrate rigidity
   c. Tetanus
   d. Severe degenerative joint disease (DJD) or rheumatoid arthritis of cervical spine
4. Comatose patients (e.g., sedative overdoses, cardiovascular accidents, head trauma
5. When paralyzing agents are contraindicated (e.g., hyperkalemia secondary to burns or renal failure)

gory includes dyspneic patients in whom the supine position is impossible or contraindicated. Second is a large group of patients in whom the oral cavity is not accessible to orotracheal intubation. Third, some patients are unable to be positioned in the proper "sniffing" position. These last two groups may include patients in whom unsuccessful orotracheal intubation attempts have been made. Fourth, certain comatose patients are candidates for the nasal technique. Last, the technique is indicated in those patients in whom paralyzing agents are contraindicated.

After evaluating the relative merits of nasotracheal vs. orotracheal intubation in a particular patient, one or the other technique has its place in the management of certain conditions. Although nasotracheal intubation has been performed in patients

with acute epiglottitis,[16] in patients with missed esophageal perforation after blunt trauma,[17] in patients with pharyngeal obstruction, and in patients with a suspected or known basilar or skull fracture,[18] the oral technique is preferred in these situations. Airway obstruction unrelieved by attempts at orotracheal intubation, however, must be managed by surgical intervention.[1]

Contraindications

Apnea or near-apnea is an absolute contraindication only in the use of the standard blind technique. However, the use of a lighted stylet fiberoptic endoscope, or tactile technique does allow nasotracheal intubation in the apneic patient.[19, 20] One report[21] described blind nasotracheal intubation in patients rendered apneic by the use of succinylcholine. The anesthesiologists relied upon movement of the endotracheal tube over and through various structures to facilitate the procedure. (See below under Procedure.) However, the technique has not been reported outside the anesthesia literature. It is not recommended to the emergency physician owing to the relatively uncontrolled environment inherent in emergency situations.

There are a number of relative contraindications to the performance of nasotracheal intubation. As with other procedures in medicine and airway management, the physician must carefully weigh the risks and benefits of performing the procedure on a case-by-case basis. Table 9–3 lists contraindications for nasotracheal intubation.

Severe nasal or maxillary facial fractures are considered a relative contraindication. This prohibition is based on the possibility of intracranial passage of a nasotracheal tube in patients with facial frac-

TABLE 9–3.

Contraindications to Nasotracheal Intubation

1. Apnea
2. Severe nasal or maxillofacial fractures
3. Blood clotting abnormalities (causing epistaxis)
4. Nasal or nasopharyngeal obstruction due to
   a. Deviated septum (congenital or acquired)
   b. Masses (e.g., cysts, polyps, tumors, abscesses.)
   c. Edema (e.g., inflammatory, angioedema, severe coryza, allergic rhinitis, inflamed adenoids)
   d. Foreign bodies (self-inserted by children; gastroenteric tubes, (e.g., the Sengstaken-Blakemore tube)
   e. Trauma (e.g., septal hematoma)
5. Closed head trauma

tures. There are two reported incidences of this complication.[22, 23] Probably, in these cases, the intubators did not understand or did not perform the technique correctly.[18] The orotracheal method is thus usually preferred in this circumstance, but nasotracheal intubation can certainly be considered.

Blood clotting abnormalities constitute another common relative contraindication. Even with vasoconstriction and gentle tube manipulation, problematic epistaxis can occur. Because nasal bleeding is not a complication of orotracheal intubation, it is the procedure of choice for patients with bleeding dyscrasias.

Nasal or nasopharyngeal obstruction is a contraindication to the performance of nasotracheal intubation. Patients with deviated septa, masses, nasal trauma, or edema are often impossible to intubate nasally. Acute epiglottitis,[24] hematomas and infections of the upper neck, and massive intraoral hemorrhage are also relative contraindications.[1] The best intubation procedure, in these cases, is one that is performed under direct visualization.[25] Obviously, the physician should never place a nasal tube into a naris that contains a foreign body, either self-inserted (e.g., a peanut) or medical (e.g., nasogastric tube).

Lastly, rapid-sequence orotracheal intubation is increasingly being used in preference to nasotracheal intubation in acute closed head trauma (see Chapter 4). Proper administration of lidocaine and paralyzing agents in conjunction with the oral route minimize the elevation of intracranial pressure associated with all intubation techniques.[26]

EQUIPMENT AND PREPARATION

Equipment

Equipment needs should be anticipated before the procedure. The physician must have endotracheal tubes, nasopharyngeal airways, nasopharyngeal vasoconstricting and anesthetic agents, lubricating agents, equipment for translaryngeal anesthesia, airway adjuncts, and so forth, on hand at all times. Equipment should be stored in a manner to ensure immediate access. Wrappings utilizing many layers of cloth or paper should be avoided.

Several adjuncts are available to prevent splashing of aspirated stomach contents or respiratory droplets into the physician's face. An adaptor called the Humid-Vent 1, (Gibeck Respiration, Sweden) may be placed on the proximal end of the endotracheal tube (Fig 9–1). This device prevents secretions

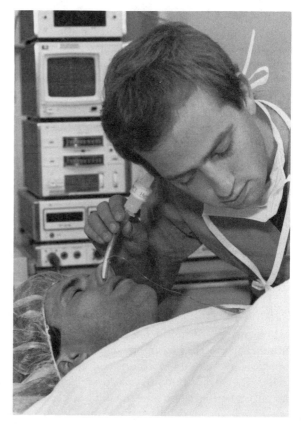

FIG 9–1.
The Humid-Vent 1: an adaptor for increasing the safety of blind nasotracheal intubation. (From Dorsey MJ, Jones BR: *Anesth Analg* 1989;69:135. Used by permission.)

containing blood and bacteria from being expelled into the air and onto the body of the operator.[27] Alternatively, a section of standard intravenous (IV) extension tubing may be used to evaluate breath sounds from a safe distance. The physician places one end of a 30-in. section of standard IV tubing approximately 2 to 3 cm into the proximal end of the endotracheal tube. The other end of the tube is then fitted into an earpiece adaptor or directly into the ear.[28]

The nasotracheal tube should be approximately 1 mm smaller in diameter than the tube used for orotracheal intubation. Usually, a tube with an inner diameter (ID) of 8.0 to 8.5 mm is appropriate for adults. It should be made of clear polyvinylchloride, since this material allows the physician to see breath condensation on the inside walls of the tube.[29] Strictly speaking, orotracheal and nasotracheal tubes are interchangeable. However, the flex-end or trigger tube (Endotrol) is now the standard of care in many emergency departments and emergency medical services systems for nasotracheal intubations.

This tube looks like a normal endotracheal tube except for a pull ring found anteriorly at the proximal end (Fig 9–2). The ring is connected to a wire contained within the wall of the tube itself. At the point of perceiving clear and distinct breath sounds, the trigger ring is pulled and the tube flexes anteriorly, thereby facilitating passage into the trachea. There is one report of airway obstruction associated with the ring.[30] Therefore, it is wise to cut off the ring after correct tube placement has been documented.

Some physicians use a nasopharyngeal airway to "prime" or test the nasal passage without actually dilating it. The airway utilized should be the same size as the endotracheal tube.[11] Several studies have investigated the effect of mechanical dilation on nasotracheal intubation. Repeated passage of dilators into the nasopharyngeal airway has been shown to increase hemorrhage and to lengthen the procedure. For these reasons it is not routinely recommended.[31]

The physician should regularly use one of three methods for assuring nasopharyngeal anesthesia and hemostasis (Table 9–4). Lidocaine and Cetacaine provide anesthesia but no vasoconstriction. Therefore, topical phenylephrine must be given concurrently to achieve vasoconstriction. Cetacaine is a mixture of benzocaine, tetracaine, butyl aminobenzoate, benzyalkonium chloride, and cetyldimethylethylammonium bromide. Cocaine is the only popular topical anesthetic agent that provides vasoconstriction as well as anesthesia.

Satisfactory lidocaine and Cetacaine anesthesia requires about 60 seconds, whereas cocaine takes 5 minutes.[11] The physician should take into account that hypertension is a relative contraindication to the use of both cocaine and phenylephrine. However, phenylephrine has been used safely in an eclamptic

TABLE 9–4.

Topical Nasopharyngeal Vasoconstricting and Anesthetic Agents

Topical or viscous 2%–4% lidocaine and 1% phenylephrine
Cetacaine solution and 1% phenylephrine
Cocaine solution, 2%–10% (not to exceed 100 mg)

woman.[32] Aqueous lidocaine jelly should be used to lubricate the nasotracheal tube in preference to ointments or creams.[18, 33]

Preparation

If the patient is conscious, he or she should receive step-by-step instructions before and during the procedure. Lack of proper psychological preparation will lead to fear, anxiety, movement, and lack of cooperation, and it is likely to cause a missed intubation.[11]

If time permits, the physician should carefully check the nose and oral cavity, the temporomandibular joint, the mandible, and the neck prior to the procedure.[34] The patency of the nostrils is determined by occluding the nares one at a time.[11] Significant septal deviation or other obstructions should be sought. The physician may need to utilize another procedure if there is significant nasal obstruction of any cause. The tube should be passed through the nostril that is least affected. Dental plates can pose a problem and should be removed. Patients with short muscular necks are more difficult to intubate, even by the nasotracheal route.[35] Listen for hoarseness or stridor, which suggests problematic laryngeal lesions. There is little information on the effect of anatomic variations in the temporomandibular joint, mandible, or neck on nasotracheal intubation.

Proper positioning of the patient is necessary. Blind nasotracheal intubation is generally performed either in the supine or the sitting position. The axes of the mouth, pharynx, and larynx should be aligned[36] by placing the patient in the "sniffing" position and by placing a folded towel under the patient's occiput. However, if cervical spine injury is suspected, the head and neck should be maintained in a neutral position. It may be necessary to utilize a different airway management technique in these patients (see Chapter 4).

There are three anesthetic techniques which may be helpful in nasotracheal intubation: nasal, pharyngeal, and translaryngeal. For nasal anesthesia either cotton swabs or a spray technique, or both, are used to anesthetize the nasal mucosa with one of the drugs listed in Table 9–4. One to two milliliters of

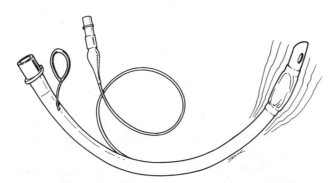

FIG 9–2.
The flex-end tube (Endotrol). (From Iserson KV, Sanders AB, Kaback K: *Am Fam Physician* 1985;31:101. Used by permission.)

solution in each naris should be sufficient.[37] For pharyngeal anesthesia a spray or two of 4% lidocaine or Cetacaine to the posterior pharynx is sufficient. It is controversial whether pharyngeal anesthesia predisposes patients to aspiration.[38] There is also the practical consideration that tube passage through the oropharynx is very rapid and anesthesia in this area may be unnecessary.[38] Translaryngeal anesthesia is not generally utilized in emergency medicine since it is unnecessary, time-consuming, and has complications.

PROCEDURE

Regardless of the technique employed, there are common features which the physician must keep in mind, particularly if he or she has limited experience with the procedure. Table 9–5 outlines the 11 steps for successful nasotracheal intubation. The exigencies of an emergent situation may permit only cursory anatomic and psychological preparation of the patient. Also, there simply may not be enough time to allow an anesthetic agent to take effect. Nonetheless, the other steps should be followed in sequence. Several steps can be performed simultaneously. While the physician is preparing and testing the equipment for the procedure, the patient should be hyperventilated using a bag valve-mask with 100% oxygen. This provides a pulmonary reservoir of O_2, lowers pulmonary carbon dioxide, and decreases intracranial pressure. Nasal anesthesia is achieved using one of the methods described above. Pharyngeal and translaryngeal anesthesia are optional.

If desired, a nasopharyngeal airway of the same diameter as the endotracheal tube is also selected and lubricated with lidocaine jelly. It is inserted into

the most widely patent nostril and left in place for approximately 1 minute. This helps to lubricate and anesthetize the nose and facilitates the eventual passage of the nasotracheal tube. It is removed after a few minutes, and the nasotracheal tube is inserted. The beveled edge of the tube is placed against the nasal septum of the nostril chosen for the procedure. This placement prevents abrasion and bleeding.[11] The tube is directed so that it enters the naris perpendicular to the facial plane with the curvature of the tube facing superiorly. A continuous forward pressure is maintained simultaneously with gentle rotation while the tube is inserted through the nasal passage and into the pharynx. The tube should never be forced! If the nasal passage appears to be obstructed, there are two alternatives: an attempt can be made to pass a smaller tube or utilize the other nostril for the procedure. Once the tube is in the pharynx, the tube should be rotated 180 degrees so that the curvature faces inferiorly. In this position, the tube serves as a nasal airway and facilitates the remainder of the procedure. The tube may impact the posterior wall of the pharynx; traction on the ring of the Endotrol will overcome this obstacle.

Upon advancing the tube forward only another inch or two, one can note air movement passing through the tube by placing a hand over the proximal end of the tube. The physician should be wary of using the mouth or ear to check for breath sounds because of patient regurgitation. As described above, a section of IV extension tubing can be used to assist in detecting breath sounds. As the physician appreciates "full" airflow, an assistant applies gentle but firm pressure on the cricoid cartilage (the Sellick maneuver). This aligns the axis of the trachea with the path of the advancing tube and also occludes the esophagus, preventing regurgitation (Fig 9–3). It is important that the tracheal pressure be applied gently and continuously throughout the procedure in order to prevent aspiration. The tube is then advanced quickly just beyond the vocal cords, preferably during inspiration. After intubation, it is necessary to inflate the tube's balloon to the point where it begins to leak, usually about 10 mm.[3] In children 7 years old or younger, an uncuffed tube is used.

The next step is to ensure correct tube placement. The radiograph should demonstrate the tip of the endotracheal tube approximately 1 to 2 cm above the carina.[1] Experienced physicians may choose to omit the confirming chest radiograph, but a clinical check should *always* be performed. The physician listens over both lungs and the epigastric

TABLE 9–5.

Steps in the Performance of Nasotracheal Intubation

1. Patient preparation, physical and psychological
2. Testing of equipment
3. Hyperventilation with 100% O_2 using bag-valve-mask ventilator
4. Anesthesia
5. Lubrication of the tube
6. Use of a nasopharyngeal airway (if desired)
7. Passage of the tube itself
8. Confirmation of correct placement of the tube
9. Fixation of the tube
10. Adjustment of the tube
11. Use of adjuncts and aids

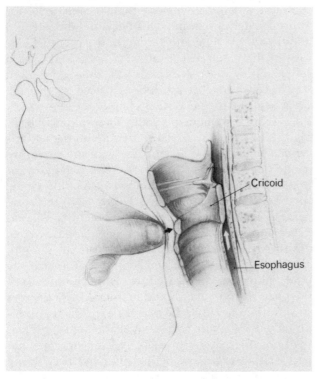

FIG 9-3.
The Sellick maneuver. (From Natanson C, Shelhamer JH, Parrillo JE: *JAMA* 1985;253:1162. Used by permission.)

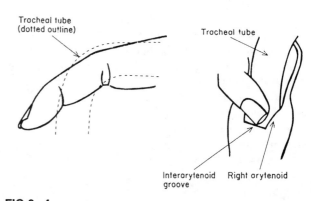

FIG 9-4.
The mid test. *Left,* the index finger reaches around the tongue to rest on the anterior surface of the tube. *Right,* the finger slides down the tube to the interarytenoid groove. (From Horton WA, Perera S, Charters P: *Anaesthesia* 1988;43:241. Used by permission.)

area. Breath sounds should be symmetric; an esophageally placed tube will result in a gurgling sound heard epigastrically upon bagging the patient. Several authors have described tactile tests to confirm tube placement. These tests are performed before the tube is affixed. One test, the mid test, requires placement of the neck in flexion with the head rotated 60 degrees to the left. The physician stands to the left side of the patient at the level of the lower chest. The right index finger is introduced into the mouth just medial to the teeth of the left lower jaw, and is hooked around the back of the endotracheal tube. The thumb and index finger of the left hand locate the thyroid cartilage and move the larynx posteriorly at the neck. These movements allow the tip of the right index finger to delineate the boundaries of the arytenoid cartilages (Fig 9-4). A positive test is obtained when the tube is felt immediately anterior to the interarytenoid groove. This test had a success rate of between 95% and 98% in physicians with small hands, and 100% in physicians with large hands.[39] Capnography is also helpful in tube placement, but only in ruling out unrecognized esophageal intubation.[40]

When placement of the tube is confirmed, it is important to affix the tube well, particularly if it is to remain in place for any length of time. The standard way to affix the tube is to wrap 10 to 15 cm of 1-in. tape close to the distal end of the endotracheal tube. A second piece of tape approximately 1 m long and 2 in. in diameter is attached as closely as possible to the patient's occiput. The tape is brought around both sides of the patient's head and face and, about at the level of the ears, each free end is wrapped around tape which has previously been affixed to the proximal end of the endotracheal tube. Another piece of 1-in. tape may be wrapped just distal to the entry of the tube into the naris to prevent the tube from slipping into a bronchus. If protracted surgery is indicated, a pericranial suture fixation can be performed.[41]

Some clinical situations render nasotracheal intubation difficult. Awake dyspneic patients—e.g., severe congestive heart failure, chronic obstructive pulmonary disease (COPD), or acute asthma—cannot remain supine long enough to allow the procedure. In these patients, sitting nasotracheal intubation is indicated. The physician should stand to the side of the patient closest to the naris being used. The remainder of the sitting intubation procedure is performed as just outlined.

Although most physicians prefer performing blind nasotracheal intubation in a breathing, alert patient, some anesthesiologists actually prefer an apneic and paralyzed patient. Maltby and his colleagues[21] have described the procedure as follows: After IV administration of methohexital and succinylcholine, the operator passes the tube as for an awake intubation. During advancement of the tube to the level of the glottis, bulging in any direction in the neck is appreciated. With anterior or lateral bulging, the tube is withdrawn and redirected. With a bulge to the right, the tube is rotated counterclockwise and advanced. With a bulge to the left, it is rotated clockwise and advanced. The patient's head is flexed slightly if the tip has entered the vallecula. If the tube has entered the esophagus, the head is extended by elevating the chin. Finally, the authors often "felt" the tip of the endotracheal tube as it passed through the tracheal rings. They confirm placement of the tube in the trachea by compressing the lower end of the patient's sternum. This pressure causes a rush of air through the tube which is audible to the anesthesiologist whose ear is pressed against the proximal end of the endotracheal tube. The authors claim that they had used this method, which is not a digital technique, in more than 20,000 cases over a 20-year period.[21] Other authors using paralysis have reported success rates ranging from 76% to 96%.[42, 43] It must be emphasized again, however, that this technique has not been examined in the uncontrolled environment of the emergency department.

Perhaps the simplest technical aid in the difficult nasotracheal intubation is redirection of the tube itself. The endotracheal tube can lie in only one of five locations outside the trachea: (1) the vocal cords outside the larynx; (2) the vallecula; (3) the left piriform fossa; (4) the right piriform fossa; and (5) the esophagus.[1] A misdirected tube at the vocal cords outside the larynx results in obstruction to passage of the tube despite good detection of breath sounds.

This problem generally occurs in a patient who has an intact airway reflex. Generally, gentle rotation or translaryngeal anesthesia, or both, will solve this difficulty. A tube that impacts in the vallecula will often cause a midline supralaryngeal bulge in the neck. Retracting the tube a few centimeters, followed by gentle pressure in the area just above the larynx or by slight flexion of the head, will generally solve this problem. Misdirection of the tube into either the left or right piriform fossa will often result in a corresponding lateral bulge in the neck. This problem is corrected by displacing the patient's larynx slightly in the direction of the bulge, by rotating the tube, or moving the head toward the side of the displacement, or by any combination of these maneuvers. Detection of esophageal intubation is difficult by inspection alone, although anterior elevation of the trachea is occasionally detectable. Cricoid pressure is applied and the patient's head is ex-

tended slightly, prior to backing the tube out and redirecting it more anteriorly.

Occasionally, as body heat begins to soften the tube, it loses some of its curvature and fails to go anteriorly enough to find the glottic opening. Placement of a tube that is cooler than room temperature into the opposite nostril often resolves this problem.[1] Substituting a tube that is a half size smaller, even though the larger tube may be anatomically correct for the patient, is sometimes successful.[11] One study found that in the compliant patient, voluntary extrusion of the tongue facilitated the procedure.[44] There are a variety of external guides which are sometimes useful as adjuncts to nasotracheal intubation. The Magill forceps,[10] Sleeman wire,[45] various introducers,[46, 47] and the retrograde technique[38] all have limited application to nasotracheal intubation.

COMPLICATIONS

Serious complications during, or as a result of, nasotracheal intubation are infrequent.[1] Nasal bleeding is by far the most common complication.[48] Fortunately, this complication is easy to avoid. First, avoid excessive force. Second, do not use an excessively large tube (>8 mm ID). Third, lubricate the tube generously. Fourth, apply vasoconstrictive agents to the nasal mucosa prior to the procedure. Tintinalli and Claffey reported their experience in 71 patients.[6] "Mild" bleeding (the presence of a small amount of blood-tinged mucus) occurred in 8 patients (11%), "moderate" bleeding in 4 (6%), and only 1 patient (1%) in the series had "severe" bleeding (requiring nasal packing). Fry[49] described a method to prevent nasal bleeding in patients receiving anticoagulants or with bleeding dyscrasias. The physician removes a finger from a size 8 surgical glove, cuts off the tip, and slits the entire length. The "finger" is lubricated inside and out and passed into the floor of the naris using a bayonet forceps. As the assistant grasps the "finger," the physician passes the nasotracheal tube. The "finger" prevents trauma to the nasal mucosa.[49]

A serious complication of nasotracheal intubation is retropharyngeal perforation with subsequent abscess and systemic infection. Fortunately, this problem is rare and easily avoided by applying gentle pressure during insertion of the tube or by utilizing an Endotrol tube.[6] The use of excessive force can also cause laryngeal injury. Laryngospasm usually results from irritation of the vocal cords by the nasotracheal tube. If this occurs, continuous positive airway pressure with a few milliliters of a local anesthetic agent (2%–4% lidocaine) should terminate the episode. Obviously, translaryngeal anesthesia would prevent the problem altogether.[11] Very rarely, the nasotracheal tube may be occluded by a thrombus.[50] This complication always occurs from bleeding and may be prevented by using the techniques described above.

One incident of nasotracheal tube aspiration has been reported. In this case, paramedical workers performed nasotracheal intubation in the field in a patient with status epilepticus. The tube's adaptor became separated and the tube could not be visualized. The physicians passed a Foley catheter, inflated the balloon beyond the distal tip of the tube, and retrieved the tube.[51]

Extubation should be done gently to avoid epistaxis. Following extubation, sore throat is common but generally clinically insignificant. One study showed a 38.2% incidence in 642 patients.[6]

By far, the major long-term complication of nasotracheal intubation is paranasal sinusitis. The majority of these infections have been reported in neurosurgical and head injury patients,[52, 53] occurring in up to 26% of such patients.[54] Sepsis occurred in 2.3% of patients in another study.[55] An aggressive approach to treatment is mandatory: replacement of the nasotracheal tube with an orotracheal tube, cultures, maxillary sinus lavage, and appropriate IV antibiotic therapy.[56]

Dinner et al. found bacteremia in three of 54 patients who were nasally intubated; since two of the three cultures were *Streptococcus viridans,* the authors postulated the need for prophylaxis in patients at risk for endocarditis.[57] Turbinate destruction and nasal necrosis have been caused by either improper technique or unrecognized anatomic variations.[58] Table 9–6 summarizes complications associated with nasotracheal intubation.

TABLE 9–6.
Complications Associated With Nasotracheal Intubation

Nasal bleeding during intubation and extubation[6, 11]
Retropharyngeal perforation[6]
Laryngospasm[11]
Laryngeal injury[16]
Turbinate or nasal necrosis[58]
Sinusitis[56]
Occlusion by thrombus[50]
Tube aspiration[51]
Kinking of pilot tube[59]
Separation of tube[60]
Sore throat[6]

PREHOSPITAL PERSPECTIVE

Nasotracheal intubation in the prehospital setting is not nearly as prevalent as orotracheal intubation, but it is used in a number of states. Some authors advocate its use over other techniques for certain indications, particularly by emergency medical systems (EMS) personnel in the management of head injuries.[61, 62] However, rapid-sequence orotracheal intubation is being used with increasing frequency for such patients in the emergency department owing to the minimal rise in intracranial pressure.[26] Prehospital nasotracheal intubation in head-injured patients should be performed only by well-trained personnel and then only if orotracheal intubation is not possible or clearly unsafe. Another major prehospital (as well as in-hospital) indication for nasotracheal intubation is acute ventilatory failure in patients with COPD, asthma, or pulmonary edema. If transport times are long, and the standard conservative oxygenation measures are ineffective, nasotracheal intubation may be lifesaving.

Despite its potential application in prehospital care, there are several reasons why nasotracheal intubation will probably never be extensively utilized in the field. First, training in the procedure is difficult since there are no good manikins or models that simulate clinical conditions. Second, medical control physicians are reluctant to utilize nasotracheal intubation because of its lower success and higher complication rates compared with the oral route. Third, field personnel lack proper analgesic and vasoconstricting agents to prepare the patient.

Some EMS jurisdictions have addressed the problems associated with field nasotracheal intubation by implementing lighted stylet and tactile techniques. These procedures are potentially extremely useful in prehospital care, but they require labor-intensive training and testing, and a high degree of physician participation and field supervision.[2] Many EMS systems simply do not have these expensive resources.

PEDIATRIC PERSPECTIVE

Pediatric nasotracheal intubation requires special attention to preparation, anatomy, and technique. Psychological preparation, relevant to the adult, is often not possible or practical for the young child. This fact often precludes the use of this procedure in the pediatric age group. Even if sufficient cooperation is possible, the technique must be modified because of the pediatric airway anatomy. Difficult pediatric intubations often require adjuncts that do not involve placement of additional equipment in the airway. Finally, tube sizes and anesthetic and vasoconstrictor doses must be modified accordingly.

In the child, the head should be in the neutral position with slight extension. Physicians should not flex the cervical spine or use the sniffing position, as for adults. There are several guidelines for determining the correct diameter of the tube. A rough rule commonly relied upon is to use a tube with the same diameter as the child's small finger. Another rule is given by the following equation:

$$\text{Size (mm)} = 16 + \text{age (yr)}/4 \qquad (1)$$

Tables are available for estimating the tube diameter in children.

The length of the tube to be utilized in the pediatric population is often troublesome. Because of the smaller anatomy involved, it is often difficult to determine the exact point at which the distal tip of the tube enters the passage through the larynx and into the trachea. Yates et al. used a regression equation to estimate nasotracheal tube length in children and infants.[63]

$$\text{Length (cm)} = 3 \times \text{ID (mm)} + 2 \qquad (2)$$

The ID of the tube is calculated as in equation (1). The length of the tube should, of course, be verified clinically and radiographically.

The physician should use a cuffed endotracheal tube in patients 7 years of age and older. Tubes in this group have an ID of 6 mm and above.

REFERENCES

1. Danzl DF, Thomas DM: Nasotracheal intubations in the emergency department. *Crit Care Med* 1980; 8:677.
2. Stewart RD: Tactile orotracheal intubation. *Ann Emerg Med* 1984; 13:175.
3. Korber TE, Henneman PL: Digital nasotracheal intubation. *J Emerg Med* 1989; 7:275.
4. Kuhn F: Die pernasale Tubage. *Muenchen Med Wochenschr* 1902; 49:1456.
5. Rowbotham S: Intratracheal anaesthesia by the nasal route for operations on the mouth and lips. *Br J Med* 1920; 2:590.
6. Tintinalli JE, Claffey J: Complications of nasotracheal intubation. *Ann Emerg Med* 1981; 10:142.
7. Magill IW: Technique in endotracheal anaesthesia. *Br Med J* 1930; 2:817.
8. Canuyt G: Les injections intratrachéales par la voie intercricothyroïdienne. *Gaz Hebd Sci Med Bordeaux* 1920; 41:266.
9. Bonica JJ: Transtracheal anesthesia for endotracheal intubation. *Anesthesiology* 1949; 10:736.
10. Simon RR, Brenner BE: Airway procedures, in Simon RR, Brenner BE (eds): *Procedures and Techniques in Emergency Medicine.* Baltimore, Williams & Wilkins, 1982, pp 30–82.
11. Pointer J: Utilizing nasotracheal intubation to full potential. *ER Rep* 1982; 3:143.
12. Depoit JP, Malbezin S, Videcoq M, et al: Oral intubation v. nasal intubation in adult cardiac surgery. *Br J Anaesth* 1987; 59:167.
13. Tahir AH: A simple manoeuvre to aid the passage of the nasotracheal tube into the oropharynx. *Br J Anaesth* 1970; 42:631.
14. Wilson RS, Rie MA: Management of mechanical ventilation. *Surg Clin North Am* 1975; 55:591.
15. Giuffrida JG, Bizzarri DV, Latteri FS, et al: Prevention of major airway complications during anesthesia by intubation of the conscious patient. *Anesth Analg* 1960; 39:201.
16. McNelis FL: Medical and legal management of adult acute epiglottitis. *Laryngoscope* 1985; 95:125.
17. Lucas CE, Splittgerber F, Ledgerwood AM: Conservative therapy for missed esophageal perforation after blunt trauma. *Am J Emerg Med* 1986; 4:520.
18. Iserson KV: Nasotracheal intubation: Myth vs. reality (letter). *Ann Emerg Med* 1985; 14:379.
19. Childress WF: New method for fiberoptic endotracheal intubation of anesthetized patients. *Anesthesiology* 1981; 14:595.
20. Verdele VP, Heller MB, Paris PM, et al: Nasotracheal intubation in traumatic craniofacial dislocation: Use of the lighted stylet. *Am J Emerg Med* 1988; 6:39.
21. Maltby JR, Cassidy M, Nanji GM: Blind nasotracheal intubation using succinylcholine. *Anesthesiology* 1988; 69:946.
22. Bovzartu WF: Intracranial nasogastric tube insertion (editorial). *J Trauma* 1978; 18:819.
23. Horellov MF, Mathe D, Feiss P: A hazard of nasotracheal intubation (letter). *Anaesthesia* 1978; 33:73.
24. Hannallah R, Rosales JK: Acute epiglottitis: Current management and review. *Can Anaesth Soc J* 1978; 25:84.
25. Karl WF: Intubation in awake debilitated geriatric patients. *Anesth Analg* 1964; 43:338.
26. Ampel L, Mott KA, Sielaff GW, et al: An approach to airway management in the acutely head-injured patient. *J Emerg Med* 1988; 6:1.
27. Dorsey MJ, Jones BR: An inexpensive, disposable adapter for increasing the safety of blind nasotracheal intubations (letter). *Anesth Analg* 1989; 69:135.

28. Young ML, Ominsky AJ: A simple aid to blind tracheal intubation (letter). *Anesth Analg* 1986; 65:825.
29. Iserson KV, Sanders AB, Kaback K: Difficult intubations: Aids and alternatives. *Am Fam Physician* 1985; 31:99.
30. Glinsman D, Pavlin EG: Airway obstruction after nasal-tracheal intubation. *Anaesthesia* 1982; 36:229.
31. Adamson DN, Theisen FC, Barrett KC: Effect of mechanical dilation on nasotracheal intubation. *J Oral Maxillofac Surg* 1988; 46:372.
32. Mokriski BLK, Malinow AM, Gray WC, et al: Topical nasopharyngeal anaesthesia with vasoconstriction in preeclampsia-eclampsia. *Can J Anaesth* 1988; 35:641.
33. Mitchell J: Value of lidocaine jelly in nasotracheal intubation (letter). *Ann Emerg Med* 1986; 15:224.
34. Rhee KJ, Derlet RW, Fung DL: Evaluating anatomical factors affecting endotracheal intubation. *J Emerg Med* 1988; 6:209.
35. Patil V, Stheling L, Zauder U: *Fiberoptic Endoscopy in Anesthesia*. St Louis, Mosby—Year Book, Inc, 1983, p 79.
36. Salem MR, Mathrubhutham M, Bennett EJ: Current concepts: difficult intubation. *N Engl J Med* 1976; 295:879.
37. Hochbaum SR: Emergency airway management. *Emerg Med Clin North Am* 1986; 4:411.
38. Denlinger JK, Ellison N, Ominsky AJ: Effects of intratracheal lidocaine on circulatory responses to tracheal intubation. *Anesthesiology* 1974; 41:409.
39. Horton WA, Perera S, Charters P: An additional tactile test: Further developments in tactile tests to confirm laryngeal placement of tracheal tubes. *Anaesthesia* 1988; 43:240.
40. Sayah AJ, Peacock WF, Overton DT: End-tidal CO_2 measurement in the detection of esophageal intubation during cardiac arrest. *Ann Emerg Med* 1990; 19:857.
41. Altemir FH: Pericranial fixation of the nasotracheal tube. *J Oral Maxillofac Surg* 1986; 44:585.
42. Fassolt A: Blind nasal tracheal intubation in the muscle-relaxed patient. *Anaesthesist* 1986; 35:505.
43. Gross JB, Hartigan ML, Schaffer DW: A suitable substitute for 4% cocaine before blind nasotracheal intubation. *Anesth Analg* 1984; 63:915.
44. Adams AL, Cane RD, Shapiro BA: Tongue extrusion as an aid to nasal intubation. *Crit Care Med* 1982; 10:335.
45. Sleeman KW: An introducer to facilitate nasotracheal intubation. *Anaesthesia Intensive Care* 1979; 7:381.
46. Dryden GE: Use of a suction catheter to assist blind nasal intubation (letter). *Anesthesiology* 1976; 45:260.
47. Gouvernew JM, Veyckemans F, Licker M, et al: Using an ureteral catheter as a guide in difficult neonatal fiberoptic intubation (letter). *Anesthesiology* 1987; 66:436.
48. Binning R: A hazard of blind nasal intubation. *Anesthesiology* 1974; 29:202.
49. Fry ENS: Letter to the editor. *Can Anaesth Soc J* 1977; 24:144.
50. Henzig D: Thrombotic occlusion of a nasotracheal tube. *Anesthesiology* 1979; 51:484.
51. McGrath RB, Einterz RM: Aspiration of a nasotracheal tube: A complication of nasotracheal intubation and mechanisms for retrieval. *Chest* 1987; 91:148.
52. Deutschman CS, Wilton PB, Sinow J, et al: Paranasal sinusitis: A common complication of nasotracheal intubation in neurosurgical patients. *Neurosurgery* 1985; 17:296.
53. Grindlinger GA, Nieoff J, Hughes L, et al: Acute paranasal sinusitis related to nasotracheal intubation of head-injured patients. *Crit Care Med* 1987; 15:214.
54. Hansen M, Poulsen MR, Bendixen DK, et al: Incidence of sinusitis in patients with nasotracheal intubation. *Br J Anaesth* 1988; 61:231.
55. Aebert H, Hunefeld G, Regel G: Paranasal sinusitis and sepsis in ICU patients with nasotracheal intubation. *Intensive Care Med* 1988; 15:27.
56. Linden BE, Aguilar EA, Allen SJ: Sinusitis in the nasotracheally intubated patient. *Arch Otolaryngol Head Neck Surg* 1988; 114:860.
57. Dinner M, Tjeuw M, Artusio JF: Bacteremia as a complication of nasotracheal intubation. *Anesth Analg* 1987; 66:460.
58. Wilkinson JA, Mathis RD, Dire DJ: Turbinate destruction—a rare complication of nasotracheal intubation. *J Emerg Med* 1986; 4:209.
59. Fagraeus L: Difficult extubation following nasotracheal intubation. *Anesthesiology* 1978; 46:43.
60. Sajjan R, Pal R: A rare accident during extubation. *J Indian Med Assoc* 1982; 80:23.
61. Green BA, Elsmont FJ, O'Heir JT: Prehospital management of spinal cord injuries. *Paraplegia* 1987; 25:229.
62. Pepe PE, Copass MK, Joyce TU: Prehospital endotracheal intubation: Rationale for training emergency medical personnel. *Ann Emerg Med* 1985; 14:1085.
63. Yates AP, Harries AJ, Hatch DJ: Estimation of nasotracheal tube length in infants and children (letter). *Br J Anaesth* 1987; 59:524.

10

Digital Intubation

Ronald Stewart, M.D.

Intubation of the trachea was recommended as the definitive technique for airway control as far back as the 18th century. A clear and concise description was given in 1796:

> . . . The Doctor who is to perform this operation placed himself on the right side of the Victim, puts his left forefinger into the right corner of the mouth along the lower row of teeth until the tip of the finger passes behind the Epiglottis. Then he takes the catheter in his right hand, passes it along the left forefingers across the glottis and turns it carefully down into the windpipe . . . .[1]

Despite the obvious disadvantage of having to insert the fingers into an unconscious patient, digital intubation continued to be described and recommended in the practice of anesthesia until well after the widespread use of the laryngoscope.[2, 3] More recent reports in the literature have usually been confined to describing the technique as a last-ditch effort to secure an airway following the failure of conventional intubation methods.[4, 5] Although the invention of the laryngoscope and other improvements in the art and science of medicine have long rendered obsolete the routine use of digital intubation, the technique can still be useful in some patients, particularly in the emergency setting.

INDICATIONS

Digital or tactile intubation can be helpful as a method of intubation when other more conventional techniques have either failed or are likely to fail. Although rarely the method of choice, it is more likely to be useful in the emergency setting in which cramped quarters, poor lighting, equipment failure, and anatomic disruption are not unusual. The technique can be particularly valuable in trauma patients, obese or short-necked patients, and in those in whom the upper airway is obscured by secretions, bleeding, or anatomic disruption.

The nature of the technique requires that the patient be deeply unconscious and relaxed so that the clinician is able to insert two fingers and an endotracheal tube into the mouth. Should these conditions be met, digital intubation should be considered in the following settings:

1. If other methods of intubation have failed.
2. In patients with anatomic disruption that renders visual identification of airway landmarks difficult if not impossible.
3. When secretions, vomitus, or blood cannot be removed with available suction techniques, so that vision is obscured.
4. In the cramped surroundings of the field setting, or in air and land transport vehicles in which space is often limited.
5. Where equipment, such as a laryngoscope, is lacking or has failed.
6. In trauma patients in whom movement of the head and neck should be limited, or in whom immobilizing devices limit vision.

In those patients in whom neuromuscular blocking agents are used, familiarity with the technique can offer the clinician added insurance against the loss of airway control that might occur should laryngoscopic intubation fail. I am aware of at least one paralyzed patient in whom the successful use of digital intubation obviated the need for a cricothyrotomy after the failure of several conventional intubation methods.

Although the technique of digital intubation is usually described for placement of endotracheal

111

tubes through the mouth, a method of nasotracheal intubation has been described using a digital technique.[6]

CONTRAINDICATIONS AND CAUTIONS

Essential to this technique is a relaxed or flaccid patient whose mouth can be opened widely without fear of loss of the clinician's fingers. The technique could possibly be carried out in cooperative patients with the use of local (topical) anesthesia, but in such patients more conventional methods would be more appropriate and likely more successful. The success of this method is largely dependent upon the relaxation of upper airway musculature (tongue, masseter, etc.) that occurs only in deep coma, cardiac arrest, or neuromuscular paralysis.

When carrying out this procedure, great care must be taken to protect the fingers of the intubator. In this era of greater awareness of disease transmission, double-gloving is recommended, since close contact with saliva, blood, or gastric contents can be expected. Even in patients with flaccid upper airway musculature the fingers and hand often contact the teeth during the digital technique, and abrasions or worse could result. The risk to the clinician should be weighed in light of the indications for the technique and the benefit to the patient.

Very small patients, or patients with small or deformed mouths may not be candidates for this procedure, although the procedure has been reported to be successful in small children and even infants.[7] Clinicians with short, stubby fingers may also have problems with the technique, although in most patients the epiglottis is readily palpated and the identification of this landmark is all that is really required for successful intubation.

Other complications of this procedure are similar to those of conventional techniques of intubation. Added to the possibility of hypoxia from prolonged attempts and trauma to the airway due to vigorous attempts at tube placement is the increased risk of unrecognized esophageal intubation. Since this technique is "blind," greater caution is advised to ensure correct intratracheal placement.

THE TECHNIQUE

Before beginning the procedure, equipment for safe intubation, including suction and ventilating devices, must be at hand and functioning.[8] While the patient is being oxygenated and ventilated, preparations can be made to carry out the technique. GLOVES MUST BE WORN. A bite-block should be placed between the patient's molars on one side to prevent injury to the clinician's fingers should the patient react to the intubation by biting. The patient's head and neck can be kept in neutral alignment, but the mouth must be able to be opened sufficient to admit the clinician's fingers and the endotracheal tube. The intubator can accomplish this by pulling and pressing forward on the tongue and lifting the tongue and jaw forward. This action not only will allow the easy introduction of the fingers and endotracheal tube into the patient's mouth but also will ensure that the epiglottis is lifted upward and away from the glottic opening—an essential maneuver in all intubation techniques.

There are several elements of the technique that are important to its success. Digital intubation is dependent upon the clinician guiding the tip of the tube through the glottic opening using the middle and index fingers of the nondominant hand. Two important factors will better ensure the success of this principle. First, the endotracheal tube should be held in an "open-J" configuration by a malleable stylet. This ensures that the tube can be directed anteriorly toward the glottis (Fig 10–1). Second, the clinician's finger must remain in contact with the tip or side hole of the tube and the epiglottis throughout the procedure. This enables the intubator to discern the position and direction of the tube tip, and will allow the tube to be guided anteriorly through the glottic opening.

Following oxygenation and proper preparation of the patient:

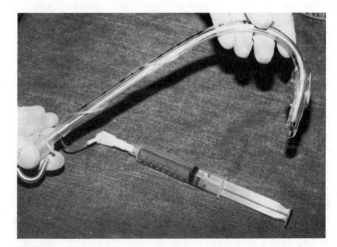

FIG 10–1.
Endotracheal tube shaped in "open-J" configuration using a stylet. Some clinicians do not use a rigid stylet for this technique.

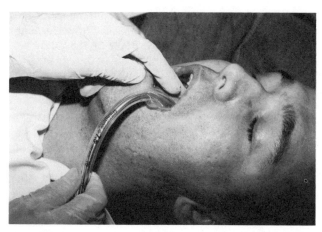

FIG 10–2.
The middle and index fingers are inserted into the patient's mouth. The middle finger presses down and pulls forward on the tongue— "walking" down the midline. The tube is inserted from the right labial angle and slid along the middle finger when that finger contacts the epiglottis. The index finger supports the tube from behind. It is important to keep the tube tip or side-hole in constant contact with the middle finger in order to identify the position of the tip.

1. The clinician stands (or kneels) facing the patient and inserts the middle and index fingers of the nondominant hand along the patient's tongue, drawing the tongue forward as the fingers "walk down" the tongue to palpate the epiglottis with the middle finger (Fig 10–2). The epiglottis feels much like a wet earlobe, in the midline at the base of the tongue. Occasionally the epiglottis will be folded down over the glottic opening, out of reach of the probing fingers. This is often due to the fact that the intubator has not pulled forward on the tongue and jaw to lift up on the epiglottis. Further pressure on the tongue will usually correct the problem. Often it is possible, particularly if the intubator has long fingers, to "hook up" the epiglottis even though it has flopped down over the glottis.

2. When the epiglottis is palpated, the lubricated tube with the stylet in place is inserted at the labial angle and is slipped along the tongue beneath the overriding index finger, with the tip sliding along the side of the middle finger which remains in contact with the epiglottis. The index finger remains above the tube, keeping the tube tip in contact with the middle finger and directing it toward the epiglottis.

3. The tube is slipped distally and held against the epiglottis by the index finger; the middle finger is then lifted to press the tube tip against the epiglottis and held there while anterior pressure is applied against the epiglottis as the tube is slipped distally toward the glottic opening (Fig 10–3).

4. Resistance will be felt as the tube enters the larynx. As the resistance increases, the tube should be held firmly in place while the stylet is withdrawn slightly in order to prevent the anterior curve from impinging on the anterior laryngeal wall.

The intubation is completed in the conventional manner, following a rigorous protocol to verify correct intratracheal placement.

An adjunct that has proved helpful in the performance of this technique is the lighted stylet or

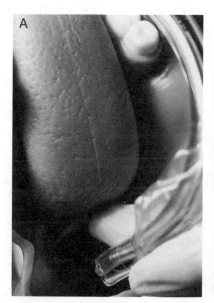
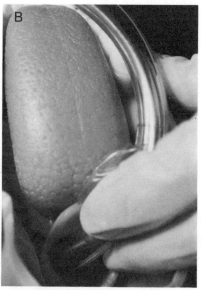

FIG 10–3.
A, cutaway (posterior) view of base of tongue, epiglottis in a mannequin. The middle finger is palpating the epiglottis, the index finger supporting the tube from behind, directing the tube tip against the epiglottis and thence through the glottic opening **(B)**.

lightwand. Its use allows the intubator to guide the tube tip by transillumination of the soft tissues of the neck, and renders the technique easier and safer. The lightwand is slipped into the endotracheal tube, bent at slightly less than a right angle, and slipped into the mouth using the technique described above. The tube-lightwand combination is used to hook up the epiglottis and a discrete, bright midline glow indicates entry of the tube into the larynx.[9]

The technique of digital intubation, while not a first-line procedure in most patients, should be known by all those familiar with conventional techniques of intubation. It offers an alternative that can provide an added safety measure when endotracheal intubation is indicated.

REFERENCES

1. Herholdt JD, Rafn CG: *Life-saving Measures for Drowning Persons.* Copenhagen, H Tikiob, 1796, pp 52–53.

2. Macewen W: Clinical observations on the introduction of tracheal tubes by the mouth instead of performing tracheotomy or laryngotomy. *Br Med J* 1880; 1:163–165.

3. Sykes WS: Oral endotracheal intubation without laryngoscopy: A plea for simplicity. *Curr Res Anesth Analg* 1937; 16:133–137.

4. Siddall WJW: Tactile orotracheal intubation. *Anaesthesia* 1966; 21:221–222.

5. Lanham HG: Tactile orotracheal intubation (letter). *JAMA* 1976; 236:2288.

6. Korber TE, Henneman PL: Digital nasotracheal intubation. *J Emerg Med* 1989; 7:275–277.

7. Woody NC, Woody HB: Direct digital intratracheal intubation for neonatal resuscitation. *J Pediatr* 1968; 73:903–905.

8. Stewart RD: Tactile orotracheal intubation. *Ann Emerg Med* 1984; 13:175–178.

9. Vollmer TP, Stewart RD, Paris PM, et al: Use of a lighted stylet for guided orotracheal intubation in the prehospital setting. *Ann Emerg Med* 1985; 14:324–328.

11

Lighted Stylet

Ronald Stewart, M.D.

Even in the emergency setting, conventional direct laryngoscopy using a metal laryngoscope is the most common method of placement of the endotracheal tube. The advantages of direct laryngoscopy include the ability to visualize the upper airway and identify any obstructions or abnormalities, as well as to correct or remove such obstructions. The disadvantages include the risk of trauma produced by the inexperienced or too vigorous instrumentation by the clinician, the need for a relaxed patient whose mouth can be opened widely, and the fact that it requires skill and practice. So important is the laryngoscope to modern anesthetic practice that the difficulty of visualizing the oral structures and the view obtained with a laryngoscope are used to classify—and predict—the success of oral intubation.[1, 2] Ideally, direct vision using the metal laryngoscope requires just that—a full view of the glottic structures obtained by positioning the patient with the neck slightly flexed (occiput elevated), head extended on the atlanto-occipital joint, and the tongue lifted forward and to the left. Although in most relaxed, anesthetized patients in the operating room this can be accomplished with varying degress of difficulty, the ideal is less frequently reached in the unprepared patient in the emergency setting. It is imperative in both settings to have alternative means of intubation available for expeditious airway control.

In 1957 Sir Robert MacIntosh and his colleague Dr. Harry Richards described the use of a malleable introducer that contained a distal light bulb connected by a wire to a proximal battery source.[3] The introducer protruded beyond the tip of the endotracheal tube and was inserted into the glottic opening, the tube then being slid distally into the larynx and trachea. The introducer simply guided the tube through the cords and helped illuminate the airway during laryngoscopy. No mention was made of transillumination as a method of guiding the tube. Two years later Yamamura et al. described the use of a flexible wire stylet with a small light bulb attached distally to assist in nasotracheal intubations.[4] During intubation, when the tip of the tube entered the larynx, the light produced by the bulb was seen clearly as a midline, circumscribed, transilluminated glow.

The possibility of using transillumination of the larynx and soft tissues of the neck to guide endotracheal tubes or the tip of a bronchoscope into the larynx was soon suggested by several sources.[5-7] A small surgical light consisting of a 25-cm coated copper wire connecting a proximal battery source and distal bulb, used by surgeons for better illumination of surgical incisions, served well as a malleable lighted stylet. A redesign of this instrument fitted it better as a stylet for orotracheal intubation,[8] and prevented the distal bulb from falling off during removal from the tube following intubation.[9]

Consistent experience for more than a decade has demonstrated light wand or light-guided intubation to be a rapid and effective intubating technique, easily acquired as a skill, and faster than conventional nasotracheal intubation (Fig 11–1).[10] It has proved to be a valuable alternative to traditional laryngoscopic intubation in prehospital care,[11] for nasotracheal intubations,[10, 12] and in the operating room.[13]

PRINCIPLES AND INDICATIONS

The use of transilluminated light to guide the tip of an endotracheal tube through the glottic opening was initially designed to solve the problem of blind

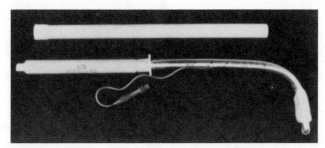

FIG 11—1.
Flexi-lum surgical light and precut endotracheal tube. Note "hockey-stick" configuration.

nasotracheal intubation.[4] With the use of a rigid wire stylet, orotracheal intubation was found to be especially useful in unusual situations in which the upper airway of some patients could not readily be visualized with the laryngoscope.[7] Owing to abnormal anatomy, orthotic appliances in place, or facial injury, some patients cannot be intubated using conventional techniques. It is those patients in whom transillumination may well be considered the first choice to aid in the placement of an endotracheal tube.

In routine general anesthesia, the use of sedatives and neuromuscular agents has made intubation by laryngoscopy relatively easy and atraumatic. Certain groups of patients tend to have a greater incidence of failed intubations, among them parturients.[14] In elective intubations, clinicians have the luxury of examining patients in an effort to predict any likely problems during the act of laryngoscopic intubation. A classification has been suggested that is based on the ability of the intubator to visualize the upper airway with the laryngoscope: grade I, full view of the glottis; grade II, view of the arytenoids; grade III, view of only the epiglottis; grade IV, not even the epiglottis is seen.[2] More recently a clinical classification has been suggested that appears predictive of difficult intubation, and which is based on a quick examination of the tongue and oral cavity.[1, 15] Although it is thought that grade III and grade IV laryngoscopic views are rare in elective intubations, in the emergency setting the opposite may hold true, particularly in trauma patients.

Therefore, despite some ability to predict problems with intubation, even elective intubations can present a significant challenge to the clinician, and can require alternative means of airway control and, if possible, intubation. In routine orotracheal intubation, transillumination can provide an added insurance against failed intubation, particularly in the grade II through grade IV laryngoscopic views.

The principle of light-guided intubation has

been expanded to include transillumination as a method of demonstrating correct intratracheal placement of an endotracheal tube.[16] The difference between the transilluminated glow from the esophagus vs. the trachea is easily discernible, and this principle can be used to rapidly confirm correct intratracheal placement. Carrying this principle further, the insertion of a light wand or lighted stylet to the distal end of an in-place tube and the adjustment of the transilluminated glow at the sternal notch will place the tube tip halfway between the cords and carina.[17]

The concept of correct placement and positioning of endotracheal tubes has not always occupied a priority in most emergency protocols even though these problems are potentially very damaging, if not life-threatening, to the patient. The principles have application not only in the emergency setting but also in the intensive care unit. The use of transillumination to solve the problem of misplaced and mispositioned tubes seeks to reduce the relatively high incidence of these difficulties found with emergency or "crash" intubations. Intubations by paramedical personnel in the adverse environment of the field have been shown to have a high rate of unrecognized esophageal and right mainstem placements.[18, 19] In the emergency department, complications as a result of intubations have been reported as higher than in elective procedures, independent of the training level, status, or specialty of the intubator.[20] In postarrest patients, 28% of patients were found to have had right mainstem intubations.[21]

In the modern practice of anesthesia, critical care, and emergency medicine, transillumination by means of a light wand or lighted stylet should be considered useful for the following:

1. As an aid to direct, routine laryngoscopic intubation.
2. For indirect visual or light-guided orotracheal intubation.[22]
3. For indirect visual or light-guided nasotracheal intubation.[12]
4. For verification of intratracheal placement of endotracheal tubes.[16]
5. For accurate and consistent positioning of the tip of an endotracheal tube.[17]

THE LIGHT WAND OR LIGHTED STYLET

The first device used to carry out orotracheal intubations in the operating room and emergency department was a flexible surgical light. Later changes in design, along with a flexible or floppy wire replacing the original rigid wire, permitted the expansion of the technique to nasotracheal intubation[12] and confirmation of placement and positioning.[16, 17] Problems with the original light wands have prompted a complete redesign of the instrument. The distal light has been increased in intensity and directed anteriorly rather than straight ahead down the airway. This allows better visualization both during the act of intubation and when the light wand is inserted into an in-place tube. The increased ability to perceive the transilluminated light provided by these design changes permits the transilluminated techniques to be carried out in normal room illumination in most patients. In addition to changes in the light, the new instrument (STL, California Medical Products, Long Beach, Calif.) can be used as either a rigid light wand for orotracheal intubation or, when the inner trocar is removed, as a flexible stylet for nasotracheal intubations and for verification of placement or accurate positioning of the tube tip.

The new light wand is designed to be used without having to cut tubes, and has both 26- and 29-cm markings clearly visible as a green band on the stylet. This allows accurate positioning of the distal bulb at the tube tip when the markings are aligned with those on the endotracheal tube. The STL also includes a solid endotracheal tube clamp to hold the light wand in place, and this is readily released after the intubation is completed. The stylet of the light wand, including the bulb, is encased in a tough plastic sheath.

TECHNIQUES

Lighting

The ability to perceive light transmitted through objects or tissues is very much dependent upon the ambient light playing on the object or tissue. In general, the lower the surrounding lighting, the easier it is to perceive transilluminated light. This is true of the technique of light wand intubation. One of the undesirable features of light wand intubation is the fact that earlier versions of the device tended to require that lights be lowered so that the transmitted light could be seen either in one of the piriform fossae or at the laryngeal prominence. By increasing the intensity of the light and directing it anteriorly, the new design of the light wand should be easily perceived in all but the brightest ambient light. Even

then, it is possible to visualize the light by shading the anterior neck with the hand or a drape.

However, increasing the intensity of the light when the ambient light is low may well increase the possibility of confusing the light transmitted from the esophagus with that emanating from the larynx. Since the brightness of the discrete intratracheal glow is even more intense in low surrounding light, it is unlikely this problem will occur. However, to further reduce the risk of any confusion, the transilluminated light seen when the tube–light wand combination is placed against the patient's cheek or in the right or left piriform fossa can be used as a standard to indicate the intensity of the light that will be transmitted when the light wand enters the patient's larynx. Using the new light wand device, it is recommended that the light level in the room *not* be reduced, but if necessary, that the neck be shielded with a hand or other object. In most patients, even this will not be needed to see the transilluminated light clearly.

Routine Laryngoscopic Intubation

Direct vision intubation using a laryngoscope can be difficult, especially in the emergency setting and in those patients in whom the mouth cannot be opened fully, or who are not sufficiently relaxed. The light wand can be inserted into an endotracheal tube, and may be helpful in illuminating the airway. In addition, should visualization be difficult, transillumination alone can place the tube quickly and reliably. Use of the stylet has the added advantage of allowing accurate positioning of the tube tip within the trachea.

Indirect Visual Orotracheal Intubation

Intubation of the trachea using the light wand has been called an "indirect visual" method, a description preferable and more accurate than "blind intubation." The technique of transillumination of the soft tissues of the neck and larynx is not proposed as a routine method in all emergency situations. However, with the accumulated experience of over a decade and with a more functional design now available, the light wand should be considered an important adjunct to intubation, as well as to verify correct placement and carry out accurate tube tip positioning. The light wand not only can serve as a reliable back-up to direct vision intubation but also may be considered as the method of choice for orotracheal intubation in selected patients by clinicians experienced in its use.

Although the technique of indirect visual orotracheal intubation is relatively simple and the skill easily acquired by most, clinicians are well advised to apply the method first to nonurgent, relatively easy intubations so that a degree of skill can be obtained before using it in the more challenging situations in which it has proved to be most useful. Continued occasional use in the nonurgent setting ensures a level of skill and comfort with the technique that can provide an added measure of confidence in the face of a difficult airway problem.

The technique of light wand intubation depends upon the transillumination of a strong light source at the end of a malleable stylet inserted into a transparent endotracheal tube. It further depends upon the fact that the position of the tip of the tube-stylet combination can be readily determined to be in either the esophagus—in which case little or no light is perceived—or in the larynx or trachea, where the relatively thin overlying tissue allows the light to be seen as a midline, circumscribed glow. The glow of intratracheal placement is readily apparent in most patients, especially if the neck is protected from bright sun or room ambient light by the hand or other object such as a towel, coat, or drape.

This method of orotracheal intubation can be particularly valuable in those patients who cannot fully open their mouths, those who may have anatomic abnormalities precluding full visualization by the laryngoscope,[23] those in cervical orthoses that restrict mouth opening,[7] and awake patients.[10]

Disadvantages of the technique include the occasional need for reduction in room lighting, and the fact that direct visualization is not possible. The complications and problems associated with the use of this method are similar to those of laryngoscopic orotracheal intubation. It should be cautioned that any technique in which the glottic opening is not directly visualized will require extra care to demonstrate correct intratracheal placement of the tube, in order to avoid the disaster of unrecognized esophageal intubation.

The technique of light wand orotracheal intubation can be readily accomplished by anyone familiar with laryngoscopic orotracheal intubation. Prior to the procedure, the patient is prepared in the same manner as with conventional methods. Oxygenation and adequate suctioning are essential to this and all other techniques.

The light wand or lighted stylet is first checked to ensure its light is bright enough by having the clinician look directly at the bulb. If the light is not uncomfortable to the eyes, the stylet should be discarded and a new one used. The rigid light wand (in the new version with trocar in place) is then lubricated and slid into the tube so that the bulb is at the level of the side hole. The light wand is then secured to the tube by the pop-off clamp provided in the body of the device. The tube–light wand combination is then bent to almost a right angle at the proximal attachment of the tube cuff. This bend is important: if it is placed too far proximal, the tube will not readily curve anteriorly, but will hit against the posterior pharyngeal wall and the distal tip will not be able to enter the glottic opening. In relaxed, prepared patients able to be placed in the "sniffing position" for conventional intubation, the tube need only be bent in a hockey stick configuration or with a slightly exaggerated pharyngolaryngeal curve.[13] In these patients the clinician is positioned at the head of the patient as with conventional laryngoscopic intubation. For patients less relaxed or whose mouth cannot be fully opened, the greater angle is recommended. That bend resembles a soup ladle, and is used to scoop up the epiglottis, thus directing the tube tip through the cords. The tube tip and cuff may be lightly lubricated in preparation for intubation.

Two positions have been described for this technique. In the first, the clinician stands at the patient's shoulder looking toward the patient's face. In the second, described by Ainsworth and Howells,[13] the intubator stands at the patient's head. The latter position is recommended if the patient is prepared and flaccid, and if the mouth is able to be fully opened. Whichever technique is used, it is recommended that the patient's cheek or piriform fossa be transilluminated in order to judge the intensity of the glow to be expected in the ambient light level when the tube tip enters the larynx.

Technique 1

The intubator opens the patient's mouth with the nondominant hand by grasping the tongue and jaw or the floor of the mouth behind the symphysis menti, and lifting gently upward and forward. This maneuver is important, as it lifts the tongue and epiglottis away from the posterior pharyngeal wall. Even if the mouth cannot be fully opened, the tongue of the patient can be protruded and the tube and light wand slipped along it. The light is turned on, and the intensity of the expected glow is estimated by placing the tube tip against the patient's cheek. The tube–light wand combination is inserted at the left labial angle, and is slipped along the tongue, directing the tip toward the right piriform fossa. A bright, circumscribed glow should be easily seen transilluminating the soft tissues overlying the right piriform fossa. The tip of the tube is then backed away from the piriform fossa and directed toward the midline; it is guided into the glottic opening by the bright, circumscribed transmitted glow evident in the midline at the laryngeal prominence. If no glow is observed, or if the glow is diffuse and weak, the tip is most likely in the esophagus and a slight withdrawal of the stylet will often cause the tip to suddenly "pop" into the glottic opening, whereupon a bright glow will result. The tube–light wand combination is then advanced slightly. With the original version of the lighted stylet the tube at this point is slipped distally off the stylet and down into the trachea. With the new STL design, the inner trocar is removed at this point, producing a flexible stylet that is still attached with the clamp to the tube, and which can now be advanced distally until the glow is located at the sternal notch. The tube tip is then properly positioned halfway between the cords and carina. The tube is held firmly in place, the clamp is released, and the light wand is removed from the tube. Ventilation can then proceed and the cuff can be inflated. The tube is then anchored firmly. Since, with this method, actual visualization of the upper airway is not accomplished, it is important that the placement of the tube be checked by auscultation and other maneuvers, including reinsertion of the

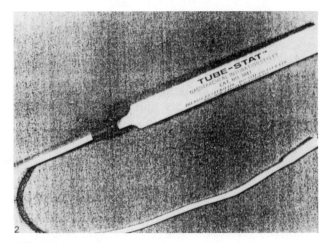

FIG 11–2.
Original Tube-Stat version of the lighted stylet.

flexible (soft) light wand to observe consistent transillumination.[16]

Technique 2

In the case of patients who can be placed in the classic sniffing position (occiput elevated, head extended on the atlanto-occipital joint) and whose mouth is easily opened, the clinician stands at the head of the patient as with laryngoscopic intubation. The following procedure is recommended[13]: The patient is oxygenated and suctioned and the intubator gloved; the light wand is prepared as described above. The clinician places a thumb in the patient's mouth behind the symphysis menti and lifts forward, pulling the jaw, tongue, and epiglottis forward and away from the posterior pharyngeal wall. The tube–light wand is inserted at the right labial angle, and the transilluminated light is observed by placing the tube tip against the opposite cheek. This allows an estimate of the intensity to be expected when the light enters the larynx. The tube tip is then directed toward the left piriform fossa, its placement indicated by the discrete glow produced there. The intensity of the light seen in the piriform fossa serves as another check of the intensity of the glow. The discrete, midline glow, as noted in technique 1, will indicate intralarygneal placement, and the intubation can be completed as described earlier.

Indirect Visual Nasotracheal Intubation

Transillumination was recommended first for nasotracheal intubation.[4] A flexible stylet designed for nasotracheal intubation was introduced following the success of the rigid version (Fig 11–2) (Concept Corp., Clearwater, Fla.). The recent introduction of the dual-purpose light wand (STL), provides the clinician with the option of using the same instrument for orotracheal (rigid) or nasotracheal (flexible) intubation. By removing an inner trocar the rigid stylet can be quickly converted to the flexible version.

An added advantage to the newer design is the fact that the flexible stylet gives some support and maintains a C curve to the nasotracheal tube which often becomes soft due to body temperature. This is particularly true of the directional-tip tube (Endotrol) the tip of which appears more readily controllable anteriorly when this light wand is in place within the tube. The principle of transillumination guides placement of the nasotracheal tube as it does with the orotracheal approach.

Technique

The technique of nasotracheal intubation is facilitated with the use of the light wand. It is recommended that the flexible light wand be used in combination with a directional-tip tube (Endotrol) that allows anterior displacement of the tube tip. The light wand is prepared and inserted into the tube in the same manner as described with the orotracheal technique, except that with the STL design, the inner trocar must be removed. The patient is prepared with oxygenation and suction, as well as with the use of cocaine or a topical anesthetic containing phenylephrine to reduce the risk of complications.[24]

The intubator stands at the head of the patient. The tube–light wand combination is passed into a nostril with the bevel of the tube along the floor or against the septum of the nasal cavity. As the tube–light wand is advanced, the tip is manipulated through the glottic opening by observing the transilluminated glow and, if necessary, directing the tip anteriorly by pulling on the drawstring of the directional-tip tube. When the typical midline glow is observed, the tube–light wand combination is advanced until the glow is located at the sternal notch. The stylet is then removed, and ventilation can begin.

Verification of Endotracheal Tube Placement

Esophageal placement and malpositioning of endotracheal tubes are more common following crash or emergency intubations.[20, 21] Auscultation appears less reliable in the emergency setting, and is particularly inadequate in the transport and prehospital environment. Rapid and reliable confirmation of intratracheal placement can be accomplished with use of the flexible light wand. It is recommended that this procedure be carried out in normal or, at most, in slightly reduced ambient light; this will help guard against an esophageal placement being mistaken for an intratracheal placement.

Technique

After ensuring adequate oxygenation of the intubated patient, the flexible light wand is inserted into the in situ tube and advanced distally. The oral cavity will initially be illuminated as the stylet is inserted into the intraoral part of the tube. As the light source passes across the cords (in the case of correct intratracheal placement), the light will suddenly dim in the oral cavity and the typical transilluminated glow will appear in the midline, first at the level of

the larynx. This is a reliable sign of correct placement.[16] If the ambient (room or outdoor) lighting is bright, the glow can be better seen by shielding the neck with the hand, or a towel or drape. The procedure should not be carried out in dim or dark lighting, since a "false-positive" result may be obtained. The higher the ambient light, the less likely is a misplaced tube in the esophagus to be mistaken for an intratracheal one. Failure to readily observe the transilluminated glow should prompt an immediate search to identify the exact placement of the tube. The improved design of the new light wand has increased the ease and reliability of this technique.

Accurate Positioning of Endotracheal Tubes

In addition to esophageal placement, endotracheal tubes can be poorly positioned within the trachea—either too high or too low. The former may lead to extrusion of the tube into the oropharynx, the latter to endobronchial intubation with all its attendant risks. These complications appear to be more common following emergency intubations.[20, 21] Since movement of the head and neck of the patient has been shown to move an endotracheal tube up and down in the airway, it is important that the tube be properly positioned. An extension of the verification technique has permitted accurate positioning of endotracheal tube tips within the tracheal lumen, approximately halfway between the carina and the cords.[17]

Technique

The flexible STL stylet is measured and marked so that when the stylet is inserted into the in situ tube, the bulb will lie at the tip of the tube when the distal edge of the green band lies opposite the 26-cm mark on the tube wall, or when the proximal edge lies opposite the 29-cm mark. As the light wand is inserted into the in-place tube, the light will illuminate the centimeter markings on the tube, and the green band can then be properly aligned. The transilluminated midline glow is then adjusted so that the maximal glow lies at or just below the sternal notch. It has been shown that at this point the tube tip will be located about halfway between the carina and the cords.[17] The light wand is then removed, ventilation is continued, and the tube is fixed in place.

Endotracheal intubation using the light wand is beginning to take its place as an accepted procedure that has been shown to be reliable, rapid, and safe in a variety of settings. It can be especially valuable in emergency settings to confirm placement, as a primary or back-up technique for intubation, and as a method of adjusting the position of endotracheal tube tips. Its future is *bright*.

REFERENCES

1. Mallampati RS, Gatt SP, Gugino LD, et al: A clinical sign to predict difficult tracheal intubation: A prospective study. *Can Anasth* 1985; 32:429–434.
2. Cormack RS, Lehane J: Difficult tracheal intubation in obstetrics. *Anaesthesia* 1984; 39:1105–1111.
3. MacIntosh R, Richards H: Illuminated introducer for endotracheal tubes. *Anaesthesia* 1957; 12:223–225.
4. Yamamura H, Yamamoto T, Kamiyama M: Device for blind nasal intubation. *Anesthesiology* 1959; 20:221.
5. Raj PP, Forestner J, Watson RD, et al: Techniques for fiberoptic laryngoscopy in anesthesia. 1974; 53:708–714.
6. Ducrow M: Throwing light on blind intubation (letter). *Anaesthesia* 1978; 33:827–829.
7. Rayburn RL: "Light wand" intubation (letter). *Anaesthesia* 1979; 34:677–678.
8. Stewart RD, Ellis DG: Lighted stylet and endotracheal intubation. I. (letter). *Anesthesiology* 1987; 66:851.
9. Stone DJ, Stirt JA, Kaplan MJ, et al: A complication of lightwand-guided nasotracheal intubation. *Anesthesiology* 1984; 780–781.
10. Fox DJ, Castro T, Rastrelli AJ: Comparison of intubation techniques in the awake patient: The Flexilum surgical light (lightwand) *versus* blind nasal approach. *Anesthesiology* 1987; 66:69–71.
11. Vollmer TP, Stewart RD, Paris PM, et al: Use of a lighted stylet for guided orotracheal intubation in the prehospital setting. *Ann Emerg Med* 1985; 14:324–328.
12. Verdile VP, Chiang JL, Bedger R, et al: Nasotracheal intubation using a flexible lighted stylet. *Ann Emerg Med* 1990; 19:506–510.
13. Ainsworth QP, Howells TH: Transilluminated tracheal intubation. *Br J Anaesth* 1989; 62:494–497.
14. Davies JM, Weeks S, Crone LA, et al: Difficult intubation in the parturient. *Can J Anaesth* 1989; 36:668–674.
15. Samsoon GLT, Young JRB: Difficult tracheal intubation: A retrospective study. *Anaesthesia* 1987; 42:487–490.
16. Stewart RD, LaRosee A, Stoy A, et al: Use of a lighted stylet to confirm correct endotracheal tube placement. *Chest* 1987; 92:900–903.
17. Stewart RD, LaRosee A, Kaplan RM, et al: Correct positioning of an endotracheal tube using a flexible stylet. *Crit Care Med* 1990; 18:97–99.
18. Stewart RD, Paris PM, Winter PM, et al: Field endotracheal intubation by paramedical personnel—Success rates and complications. *Chest* 1984; 85:341–345.
19. Pointer JE: Clinical characteristics of paramedics' performance of endotracheal intubation. *J Emerg Med* 1988; 6:505–509.
20. Taryle DA, Chandler JE, Good JT, et al: Emergency room intubations—Complications and survival. *Chest* 1979; 5:541–543.
21. Dronen S, Chadwick O, Nowak R: Endotracheal tip position in the arrested patient (letter). *Ann Emerg Med* 1982; 11:116–117.
22. Weis FR, Hatton MN: Intubation by use of the light wand: Experience in 253 patients. *J Oral Maxillofac Surg* 1989; 47:577–580.
23. Holzman RS, Nargozian CD, Florence FB: Lightwand intubation in children with abnormal upper airways. *Anesthesiology* 1988; 69:784–787.
24. Gross JB, Hartigan ML, Schaffer DW: A suitable substitute for 4% cocaine before blind nasotracheal intubation: 3% lidocaine–0.25% phenylephrine nasal spray. *Anesth Analg* 1984; 63:915–918.

12

Fiberscopic Assisted Intubation

Thomas Purcell, M.D.

During the late 1960s, a new era of endotracheal intubation (ET) followed early reports of the use of the fiberoptic choledocoscope to facilitate nasotracheal intubation.[1] The clinical potential of this technique was quickly appreciated, and in 1972 use of the bronchofiberscope was described to facilitate nasotracheal intubation.[2] Subsequently, a specifically designed fiberoptic laryngoscope as well as pediatric fiberscopes have been marketed and have gained wide acceptance.[3]

Fiberscopic assisted intubation has several advantages. The operator has a direct view of the airway, allowing a more controlled and orderly placement of an ET tube through the glottis. The patient may be awake during the procedure, and may even be sitting up, making this technique more acceptable to the patient, and safer in that vomiting is less likely and the protective gag reflex is maintained. The suction channel present on most devices allows the removal of blood and excessive secretions from the field during the procedure, which in turn reduces the risk of aspiration and improves visibility. In the awake patient, intubation by means of fiberoptic laryngoscopy appears to have a higher success rate than rigid laryngoscopy, even in patients who are not judged to be potentially difficult intubations.[4] Finally, fiberoptic intubation may offer a particular advantage in selected patients with multiple injuries, in that placement of an ET tube using this technique may be accomplished without manipulation of the cervical spine.[5]

INDICATIONS AND CONTRAINDICATIONS

Indications

Fiberoptic intubation should be considered in any patient in whom more expeditious standard techniques of endotracheal intubation are either contraindicated or impossible, or when exposure of the vocal cords is anticipated to be difficult owing to anatomic limitations. Among the clinical situations in which fiberoptic intubation has proved to be the procedure of choice, the following have been reported:

1. Patients with limited ability or inability to open or protrude the mandible, as in Ludwig's angina,[6] temporomandibular arthritis,[7] trismus, or status epilepticus (actively seizing patients are relatively easy to intubate using this method).[6]
2. Congenital or acquired anatomic abnormalities that render visualization of the glottis difficult, e.g., kyphosis; protruding upper incisors; morbid obesity; a short, thick neck or large tongue[7]; retropharyngeal abscess; or in the case of encroachment of the airway by intrinsic or extrinsic hematoma[8] or other mass effect.[9]
3. Restricted motion of the cervical spine due to cervical arthritis,[7] patients in halo traction, or potential or actual unstable injuries of the cervical spine.
4. Severe facial fractures,[8] or penetrating neck injuries.[10]

5. Failed nasotracheal intubation[7, 10] or patients with known previous difficult intubation.[7]

6. Overdose patients requiring airway protection prior to gastric lavage.[6, 10, 11]

7. Patients with respiratory failure from chronic obstructive pulmonary disease (COPD), asthma, or pulmonary edema, and patients with superior vena cava syndrome. The ability to intubate these patients while awake and sitting up is particularly useful.[6, 12]

When a difficult intubation can be anticipated, fiberoptic intubation should be used as a first-line approach rather than a last-ditch effort in a crisis situation. If conventional means have been attempted numerous times beforehand, a sometimes bloody field may make fiberoptic intubation much more difficult.[6, 8, 13]

Contraindications and Caveats

Patients in extremis requiring intubation by the quickest possible means (such as the apneic patient) are seldom candidates for fiberoptic intubation unless more direct methods fail and the required instrumentation is immediately at hand. In most instances, setup of equipment alone may take several minutes.[14] Brisk bleeding and copious secretions will frequently make use of the fiberoptic method difficult. A foreign body in the airway may be further impacted by the tip of the scope.[14, 15] Intubation with the fiberscope produces a significantly greater and more sustained tachycardia than that associated with conventional intubation techniques, and thus should be used with caution in patients known to have significant cardiovascular disease.[16]

EQUIPMENT

General

Oxygen, suction, and a cuffed ET tube and equipment for bag-mask ventilation should be at hand prior to initiating the procedure. Most devices intended for use on adult patients will require the use of an ET tube with an inside diameter of no less than 7 mm. A water-soluble lubricant, a topical mucosal anesthetic spray (such as benzocaine or lidocaine), and for nasal intubations, a mucosal vasoconstrictor (such as 0.25% phenylephrine), will be needed.

Fiberoptic Bronchoscope and Laryngoscope

The fiberscope usually consists of a light source, handle, body with control knob, and the fiberoptic bundle in an elongated flexible shaft (Fig 12–1). The image is transmitted from the objective lens within the optic tip to the eyepiece through thousands of glass fibers.

A small knob on the side of the body (Fig 12–2) controls the movement at the distal end of the shaft, which can be flexed and extended through a range of more than 180 degrees. This movement is in one plane only. In order to change the plane of tip movement, the entire instrument is simply rotated around its long axis.

The deflecting mechanism is not strong enough to bend an ET tube. If the tip is forcibly deflected by turning the control knob while it is within the tube, the fine-gauge control wires may rupture. In addition, bending the shaft in excessively sharp curves (radius less than 2 in.) may break some of the glass fibers, resulting in minute "black spots" within the viewing field.

The ideal fiberscope should reach the carina before the tip of a threaded ET tube enters the nose. This allows maximum flexibility and maneuverability of the scope and reduces nasal hemorrhage.[6] Fiberoptic bronchoscopes have a slightly longer working shaft than laryngoscopes (Fig 12–3) and consequently are preferred by some clinicians.[17, 18] Simplified fiberoptic laryngoscopes generally have a working length of 45 to 50 cm and an outside shaft diameter of 6.4 mm. A suctioning lumen (Figs 12–4 and 12–5), absent in early models, is highly desirable.[6] Battery-powered models are available having

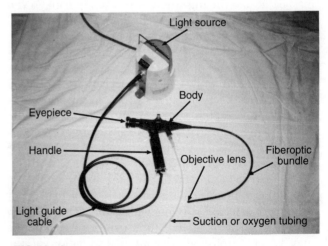

FIG 12–1.
Operational fiberscope.

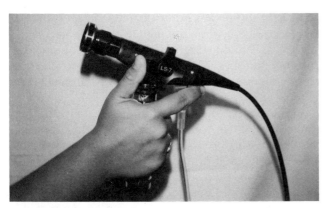

FIG 12–2.
Tip deflection control knob.

the advantages of speed of setup and ease of conveyance, but lack the suctioning lumen.

TECHNIQUE

The success of fiberoptic intubation depends largely upon the proficiency of the intubator. It has been suggested that 30 successfully performed fiberoptic intubations in awake and unconscious patients are essential to attain the requisite competence.[19, 20] Delaney and Hessler found that the experience gained from ten cases ensured that the procedure could be accomplished quickly and reliably.[6] Others have found that instruction utilizing manikins provided an acceptable degree of familiarity with the procedure.[10]

In experienced hands, under ideal controlled

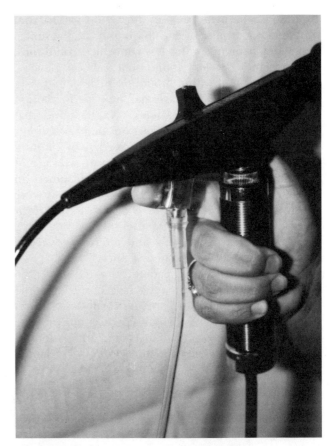

FIG 12–4.
Operation of suction bypass.

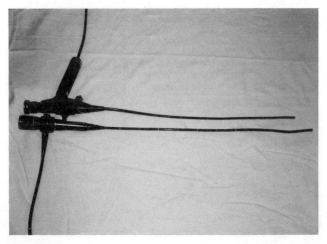

FIG 12–3.
Fiberoptic laryngoscope *(above)* and bronchoscope *(below).*

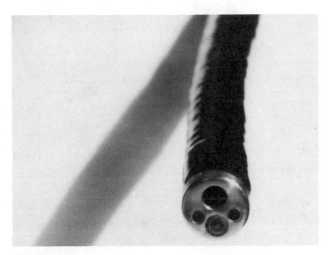

FIG 12–5.
Magnified view of fiberscope tip showing working (suction) channel *(superior)*, lens *(inferior)*, and two light source bundles.

conditions, the mean time to intubation varies from 37 seconds[16] to just over 2 minutes.[21] In the emergency department, under less controlled conditions, Delaney and Hessler[6] found that 70% of patients may be intubated within 3 minutes or less, and 97% within 6 minutes. The average time to intubation was 3.0 ±2.4 minutes.[6] Mlinek et al.[10] found that successful fiberoptic intubations on medical patients could be accomplished within an average of 1.8 minutes, and on trauma patients, within an average of 3.0 minutes, whereas failed attempts consumed an average of 7.8 minutes before other techniques were substituted. This led to the conclusion that if fiberoptic intubation is not accomplished within 2 to 3 minutes, success is unlikely and alternative airway techniques should be initiated at once.[10]

In the unconscious patient, the tonus of the tongue disappears, the tongue sags posteriorly, the epiglottis falls back, and the piriform fossa is relaxed, all of which greatly limit visualization with the fiberoptic laryngoscope. Fiberoptic intubation is therefore easier in the conscious patient,[19, 20] and if

a difficult intubation is anticipated, the procedure is best carried out while the patient is still awake, using topical anesthesia. Light sedation is recommended by some authors,[19, 20] but this may compromise patient cooperation and depress airway protective reflexes.[9]

The patient may be either supine or sitting upright (Figs 12–6,A and B). Patients with respiratory distress due to bronchospasm or pulmonary edema may be intubated in the sitting position without preintubation sedation, thus allowing them to maintain their gag reflex, maximum respiratory effort, and cooperation until the procedure can be completed.[6]

The choice of route will be influenced by several factors. The oral route is often less desirable than the nasal route because the optic tip enters the glottis at a more acute angle than via the nasal route[19–21] (Fig 12–7). Use of the oral route in the awake patient also requires excellent patient cooperation, because a single inadvertent bite on the fiber shaft may destroy the instrument. Further, the oral route often requires the presence of an assistant to apply

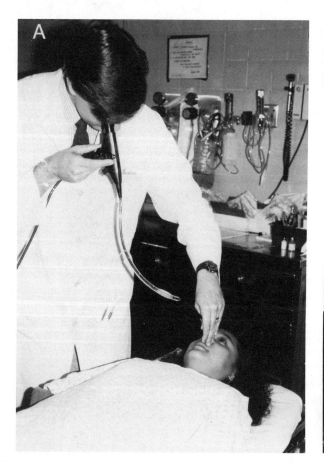 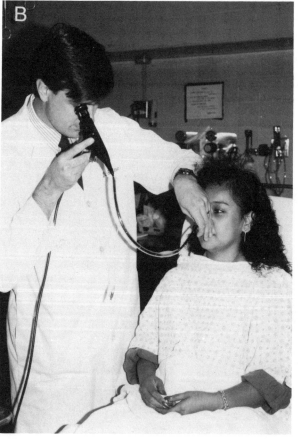

FIG 12–6.
Fiberscopic assisted intubation, single operator. **A,** patient in supine position. **B,** patient in sitting position.

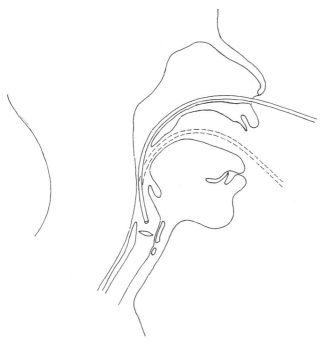

FIG 12–7.
The optic tip passed through the mouth approaches the glottis at a more acute angle than via the nasal route.

forward traction on the mandible and tongue.[22]

On the other hand, the nasal route requires considerable skill in maneuvering the tip of the scope through the nasal passage and the nasopharynx. Nasal anatomy may also limit the size of ET tube used.[22]

Nasotracheal Route

The use of cardiac and blood pressure monitoring during the procedure, as well as pulse oximetry, is advisable. A nasal ET tube is cut to the desired length as determined by measuring the distance from the suprasternal notch to the mandibular angle to the alar base of the nose.[8] Removal of any excess length from the ET tube prior to threading it over the fiberoptic shaft allows maximum unimpeded penetration of the respiratory tract by the fiberscope.

The nasal fiberoptic intubation technique requires particular attention to protection of the nasal mucosa with preoperative sprays and lubricants.[8] If the procedure is semielective, beclomethasone and oxymetazoline nasal sprays shrink the nasal mucosa, minimize hemorrhage, and improve visibility.[8] Other authors recommend that cocaine (in concentrations ranging from 4%–10%) be instilled or sprayed into each nostril as a vasoconstric-

tor.[9, 17, 21, 23] As an alternative, 2% phenylephrine with 4% lidocaine has also been recommended.[6] Careful preparation of the nasal mucosa with these agents requires at least 2 to 3 minutes.[6]

A preserved gag reflex makes fiberoptic laryngoscopy difficult[23] and a viscous lidocaine gargle or a topical anesthetic spray of the oropharynx and hypopharynx is advisable.[9, 23] Percutaneous translaryngeal injection of 4% lidocaine effectively anesthetizes the cords[8, 17] but this is generally not necessary for provision of adequate anesthesia[8, 9] and may increase the potential for aspiration in patients with a full stomach.[23]

Oxygen tubing may be attached to the suction port on the handle of the scope for insufflation of oxygen during intubation. A constant flow of oxygen of 1 L/min is advisable for supplementation during the procedure,[18] while intermittent insufflations of high-flow oxygen (10–15 L/min) will keep debris and secretions away from the optic tip.[6, 10, 14] If copious secretions or bleeding is encountered, the oxygen tubing may be replaced with suction tubing. Suctioning is then performed by covering the suction bypass hole with the index finger (see Fig 12–4).

If high-flow oxygen is insufflated during the procedure, adequate clearance is essential between the outside of the scope shaft and the inside of the ET tube to allow escape of gases and to prevent barotrauma. The smallest tube that can be used with the 6.0-mm scope with high-flow oxygen is 7.5 mm inside diameter (ID).[6]

A water-soluble jelly lubricant is applied to the mucosa of the nostril to be intubated and to the shaft of the scope, taking care not to allow the lubricant to cover the lens at the tip of the scope, as it will cloud the image. A cuffed endotracheal tube, with the nasal tip adaptor removed, is then passed over the fiberoptic bundle shaft until it abuts the body, leaving the distal portion of the shaft exposed.[8] Before using the scope, the optic tip is held near printed matter and the eyepiece is adjusted for best focus. To prevent fogging, the optic tip may be immersed briefly in warm water or dilute hexachlorophene solution just before using.[23]

The thumb of the hand holding the control section of the scope manipulates the knob that regulates angulation of the tip of the scope, and the index finger controls the suction bypass (see Figs 12–2 and 12–4). The bronchoscope tip is advanced through the anesthetized nostril and pharynx and into the supraglottic region by direct visualization through the scope (Fig 12–8). Suctioning of mucus,

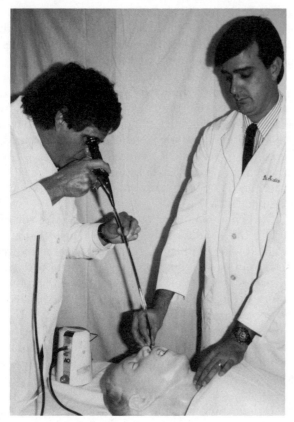

FIG 12—8.
Advancing the fiberscope through the nasopharynx under direct vision.

secretions, and blood allows a clear view. While advancing the scope, if a "veil of red" or "red-out" is seen, it means that the tip of the scope has abutted against a mucosal surface. In this case, the scope is withdrawn a few centimeters until the airway is again visualized, and then advanced. Once the vocal cords are seen, the patient is asked to inhale deeply (to abduct the cords). The control knob on the handle aids in directing the optic tip through the glottis and the scope is advanced a few centimeters further until the tracheal rings are identified. Some authors advise that once in view, the vocal cords be sprayed with 2 mL of 2% lidocaine through the working channel of the fiberscope prior to advancing through the glottis.[7, 9, 24] However as noted above, this may increase the risk of aspiration in some patients.

Alternatively, if sufficient time (2–3 mins) is available for topical preparation of the nasal mucosa to decrease bleeding, blind nasal intubation to the level of the hypopharynx may first be conducted in the usual manner (Fig 12–9,A and B). When breath sounds are heard through the tube, the lubricated fi-

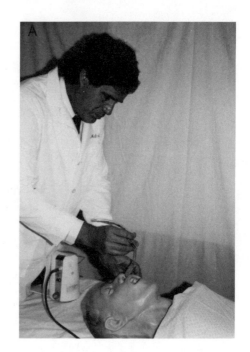

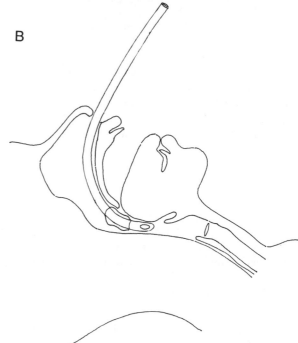

FIG 12—9.
A, blind nasopharyngeal intubation. **B,** the ET tube is advanced to the hypopharynx.

beroptic bundle is passed through the immobilized ET tube until the cords are visualized[1, 6, 10, 14] (Fig 12–10,A and B), and then advanced through the glottis as described above (Fig 12–11, A and B). In urgent cases, when adequate nasal mucosal preparation cannot be achieved, this approach may stimulate

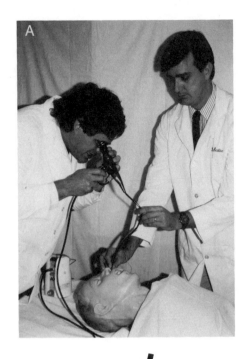

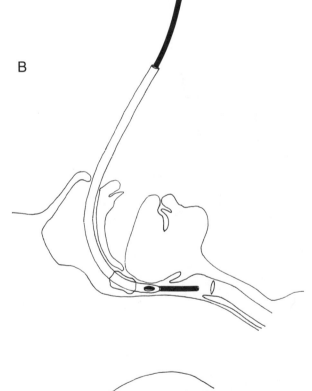

FIG 12–10.
A and **B,** the fiberscope is advanced through the ET tube to visualize the vocal cords.

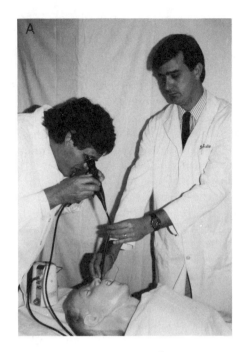

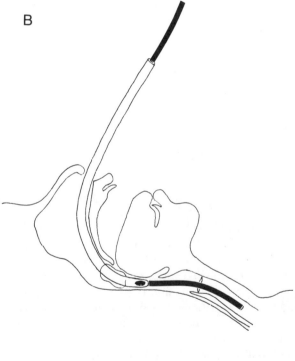

FIG 12–11.
A and **B,** While the ET tube is held in position, the fiberscope is advanced through the glottis and into the trachea.

bleeding and contribute to delay or failure of intubation.[10]

Occasionally, as a result of copious secretions or blood, visualization of the glottis is difficult or impossible. In this case, the room lights may be momentarily turned down and the fiberscope used as a lighted stylet. Entry into the trachea is then facilitated by following the midline glow of light transilluminated through neck tissues. This technique is described more fully below.

When the instrument tip is within the trachea just above the carina, the scope is held stationary while the ET tube is advanced over the bronchoscope (Fig 12–12,A and B). Proper final position of the ET tube is confirmed by direct visualization of the edge of the tube as it advances beyond the end of the scope.

When the ET tube is in its proper position, it is then held in place while the bronchoscope is withdrawn (Fig 12–13). The nasal tip adaptor is now replaced and firmly seated, the cuff inflated (Fig 12–14,A and B), the tube secured by the usual means, and the patient ventilated. Placement can then be reconfirmed by auscultation of breath sounds.

Tube placement may be assessed by the chest film, but if placement has previously been confirmed by physical examination and direct vision through the fiberscope, this will generally not be required.[25, 26]

Orotracheal Route

The ET tube is prepared as described above and the fiberscope is lubricated and inserted through the tube lumen until the optic tip is protruding from the distal end of the tube. A bite-block is used to prevent closure of the teeth on the instrument.

This method, as described by Clinton and Ruiz,[14] is best accomplished with an assistant. After anesthetizing the oropharynx and hypopharynx and preoxygenating the patient, the first operator retracts the tongue with a standard rigid laryngoscope as for direct laryngoscopy, grasps the fiberscope–ET tube combination, and advances the optic tip toward the larynx. The second operator then visualizes the glottis through the scope, instructs the patient to inhale deeply, and advances the tip between the cords.[14] Alternatively, the patient may be asked to protrude the tongue, or the tongue may be grasped by an assistant with thumb and index finger over gauze, and pulled anteriorly. This decreases the angle to be negotiated by the shaft of the scope as it enters the glottis.

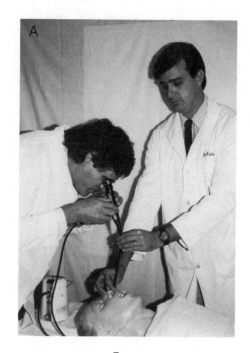

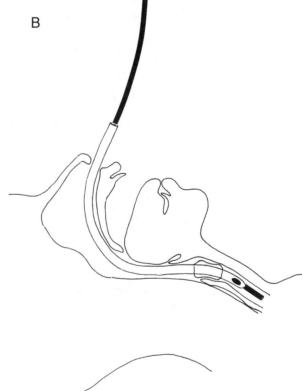

FIG 12–12.
A and **B,** the fiberscope is held stationary while the ET tube is passed into the trachea.

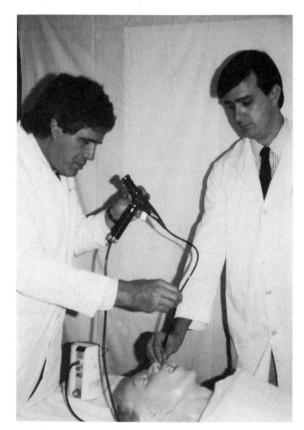

FIG 12–13.
The ET tube is held in position while the fiberscope is withdrawn.

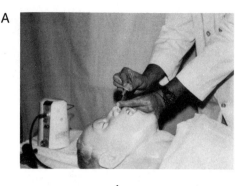

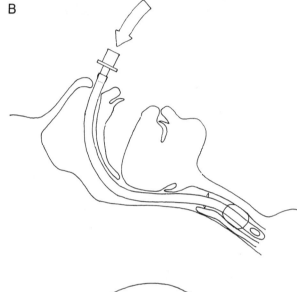

FIG 12–14.
A and **B,** the nasal tip adaptor is replaced and firmly seated. The cuff is inflated.

Rogers and Benumof[22] described a third method utilizing a specially designed oral Airway Intubator (Airway Intubator, Ltd., Calgary, Alta., Canada). Described earlier by Williams and Maltby,[27] this device consists of an oropharyngeal airway adapted to serve as a combination bite-block and intubation guide (Fig 12–15). The Airway Intubator is inserted through the mouth reaching the hypopharynx (Fig 12–16). The fiberscope is lubricated, and passed through the cuffed ET tube in the manner described above. The scope is then advanced through the Airway Intubator and, under direct vision, between the vocal cords. At this point, the ET tube is advanced over the fiberscope, through the Airway Intubator, and into the trachea. After visually confirming tube placement, the fiberscope is withdrawn (Fig 12–17). The Airway Intubator may either be removed over the ET tube, or left in place. The ET tube adaptor is reconnected, the cuff inflated, and the patient ventilated while the lungs are auscultated to verify placement.

PREHOSPITAL PERSPECTIVE

To date, this technique has not been applied in the prehospital setting. High equipment cost, significant potential for instrument damage in the uncontrolled field setting, requirements for bedside suction, power source and oxygen, associated time delays, space limitations, and lack of familiarity with the potential and technique of fiberoptic intubation have likely restricted its application by prehospital care providers. It is foreseeable that these obstacles may be overridden by the absolute necessity of obtaining a protected airway in selected patients, especially where very long transport times are involved. Further, fiberoptic verification of correct ET tube placement may prove invaluable in the noisy environment of the mobile unit where auscultation of breath sounds is difficult and frequently unreliable.

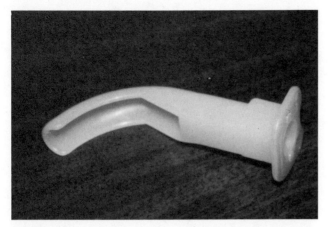

FIG 12–15.
The Airway Intubator.

PEDIATRIC PERSPECTIVE

As recently as 1985 the smallest pediatric fiberscopes required the use of a 4.0- to 4.5-mm ID ET tube or larger.[17] Newer pediatric models currently are available with an outside shaft diameter as small as 2.1 mm, allowing passage of ET tubes down to 3.0 mm ID.[26] Once in place, verification of the position

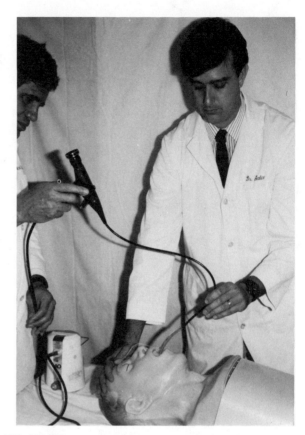

FIG 12–17.
The ET tube is positioned through the Airway Intubator into the trachea. The fiberscope is being withdrawn.

of the tip of the ET tube by the fiberscope, combined with a good physical examination, is safe, and as accurate as a conventional chest film.[26]

COMPLICATIONS

Complications associated with fiberoptic intubation via the nasal route are chiefly those due to nasotracheal intubation and include nasal mucosal injury, hemorrhage, and esophageal intubation.[6, 28] Notably, excessive delay of intubation while executing repeated attempts may be a much greater hazard with fiberoptic intubation owing to the novelty and intricacy of the technique. Accordingly, very close attention to procedure duration and strict adherence to time limits, and careful monitoring, which may include pulse oximetry, are critical to avoid iatrogenic hypoxic insult.[14]

While fiberoptic orotracheal intubation causes less of a hypertensive response than does conventional intubation, it does provoke significantly greater tachycardia, which persists for up to 5 minutes following completion of the procedure. Accord-

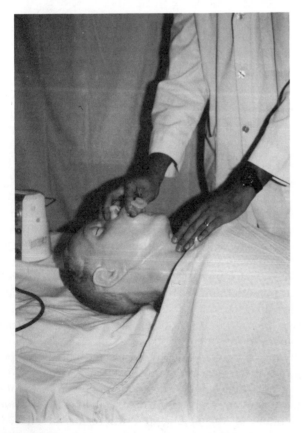

FIG 12–16.
Insertion of the Airway Intubator.

ingly, the technique must be used with caution (if at all) in patients with cardiovascular disease.[16] Iatrogenic introduction of a foreign body during the procedure (e.g., the diaphragm from the anesthesia mask) has been reported,[15] as has inability to withdraw the fiberoptic scope from the ET tube owing to intussusception of the tip of the unit into the covering sleeve of the scope.[29] Inadvertent passage of the scope through the lateral opening (Murphy's eye) of the ET tube with subsequent inability to withdraw the fiberscope from the ET tube,[30] and failure to intubate the patient because of inability to pass the ET tube through the naris[6] have also been described.

Fiberoptic intubation should be considered in selected patients in whom exposure of the vocal cords is anticipated to be difficult owing to anatomic limitations. When its use is indicated, it should be employed as a first-line approach rather than as a last-ditch effort after other methods have failed.

REFERENCES

1. Murphy P: A fibre-optic endoscope used for nasal intubation. *Anaesthesia* 1967; 22:489.
2. Taylor PA, Towey RM: The broncho-fiberscope as an aid to endotracheal intubation. *Br J Anaesth* 1972; 44:611.
3. Stiles CM, Stiles QR, Denson JS: A flexible fiber-optic laryngoscope. *JAMA* 1972; 221:1246.
4. Schrader S, Ovassapian A, Dykes MHM, et al: Cardiovascular changes during awake rigid and fiberoptic laryngoscopy. *Anesthesiology* 1987; 67:A28.
5. Mulder DS, Wallace DH, Woolhouse FM: The use of the fiberoptic bronchoscope to facilitate endotracheal intubation following head and neck trauma. *J Trauma* 1975; 15:638.
6. Delaney KA, Hessler R: Emergency flexible fiberoptic nasotracheal intubation: A report of 60 cases. *Ann Emerg Med* 1988; 17:919.
7. Ovassapian A, Krejcie TC, Yelich SJ, et al: Awake fibreoptic intubation in the patient at high risk of aspiration. *Br J Anaesth* 1989; 62:13.
8. Stella JP, Kageler WV, Epker BN: Fiberoptic endotracheal intubation in oral and maxillofacial surgery. *J Oral Maxillofac Surg* 1986; 44:923.
9. Rashid J, Warltier B: Awake fibreoptic intubation for a rare cause of upper airway obstruction—an infected laryngocoele. *Anaesthesia* 1989; 44:834.
10. Mlinek EJ, Clinton JE, Plummer D, et al: Fiberoptic intubation in the emergency department. *Ann Emerg Med* 1990; 19:359.
11. Messeter KH, Pettersson KI: Endotracheal intubation with the fibre-optic bronchoscope. *Anaesthesia* 1980; 35:294.
12. Shapiro HM, Sanford TJ, Schaldach AL: Fiberoptic stylet laryngoscope and sitting position for tracheal intubation in acute superior vena caval syndrome. *Anesth Analg* 1984; 63:161.
13. Witton TH: An introduction to the fiberoptic laryngoscope, *Can Anaesth Soc J* 1981; 28:475.
14. Clinton JE, Ruiz E. Emergency airway management procedures, in Roberts JR, Hedges JR (eds): *Clinical Procedures in Emergency Medicine.* Philadelphia, WB Saunders Co, 1985, pp 2–29.
15. Zornow MH, Mitchell MM: Foreign body aspiration during fiberoptic-assisted intubation (letter). *Anesthesiology* 1986; 64:303.
16. Smith JE, Mackenzie AA, Sanghera SS, et al: Cardiovascular effects of fibrescope-guided nasotracheal intubation. *Anaesthesia* 1989; 44:907.
17. Berthelsen P, Prytz A, Jacobsen E: Two-stage fiberoptic nasotracheal intubation in infants: A new approach to difficult pediatric intubation. *Anesthesiology* 1985; 63:457.
18. Wei WI, Siu KF, Lau WF, et al: Emergency endotracheal intubation under fiberoptic endoscopic guidance for malignant laryngeal obstruction. *Otolaryngol Head Neck Surg* 1988; 98:10.
19. Sia RL, Edens ET: How to avoid problems when using the fibre-optic bronchoscope for difficult intubations (letter). *Anaesthesia* 1981; 36:74.
20. Edens ET, Sia RL: Flexible fiberoptic endoscopy in difficult intubations. *Ann Otol Rhinol Laryngol* 1981; 90:307.
21. Coe PA, King TA, Towey RM: Teaching guided fibreoptic nasotracheal intubation: An assessment of an anesthetic technique to aid training. *Anaesthesia* 1988; 43:410.
22. Rogers SN, Benumof JL: New and easy techniques for fiberoptic endoscopy-aided tracheal intubation. *Anesthesiology* 1983; 59:569.
23. Mishkel L, Wang JF, Gutierrez F, et al: Nasotracheal intubation by fiberoptic laryngoscope. *South Med J* 1981; 74:1407.
24. Ovassapian A, Yelich SJ, Dykes MHM, et al: Fiberoptic nasotracheal intubation: Incidence and causes of failure. *Anesth Analg* 1983; 62:692.
25. O'Brien D, Curran J, Conroy J, et al: Fibre-optic assessment of tracheal tube position. A comparison of tracheal tube position as estimated by fibre-optic bronchoscopy and by chest x-ray. *Anaesthesia* 1985; 40:73.
26. Dietrich KA, Strauss RH, Cabalka AK, et al: Use of flexible fiberoptic endoscopy for determination of endotracheal tube position in the pediatric patient. *Crit Care Med* 1988; 16:884.
27. Williams RT, Maltby JR: Airway intubator (letter). *Anesth Analg* 1982; 61:309.
28. Moorthy SS, Dierdorf SF: An unusual difficulty in fiberoptic intubation. *Anesthesiology* 1985; 63:229.
29. Siegel M, Coleprate P: Complication of fiberoptic bronchoscope. *Anesthesiology* 1984; 61:214.
30. Ovassapian A: Failure to withdraw flexible fiberoptic laryngoscope after nasotracheal intubation (letter). *Anesthesiology* 1985; 63:124.

13

Retrograde Tracheal Intubation

Thomas Purcell, M.D.

HISTORY

In 1960 Butler and Cirillo[1] described a new technique for passing an endotracheal tube which involved an initial retrograde introduction of a catheter through a tracheostomy into the pharynx, and the subsequent use of this catheter as a guide for the distal passage of the endotracheal tube. Subsequent reports in 1963 by Waters[2] and in 1967 by Powell and Ozdil[3] modified the technique for application to patients without a tracheostomy by introducing a large-bore needle through the cricothyroid membrane (CTM), which in turn channeled a catheter retrograde in the manner described by Butler and Cirillo. The technique has endured, with small modifications, as an option in selected patients for the establishment of an endotracheal airway.

The proliferation of names for this procedure may lead to some confusion. The terms "retrograde tracheal intubation,"[1, 4, 5] "retrograde transtracheal intubation,"[6] "retrograde guide for endotracheal intubation,"[7] and "retrograde intubation"[8-11] have all been used. Some authors[12-14] have correctly noted that "retrograde intubation" is technically a misnomer. While the guide wire or catheter is threaded in a retrograde manner, the endotracheal tube itself is passed in the normal direction. This fact has given rise to a second school of nomenclature embracing such terms as "translaryngeal guided intubation,"[13-15] "translaryngeal guided retrograde intubation,"[16] and "guided blind oral intubation."[2, 17] Lacking a consensus on terminology, the simple, albeit admittedly flawed, designation of "retrograde tracheal intubation" (RTI) is used in this chapter.

INDICATIONS AND CONTRAINDICATIONS

When properly performed, RTI is one of the most effective emergency techniques for securing an airway should conventional means of endotracheal intubation fail.[13] Nevertheless, the technique has not yet gained wide clinical acceptance, possibly because of its invasive nature and the potential difficulties associated with cricothyroid puncture[13] and because it is rarely taught in the clinical setting.[13, 16] RTI requires minimal operator experience and can be performed without head or neck movement.[5, 13]

Indications

Patients requiring endotracheal intubation in whom conventional techniques are unsuccessful or inappropriate owing to inability to visualize the vocal cords should be considered candidates for this approach. Stable, cooperative patients, and comatose patients with free access to the posterior pharynx and spontaneous respiratory efforts are the most suitable candidates.[11] RTI has proved effective in patients with abnormal anatomic or pathologic conditions of the upper airway, including congenital orofacial lesions,[6, 8] tumors, and infections, including acute epiglottitis.[2, 5] RTI has also been useful in patients with other conditions limiting visualization of the glottis, such as cervical spondylosis or trauma[10] and severe kyphosis.[5, 18] Patients sustaining severe orofacial trauma in whom distortion of normal anatomy and a bloody field precludes conventional endotracheal intubation are also candidates for RTI.[4, 5, 13, 16] Generally, in those clinical predicaments in which cricothyrotomy or transtracheal ventilation is considered, RTI may be a reasonable alternative.[5]

Contraindications

Retrograde tracheal intubation may not be suitable for patients requiring immediate intubation and ventilation, since the procedure can be expected to take up to 5 minutes for completion.[4] Other situations in which RTI may be inadvisable include the uncooperative patient, coagulation abnormalities (owing to the associated danger of severe endotracheal bleeding),[16] involvement of the puncture site by tumor[16, 19] or overlying infection,[19] inability to open the mouth for catheter retrieval,[5] and the presence of an enlarged thyroid gland.[19]

EQUIPMENT

The length of the catheter or wire must be sufficient to span the distance from the CTM to the lips or external nares, and the entire length of the endoctracheal tube. Generally a length of 70 cm is adequate in adults.[5]

A long (75 cm) central venous catheter may be preferable to a guide wire in patients with severe maxillofacial trauma or other conditions resulting in a bloody field because it allows air injection as an aid to locating the catheter tip in the mouth.[4]

The use of a wire instead of a long plastic catheter decreases the elasticity of the guide while the nasotracheal tube is being inserted, thereby minimizing the chance of breaking the introducing catheter.[6] A Seldinger wire FC101, 75 cm long, 0.8 mm external diameter (Extracorporeal, King of Prussia, Pa.), using an 18-gauge 1.3-mm introducing needle, is effective for this purpose.[4]

Several technical problems associated with the use of straight catheters and wires have been reported. Difficulty passing the wire through the vocal cords has been encountered, as well as problems in visualizing the catheter in the oropharynx because of its transparency or immersion in a bloody field. Surface tension causes the straight tip of the plastic catheter to cling to the posterior pharynx, and consequently it may be difficult to retrieve without damaging the surrounding mucosa.[15] As a solution to these difficulties, Gerenstein and Arria-Devoe proposed the use of a J-wire similar to that used for central venous catheterization. The J shape facilitates the passage of the guide proximally without injury. When the J lies in the oropharynx, rotating the wire back and forth along its long axis produces a twisting motion of the tip, making it easier to see, even in a bloody field. Finally, this same twisting motion turns and elevates the curved tip of the J away from the mucosal surface, making it easier to pick up with the forceps without injury.[15]

A rigid needle, long enough to enter the larynx, is required. The inside diameter of the needle is dictated by the type of guide wire or catheter chosen. Needed also will be: a syringe, a no. 11 blade and handle, forceps, scissors (or wire cutter), clamp, and materials for local anesthesia, sterile preparation, and draping of the field. Suction equipment, bag-mask ventilation equipment, and oxygen should be available at the bedside.

TECHNIQUE

Regardless of whether the oral or nasal route is employed, the patient must be oxygenated, and, if necessary, ventilated, to the maximum extent possible. The use of RTI allows unimpeded upper airway management up to the point of retrieval of the guide catheter or wire from the posterior pharynx. Until then, oxygen supplementation by mask is advisable in all patients. Bag-mask ventilation may also be added if spontaneous respirations are deemed inadequate.

Orotracheal Route

After preoxygenation of the patient and equipment preparation, the posterior pharynx is sprayed with topical anesthetic. Sterile technique is advisable, time permitting. The skin overlying the cricothyroid space is disinfected with 10% providone-iodine, and then 1 mL of 1% lidocaine is injected into the skin overlying the CTM and another 2 mL is injected into the glottic space and subglottic lumen.[4] In the awake patient, care should be taken to remove the needle quickly after this maneuver to avoid injury from subsequent coughing.[5, 19]

The introducing needle is connected to a syringe half-filled with saline, and the bevel of the needle is aligned with the scale marked on the barrel of the syringe. This allows direction of the bevel once inside the larynx. The thyroid cartilage is stabilized with the thumb and middle finger of one hand. The index finger identifies the thyroid prominence and is slid caudad to locate the depression of the CTM. A small stab incision with a no. 11 blade may facilitate

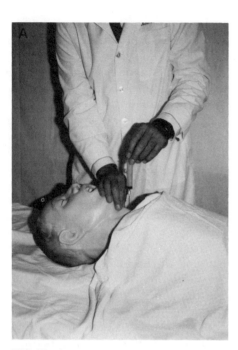

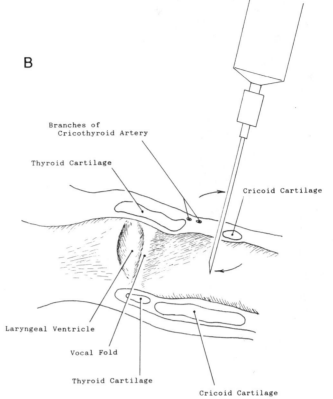

B

Branches of
Cricothyroid Artery

Thyroid Cartilage

Cricoid Cartilage

Laryngeal Ventricle

Vocal Fold

Thyroid Cartilage

Cricoid Cartilage

FIG 13–1.
A and **B,** needle cricothyrotomy.

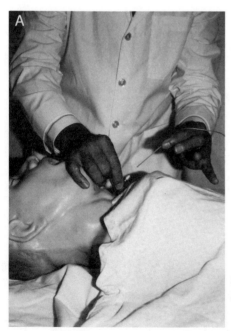

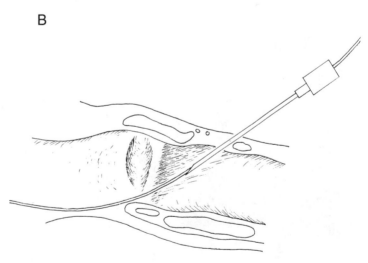

B

FIG 13–2.
A and **B,** passing the guide catheter through the introducing needle.

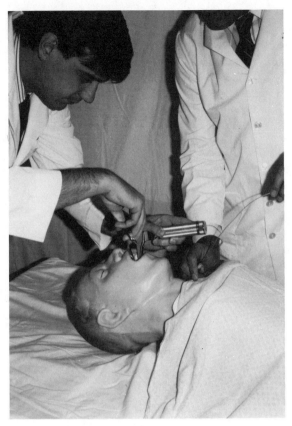

FIG 13–3.
Retrieval of the catheter from the oropharynx.

entrance of the needle through the skin. With the index finger as a guide, the needle with syringe is used to pierce the skin overlying the CTM. The needle is then angled 30 to 40 degrees caudad and the inferior aspect of the CTM is punctured to avoid the superiorly placed cricothyroid arteries[5, 20] (Fig 13–1,A and B). Free aspiration of air signals entrance into the laryngeal space. Without further advancement, the needle point is now angled cephalad at 30 to 45 degrees, and the barrel is rotated so that the bevel is directed proximally. Repeated aspiration of air confirms continued intraluminal placement.[11]

Holding the needle in this position, the syringe is removed from the hub and the guide wire or catheter is passed through the needle (Fig 13–2,A and B) and retrieved from the mouth under direct vision (Figs 13–3 and 13–4,A and B). The introducing needle is removed and a clamp is placed on the trailing end of the guide wire or catheter to prevent pulling it inadvertently through the puncture site. The proximal end of the guide wire is then passed through a lubricated, cuffed endotracheal tube via the side hole. Originally, the technique called for threading the guide through the bevel of the endotracheal tube. As a result, frequently either the tip of the endotracheal tube did not pass between the cords or flipped out of the trachea when the catheter was withdrawn, resulting in esophageal intubation.

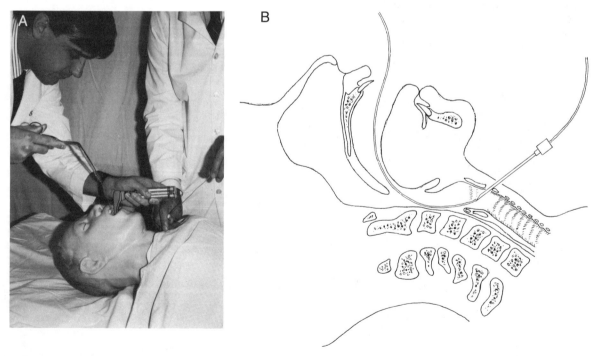

FIG 13–4.
A and **B,** retrograde passage of the guide catheter out of the mouth.

B

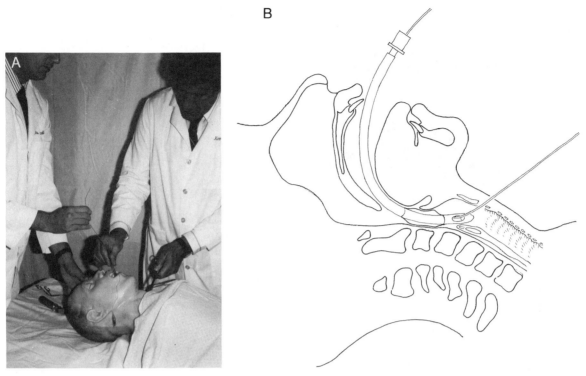

FIG 13–5.
A and **B,** the endotracheal tube is passed over the guide catheter to the puncture site.

Bourke and Levesque[7] found that placement of the guide wire through the side hole of the endotracheal tube (Murphy's eye), previously described by Powell and Ozdil,[3] allows an additional 10 to 11 mm of endotracheal tube to be within the trachea prior to removal of the guide wire (see Fig 13–6), thereby increasing the chance of its subsequent passage into the trachea.[3, 6, 7]

With the guide wire or catheter under slight tension (an assistant may be of value here) the endotracheal tube is moved past the hypopharynx into the trachea and advanced until it will pass no further (Fig 13–5,A and B). The endotracheal tube now abuts against the wire or catheter at the level of the CTM (Fig 13–6).

At times, using this technique, the advancing beveled edge of the endotracheal tube may strike against the vocal cord. If so, the use of force to move the tube through the glottis must be avoided. Rather, simple counterclockwise rotation of the endotracheal tube 90 degrees brings Murphy's eye anterior and aligns the bevel perpendicular to the glottic slit, allowing the tube to pass.[8]

While applying gentle distad pressure on the endotracheal tube, the guide catheter or wire is cut flush with the skin overlying the CTM (Fig 13–7), and the endotracheal tube is immediately slid distally

into the trachea as the wire tension is released. The wire is withdrawn from the mouth in a retrograde direction (cephalad) to prevent contamination of cervical soft tissues at the puncture site.

Keeping the guide wire taut minimizes the risk of the tube kinking or passing into the esophagus. However, in so doing, the wire introducer moves anteriorly toward the narrowest portion of the glottis which may impede passage of the tube. King et al.[13] addressed this problem with a slight modification in technique. First, retrograde passage of the guide wire is accomplished as described above. Then,

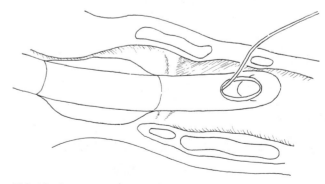

FIG 13–6.
The tip of the endotracheal tube is just inferior to the puncture site, the guide catheter exiting from Murphy's eye.

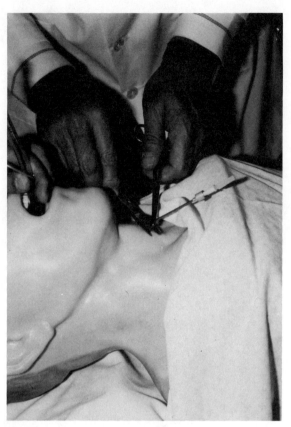

FIG 13–7.
The guide catheter is cut flush with the skin while downward pressure is maintained on the endotracheal tube.

rather than immediately threading the endotracheal tube, the plastic sheath protector that comes with the wire is cut to a length of 60 to 65 cm, straightened slightly, passed over the proximal end of the wire, and advanced toward the larynx. When the plastic sheath passes into the larynx and reaches the puncture point, it is immobilized while the wire is cut and withdrawn, as described above. The sheath is then advanced into the trachea, a lubricated endotracheal tube is inserted to the desired distance using the plastic sheath as a stylet, and the sheath is then withdrawn. Recently, a prepackaged set has become available which uses a 4-mm Teflon catheter-over-wire introducer to facilitate passage of the tube (see Fig 13–8: Cook Critical Care, Bloomington, Ind.).

Nasotracheal Route

Should nasal intubation be desired, and time is not a limiting factor, a small lubricated rubber urethral catheter may be inserted through the nose and retrieved through the mouth. The retrograde laryngeal wire is then secured to the urethral catheter and pulled through the nasal opening (Fig 13–9,A–C). The wire may then be threaded through the endotracheal tube and used as a guide in the manner described above.[3]

PREHOSPITAL PERSPECTIVE

Barriot and Riou[4] reported their experience in applying this procedure to trauma patients in the field within a prehospital mobile emergency care unit staffed by a nurse and a physician. A guide wire was delivered via needle cricothyrotomy through the mouth and a cuffed endotracheal tube was then advanced over the wire into the trachea. Rigid laryngoscopy was used to assist in retrieval of the wire in

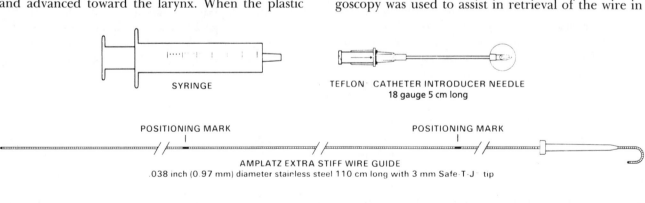

SYRINGE

TEFLON CATHETER INTRODUCER NEEDLE
18 gauge 5 cm long

POSITIONING MARK

POSITIONING MARK

AMPLATZ EXTRA STIFF WIRE GUIDE
.038 inch (0.97 mm) diameter stainless steel 110 cm long with 3 mm Safe-T-J tip

CATHETER
Radiopaque Teflon

FIG 13–8.
The Cook retrograde intubation set. (Courtesy of Cook Critical Care, Bloomington, Ind.)

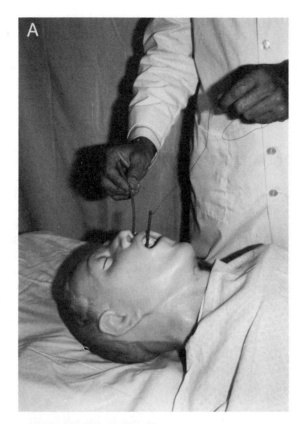

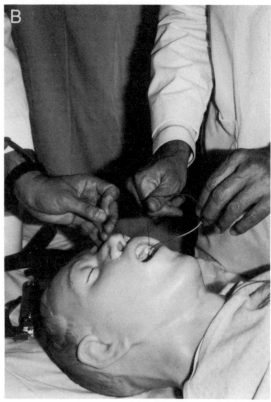

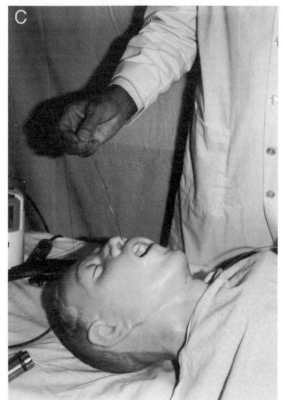

FIG 13–9.
A, the urethral catheter is passed through the nose and out the mouth. The silk suture is attached. **B,** the suture is attached to the retrograde laryngeal wire. **C,** the retrograde laryngeal guide wire is delivered through the nose.

the mouth. In patients with a grossly bloody field due to severe maxillofacial wounds, a central venous catheter was used as a guide, and air was injected through the catheter to facilitate location of the bubbling tip within the mouth. The procedure was attempted on 19 trauma patients in the field. All patients were intubated successfully on one attempt within 5 minutes and there were no serious complications.[4] While there are no data documenting the use of this procedure by nonphysician health care workers in the field, the technique is easily taught and quickly performed, and may have potential future application in this arena.[14]

PEDIATRIC PERSPECTIVE

Successful application of this technique in the pediatric population has been described in a 14-month-old infant with Pierre Robin syndrome,[21] in a 20-month-old infant with a retropharyngeal abscess,[22] and in a 30-month-old child with micrognathia.[6]

Borland et al.[6] successfully employed the following protocol. A 16-gauge red rubber catheter with a no. 2 silk suture tied to the trailing end is passed through the naris into the posterior pharynx and retrieved from the mouth. A 20-gauge needle attached to a saline-filled syringe is introduced through the CTM and its position confirmed by aspiration of air. A 0.021-extra-long flexible tip guide wire (Becton-Dickinson, 100-cm Safe guide, stainless steel guide wire) is threaded via this needle superiorly through the larynx, into the pharynx, and retrieved via the mouth. The wire and no. 2 silk suture are spliced and retrieved through the left naris. A lubricated 4.5-mm nasotracheal tube is threaded through the side hole over the wire, and while maintaining tension on the wire from both ends is advanced through the glottis. While applying gentle downward pressure on the nasotracheal tube, the guide wire is withdrawn and the tube advanced further into the trachea.

Cooper and Murray-Wilson[8] describe an oral approach used successfully on a 5-month-old, 4.8-kg infant. An 18-gauge needle is passed into the trachea and its position confirmed as above. A 25-gauge, 30-cm polyvinylchloride catheter with introducing wire is then passed through the needle and advanced through the mouth. The needle is then removed and a lubricated endotracheal tube of 2.5 mm inner diameter is passed over the catheter, through the glottis, and into the trachea.

Even in the adult population, puncture of the

CTM may be associated with significant complications (discussed below). In infants and small children, the small scale and close proximity of important neck structures add to the difficulty of this procedure. Therefore, corresponding caution and meticulous technique must be employed in this age group.

COMPLICATIONS

Potential complications associated with RTI in all age groups are mainly those related to CTM puncture, i.e., subcutaneous and mediastinal emphysema, vocal cord damage, bleeding, aspiration, esophageal puncture, bradycardia, and cardiac arrest.[5, 11, 19, 23, 24] Barriot and Riou[4] reported the use of the technique on 19 trauma patients in the field with no major complications. There was minor bleeding at the puncture site in 3 patients.[4] Guggenberger and Lenz[16] described their experience with 70 patients. There were no serious injuries of the mucous membranes or cartilage and no posterior laryngeal damage or penetration. One patient experienced significant bleeding at the puncture site.[16]

REFERENCES

1. Butler FS, Cirillo AA: Retrograde tracheal intubation. *Anesth Analg* 1960; 39:333.
2. Waters DJ: Guided blind endotracheal intubation: For patients with deformities of the upper airway. *Anaesthesia* 1963; 18:158.
3. Powell WF, Ozdil T: A translaryngeal guide for tracheal intubation. *Anesth Analg* 1967; 46:231.
4. Barriot P, Riou B: Retrograde technique for tracheal intubation in trauma patients. *Crit Care Med* 1988; 16:712.
5. McNamara RM: Retrograde intubation of the trachea. *Ann Emerg Med* 1987; 16:680.
6. Borland LM, Swan DM, Leff S: Difficult pediatric endotracheal intubation: A new approach to the retrograde technique. *Anesthesiology* 1981; 55:577.
7. Bourke D, Levesque PR: Modification of retrograde guide for endotracheal intubation. *Anesth Analg* 1974; 53:1013.
8. Cooper CMS, Murray-Wilson A: Retrograde intubation: Management of a 4.8 kg, 5-month infant. *Anaesthesia* 1987; 42:1197.
9. Freund PR, Rooke A, Schwid H: Retrograde intubation with a modified Eschmann stylet (letter). *Anesth Analg* 1988; 67:596.
10. Harrison CA, Wise CC: Retrograde intubation (letter). *Anaesthesia* 1988; 43:609.

11. Yealy DM, Paris PM: Recent advances in airway management. *Emerg Med Clin North Am* 1989; 7:83.
12. Cossham PS: Letter to the editor. *Anaesthesia* 1988; 43:609.
13. King HK, Wang LF, Khan AK, et al: Translaryngeal guided intubation for difficult intubation. *Crit Care Med* 1987; 15:869.
14. King HK, Wang LF, Wooten DJ: Endotracheal intubation using translaryngeal guided intubation vs. percutaneous retrograde guidewire insertion (letter). *Crit Care Med* 1987; 15:183.
15. Gerenstein RI, Arria-Devoe G: J-wire and translaryngeal guided intubation (letter). *Crit Care Med* 1989; 17:486.
16. Guggenberger H, Lenz G: Training in retrograde intubation (letter). *Anesthesiology* 1988; 69:292.
17. Harmer M, Vaughan R: Guided blind oral intubation (letter). *Anaesthesia* 1980; 35:921.
18. Lechman MJ, Donahoo JS, Macvaugh H: Endotracheal intubation using percutaneous retrograde guidewire insertion followed by antegrade fiberoptic bronchoscopy. *Crit Care Med* 1986; 14:589.
19. Gold MI, Buechel DR: Translaryngeal anesthesia: A review. *Anesthesiology* 1959; 20:181.
20. Kress TD, Balasubramaniam S: Cricothyroidotomy. *Ann Emerg Med* 1982; 11:197.
21. Manchester GH, Mani MM, Master FW: A simple method for emergency orotracheal intubation. *Plast Reconstr Surg* 1972; 49:312.
22. Payne KA: Difficult tracheal intubation. *Anaesth Intensive Care* 1980; 8:84.
23. Lyons GD, Garrett ME, Fourier DG: Complications of percutaneous transtracheal procedures. *Am J Otolaryngol* 1977; 86:633.
24. Spencer CD, Beaty HN: Complications of transtracheal aspiration. *N Engl J Med* 1972; 286:304.

14

Pharmacologic Aids in Airway Management

Barry Simon, M.D.

The history of anesthesia is a fascinating chronology of events that extends back to the writings of Hippocrates and Galen. Even Homer's writings include passages about infusions of herbs and various drugs that were used to induce sleep. Hundreds of years before Christ it is recorded that the sap of various seeds was used to produce euphoria, forgetfulness, and inebriation. Opium from the poppy seed was known to alleviate pain and induce sleep and is commonly discussed in much of the ancient history of medicine. One of the more unusual methods of anesthesia was used by the Assyrians for circumcision of their young male children. They describe strangulation to the point of unconsciousness to relieve the "moment" of pain. This method was used by the Italians as recently as the 17th century. In the 18th century alcohol was frequently used to produce a state of stupor prior to the onset of painful procedures.

Modern methods of anesthesia possibly begin with the use of nitrous oxide by a Connecticut dentist, Horace Wells, in the early 1840s. However, the agent, and Dr. Wells, fell into disrepute after a demonstration at the Massachusetts General Hospital failed. Crawford W. Long and William T.G. Morton, in the mid-1840s, were the first to study the effects of ether. Long frightened the community and was forced to give up his work or risk a public lynching. Morton's experiments led to a demonstration given on November 18, 1946 at Harvard Medical School. The successful induction was described by Dr. Henry Bigelow. Bigelow's and subsequent papers served to establish Morton as the discoverer of surgical anesthesia.[1]

The emergence of emergency medicine as a growing specialty led to the first major move for the use of anesthesia out of the operating room arena. Needs that are unique to the emergency department will help shape subsequent development of the drugs and techniques of anesthesia. Emergency medicine literature is replete with studies and case reports of the uses of nitrous oxide, ketamine, and neuromuscular blocking drugs. Ideal drugs and methods for techniques such as rapid-sequence intubation (RSI) are being debated and challenged. The growth of emergency medicine will continue to generate more questions and, it is hoped, some answers.

Anesthesia is defined as total loss of sensation, especially the sense of touch, in skin or mucous membrane. When loss of consciousness is added to the definition this is referred to as *general anesthesia*. *Induction* alludes to the period of time from the start of anesthesia to the attainment of the third stage. This stage is the period when there is total loss of consciousness, loss of sensation, and complete muscle paralysis. With the exception of topical cocaine and lidocaine this chapter discusses only intravenous (IV) anesthesia. Following a detailed discussion of topical anesthesia the next major section discusses the myriad drugs which may be used alone or in combination as induction agents. There is a great deal of overlap among these medications but they all may be classified as sedatives, hypnotics, or analgesics, or having a combination of these properties. Fentanyl and alfentanil have both sedative and analgesic properties whereas droperidol and haloperidol are basically sedatives. The rest of the drugs that will be discussed are all induction agents that have potent

145

sedative or hypnotic properties or both. Table 14–1 is a list of these drugs. Ketamine is unique and is discussed at length. It is the only medication that has all three properties: sedation, hypnosis, and analgesia. The last major section is an in-depth look at the neuromuscular blocking agents. The physiology of neuromuscular transmission is reviewed and followed by a detailed look at each of the drugs that have clinical significance. The chapter ends with a study of RSI.

All emergency physicians should maximize their knowledge of the drugs discussed in this chapter. Nowhere else in medicine are so many potentially dangerous drugs used in often frenzied emergent situations. Unlike the controlled confines of the operating room where time is available to check and double-check, examine and reexamine, etc., the emergency department rarely allows such luxury. Physicians who use these agents must have a ready working knowledge of the options available, their indications, contraindications, dosages, and complications.

TOPICAL ANESTHETICS

Local anesthetics are probably the most underutilized pharmacologic adjuncts for airway management. Proper application of these agents may be an

TABLE 14–1.

Pharmacology in Emergency Anesthesia

 I. Preparation
   A. Oxygen
 II. Topical anesthetics
   A. Cocaine
   B. Lidocaine
III. Induction*
   A. Thiopental (Pentothal) S,H
   B. Methohexital (Brevital) S,H
   C. Propofol (Diprivan)   S,H
   D. Etomidate (Amidate)   S,H
   E. Fentanyl   S,A
   F. Alfentanil   S,A
   G. Diazepam (Valium)   S,H
   H. Midazolam (Versed)   S,H
   I. Haloperidol (Haldol)   S
   J. Droperidol (Inapsine)   S
   K. Ketamine (Ketalar)   S,A,H
IV. Neuromuscular blocking drugs
   A. Succinylcholine (Anectine, Quelicin)
   B. Vecuronium (Norcuron)
   C. Pancuronium (Pavulon)
   D. Atracurium (Tracrium)
   E. Tubocurarine (Tubarine)

*S = sedation; H = hypnosis; A = analgesia.

---

invaluable aid for successful intubation and for patient comfort. The most commonly used local drugs are cocaine and lidocaine. Cocaine is used exclusively as a liquid applied to the nasal mucosa for nasotracheal intubation. Lidocaine is more versatile and is available as a jelly or liquid for nasal anesthesia or as a spray or liquid for topical or injected anesthesia of the oropharynx or the larynx.

Cocaine

The "caine" family of anesthetic drugs includes both esters and amides. Cocaine is an ester similar to procaine and tetracaine. It is unique in that it produces vasoconstriction in addition to topical anesthesia. Hence it is the preferred agent to provide analgesia of the nasal mucosa. Despite this clinical benefit cocaine is a potentially dangerous drug with numerous serious side effects.

Systemic toxicity may involve all organ systems. Yet its most striking effects may be in the central nervous system (CNS) and the cardiovascular system. The CNS is stimulated from higher cortical centers first and then down through the brainstem. Initial stimulation results in restlessness, excitement, and a greater capacity for work. With toxicity, patients manifest agitation, tremulousness, delirium, and eventually seizure activity. Cardiovascular toxicity is manifested by increased heart rate and blood pressure secondary to central and peripheral stimulation of the sympathetic nervous system. Large IV doses of cocaine can cause immediate death from cardiac failure due to a direct toxic action on heart muscle. Systemic toxicity may also result in death from respiratory depression. Cocaine is well absorbed from mucous membranes and exposure to large amounts or high concentrations may result in life-threatening toxicity.[2–5]

Cocaine is available in concentrations of 4% to 10% (40–100 mg/mL). The maximum safe dose is variable and ranges from 1 to 4 mg/kg. The 4% solution is highly effective and is preferred because of the drug's low safety index. Toxic reactions have occurred after administration of as little as 20 to 30 mg (less than 1 mL of the 4% solution). A dose of 1.2 g is considered fatal to most human adults yet death has been reported after ingesting significantly less. It can be applied to the nose via saturated (but not dripping wet) cotton pledgets or cotton-tip applicators. Onset of anesthesia is immediate while vasoconstriction may require 5 to 10 minutes of exposure. The duration of anesthesia is 30 to 90 minutes. Great caution should be exercised in patients with a history of hypertension, coronary artery disease, or cerebrovascular disease.[1–3]

In summary, cocaine is a drug that is to be used with a great deal of caution. With respect to airway management it can be used to anesthetize the nasopharynx in preparation for nasotracheal intubation. Small doses are effective, and therefore minimal amounts of the lowest concentration available should be used.

Lidocaine

Lidocaine is an amide similar to bupivacaine. Concentrations of 2% to 4% (20–40 mg/mL) are most effective for airway anesthesia. The maximum safe dose is 3 to 4 mg/kg. Lidocaine without epinephrine produces mucous membrane anesthesia within 1 minute and reaches maximum intensity in 2 to 5 minutes. The analgesic effect will last from 30 to 90 minutes.[3, 6]

Lidocaine may be administered in a number of ways. As with cocaine it can be applied to the nasal mucosa with cotton pledgets or applicators. Lidocaine jelly may also be placed in the nares for lubrication as well as anesthesia. More complete anesthesia of the nasopharynx can be accomplished with inhaled lidocaine in cooperative patients who require elective nasotracheal intubation.[7] Three to 5 mL of 2% lidocaine is placed in an atomizer which is attached to an oxygen source via tubing with a hole cut into the side. The patient intermittently covers the hole while inhaling the solution into each naris. Complete anesthesia from the nose to the vocal cords is achieved in about 5 minutes. The same technique may be used for anesthesia of the oropharynx by using 4 mL of 4% lidocaine administered by a hand-held nebulizer. Once again complete anesthesia past the cords is accomplished within 5 minutes. The oropharynx may also be anesthetized with commercially available lidocaine spray or by having the patient gargle several times with viscous lidocaine. Another method of achieving effective anesthesia is via direct nerve block of the glossopharyngeal or superior laryngeal nerves. The former will provide anesthesia of the mouth and pharynx while the latter blocks the larynx and superior surface of the epiglottis. These blocks may be effective but require considerable physician skill and patient cooperation.

The literature has addressed the question of how effective alternative methods are at providing airway anesthesia. Efficacy is judged by how well the cardiovascular response to intubation is blunted. Following years of study and innumerable publications,

the answer is still not clear. Various methods and solutions of lidocaine have been investigated, including direct topical application, nebulized solutions, local injection, and IV administration. Preparations have included various concentrations of viscous, IV, and nebulized solutions. Out of three studies that compared IV with topical lidocaine, two found that IV lidocaine was more effective[8, 9] and one noted greater benefit with topical lidocaine.[10] Of six studies that simply looked at the effectiveness of topical lidocaine, four found the method to be of benefit[4, 11–13] while two found the technique to be ineffective.[14, 15]

Summary

Topical lidocaine can be administered using many different methods. Patient comfort is enhanced when the drug is delivered effectively. The cardiovascular response to intubation may also be ameliorated. Intravenous lidocaine may be effective at blunting the rise in blood pressure and heart rate. The effect of IV lidocaine on intracranial pressure is discussed in Chapter 24.

INDUCTION AGENTS

Pharmacologic sedation in the context of airway management should be considered in two distinct forms. Intervention may be necessary to facilitate endotracheal intubation or to provide control of the patient for the clinician to assess and then appropriately manage the airway. The sedative-hypnotic properties desired for RSI may be obtained with drugs such as midazolam, methohexital, propofol, and others. An agitated, combative patient may need to be controlled to have the airway assessed, to have oxygen administered, or perhaps to have airway assistance with a bag and mask. Haloperidol or droperidol may be acceptable or preferred under these circumstances. Each of the drugs available has its unique pharmacologic actions and activities. Some produce significant respiratory depression and greater risk of further airway compromise. Others provide excellent sedation but render little or no analgesia. The clinical considerations are complex, yet the aid of these medications is essential.

Haloperidol

Haloperidol (Haldol), a butyrophenone, is most commonly used in the emergency department setting for the control of agitated and combative patients. Its sedative and antipsychotic properties are useful in a number of clinical situations. The efficacy of haloperidol in the management of severe alcohol withdrawal, agitated trauma patients, and acute psychosis is well described. The drug may also be used to help gain control of the airway in agitated patients. It has not been studied as an adjunct to RSI. The effect of haloperidol on intracranial pressure is not known.

Clinical Considerations

Serious acute complications are rare. Cardiovascular changes include tachycardia, transient hypotension, and occasionally hypertension. These sequelae have not been found to be clinically significant, even in critically ill patients. Haloperidol will lower the seizure threshold and therefore should be used with added caution in patients with a seizure history. Extrapyramidal reactions are the most common side effects.[16] These reactions are readily treated with anticholinergic or antiparkinsonian drugs with rapid resolution. Sudden death has been reported in patients receiving haloperidol. The incidence is extremely rare and a true causal relationship has not been proved. Another rare but potentially life-threatening complication is neuroleptic malignant syndrome. This entity is more common in patients on chronic therapy but has been reported after a single dose. The syndrome consists of diffuse muscular rigidity, akinesia, and fever. Laboratory studies usually document leukocytosis, elevated liver enzymes, and myoglobinuria from rhabdomyolosis. Treatment is generally supportive, often with less than satisfying results.[17-20]

Pharmacokinetics

Haloperidol can be given orally, intramuscularly (IM), or IV. Intravenously, onset of sedation begins within 5 minutes and can be repeated every 5 to 60 minutes as necessary. Aliquots of 5 to 10 mg IV, given to combative, out-of-control patients, may result in impressive calming within minutes. However, some severely agitated patients may need much higher doses before adequate control is achieved. It is not unusual to administer 30 or 40 mg and reports of using more than 100 mg in a 24-hour period have been recorded.[21] Intramuscular injection results in peak plasma concentrations within 10 to 20 minutes and peak pharmacologic effect in 30 to 45 minutes.[17]

Practical Airway Considerations

The use of haloperidol in airway management is recommended for its ability to calm and sedate patients. This may be to facilitate preoxygenation or active airway management short of endotracheal intubation. The drug will not produce apnea and has minimal effect on the cardiovascular system. Haloperidol is not recommended for induction.

Droperidol

The indications for droperidol (Inapsine), another butyrophenone, concerning airway management are the same as for haloperidol. Droperidol has been used mostly as a preoperative medication to achieve sedation and for its antiemetic effects. It is frequently used in conjunction with opiates as it serves to potentiate their analgesic effect and to act as an anxiolytic.

Clinical Considerations

The benefits of droperidol over haloperidol include its rapid onset, more potent sedation, and a lower incidence of dystonic reaction. In addition, it may actually raise the seizure threshold as it will return electroencephalogram (EEG) patterns to normal following its administration. The cardiovascular effects are rarely clinically significant. Yet droperidol does have some α-adrenergic blocking properties that can occasionally result in significant hypotension. This response is rare and is more common in patients who are also hypovolemic when they receive the drug. When used to premedicate patients prior to induction, droperidol will help to blunt the cardiovascular response to intubation.[22, 23]

Pharmacokinetics

The pharmacokinetics of droperidol are similar to haloperidol although the onset of action for droperidol is faster. When droperidol is used concomitantly with other CNS depressants, such as opiates, the dose of each medication should be reduced. The sedative and respiratory depressant properties of the combined drugs are cumulative. In agitated patients its calming and sedative properties are impressive. Intravenously, results may be obtained within minutes but when administered IM it may take up to 30 minutes to produce desired effects.

The dose of droperidol is 2.5 to 10.0 mg IV or IM. For the control of agitated patients, 7.5 or 10.0 mg can be used initially. When used as an antiemetic, an anxiolytic, or in conjunction with a narcotic, the starting dose should be no greater than 5 mg. It is also recommended that in elderly or debilitated patients smaller doses be used.[22-24]

Practical Airway Considerations

The use of droperidol in airway management is the same as with haloperidol, yet the more rapid and more potent qualities of droperidol make it preferable. Patients undergoing elective intubation may benefit from premedication with droperidol.

Diazepam

Diazepam (Valium) is the prototypal benzodiazepine. It is basically an anxiolytic but also provides muscle relaxation and mild sedation. In addition, it provides antegrade amnesia and has potent anticonvulsant properties. With respect to airway management, diazepam is most useful as a sedative once definitive control has been secured. It can also be used to help control agitated patients who may require less invasive airway management. It cannot be used alone to produce profound anesthesia unless very large doses are used (800 µg/kg). This use is further limited by its relatively slow onset and recovery compared with other available drugs.[25, 26]

Clinical Considerations

Benzodiazepines have been proved to be teratogenic in the first trimester and therefore must be avoided early in pregnancy or when pregnancy may be suspected. Although the respiratory depressant effects are mild, caution should be great when diazepam is administered to patients with chronic obstructive pulmonary disease (COPD). In addition, diazepam is very irritating to veins. Extravasation is likely to produce venous thrombosis or phlebitis. The IV catheter should be secured in a large vein and the solution should be injected slowly.[25, 26]

Pharmacokinetics

The usual adult dose of diazepam is 2 to 10 mg slow IV bolus injection (0.2–0.3 mg/kg in children), yet there is a great deal of interpatient variability. Sedation occurs in 1 to 2 minutes and lasts 2 to 4 hours. Hypotension and apnea are rare complications unless associated with rapid IV injection. The drug may be administered IM but absorption tends to be erratic. Benzodiazepines will potentiate the actions of other CNS depressants and can cause cardiovascular and respiratory depression when used in combination. The desired effect can be obtained by titrating the dose with 2.5- to 5.0-mg aliquots.[25, 26]

Practical Airway Considerations

Diazepam should not be used as an induction drug. In an emergency, very large doses may produce the desired effect but it would not be the drug of choice. Its greatest role in airway management is to provide moderate sedation subsequent to or following active airway management. The role of diazepam may become greater once reversal drugs are approved for use in the United States.

Midazolam

Midazolam (Versed) is a water-soluble benzodiazepine that is two to four times as potent as diazepam. It is a rapid-acting drug with a much shorter duration of action. Like diazepam, it has potent amnestic properties as well as sedative and anticonvulsant activity. It can be used for conscious sedation or it can be administered along with an analgesic for induction of anesthesia. The hypnotic, anxiolytic effects of midazolam make it an excellent adjunct in IV anesthesia.[26-30]

Clinical Considerations

The undisturbed patient will have a slight decrease in intracranial pressure following the administration of midazolam. However, midazolam will not block the rise of intracranial pressure associated with intubation. The drug will depress the ventilatory response to carbon dioxide and can produce apnea. Care should be taken never to use rapid IV administration and to be extracautious when other sedatives have been used concurrently. A slight to moderate fall in blood pressure can be anticipated. The change in heart rate is variable and has not been found to be clinically significant.[26, 27, 30, 31]

Pharmacokinetics

Midazolam is not irritating to the veins and will not produce phlebitis. It is well absorbed IM. The drug is metabolized in the liver with most of its metabolites being excreted in the urine. The pharmacokinetics depend on the dose and method of administration. Generally, following an IV injection, onset of sedation begins in 1 to 2 minutes and functional recovery occurs in 30 to 120 minutes.[26, 27, 29]

The dose required for conscious sedation ranges from 1 to 5 mg. The amount should be titrated with 0.5-mg increments every 2 minutes until the desired effect is reached. Lower doses should be used in the elderly, when other CNS depressants are being administered, and in patients with COPD. To provide sedation and hypnosis for induction prior to intubation, the recommended dose varies from 0.07 to 0.3 mg/kg.[26–29, 31]

Practical Clinical Considerations

Midazolam is a much more effective induction drug than diazepam and is excellent for sedation. Its relatively long duration of activity limits its usefulness in short procedures but may be of benefit when prolonged sedation is desired.

Flumazenil

Flumazenil is a benzodiazepine antagonist that has been available in Europe since the early 1980s. It has been found to be a safe and effective reversal drug that should be available in the United States soon. The drug is a highly specific competitive antagonist acting at the benzodiazepine receptor site. The minimum effective dose is 0.2 mg IV and the maximum dose needed is 1 mg. Flumazenil has no independent effect on the pulmonary or cardiovascular system and doses up to 3,000 times the therapeutic dose are well tolerated. The half-life is about 1 hour, and therefore caution must be exercised before discharging patients who may have received or ingested longer-acting benzodiazepines. Clinical studies and reports in the United States have found the drug to be effective as a diagnostic and therapeutic tool.[32–34]

Propofol

Propofol (Diprivan) is a 2,6-diisopropylphenol with potent sedative-hypnotic properties. The drug is a proposed alternative to benzodiazepines and barbiturates such as thiopental for induction of anesthesia. Investigators have been studying propofol because of its rapid onset of action, rapid recovery with little hangover effect, powerful amnestic properties, and minimal effect on heart rate.

Clinical Considerations

Propofol may have profound cardiopulmonary effects. It will attenuate the rise in blood pressure and intracranial pressure in response to endotracheal intubation. Yet, when the airway is not being manipulated it results in a fall in systolic, diastolic, and cerebral perfusion pressures of 20% to 30%. This concern of hypotension, especially in hypovolemic patients, is the greatest contraindication to the use of propofol. It also blunts the respiratory response to CO_2. The response is more potent than the effect seen with diazepam and frequently causes

apnea when administered as a rapid bolus injection. When administered as an IV bolus slowly or as an infusion, apnea has not been noted to be a clinically significant concern. Less serious adverse effects include a burning, stinging pain on injection, and nausea with occasional emesis.[35]

Pharmacokinetics

Given as a bolus of 2.0 to 2.5 mg/kg IV for induction during RSI, loss of consciousness occurs in less than 1 minute and lasts for about 5 minutes. Propofol can also be given as an infusion for longer procedures. The average initial dose is about 1 mg/kg followed by a continuous infusion of 2 to 9 mg/kg/hr. Time to recovery after continuous infusion is swift, with eye opening in about 5 minutes and complete recovery in 10 to 30 minutes. A lower induction dose (up to 50% lower) and a slower rate of administration should be used in elderly or debilitated patients. Although the drug is primarily metabolized by the liver, its pharmacokinetics do not appear to be altered in patients with chronic liver disease or renal failure. Propofol is only slightly soluble in water and is formulated in a white, oil-in-water emulsion. Because it is difficult to keep the drug in solution it is recommended that the ampule be shaken well prior to injection.[26, 35–40]

Practical Airway Considerations

Propofol can be used as an induction agent for endotracheal intubation but must be followed by an infusion or by the administration of a longer-acting sedative. Compared with most of the alternative induction agents, propofol has the most rapid recovery period. In the emergency department setting, the rapid recovery of patients receiving propofol makes propofol an attractive alternative for the short procedures often performed. Unlike barbiturates, propofol is not contraindicated in patients with a history of asthma or porphyria. Its use as a continuous infusion is limited because most emergency departments are not set up for the close monitoring that would be required. This is an increasingly popular drug that has great potential in the emergency and outpatient setting.

Thiopental

Thiopental (Pentothal) is a short-acting barbiturate that is most commonly used as an induction agent to provide sedation during anesthesia. Its greatest advantages are its rapid onset of action, short duration of activity, and profound sedation.

Clinical Considerations

Cardiopulmonary effects of thiopental include a fall in blood pressure of about 10% during induction which may be more pronounced in hypovolemic patients. Thiopental does not attenuate the rise in heart rate and blood pressure that occurs during intubation. Apnea lasting greater than 10 seconds occurs in about 80% of patients receiving induction doses. Slow IV injection may prevent or minimize the extent of apnea. As with all barbiturates extravasation can cause tissue damage and accidental arterial injection may produce an arteritis that may progress to gangrene. Consider injecting 40 to 80 mg of papaverine locally if there is extravasation or accidental intraarterial injection. Local infiltration of an α-adrenergic blocking agent such as phentolamine may also be attempted. Barbiturates are also contraindicated in patients with porphyria.[26, 41]

Pharmacokinetics

Administration of thiopental as an IV bolus of 3 to 5 mg/kg will induce unconsciousness within 20 to 40 seconds which lasts for 5 to 10 minutes. Sedation can be maintained with intermittent boluses of 25 to 50 mg or by titrating an infusion with a drug concentration of 0.2% to 0.4%. Recovery is delayed after repeated doses because the drug accumulates in fatty tissue and is slowly released. It is metabolized in the liver and its degradation products are excreted by the kidneys.[26, 41–45]

Practical Airway Considerations

Thiopental is one of the most common drugs used for induction. It has a long history of being safe and effective. Newer drugs have little benefit over thiopental and it has few major contraindications. Physicians that are comfortable with the drug have no reason to change. All clinicians should become comfortable with at least one other drug from a different class.

Methohexital

Methohexital (Brevital) is an ultrashort-acting barbiturate that is at least twice as potent as thiopental with a duration of action that is about half as long. Clinical indications and contraindications are similar to thiopental.

Clinical Considerations

Precautions are generally directed toward the cardiopulmonary system and CNS. Methohexital will cause a moderate fall in systolic blood pressure and a significant increase in heart rate. Respiratory drive may be reduced by up to 50% for several minutes and should be anticipated, especially in patients with compromised respiratory function. Methohexital must also be used with great caution or avoided altogether in patients with a history of seizure disorder. The seizure threshold is reduced and status epilepticus is a reported complication. Intraarterial injection may cause thrombosis and gangrene distal to the injection site. Treatment considerations are discussed under Thiopental. Rapid injection of induction doses can cause respiratory depression and apnea.[26, 46–50]

Pharmacokinetics

Methohexital does not appear to concentrate in fatty tissue as much as other barbiturates and therefore has less cumulative effect. The induction dose of 1 to 2 mg/kg IV produces loss of consciousness in less than 30 seconds and this persists for 4 to 7 minutes. Sedation may be maintained with boluses of 20 to 40 mg every 5 minutes as needed or with an infusion of a 0.2% solution. Methohexital is generally administered IV, but pediatric studies have found it to be safely and effectively administered rectally in a 2% solution for induction of anesthesia. As with other barbiturates methohexital is metabolized in the liver. In patients with severe liver failure its duration of activity may be greatly prolonged.[46]

Practical Airway Considerations

Methohexital is similar to thiopental. Rapid recovery offers added safety with difficult intubations but practical differences are minimal.

Etomidate

Etomidate (Amidate) is a nonnarcotic, nonbarbiturate hypnotic agent that was introduced in the early 1980s as an alternative induction drug. Chemically, etomidate is the ester of a carboxylated imidazole and is unique. The purpose of introducing another rapid-acting, short-duration compound was to improve upon the cardiopulmonary complications of the other drugs that are available.

Clinical Considerations

The major disadvantages of etomidate include the development of uncomfortable myoclonic muscle movements during induction in up to 33% of patients. The drug can be painful during injection and may produce nausea or vomiting in a large number of patients. Unlike barbiturates, etomidate failed to attenuate succinylcholine-induced hyperkalemia. Plasma cortisol and aldosterone levels are reduced for 6 to 8 hours after induction with etomidate. Exogenous replacement is necessary under the appropriate clinical circumstances.[45, 51–53]

Pharmacokinetics

The induction dose of 0.2 to 0.4 mg/kg produces loss of consciousness and a duration of action similar to propofol. Etomidate has relatively minimal cardiovascular effects and produces less respiratory depression. Tachycardia and apnea may occur but to a lesser extent than with most of the other induction agents. Cerebral perfusion pressure, intracerebral pressure, cerebral oxygen consumption, and intraocular pressure are all decreased. In addition, etomidate does not cause histamine release and bronchospasm.[45, 51, 52]

Practical Airway Considerations

Etomidate should be considered an alternative induction drug (after all the other induction drugs discussed here). It may be considered most seriously in patients with coronary artery disease or elevated intracranial pressure.

Opioids

Opioids are potent analgesics which also produce significant sedation. These two properties make the drugs discussed below, fentanyl and alfentanil, excellent induction agents. In addition, their rapid onset, brief duration, and ability to be reversed make them nearly ideal in the emergency department setting.

Fentanyl

Fentanyl is a narcotic analgesic with a potency that is 70 to 150 times that of morphine. It is most often used to provide sedation and analgesia as an adjunct to general anesthesia. It can be used as premedication, during induction, in maintenance, or postoperatively. In the emergency department its use is primarily restricted to sedation and analgesia during RSI and as maintenance while the patient remains paralyzed.[54]

Clinical Considerations.—Respiratory depression, excessive sedation, and nausea are the primary concerns when using fentanyl. These effects can rapidly be reversed by naloxone. Parasympathetic stimulation may produce profound bradycardia and hypotension that does respond to atropine. How-

ever, added caution should be exercised in patients who have preexisting bradyarrhythmias. Other CNS depressant drugs such as barbiturates, benzodiazepines, and butyrophenones potentiate the effects of fentanyl and the dose should be adjusted accordingly. Skeletal muscle rigidity can occur and on rare occasions may be severe enough to cause management problems. The incidence is related to the dose and speed of injection. The concomitant use of neuromuscular blocking drugs will prevent this complication. Fentanyl has been noted to blunt the hemodynamic reactions to intubation.[55, 56]

Pharmacokinetics.—Fentanyl is provided in solution at a concentration of 50 μg/mL. It may be stored at room temperature but must be protected from light. The recommended dose varies depending on the indication, age of the patient, etc. A low initial dose of 2 μg/kg may be used for mild sedation or for minor but painful surgical procedures. For severe persistent pain and stressful circumstances, doses of up to 20 μg/kg may be needed. Intravenously, the onset of effect is in less than 1 minute with a peak effect at 2 to 4 minutes. The duration of action is 30 to 60 minutes. Intramuscularly, the onset is in 7 to 8 minutes and the duration of action is 1 to 2 hours. The duration of respiratory depression may be longer than the analgesic effect. The drug is primarily metabolized in the liver and the majority is excreted as various metabolites in the urine. Fentanyl is highly fat-soluble and repeat doses will accumulate in fatty tissue. Under these circumstances the effective half-life may be significantly prolonged.[55]

Practical Airway Considerations.—Fentanyl is a practical drug for use in emergency department anesthesia. It has been found to be safe and effective as an adjunct to RSI as it attenuates the circulatory responses to airway manipulation.[56] It also satisfies several other practical concerns that often are of importance to emergency physicians. The drug is rapid-acting with an onset of action of less than 1 minute. It is readily reversible, yet can last long enough for most emergency procedures and studies.[57]

Alfentanil

A newer opioid analgesic has been introduced and is worthy of a brief discussion. Alfentanil is a derivative of fentanyl that is pharmacologically similar to the parent drug but is notable for a more rapid onset of action and a shorter duration. Significant drug effect occurs within 30 seconds and peaks in less than 2 minutes. The duration of action is less than 15 minutes when small doses are used. Alfentanil is one fourth to one tenth as potent as fentanyl and this is reflected in the recommended induction dose of 20 to 40 μg/kg. In addition, it is less fat-soluble than the parent compound and its volume of distribution is less than 25% that of fentanyl. Although the hepatic clearance of alfentanil is actually slower than fentanyl, its half-life is much shorter because of its relatively small volume of distribution. Faster elimination means that alfentanil is less likely to produce the cumulative effects seen with fentanyl. Prolonged respiratory depression is less likely to occur even when large doses are used. Other clinical concerns and complications are nearly identical to those of the parent drug. For longer procedures fentanyl would be preferred, yet when rapid onset may be advantageous, such as with RSI, alfentanil may be the better choice.[58-60]

Practical Airway Considerations.—Fentanyl and alfentanil are excellent induction choices. For patients who need analgesia in addition to sedation, these drugs are preferable to barbiturates or benzodiazepines. Fentanyl may be preferred over alfentanil as noted above. However, their characteristics are such that the clinician can effectively choose the drug he or she is most comfortable with.

Ketamine

Ketamine (Ketalar) was produced in the laboratory in 1963 as a result of manipulations of the drug phencyclidine (PCP). Its sedative, amnestic, and analgesic properties make it unique. Acceptance by emergency medicine physicians has not been widespread, yet it has characteristics which suggest it may be useful and at times lifesaving. Reluctance to use ketamine may derive from its notoriety as a street drug or perhaps from reports of nightmares, often referred to as the emergence phenomenon. Despite past hesitation, the increase in the number of studies documenting its advantages, and which appear to show few serious side effects, has renewed interest in the drug.

Ketamine is not a true general anesthetic because protective airway reflexes are maintained and there is no clinically significant respiratory depression. Muscle tone is maintained and purposeful movements may occur unrelated to painful stimuli. However, sedation, analgesia, and amnesia are profound, allowing for the performance of invasive procedures often without any adjunctive medication.

The effect produced has been described as "dissociative anesthesia." Ketamine actually produces a functional and electrophysiologic dissociation between the cortical and limbic systems. The result is a trancelike state in which the patient's eyes are open yet the patient is totally unaware of his or her surroundings and of the manipulation or procedure he or she is undergoing.[61, 62]

Clinical Considerations
Airway.—Active airway intervention, such as endotracheal intubation, is rarely needed when ketamine is used. Protective airway reflexes—cough, sneeze, and gag—are maintained. Respiratory drive remains intact despite a mild dose-related depression. Minute ventilation is unaffected but there appears to be a slightly decreased response to hypercapnia. Very high doses of ketamine have been associated with case reports of respiratory depression. It is postulated that this may have been from a loss of response to a rising carbon dioxide partial pressure (PCO_2). Regardless of the risk, intubation paraphernalia should be on hand and prepared for use should the need arise.[63]

Risk of aspiration is one of the basic concerns of airway management. Several studies have looked at the risk with ketamine and reported varying results. Barium studies have shown that aspiration does occur in a significant number of patients but the clinical importance of these data is questioned. Perhaps the most practical data come from a paper that reviewed 97 series of over 11,000 pediatric patients in which no cases of aspiration were reported. As with any drug that may depress the level of consciousness, ketamine should be avoided in patients with a full stomach. Yet, clinically, the risk appears to be minimal and is certainly unavoidable in most emergency department settings.[62]

Laryngospasm is another feared complication of all drugs involved with anesthesia and airway management. With ketamine the cause may be related to stimulation of hypersensitized laryngeal reflexes or from the irritation caused by excessive secretions. Ketamine stimulates the release of salivary and tracheobronchial secretions. Most authors recommend the concurrent use of an anticholinergic drug such as atropine to help limit the amount of these secretions, yet ketamine has been used safely in a large number of patients without adjunctive therapy. Although laryngospasm has been reported in patients receiving ketamine, the incidence appears to be significantly less than the reported incidence associated with traditional general anesthesia. The pediatric series noted above reported 2 patients in 11,589 (0.017%) who had spasm that was severe enough to require endotracheal intubation. In general anesthesia, the overall incidence has been noted to be 0.87% and in children less than 10 years of age, 1.74%. Laryngospasm has been noted to be more common in infants 3 months old or younger and in patients of all ages who have active respiratory infection. The presence of respiratory infection should be considered a relative contraindication to the use of ketamine and until more information is available, its use in infants 3 months old or younger should be avoided.[62]

Pulmonary.—There is evidence that ketamine is a potent bronchodilator and thus helpful in patients with status asthmaticus. This effect may be the result of increased circulating catecholamines, a direct relaxation of smooth muscle, inhibition of vagal impulses, or a combination of the three. There are several papers that report marked improvement in asthmatics who received ketamine after failure with all standard treatment modalities. Similar beneficial responses have been noted in patients with bronchospasm from inhalational anesthesia and in ventilator patients with refractory bronchospasm. Ketamine should be seriously considered for emergency department asthmatic patients who have been refractory to other forms of treatment. With the incidence of asthma increasing, the role of ketamine may become much greater as emergency physicians become more familiar with the drug.[64–66]

Cardiovascular.—Ketamine acts on the cardiovascular system to increase heart rate, blood pressure, and cardiac output. It also increases coronary artery perfusion and myocardial contractility, ultimately increasing myocardial oxygen consumption. All of these effects are more pronounced when the drug is given by rapid IV injection. The responses are minimal when administered IM. These properties have helped to make ketamine a popular drug in the sedation and anesthesia of hypovolemic patients. Ketamine should be used with caution in patients with coronary artery disease and in those with hypertension.[62]

Neuromuscular.—Hypertonicity is commonly reported when ketamine is used. The degree of increased tone is dose-related and may become excessive at very high doses. Myoclonic movements have been noted and occasionally mistaken for seizure activity. However, the movements are benign and are

not associated with EEG changes. There are case reports of ketamine being used successfully to treat seizures. Ketamine will raise intracranial pressure through vasodilation and increased systemic vascular resistance. The effect may be substantial and head trauma should be considered a strong relative contraindication. Animal studies have shown that the administration of benzodiazepines will blunt the rise of intracranial pressure.

Emergence Phenomenon.—The emergence phenomenon refers to the hallucinations or unusual dreams that may be experienced following the administration of ketamine. Experiences have been described as nightmares, out-of-body states, visualizing vivid or psychedelic colors, etc. This phenomenon is presumably one of the major reasons for the reluctance of emergency physicians to become more familiar with the use of this drug. A number of studies have explored the causes for these unusual reactions. The dissociative state, which literally divides the connections between the cortical and limbic systems, undoubtedly plays an integral role. It is of interest, however, that patients who are well prepared with verbal instructions to anticipate pleasant dreams have far fewer uncomfortable experiences, whereas patients with personality disorders or psychiatric disease have a significantly higher rate of unpleasant reactions. Emergence reactions are more common in adults, women, in those who receive rapid IV injection, and where there was excessive noise or stimulation during recovery. Administration of benzodiazepines or narcotics along with ketamine will ameliorate the emergence experience. Although there is a case report of two 3-year-old children who apparently had personality changes for as long as 12 months, other studies suggest that it is highly unlikely that ketamine causes permanent change in personality or intellectual function.[62]

Pharmacokinetics

Ketamine is water-soluble at commercial concentrations and yet maintains lipid solubility that allows it to quickly pass the blood-brain barrier. In the CNS ketamine blocks association of the limbic system from the higher cortical centers, preventing the perception of visual, auditory, or painful stimuli. The mechanism of this action is unknown. Intravenously administered, peak concentration occurs in the CNS within 1 minute. The drug will redistribute in the peripheral tissue fairly rapidly as the average patient will regain coherence in about 15 minutes. Intramuscular injection will produce peak levels in about

5 minutes. Return of coherence is variable and ranges from 30 to 120 minutes. The half-life in adults is 2 to 3 hours and closer to 2 hours in children. Although little is known about the detailed metabolism of ketamine, the liver begins breakdown via methylation in the cytochrome P-450 system to a weakly active metabolite. The majority of breakdown products are eventually excreted in the urine.

Ketamine may be administered IV or IM. It is prepared as a water-soluble solution that does not need to be refrigerated. It may also be given orally or rectally but induction and recovery times are slower. Dosing schedules are confusing and depend on the method of administration, the goal one wishes to attain, and the age of the patient. Some physicians have described using subdissociative amounts in the belief that it will decrease the occurrence of side effects. This has not been shown to be true and full dissociative doses appear to have as wide a safety margin as subdissociative doses. In addition, doses of ketamine sufficient to produce dissociation provide better immobilization and eliminate the need for adjunctive analgesia or anesthesia.

The range of IV dosing reported in the literature is 0.25 to 11 mg/kg. To achieve dissociation the recommended dose is 1 to 2 mg/kg. Continuous IV infusions may result in fewer emergence reactions and a shorter recovery period. It is recommended that a bolus of 1 mg/kg be followed with an infusion of 0.5 to 1.0 mg/kg/hr. Continuous therapy has not been studied in children. Single doses can be supplemented with an additional 5 to 10 mg IV as needed. The range of IM dosing reported is 0.5 to 17 mg/kg. To achieve dissociation the range was 4 to 13 mg/kg. There does not seem to be a greater incidence of side effects from higher dosing (7–17 mg/kg), yet lower doses (4–7 mg/kg) were equally efficacious.[61, 62, 67]

Practical Airway Considerations

Ketamine has been studied mostly in the pediatric population as an agent to be used in situations where analgesia or immobilization is needed. It has been proved safe and effective under these circumstances. In adults, in whom the emergence phenomenon is of greater concern, it should be used with more caution. Although more studies need to be done it appears that ketamine may be a potentially lifesaving treatment for refractory status asthmaticus. Ketamine may also be considered an induction adjunct for endotracheal intubation, especially for the asthmatic patient in respiratory failure.

Because ketamine has been shown to support the cardiovascular system it has a role in providing analgesia and anesthesia in patients who are hypovolemic. In military surgery, ketamine is considered an excellent drug for use in trauma patients for this reason. In addition, the flexibility with methods of administration, the fact that it does not need to be refrigerated, and its short half-life are also beneficial. It must, however, be avoided in patients with head trauma because of its potential to raise intracranial pressure. This sequela prevents ketamine from being used to sedate most patients for radiographic studies such as computed tomography (CT) of the head.

Summary

The variety of induction drugs available affords the clinician the opportunity to become familiar with at least one from each class. Emergency physicians should be comfortable with a number of different drugs in order to deal expeditiously with a myriad of clinical circumstances. Any one of the drugs discussed is acceptable under most clinical situations. Thiopental and methohexital are excellent medications but alternatives must be available for the patient who has an allergy to barbiturates or has porphyria. Propofol may be the preferred agent because it has the most rapid onset of action and the shortest duration. In comparison with other drugs, patients often preferred propofol and it has been shown to be effective at blunting the cardiovascular responses to intubation. Yet options must be available for the hypotensive or hypovolemic patient who might not fare well with a drug that will cause a further reduction in blood pressure. Under these circumstances ketamine may be the optimal selection. Etomidate does not offer any major advantages compared with the other induction agents and should be considered only if there are significant contraindications to the other drugs.

The opioids, fentanyl and alfentanil, may also be considered effective induction agents, especially in circumstances when pain control is of significant benefit. Haloperidol and droperidol may be used primarily for sedation of the agitated patient. Diazepam may be used for sedation but is not an effective induction drug. Midazolam should replace diazepam for most emergency situations. It can be used for most of the same indications and is a much better induction drug. With the development of reversal drugs, the benzodiazepines will become more valuable emergency medications.

The sedation and induction drugs are summarized in Table 14–2.

TABLE 14–2.

Sedation and Induction Drugs

Drug	Dose	Onset	Duration	Comments*	Indications
Benzodiazepines					
Diazepam	2–10 mg	1–2 min	2–4 hr	Respiratory depression, hypotension, phlebitis, apnea	Used for induction but the effective dose is variable; better for sedation
Midazolam	1–5 mg; 0.07–0.3 mg/kg for induction	<1 min	30–60 min	Apnea, no phlebitis	Better than diazepam for induction; short duration is most valuable asset; may be given IM
Narcotics					
Fentanyl	2–20 µg/kg	<1 min	30–60 min	Respiratory depression; hypotension; decreased HR; reverse with naloxone; muscle rigidity	May be used for sedation, analgesia, induction; can administer IM
Alfentanil	20–40 µg/kg	<30 sec	<15 min	Same as fentanyl, but less accumulation in fatty tissue	Excellent for short procedures
Barbiturates					
Thiopental	3–5 mg/kg	20–40 sec	5–10 min	Respiratory depression; decreased BP; phlebitis; porphyria	The gold standard induction agent
Methohexital	1–2 mg/kg	<1 min	4–7 min	Same	Benefit is its short duration; good induction drug
Butyrophenones					
Droperidol	2.5–10.0 mg	5 min	60–120 min	Dystonic reactions rare; may be given IM; potent sedation	Best as premedication; potent antiemetic
Haloperidol	5–10 mg IV	5–10 min	60–120 min	Dystonic reactions common; decreased seizure threshold; decreased BP; tachycardia	Best to control severe agitation
Miscellaneous					
Propofol	2.0–2.5 mg/kg	<1 min	4–6 min	Significantly decreased BP; no tachycardia; apnea	Excellent induction drug
Etomidate	0.2–0.3 mg/kg	<1 min	4–6 min	Less cardiac and respiratory depression; myoclonus	Adequate alternative induction agent
Ketamine	1–2 mg/kg IV 4–7 mg/kg IM	1 min IV 3–5 min IM	5–15 min 30–120 min	Increased BP and HR; bronchodilation; myoclonus; lowers seizure threshold	Excellent induction drug; good for short procedures in children; for status asthmaticus in adults.

*HR = heart rate; BP = blood pressure.

NEUROMUSCULAR BLOCKADE

There can be little argument that neuromuscular blockers are powerful drugs with incredible potential to save or to harm. One should never consider their use unless he or she is intimately familiar with their pharmacologic actions and the indications are absolute. Practitioners must remember that paralyzing a patient may convert a compromised airway to no airway. When used safely, these drugs are invaluable adjuncts to endotracheal intubation. According to a survey, 95% of emergency medicine residency programs and 89% of community emergency physicians use these drugs.[68]

An understanding of the neuroanatomy and physiology of neuromuscular transmission is essential for the complete appreciation of the actions of neuromuscular blocking agents. The neuromuscular junction is the site of action for all the drugs that are discussed in this section. Their mechanisms of action, however, differ, as do their interactions with other systems of the body (Fig 14–1).

The site (synapse) where the motor end plate approximates the nerve terminal is the neuromuscular junction. As an impulse arrives at the motor nerve terminal, acetylcholine (ACh) is released and diffuses across the synaptic cleft to the cholinergic receptor on the motor end plate. Acetylcholine is the

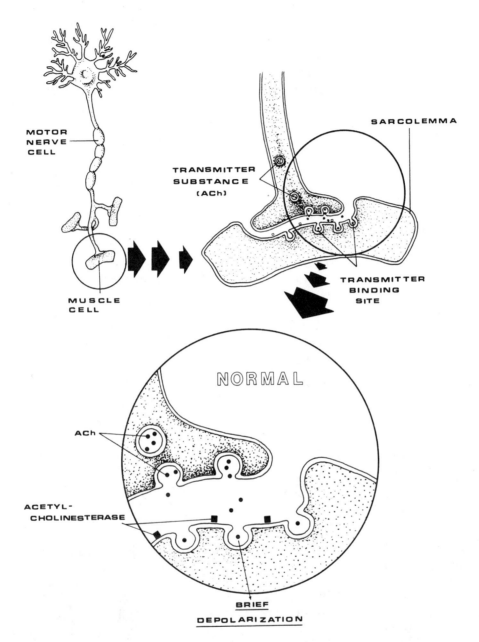

FIG 14–1.
Normal physiology of the neuromuscular junction. There is uninhibited access for ACh at the postjunctional receptors.

neurotransmitter that is stored in synaptic vesicles at the nerve terminal. Once the neurotransmitter traverses the cleft and attaches to the postjunctional receptor, the membrane permeability to sodium and potassium increases, resulting in depolarization. The depolarization of individual ACh receptors produces an end-plate potential. When sufficient ACh is released, multiple end-plate potentials are created which can summate to reach threshold and trigger a propagated action potential resulting in contraction of the skeletal muscle fiber. The event is termed *excitation-contraction coupling*. The ACh is removed by diffusion from the cleft and metabolized by the hydrolyzing action of acetylcholinesterase. The ACh metabolized at the cleft produces choline which is then available for reuptake and resynthesis of the original neurotransmitter by the motor nerve. The remainder of the ACh diffuses away from the receptor site to be hydrolyzed in the bloodstream.

As the motor nerve approaches the muscle it arborizes into smaller and smaller branches which ultimately innervate individual muscle fibers. Muscles that are intended to perform fine, delicate maneuvers have relatively few muscle fibers innervated by each nerve branch. In contrast, the large muscle groups required for power and strength may have hundreds of muscle fibers innervated by each nerve branch. Because each of these motor units responds in an all-or-none fashion, finely controlled responses can only be achieved in those units containing relatively few muscle fibers.[69–71]

As with most physiologic systems in nature, there is a wide margin of safety in the functioning of the neuromuscular junction. In healthy patients it is not possible to measure a decrease in skeletal muscle strength until 70% of the ACh receptors are blocked. Anesthesiologists generally use devices to stimulate the ulnar nerve to monitor the extent of receptor blockade. The nerve is stimulated at 2 cps (2 Hz) and the fingers are observed for 2 seconds. In the normal, nonparalyzed patient four twitches of the fingers should be noted during that period of time. The physician can assume about 75% blockade when the fourth twitch is lost. Abolition of subsequent finger responses correlate with 80%, 90%, and 100% blockade, respectively.

Return of function can be monitored in much the same way. However, from a practical standpoint it is more useful to the clinician to be able to assess when it is safe to extubate a patient. The ability to raise one's head off the pillow is an indicator of sufficient return of muscle strength to sustain respiration. This bedside test actually offers an extra measure of safety because the ability to raise one's head will lag behind the return of respiratory muscle power. The patient must be alert enough to be able to protect his or her own airway. Adequate ventilatory function for extubation can be assessed with three weaning criteria: tidal volume should be 7 to 10 mL/kg with a rate of 12 to 15 breaths per minute. Vital capacity must be greater than 15 mL/kg to generate an effective cough. Inspiratory force should exceed −20 cm H_2O pressure.[69]

Historical observation of the actions of various paralyzing agents have led to the understanding of three classes of neuromuscular blockade. One group was noted to cause opisthotonos and spasticity, while another caused a flaccid paralysis. The third phenomenon observed was the occurrence of initial spastic paralysis followed by the development of flaccidity. These three types of neuromuscular blockade are classified as depolarizing, nondepolarizing, and desensitization.

The depolarizing drugs are also called noncompetitive, nonreversible relaxants. This group of paralyzing agents includes succinylcholine and decamethonium. Initially, these drugs will bind to the postsynaptic receptors much the same as ACh. The resulting depolarization produces a brief period of repetitive excitation manifested by transient muscular fasciculations. This phase is followed by a block of neuromuscular transmission and flaccid paralysis. The mechanism of the blockade is not completely understood but some theories have been offered to explain the phenomenon. One hypothesis suggests that there is a period of desensitization during which the membrane potential is restored but the postsynaptic region remains unexcitable. Alternative explanations suggest that there is a presynaptic effect of the drugs on the cholinoceptors of the motor nerve terminal.[69–71]

Nondepolarizing, competitive, reversible, neuromuscular blockers act by competing with ACh for the postsynaptic receptors, but do not activate them. Commonly used agents in this classification include pancuronium, vecuronium, tubocurarine, and atracurium. Once the concentration of these drugs is sufficient, an action potential can no longer be generated and transmission will fail. Characteristics of this blockade include absence of fasciculations prior to paralysis, decreasing strength of contraction (fade on successive twitches), and eventual antagonism by acetylcholinesterase inhibitors (neostigmine, pyridostigmine, and edrophonium) (Fig 14–2).[69–72]

A phase II or mixed block has been referred to as a desensitization-type block. The exact mechanism is unknown but its clinical characteristics are similar to those produced by nondepolarizing drugs. The block is a common result of prolonged or repeated exposure to depolarizing agents. If well-established, it may not be possible to reverse the block with neostigmine or other acetylcholinesterase inhibitors.[72]

A number of factors may potentiate or antagonize neuromuscular blockade. The list of influences is long and confusing because their effects may be different depending on which class of drugs is being used. For example, respiratory acidosis and hypokalemia will augment nondepolarizing blockade but will oppose the action of depolarizing agents. However, factors such as hypothermia and dehydration will potentiate the actions of both groups.[70, 73] A complete list of factors influencing neuromuscular blockage is shown in Table 14–3.

Neuromuscular blocking drugs are most commonly used to provide muscle relaxation to facilitate endotracheal intubation in the operating room and

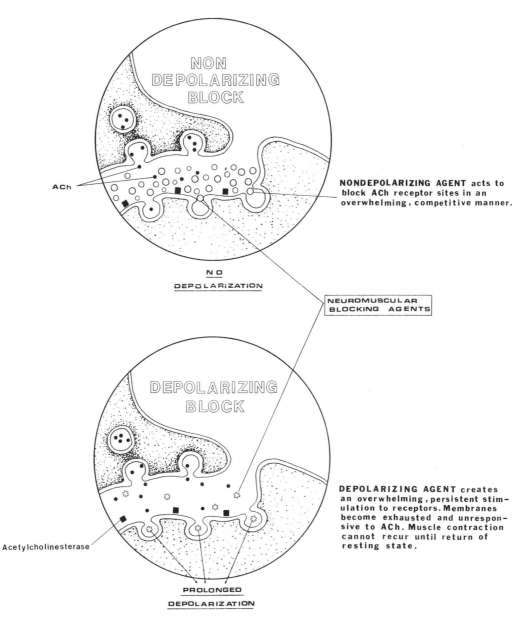

FIG 14–2.
Illustrations of the proposed mechanisms of action for the two major classes of neuromuscular blocking drugs.

in the emergency department. Recent studies have also investigated their use in prehospital settings. One study documented the safety and efficacy of succinylcholine-assisted intubation in 95 patients over a 2-year period.[74] Another looked at the use of succinylcholine and pancuronium in a helicopter ambulance program and found that the drugs could be used safely and effectively.[75] There are other medicinal uses for these drugs in intensive care unit (ICU) and emergency department settings. Patients who are excessively combative may need complete muscle relaxation to permit efficient airway control,

for performance of invasive procedures, or for control of these patients during studies such as CT scanning. Patients requiring mechanical ventilation may achieve better oxygenation at lower inspiratory pressures when they are paralyzed. The same is true for patients with refractory status asthmaticus after they are intubated. Disorders of severe muscle hypertonicity, such as tetanus and strychnine poisoning, may also benefit from complete skeletal muscle paralysis. A detailed discussion of the role of paralytic drugs in these entities as well as in other clinical situations is beyond the scope of this chapter.

TABLE 14–3.

Factors Influencing Neuromuscular Blockade

Depolarization	Nondepolarization
Potentiators	
Decreased cholinesterase	Myasthenic syndromes
Hypothermia	Hypothermia
Respiratory alkalosis	Respiratory acidosis
Dehydration	Dehydration
Hyperkalemia	Hypokalemia
Hypermagnasemia	Hypermagnasemia
Drugs	Drugs
Anticholinesterase	Sedative hypnotics
Aminoglycosides	Lidocaine, other "caines"
Tetracyclines	Quinidine
Polymyxins	Aminoglycosides
Lidocaine, other "caines"	Tetracyclines
Quinine	Polymyxins
Antagonists	
Respiratory acidosis	Respiratory alkalosis
Shock	Shock
Hypokalemia	Hypernatremia
Hypocalcemia	Anticholinesterases

Each neuromuscular blocking drug differs in its pharmacology, indications, contraindications, and so forth. Yet, because the net effect of all the drugs is the same, there are generic concerns and complications that should be considered. Paralysis prevents any further useful physical examination. This may lead to a delay in diagnosis and the discovery of additional injures. Failure to adequately sedate these patients is a common problem which can be devastating to the patient. Inadequate dosing resulting in incomplete relaxation can be dangerous if invasive procedures are underway and can delay therapeutic maneuvers. Aspiration and failed intubation requiring a surgical airway are always potential concerns.

Reversal of Neuromuscular Blockade

Emergency department physicians are rarely confronted with the need to reverse the effect of paralytic drugs. Yet an understanding of the mechanism and the pharmacology is important for better appreciation of this subject.

The mechanism of action of these drugs is related to their anticholinesterase activity. All of these reversal agents basically act by blocking the activity of both types of the cholinesterase enzyme. This action permits the local concentration of ACh molecules to rise. In addition, there is evidence that the reversal drugs may facilitate mobilization of ACh from the nerve ending. Neostigmine, edrophonium chloride, and pyridostigmine are the three most common reversal drugs used. Atropine must always be used with neostigmine because it has potent muscarinic action that results in significant bradycardia. The muscarinic effects are less when the last two drugs are used. Atropine should be on hand but may be administered as needed. The dose of neostigmine is 0.01 to 0.035 mg/kg IV; of edrophonium, 0.3 to 1.0 mg/kg; and of pyridostigmine, 0.1 to 0.25 mg/kg. Edrophonium has the most rapid onset followed by neostigmine and then pyridostigmine. Their duration of action increases in the same order. These drugs should not be used when total neuromuscular blockade is present. Peripheral nerve stimulators must document some amount of spontaneous recovery prior to their administration.[76–78]

Neuromuscular Blocking Drugs

Curare

Curare was the original nondepolarizing neuromuscular blocker and was first used for medicinal purposes in 1942. The popular literature romanticized curare for centuries and the word "curare" became associated with all poisonous arrows used in Africa and South America. Crude curare contains a number of closely related alkaloids that exert similar pharmacologic actions. The alkaloid, *d*-tubocurarine, was ultimately used to produce a semisynthetic derivative, dimethyl tubocurarine (Tubarine), that has since been used clinically. Although it has been used successfully for many years, curare has a number of clinically significant side effects that make newer agents preferable. Curare causes more release of histamine than any of the other neuromuscular blocking drugs. It can cause severe bronchospasm and is contraindicated in any patient with a history of asthma. It also produces hypotension owing to ganglionic blockade and histamine release.[70]

Pharmacokinetics.—Curare is largely excreted unchanged in the urine but biliary excretion increases significantly in patients with renal failure. The dose is 0.2 to 0.4 mg/kg IV, it provides good muscle relaxation for 45 to 75 minutes, and it can be used for complete paralysis or as a defasciculating drug prior to administering succinylcholine. Although curare is still available, it has been replaced by more refined agents that have less side effects and more predictable results.[70–72]

Succinylcholine

Succinylcholine (Anectine, Quelicin) is a synthetic depolarizing neuromuscular blocking agent. It was first described by Bovet in 1949 and later by Castillo and de Beer in 1950. The drug has retained a great deal of popularity because of its rapid onset and brief duration of action despite the risk of numerous serious complications.[72]

Clinical Considerations.—There are several potentially life-threatening complications that can result from the use of succinylcholine. Physicians who use the drug must be well versed in the potential hazards and their treatments before considering its use. Cardiac arrhythmias, hyperkalemia, increased intracranial pressure, increased intragastric pressure, rhabdomyolosis, and malignant hyperthermia are some of the more serious dangers to consider.

Succinylcholine will produce a rise in serum potassium of less than 0.5 mEq/L in healthy adults. Intracellular potassium is released as neuromuscular depolarization leads to action potential propagation. In patients with neuromuscular disease where there is functional denervation, the rise in potassium may greatly exceed 0.5 mEq/L and can approach or exceed life-threatening levels. Physicians should be aware of the dangers of succinylcholine-induced hyperkalemia under the following circumstances: extensive burns, massive trauma (especially when there is significant crush injury), lower motor neuron disease (traumatic or viral), and upper motor neuron diseases including trauma, cerebrovascular accidents, and encephalitis. Investigation into the phenomenon of hyperkalemia associated with succinylcholine administration has discovered a time relationship to many of the above diseases. Patients with upper motor neuron disease appear to be at risk from 5 to 14 days after the onset of illness and for up to 6 months after the condition stabilizes. Patients with burns and massive muscle injury are at risk from 2 to 3 days post trauma and for up to 2 to 3 months. Pretreatment with competitive blockers may prevent the rise of potassium in trauma patients but will not be helpful in postburn patients.[70–72, 79]

Cardiovascular instability may develop from the rise in serum potassium, from the vagal effects produced by succinylcholine, or from the release of histamine. The risk of bradydysrhythmia and cardiac standstill is greater in children but may be seen in adults, especially when a second dose must be administered during a prolonged intubation. In one study of 48 patients who received succinylcholine to aid intubation, 1 patient, a 53-year-old man with COPD, developed transient asystole that was easily treated with atropine and epinephrine.[79] Pretreatment with atropine or a nondepolarizing drug will

prevent this complication.[71] Histamine-induced bronchospasm and hypotension is rare.

Rhabdomyolosis can occur with clinically significant myoglobinuria and eventual renal failure. Postoperative myalgias will be present in 20% to 50% of patients. Although the muscle pain is usually mild, it may be severe and debilitating. In some patients it may require several days of bed rest and the use of analgesics. Fasciculations and muscle breakdown may be prevented or ameliorated by pretreatment with a nondepolarizing drug. This is discussed in more detail under Administration below. Increased intraocular pressure is well documented. Succinylcholine should be avoided or used with caution in patients with glaucoma or trauma to their globe. Intragastric pressure is also elevated, increasing the risk of emesis and aspiration that is always a concern during RSI. Intracranial pressure is an area of great concern for the clinician. Succinylcholine alone will increase the intracranial pressure. Many drugs are available to help blunt this effect and are discussed at length in Chapter 24.[70–72, 79–82]

There are additional complications which may be serious. Some can be avoided, while others must be anticipated to treat effectively. Powerful muscle contractions can produce additional trauma in patients with skeletal fractures. This may be avoided by using defasciculating drugs or by choosing an alternative to succinylcholine . Malignant hyperthermia, the result of fulminant hypermetabolism of skeletal muscle, has been associated with the use of succinylcholine. Clinical manifestations include generalized rigidity, tachycardia, tachypnea, and profound hyperthermia. As the syndrome progresses, the patient develops hypotension, coagulopathies, and severe metabolic acidosis. Successful treatment requires early recognition of the entity. The offending agent is stopped, the patient is supported with oxygen, fluids, cooling measures, etc., and dantrolene (a skeletal muscle relaxant) is administered.[73]

Physiology and Pharmacokinetics.—Succinylcholine acts at the neuromuscular junction to produce depolarization and the propagation of action potentials. The initial result is the stimulation of all cholinergic autonomic receptors, nicotinic and muscarinic. Skeletal muscle throughout the body contracts and may be observed as fasciculations. Smooth muscle and myocardium are not affected but arrhythmias can occur from vagal stimulation or from local changes in potassium concentration.

Complete skeletal muscle paralysis occurs in 30 to 45 seconds with complete paralysis by 2 minutes.

The duration of action is from 4 to 6 minutes. Succinylcholine is metabolized in the liver by hydrolysis and in the plasma by pseudocholinesterase to succinylmonocholine and then to succinic acid and choline. About 10% of the drug is excreted unchanged in the urine. The duration of neuromuscular blockade is not significantly altered by renal insufficiency. There are many factors which can alter the onset and duration of action of succinylcholine. Prolongation of the block may occur if the patient has low levels of plasma pseudocholinesterase. Deficiency of this enzyme may be found in patients with a homozygous complement of this recessive hereditary trait (1/3,000), and in liver disease, burns, severe anemia, pregnancy (decreased about 24%), malnutrition, or in patients receiving antimalarial drugs. Patients who demonstrate a prolonged response to succinylcholine should be ventilated with 50% nitrous oxide and oxygen until neurologic recovery occurs. Fluid infusions may help recovery by increasing the distribution volume and promoting diuresis. The block may also be prolonged in patients who have received very large (>4 mg/kg) or repeated doses of succinylcholine over a prolonged period of time. In this instance the block changes from the characteristic depolarization block to a nondepolarizing block. Under these circumstances small repeated doses of a neuromuscular antagonist such as neostigmine may be effective as a reversal agent. Table 14–3 has a more complete list of factors which may effect neuromuscular blockade but in general blockade is potentiated by quinine and magnesium and antagonized by hypokalemia or hypocalcemia.[70, 72, 79, 84]

Administration.—Succinylcholine is usually administered IV in a dose of about 1.0 to 1.5 mg/kg. The dose in children is 1.5 to 2.0 mg/kg. In emergent situations where IV access is not readily available, succinylcholine can be given IM or subcutaneously (SC). The IM and SC dose in adults and children is 2.5 mg/kg not to exceed 150 mg. Failure to achieve complete relaxation may be a result of inadequate dosing or from mixing succinylcholine with an alkaline solution. Refractory spasm of the masseter muscle has also been described in patients who develop malignant hyperthermia. The cause is unknown. Premedication is used when time allows and the situation calls for it. Atropine 0.015 mg/kg IV will prevent bradyarrhythmias and should always be given to young children. Use of a nondepolarizing drug such as pancuronium 0.02 mg/kg IV or vecuronium 0.02 mg/kg IV will alleviate many of the

complications and block the fasciculations.[84] Some evidence exists that a small dose of succinylcholine, 0.15 mg/kg, may be used as pretreatment to prevent fasciculations. This "self-taming" dose appears to decrease the incidence and severity of fasciculations but does not eliminate the myalgias that occur.[85, 86]

Practical Airway Considerations.—Succinylcholine continues to be the neuromuscular blocker of choice in most emergent situations. The fact that it produces paralysis rapidly and is then metabolized within minutes is invaluable to the clinician. No other drug is available which comes close to these two properties. Vecuronium, discussed later, will work almost as rapidly if given in high doses, but its duration of action increases with the dose. In patients with a severely unstable airway, physicians want a drug that works quickly and lasts only as long as necessary. Should intubation be unsuccessful after paralysis with succinylcholine, the patient may be able to assist with his or her own respiration within minutes. With vecuronium the patient will be unable to assist for at least 30 minutes and perhaps longer if higher doses had been used. Despite the rare serious complications that can result from its use, succinylcholine continues to be an essential drug in the emergency physician's armamentarium.[87] Other drugs should be considered when there are minutes to spare or when circumstances are more controlled.

Control of the airway will always take precedence over all other considerations. In other words, in emergent situations, the physician must use whatever is available and will be most efficacious in aiding airway control at that moment. Therefore, there may not be any absolute contraindications to the use of succinylcholine. The decision to avoid the drug must be based on the degree of need vs. the relative importance of the contraindication. Administration of succinylcholine will cause the release of a small amount of histamine into the systemic circulation and can result in bronchospasm. Clearly, if time allows, succinylcholine should be avoided in patients with asthma or COPD. However, the risk of producing severe or even clinically significant bronchospasm is small. Therefore, if rapid control of the airway is needed, succinylcholine should not be withheld. The patient who has suffered extensive burns in recent weeks risks life-threatening hyperkalemia from the use of succinylcholine which cannot be blocked with any form of pretreatment. Under these circumstances, succinylcholine should be avoided if at all possible. The other relative contraindications noted above include: recent major trauma or neurologic disease, hyperkalemia, globe trauma or glaucoma, long-bone fractures, elevated intracranial pressure, pseudocholinesterase deficiency, etc. The use of premedication in the form of sedatives, analgesics, anxiolytics, and nondepolarizing blocking drugs may help to eliminate or alleviate many of the complications.

Pancuronium

Pancuronium (Pavulon), first available in 1964, had been the nondepolarizing neuromuscular blocking agent of choice until the mid 1980s. It is preferred over curare because it causes little or no histamine release and no cardiac depression. It is about one third less potent than vecuronium but five times more potent than curare. Pancuronium may be used as a defasciculating drug prior to succinylcholine or by itself for complete paralysis.[88, 89]

Clinical Considerations.—Pancuronium will not cause a rise in intracranial pressure. In addition, histamine effects such as bronchospasm and flushing are rare. However, it may produce some cardiovascular effects that can be undesirable. A dose-related response may result in an increased heart rate and an increase in peripheral vascular resistance. The former is secondary to an atropine-like effect on the sinoatrial node. The increased vascular resistance may be associated with inhibition of the reuptake of catecholamines by heart muscle. This propensity to increase the heart rate and afterload make it an undesirable choice in patients with coronary artery disease.[70–72, 90]

Pharmacokinetics.—Pancuronium is principally excreted in the urine. Renal failure results in variable prolongation of the neuromuscular block. Varying amounts of pancuronium are also recovered from the bile. In patients with hepatic or biliary disease the elimination half-life is doubled and plasma clearance is reduced. The result is a delay in onset and prolongation of paralysis. Although animal reproductive studies have not been performed it is known that only very small amounts of pancuronium cross the placental circulation. The drug is therefore a reasonable choice when complete paralysis is needed in a pregnant patient. Caution must be exercised in toxemic patients because magnesium will enhance the neuromuscular block. The pharmacokinetics in infants and children are similar to those in adults. Neonates, however, are more sensitive to neuromuscular blockers. The dose must be de-

creased and prolonged blockade anticipated in these patients.[70–72, 90]

The full paralyzing dose is about 0.1 mg/kg IV, onset to effective paralysis is 2 to 5 minutes, and duration of apnea is 60 to 90 minutes. Onset and duration of action is dose-dependent. Pancuronium is a cumulative drug resulting in progressively longer durations of action with subsequent doses. It is recommended that repeated doses be 5% to 10% of the initial dose. When used as a pretreatment to succinylcholine, the recommended dose is 0.01 mg/kg.[71, 72, 90]

Practical Airway Considerations.—The only advantage pancuronium may have over alternative nondepolarizing blockers is its longer duration of action. Vecuronium has fewer side effects and greater dosing flexibility. In patients who need prolonged paralysis, repeat doses of vecuronium can be safely administered without the cumulative properties of pancuronium. Vecuronium is also preferred in patients with renal disease. Atracurium is the preferred agent in patients with severe liver disease. Given the choices available, pancuronium should only be considered as an alternative to vecuronium in most clinical settings.

Vecuronium

Vecuronium (Norcuron) is a nondepolarizing neuromuscular blocking drug that was developed in a search to find an agent that had an onset of action more rapid, and a duration of activity shorter than pancuronium. Structurally, it is similar to pancuronium, differing only by the addition of one methyl group. The ultimate result was a drug that satisfied both of those requirements and had other characteristics which in many ways makes vecuronium the preferred paralytic.

Clinical Considerations.—The cardiovascular effects of vecuronium are minimal, which may be one of its greatest benefits over other neuromuscular blocking drugs.[91] Even when doses which far exceed recommendations are used, there is little change in heart rate. One study looked at the effect of giving 0.28 mg/kg (12 times the effective dose for 90% of the population) to patients about to undergo coronary artery bypass grafting. There was no change in heart rate or blood pressure.[92] Another study looked at the effects of large dosages and found a mean heart rate decrease of three beats per minute and a mean arterial pressure drop of 6.7 mm Hg. There were no clinically significant changes in cardiac output.[93] Histamine is not released and hypersensitivity reactions such as bronchospasm and flushing have not been noted.[72, 92]

Pharmacokinetics.—The pharmacokinetics of vecuronium vary depending on the dose used. Onset of action (the time required for good to excellent intubation conditions) may be as rapid as 1 minute when large doses are used. However, the duration of action at these dosages may be greater than 2 hours. When standard doses are used, the onset of action is 2.5 to 3.0 minutes, but time to recovery is reduced to 25 to 40 minutes. The metabolism of vecuronium is not yet completely known. It appears that about 10% of the drug is excreted in the urine. Vecuronium has been used in renal transplant surgery with little change in the duration of action. In animal studies about 50% of the metabolites have been found in the bile and human studies in patients with liver disease have noted a recovery period of up to twice as long as in healthy patients. Age does not appear to have clinically significant effects on the pharmacokinetics of vecuronium. Potency is the same in all age groups. Duration of action, given equal doses, was longest in infants: 73 minutes (mean); in children, 35 minutes; and in adults, 53 minutes. The mean duration in pregnancy is reduced and very little of the drug crosses the placental barrier.[72, 92, 94–96] The recommended initial dose is 0.08 to 0.10 mg/kg IV with an expected effective time to onset of 2.5 to 3.0 minutes. The drug may also be an alternative to succinylcholine for RSI at doses of 0.25 mg/kg. Effective paralysis will occur in about 60 seconds.[97, 98]

Practical Airway Considerations.—Vecuronium should replace pancuronium for all of its current uses in the emergency department. Vecuronium is safer with fewer side effects and has greater dosing flexibility. It may be used for procedures or clinical situations that call for relatively short periods of paralysis. Larger doses or repeat doses may be safely given for longer durations of action. In patients requiring RSI, vecuronium may be used alone or as a defasciculating agent prior to succinylcholine. The only significant clinical concern when using it for RSI is that the large doses needed result in a duration of action that may exceed 90 minutes. The lengthy period of paralysis may be undesirable in certain clinical settings and should be taken into consideration before using it in this manner.

Atracurium

Like vecuronium, atracurium (Tracrium) was produced as a result of the search to discover neuromuscular blocking drugs with fewer side effects, rapid onset, and brief duration of action. Unlike vecuronium, atracurium represents a structurally new class of nondepolarizing agents. The result is that some of its properties may make it more advantageous than pancuronium but may not offer as much safety as vecuronium.[92, 94]

Clinical Considerations.—The cardiovascular effects of atracurium are minimal at standard recommended doses. Yet at the large doses which have been studied for RSI, the heart rate increases significantly and moderate hypotension occurs. Atracu-

TABLE 14–4.

Neuromuscular Blocking Drugs

Drug	Dose Paralyzing	Dose Pretreat	Onset	Duration of Action	Refrigeration
Succinylcholine (Anectine, Quelicin)	1.0–1.5 mg/kg IV adult 1.5–2.0 mg/kg IV children 2.5 mg/kg IM	0.15 mg/kg IV	30–60 sec IV 2–3 min IM	4–6 min IV 8–20 min IM	Yes, but may be kept 24 hr at room temperature
Vecuronium (Norcuron)	0.1 mg/kg IV standard dose 0.25 mg/kg IV rapid-sequence intubation	0.01 mg/kg IV	2.5–3.0 min standard dose; 60 sec with larger dose	25–40 min >90 min with larger dose	Not necessary
Pancuronium (Pavulon)	0.1 mg/kg IV	0.01 mg/kg IV	2–5 min	60–90 min	Not necessary; 6 mo at room temperature
Atracurium (Tracrium)	0.4 mg/kg IV	0.04 mg/kg IV	2–3 min	25–35 min	Yes, but may be kept up to 14 days at room temperature
Tubocurarine (Tubarine)	0.3 mg/kg IV	0.03 mg/kg	3–5 min	45–75 min	?

rium does cause the release of histamine which may account for these cardiovascular changes. Facial flushing has also been documented when higher doses are used.

Age, including studies in infants, has not been shown to affect the duration of action. Pregnancy does not appear to alter the pharmacokinetics, nor does atracurium cross the placental circulation appreciably, as concentrations of the drug were undetectable in the umbilical cord blood of women undergoing cesarean section. Atracurium is safe in patients with renal and liver disease as studies have not found a significant change in the onset or duration of action.[72, 92, 94, 98, 99]

Pharmacokinetics.—Atracurium is about 25% to 33% as potent as pancuronium. At recommended doses the time to onset of effective paralysis is about 3 minutes. Using much larger doses, the time to onset could be decreased to about 60 seconds. The duration of action was 30 to 40 minutes when low doses were used and 71 minutes on average when larger doses were administered. Repeat doses had minimal cumulative effect. Atracurium undergoes spontaneous decomposition via a process called Hofmann elimination. In addition, it is hydrolyzed by plasma esterases other than pseudocholinesterase. Significant renal and liver disease do not appear to affect metabolism.

The standard intubating dose is 0.4 mg/kg IV, with effective relaxation in 2 to 3 minutes and a duration of effectiveness of 25 to 35 minutes. Larger doses of about 1.5 mg/kg can be used with a decreased time to onset of about 60 seconds. However,

this has been associated with more cardiovascular complications and a longer duration of action.[92, 98]

Practical Airway Considerations.—The availability of vecuronium limits the clinical usefulness of another blocking agent such as atracurium. Because the two drugs have similar pharmacokinetics and vecuronium has fewer side effects, the latter is the preferred agent. The only practical use for atracurium may be in the patient with serious liver disease who needs only a brief period of paralysis.

Summary

Succinylcholine must be considered an essential drug to have available. In situations which call for immediate control of the airway, it produces rapid complete paralysis. The effect usually lasts less than 5 minutes, which is another important advantage in emergency settings. The only absolute contraindications are in patients with known previous adverse reactions to the drug and those at serious risk of developing hyperkalemia. The dose is 1.0 to 1.5 mg/kg and can be given IV or IM.

Vecuronium must be considered the longer-acting agent of choice. In many settings it can replace succinylcholine as a safer alternative. When given in large doses it can become effective in about 60 seconds and therefore can be used in RSI. It should replace pancuronium in all clinical situations. No serious complications specific to vecuronium have been identified. The dose is about 0.1 mg/kg IV for standard intubation and 0.25 mg/kg for RSI.

Curare should no longer be considered as an alternative agent in airway management.

Metabolism	How Supplied	Indications	Concerns
Liver hydrolysis and plasma pseudocholinesterase	Single or multidose vials with or without preservatives	Rapid-sequence intubation (RSI)	Burns, crush trauma, neuromuscular disease, hyperkalemia, increased intracranial pressure
10% renal and up to 50% liver	Provided as a powder that needs reconstitution	Routine paralysis and RSI	Long paralysis when large doses are used
Primarily liver	Premixed solution 1 or 2 mg/mL	Routine paralysis	Increases heart rate and peripheral vascular resistance
Hofmann elimination	Premixed solution 10 mg/mL	Routine paralysis, severe liver and renal disease	Cardiovascular instability at high doses
Primarily renal	?	Only if other noncompetitive drugs are unavailable	Severe bronchospasm, marked hypotension

Pancuronium is a drug that emergency physicians should be familiar with. Many emergency departments do not stock vecuronium and it should be considered as an alternative drug. It cannot be used in RSI because the time to effective paralysis is too long. The dose is 0.1 mg/kg IV.

Atracurium may be an acceptable alternative to vecuronium. It has been shown to produce more tachycardia and histamine-related sequelae. Renal failure and liver disease do not effect the metabolism. The dose is about 0.4 mg/kg IV. Larger doses can be used for RSI but have been associated with more tachycardia and hypotension.

The neuromuscular blocking drugs, their dosage, metabolism, indications, etc. are summarized in Table 14–4.

RAPID-SEQUENCE INTUBATION

Rapid sequence intubation refers to a specific method of inducing general anesthesia while securing active airway control. The technique was intended to deal specifically with the concerns of administering induction and paralyzing drugs to patients with a full stomach and thus a greater risk of aspiration. The technique of RSI was first described in obstetric patients in 1946. A significant contribution was added by Sellick in 1961.[100] The Sellick maneuver was planned to further diminish the chance of aspiration. As consciousness is lost on induction (loss of the lash reflex) the practitioner applies firm pressure on the cricoid cartilage, occluding the esophagus in the process. The degree of backward pressure is the pressure that would produce discomfort if applied to the bridge of the nose.[101] A key to the method is that pressure must be maintained until the tube has been successfully placed and the balloon inflated. Application of cricoid pressure to the awake or lightly unconscious patient may induce vomiting. Moreover, premature release of pressure may make vomiting and aspiration more likely. Recent studies have documented the effectiveness of cricoid pressure but suggest that the technique not be used universally, that inadequate pressure is often applied, and that premature release of force is common.[101, 102] Sellick recommends that pressure be released in the event that emesis occurs to avoid the risk of esophageal perforation.

The rapid-sequence method is commonly used in the emergency department because all patients are assumed to have a full stomach. The approach, followed by oral endotracheal intubation, is a rapid and safe method of achieving airway control.[103, 104] Yet the approach does not always need to be performed in a hurried manner. It is preferable to preoxygenate the patient with 100% oxygen for at least 2 minutes. Every attempt should be made to avoid bag-mask positive pressure ventilation, which will result in gastric distention. All necessary equipment and medication should be made available and verified to be in working order. This preparation, especially preoxygenation, is the first step in RSI.

The medication choices that can be used subsequently have been discussed above. The following description includes just a few of the many alternatives available. Following oxygenation, a defasciculating dose (0.01 mg/kg) of a drug such as vecuronium or pancuronium is administered. Atropine or glycopyrrolate may be given to attenuate potential bradycardia. Two to 3 minutes later, general anesthesia is induced with 3 to 4 mg/kg of thiopental given by rapid IV injection. This is followed immediately by 1 to 2 mg/kg of succinylcholine administered as an IV bolus. As consciousness is lost cricoid pressure is applied by an assistant. Thirty to 60 seconds after the thiopental and succinylcholine are given, the trachea is intubated and the cuff is inflated. Cricoid pressure is relaxed once successful tube placement is confirmed. Vecuronium may be used in place of succinylcholine for muscle relaxation. The dose of vecuronium will be 0.25 mg/kg and a defasciculating drug will not be necessary. The induction drug is given immediately prior to the injection of the paralytic agent. The patient will be ready for intubation in about 60 seconds.[105, 106]

Rapid-sequence intubation and an alternative are summarized in Table 14–5.

SUMMARY OF DRUGS IN ANESTHESIA

I. A. Topical anesthesia.
   1. Lidocaine may be used to anesthetize the entire nasopharynx and oropharynx down to the vocal cords.
   2. Cocaine is used exclusively in the nose.
II. Sedation and induction drugs.
   A. Butyrophenones (haloperidol and droperidol) are generally used for sedation and premedication, not for induction.
   B. Benzodiazepines (diazepam and midazolam) are generally used for sedation, but can be used for induction as second-line agents.
   C. Opioids (fentanyl and alfentanil) are good induction agents that also provide potent analgesia.
   D. Propofol is an excellent induction drug. It

TABLE 14–5.

Rapid-Sequence Intubation

1. Preoxygenate with 100% oxygen (no positive pressure ventilation)
2. Equipment preparation (suction, endotracheal (ET) tube, bag, mask, laryngoscope, etc.)
3. Pretreat with a defasciculating dose (0.01 mg/kg) of vecuronium or pancuronium
4. Induction with thiopental, 3–4 mg/kg rapid IV bolus injection
5. Sellick maneuver (cricoid pressure) to be applied as consciousness is lost
6. Follow thiopental immediately with 1–2 mg/kg succinylcholine IV bolus injection
7. Intubate the trachea and verify position
8. Release cricoid pressure

Alternative

1. Preoxygenate with 100% oxygen (no positive pressure ventilation)
2. Equipment preparation (suction, ET tube, bag, mask, laryngoscope, etc.)
3. Induction with thiopental, 3–4 mg/kg rapid IV bolus injection
4. Vecuronium 2.5 mg/kg IV bolus injection
5. Sellick maneuver (cricoid pressure) to be applied as consciousness is lost
6. Intubate the trachea and verify position
7. Release cricoid pressure

---

may also be used to provide sedation for brief procedures.

E. Thiopental is the prototypal induction drug.

F. Methohexital is another excellent choice for induction or brief, potent sedation.

G. Etomidate is an induction agent that should be considered as an alternative to the above drugs.

H. Ketamine is an interesting drug that can be used for bronchodilation, sedation, immobilization, or induction.

III. Neuromuscular blockers.

A. Curare was the original paralytic but has since been replaced with safer agents.

B. Succinylcholine continues to be the preferred drug for RSI despite potentially serious complications.

C. Vecuronium has replaced pancuronium as the longer-acting agent of choice because of its fewer side effects. It may also be used for RSI.

D. Pancuronium is an acceptable alternative to vecuronium for prolonged paralysis.

E. Atracurium is similar to vecuronium but with more cardiovascular effects.

REFERENCES

1. Collins VJ: *Principles of Anesthesiology*, ed 2. Philadelphia, Lea & Febiger, 1984.
2. *AMA Drug Evaluations*, ed 4. New York, American Medical Association, 1980, pp 386–396.
3. Goodman LS, Gilman A: *The Pharmacologic Basis of Therapeutics*, ed 8. New York, Macmillan Publishing Co, 1990, pp 539–545.
4. Rector F, Denuccio DJ, Aloen MA, et al: A comparison of cocaine, oxymetazoline, and saline for nasotracheal intubation. *J Am Assoc Nurs Anesth* 1987; 55:49–54.
5. Dailey RH: Fatality secondary to misuse of TAC solution. *Ann Emerg Med* 1988; 17:117–120.
6. Xylocaine (lidocaine hydrochloride) package insert. Westboro, Mass., Astra Pharmaceutical Products, Inc, 1989.
7. Isaac PA, Barry JE, Vaughan RS, et al: A jet nebuliser for delivery of topical anesthesia to the respiratory tract. A comparison with cricothyroid puncture and direct spraying for fiberoptic bronchoscopy. *Anaesthesia* 1990; 45:46–48.
8. Hamill JF: Lidocaine before endotracheal intubation: Intravenous or Laryngotracheal? *Anesthesiology* 1981; 55:578–581.
9. Youngberg JA, et al: Comparison of intravenous and topical lidocaine in attenuating the cardiovascular responses to endotracheal intubation. *South Med J* 1983; 76:1122–1124.
10. Kraut RA: A comparison of intravenous and laryngotracheal lidocaine before endotracheal intubation. *Anesth Prog*, Mar/Apr 1983, pp 34–36.
11. Dyson DH: Efficacy of lidocaine hydrochloride for laryngeal desensitization: A clinical comparison of techniques in the cat. *J Am Vet Med Assoc* 1988; 192:1286–1288.
12. Sutherland AD, Williams RT: Cardiovascular responses and lidocaine absorption in fiberoptic-assisted awake intubation. *Anesth Analg* 1986; 65:389–391.
13. Venus B, et al: Effects of aerosolized lidocaine on circulatory responses to laryngoscopy and tracheal

intubation. *Crit Care Med* 1984; 12:391–394.

14. Kautto UM, Heinonen J: Attenuation of circulatory response to laryngoscopy and tracheal intubation: A comparison of two methods of topical anaesthesia. *Acta Anaesthesiol Scand* 1982; 26:599–602.

15. Derbyshire DR, et al: Effect of topical lignocaine on the sympathoadrenal responses to tracheal intubation. *Br J Anaesth* 1987; 59:300–304.

16. Magliozzi JR, et al: Mood alteration following oral and intravenous haloperidol and relationship to drug concentration in normal subjects. *J Clin Pharmacol* 1985; 25:285–290.

17. Haloperidol package insert. Franklin Park, Ill, Smith & Nephew, 1989.

18. Frey S, et al: Spontaneous motor activity in healthy volunteers after single doses of haolperidol. *Int Clin Psychopharmacol* 1989; 4:39–53.

19. Rosenbloom A, et al: Emerging treatment options in the alcohol withdrawal syndrome. *J Clin Psychiatry* 1988; 49(suppl):28–32.

20. Clinton JE, et al: Haloperidol for sedation of disruptive emergency patients. *Ann Emerg Med* 1987; 16:319–322.

21. Tesar GE, et al: Use of high dose intravenous haloperidol in the treatment of agitated cardiac patients. *J Clin Psychopharmacol* 1985; 5:344–347.

22. Curran J, et al: Droperidol and endotracheal intubation. *Anaesthesia* 1980; 35:290–294.

23. Balfors E, et al: Droperidol inhibits the effects of intravenous ketamine on central hemodynamics and myocardial oxygen consumption in patients with generalized atherosclerotic disease. *Anesth Analg* 1983; 62:193–197.

24. Droperidol package insert. Piscataway, NJ, Janssen Pharmaceutica, 1988.

25. Diazepam package insert. Cherry Hill, NJ, Elkins-Sinn, 1988.

26. Churchill-Davidson HC: *A Practice of Anaesthesia.* London, Henry Kimptom Publishers, 1978, pp 626–639.

27. Persson P: Pharmacokinetics of midazolam in total IV anesthesia. *Br J Anaesth* 1987; 59:548–556.

28. Wright SW, et al: Midazolam use in the emergency department. *Am J Emerg Med* 1990; 8:97–100.

29. Restall J, et al: Total intravenous anaesthesia for military surgery. *Anaesthesia* 1988; 43:46–49.

30. Conrad B, et al: Propofol infusion for sedation in regional anesthesia. A comparison with midazolam. *Anasth Intensivther Notfallmed* 1990; 25:186–192.

31. Versed (midazolam) package insert. Nutley, NJ, Hoffmann-La Roche Inc., 1987.

32. Amrein R, et al: Clinical pharmacology of flumazenil. *Eur J Anaesthesiol Suppl* 1988; 2:65–80.

33. Philip BK, et al: Flumazenil reverses sedation after midazolam-induced general anesthesia in ambulatory surgery patients. *Anesth Analg* 1990; 71:371–376.

34. Rosenbaum NL, Hooper PA: The use of flumazenil as an antagonist to midazolam in intravenous sedation for dental procedures. *Eur J Anaesthesiol Suppl* 1988; 2:183–190.

35. Diprivan (profofol) package insert. Wilmington, Del, Stuart Pharmaceuticals, 1989.

36. Valtonen M, et al: Propofol infusion for sedation in outpatient oral surgery, a comparison with diazepam. *Anaesthesia* 1989; 44:730–734.

37. Patterson KW: Propofol sedation for out-patient endoscopy—a comparison with midazolam. 1989; 68:S222.

38. Skues MA, Prys-Roberts C: The pharmacology of propofol. *J Clin Anesth* 1989; 1:387–400.

39. Kanto J, Gepts E: Pharmacokinetic implications for the clinical use of propofol. *Clin Pharmacokinet* 1989; 17:308–326.

40. Dubois A, et al: Use of propofol for sedation during gastrointestinal endoscopies. *Anaesthesia* 1988; 43(suppl):75–80.

41. Pentothal (thiopental) package insert. North Chicago, Ill, Abbott Laboratories, 1988.

42. White PF: Comparative evaluation of intravenous agents for rapid sequence induction—thiopental, ketamine, and midazolam. *Anesthesiology* 1982; 57:279–284.

43. Bassil A, et al: Propofol versus thiopentone for induction of anesthesia in patients undergoing outpatient surgery. *Middle East J Anesthesiol* 1989; 10:307–314.

44. Kashtan H: Comparative evaluation of propofol and thiopentone for total intravenous anaesthesia. *Can J Anaesth* 1990; 37:170–176.

45. Harris CE, et al: Effects of thiopentone, etomidate and propofol on the haemodynamic response to tracheal intubation. *Anaesthesia* 1988; 43(suppl):32–36.

46. Brevital sodium (methohexital) package insert. Indianapolis, Ind, Eli Lilly & Co., 1989.

47. Doze VA, et al: Comparison of propofol with methohexital for outpatient anesthesia. *Anesth Analg* 1986; 65:1189–1195.

48. Boysen K, et al: Comparison of induction with and first hour of recovery from brief propofol and methohexital anesthesia. *Acta Anaesthesiol Scand* 1990; 34:212–215.

49. Gold MI, et al: A controlled investigation of propofol, thiopentone and methohexitone. *Can J Anaesth* 1987; 34:478–483.

50. Knell PJ: Total intravenous anaesthesia by an intermittent technique. Use of methohexitone, ketamine and a muscle relaxant. *Anaesthesia* 1983; 38:586–587.

51. Amidate (etomidate) package insert. North Chicago, Ill, Abbott Laboratories, 1988.

52. Giese JL, Stanley TH: Etomidate: A new intravenous anesthetic induction agent. *Pharmacotherapy* 1983; 3:251–258.

53. Boysen K, et al: Induction and recovery characteristics of propofol, thiopental and etomidate. *Acta Anaesthesiol Scand* 1989; 33:689–692.

54. Randall CC, et al: Fentanyl preloading for rapid sequence induction of anesthesia. *Anesth Analg* 1984; 63:60–64.
55. Fentanyl package insert. Cherry Hill, NJ, Elkins-Sinn, Inc, 1989.
56. Martin DE, et al: Low-dose fentanyl blunts circulatory responses to tracheal intubation. *Anesth Analg* 1982; 61:680–684.
57. Chudnofsky CR, et al: Safety of fentanyl use in the emergency department. *Ann Emerg Med* 1989; 18:635–639.
58. Larhani GE, Goldberg ME: Alfentanil hydrochloride: A new short-acting narcotic analgesic for surgical procedures. *Clin Pharm* 1987; 6:275–282.
59. Persson MP, et al: Pharmacokinetics of alfentanil in total I.V. anesthesia. *Br J Anaesth* 1988; 60:755–761.
60. Rosow CR: Newer opioid analgesics and antagonists. *Anesthesiol Emerg Med Clin North Am* 1988; 6:319–333.
61. Green SM, et al: Ketamine sedation for pediatric procedures: Part 1, a prospective series. *Ann Emerg Med* 1990; 19:1024–1032.
62. Green SM, Johnson NE: Ketamine sedation for pediatric procedures: Part 2, review and implications. *Ann Emerg Med* 1990; 19:1033–1046.
63. Hamza J, et al: Ventilatory response to CO_2 following intravenous ketamine in children. *Anesthesiology* 1989; 70:422–425.
64. Rock MJ, et al: Use of ketamine in asthmatic children to treat respiratory failure refractory to conventional therapy. *Crit Care Med* 1986; 14:514–516.
65. L'Hommedieu CS: The use of ketamine for the emergency intubation of patients with status asthmaticus. *Ann Emerg Med* 1987; 16:568–571.
66. Park GR, et al: Ketamine infusion. *Anaesthesia* 1987; 42:980–983.
67. Ketalar (ketamine) package insert. Morris Plains, NJ, Parke-Davis, 1982.
68. Bessen HA, Rothstein RJ. NMB Usage Survey (letter). *Ann Emerg Med* 1986; 15:1251–1252.
69. Churchill-Davidson HC: *A Practice of Anaesthesia.* London, Henry Kimptom Publishers, 1978, pp 660–675.
70. DeGarmo BH, Dronen S: Pharmacology and clinical use of neuromuscular blocking agents. *Ann Emerg Med* 1983; 12:48–54.
71. Batlan DE: Neuromuscular blockade in the emergency department. *J Emerg Med* 1987; 5:225–232.
72. Churchill-Davidson HC: *A Practice of Anaesthesia.* London, Henry Kimptom Publishers, 1978, pp 676–707.
73. Churchill-Davidson HC: *A Practice of Anaesthesia.* London, Henry Kimptom Publishers, 1978, pp 708–726.
74. Hedges JR, et al: Succinylcholine-assisted intubations in prehospital care. *Ann Emerg Med* 1988; 17:469–472.
75. Syverud SA, et al: Prehospital use of neuromuscular blocking agents in a helicopter ambulance program. *Ann Emerg Med* 1988; 17:236–242.
76. Churchill-Davidson HC: *A Practice of Anaesthesia.* London, Henry Kimptom Publishers, 1978, pp 727–734.
77. Geller E, et al: Reversal agents in anaesthesia. *Acta Anaesthesiol Scand Suppl* 1988; 87:28–32.
78. Buzello W: Postoperative care: Antagonism of drugs used in anaesthesia: Muscle relaxants. *Acta Anaesthesiol Scand Suppl* 1988; 87:25–27.
79. Thompson JD, Fish S: Succinylcholine for endotracheal intubation. *Ann Emerg Med* 1982; 11:526–529.
80. Laurence AS: Myalgia and biochemical changes following intermittent suxamethonium administration. *Anaesthesia* 1987; 42:503–510.
81. Stirt JA, et al: "Defasciculation" with metocurine prevents succinylcholine induced increases in intracranial pressure. *Anesthesiology* 1987; 67:50–53.
82. Minton MD, et al: Increases in intracranial pressure from succinylcholine: Prevention by prior nondepolarizing blockade. *Anesthesiology* 1986; 65:165–169.
83. Churchill-Davidson HC: *A Practice of Anaesthesia.* London, Henry Kimptom Publishers, 1978, pp 735–737.
84. Quelicin (succinylcholine) package insert. North Chicago, Ill, Abbott laboratories, 1989.
85. Brodsky JB, Brock-Utne JG: Does "self taming" with succinylcholine prevent postoperative myalgia? *Anesthesiology* 1979; 50:265–267.
86. Baraka A: Self-taming of succinylcholine-induced fasciculations. *Anesthesiology* 1977; 46:292–293.
87. Bonneru MC, et al: Vecuronium or suxamethonium for rapid sequence intubation: Which is better? *Br J Anaesth* 1987; 59:1240–1244.
88. Mehta MP, et al: Accelerated onset of nondepolarizing neuromuscular blocking drugs: Pancuronium, atracurium and vecuronium. A comparison with succinylcholine. *Eur J Anaesthesiol* 1988; 5:15–21.
89. Mehta MP: Facilitation of rapid endotracheal intubation with divided doses of nondepolarizing neuromuscular blocking drugs. *Anesthesiology* 1985; 62:392–395.
90. Pancuronium package insert. Cherry Hill, NJ, Elkins-Sinn, Inc, 1989.
91. Wierda JM, et al: Hemodynamic effects of vecuronium. *Br J Anaesth* 1989; 62:194–198.
92. Miller RD, et al: Clinical pharmacology of vecuronium and atracurium. *Anesthesiology* 1984; 61:444–453.
93. Tullock WC, et al: High dose vecuronium: Onset and duration, *Anesth Analg* 1988; 67:S1–S266.
94. Hilgenberg JC: Comparison of the pharmacology of vecuronium and atracurium with that of other currently available muscle relaxants. *Anesth Analg* 1983; 62:524–531.
95. Feldman SA, Liban JB: Vecuronium—a variable dose technique. *Anaesthesia* 1987; 42:199–201.

96. Norcuron (vecuronium) package insert. West Orange, NJ, Organon Inc, 1989.

97. Kunjappan VE, et al: Rapid sequence induction using vecuronium. *Anesth Analg* 1986; 65:503–506.

98. Lennon RL, et al: Atracurium or vecuronium for rapid sequence endotracheal intubation. *Anesthesiology* 1986; 64:510–513.

99. Tracrium (atracurium) package insert. Triangle Park, NC, Burroughs Wellcome Co, 1989.

100. Sellick BA: Cricoid pressure to control regurgitation of stomach contents during induction of anesthesia. *Lancet* 1961; 2:404–406.

101. Howells TH, et al: The application of cricoid pressure. *Anaesthesia* 1983; 38:457–460.

102. Wraight WK, et al: The determination of an effective cricoid pressure. *Anaesthesia* 1983; 38:461–466.

103. Talucci RC, Schwab CW: Rapid sequence induction with oral endotracheal intubation in the multiply injured patient. *Am Surg* 1988; 54:185–187.

104. Yamamoto LG, et al: Rapid sequence anesthesia induction for emergency intubation. *Pediatr Emerg Care* 1990; 6:200–213.

105. Morris IR: Pharmacologic aids to intubation and the rapid sequence induction. *Emerg Med Clin North Am* 1988; 6:753–768.

106. Stept WJ, Safar P: Rapid induction/intubation for prevention of gastric-content aspiration. *Anesth Analg* 1970; 49:633–635.

15

Manual Translaryngeal Jet Ventilation

Ronald Stewart, M.D.

Clinicians responsible for the care of seriously ill or injured patients must have a well-defined plan to maintain in each patient a patent airway, and ensure adequate oxygenation and ventilation. Although most airway problems can be managed with basic maneuvers, at times a patient will present with a unique problem that will require the application of a defined "drill" or plan to deal with the difficult airway. Among the tools and techniques necessary to skilled clinicians are bag-mask ventilation, and orotracheal and nasotracheal intubation using conventional and light-guided techniques. However, rarely, a patient will present in whom these measures may not suffice. Those who, for whatever reason, cannot be intubated, or who may require ventilation below the level of the cords, can present an alarming challenge, even to clinicians who are experienced and well versed in airway management. When carried out using the appropriate equipment and technique, manual translaryngeal jet ventilation offers a rapid, relatively safe, and effective method of oxygenation *and* ventilation that can be lifesaving in selected patients.

DEFINITIONS AND MISCONCEPTIONS

The modern technique of translaryngeal jet ventilation (TLJV) is based upon work done at the beginning of this century that demonstrated animals could be ventilated via pressurized air delivered through an incision in the tracheal wall.[1] Further data indicated that both oxygenation *and* ventilation could be achieved in apneic animals, but high pressure oxygen was required to produce ventilatory movements and maintain normocapnia.[2] Over several years the manual jet ventilation technique for emergency airway control was demonstrated in both animals and patients to provide rapid access to the airway below the level of the cords.[3, 4]

Confusion has arisen regarding the technique of translaryngeal oxygenation and ventilation, despite early and consistent evidence that ventilation required the insufflation of *high pressure* oxygen. This has arisen because of the confusion of terms and circumstances surrounding reports in the literature. While *oxygenation* could be accomplished with low flow rates of oxygen being delivered via a cannula inserted through the cricothyroid membrane,[5] ventilation could not.[6, 7]

The later introduction of *high frequency* jet ventilation has led to more confusion about the manual method of jet ventilation. High frequency jet ventilation delivers rapid (e.g., 100–200/min) but small-volume bursts of oxygen to the airway through a transcricothyroid membrane cannula.[8] Manual TLJV delivers large (up to 1,200 mL/sec) volumes to the airway under high pressure (50 psi), but at normal ventilatory rates (12–20/min). The use of TLJV in patients who required ventilation below the level of the cords has demonstrated that emergency manual TLJV requires three conditions[9]:

1. A high-pressure source of oxygen (50 psi).
2. A translaryngeal cannula of at least 16 gauge.
3. A method of interrupting the burst of oxygen to the cannula to allow for exhalation.

MECHANICS AND PHYSIOLOGY

Manual TLJV can provide emergency oxygenation and ventilation below the level of the cords.

The technique requires puncture of the cricothyroid membrane, a relatively avascular structure that usually can be palpated just above the cricoid cartilage.[10] Puncture of this membrane by a 14- or 16-gauge cannula is considered to be quicker and safer than the incision of the same membrane required for emergency cricothyroidotomy.[11]

Manual TLJV can be regarded as a positive pressure ventilation technique. Ventilation is achieved by the large volume of oxygen delivered to the airway—up to 1,200 mL/sec, delivered from a 50-psi source of oxygen. The delivered volume inflates the lungs, the diaphragm descends, and the chest wall expands. When the flow of oxygen is interrupted (expiratory phase), this process is reversed and the patient exhales. Normocarbia—i.e., ventilation—is maintained as long as the high volume oxygen is insufflated through the cannula.

There are several important differences between positive pressure ventilation produced by bag-valve-mask or bag–endotracheal tube and TLJV. The former methods deliver volumes under relatively low pressures to a closed, or relatively closed, airway. Intratracheal pressures can vary from 10 to 60 cm H_2O, depending on the vigor with which the bag is squeezed or the effectiveness of the seal achieved by the mask or tube. The technique of TLJV delivers high volume oxygen from a high pressure (50 psi) source into an *open* airway. The intratracheal pressures generated by high pressure (50 psi) intermittent oxygen insufflation through a 16- or 14-gauge transcricothyroid membrane cannula will average 15 cm H_2O.[12] Such pressures are reached with an open proximal airway into which large volumes (1,200 mL/sec) are delivered through the laryngeal cannula. Of the total volume of oxygen delivered to the trachea, 30% to 60% will escape[12] proximally through the open glottis. This not only prevents high airway pressures from being reached but also can remove upper airway secretions and guard against aspiration.[13]

It has been shown repeatedly that driving pressure and cannula size are crucial elements for ventilation through a transcricothyroid membrane cannula.[14, 15] Despite this, recommendations have been made and continue to be made suggesting that oxygenation and even ventilation can be achieved through low flow, low pressure oxygen delivered through a cannula by continuous flow, or by a resuscitator bag connected to the cannula.[16] A resuscitator bag connected to a cannula can generate pressures of only 1 to 2 psi,[14] with flows reaching only 150 to 200 mL/sec through a 16- to 14-gauge cannula.[9] While baseline *oxygen* requirements may be met

with such a setup, ventilation cannot be achieved, and respiratory acidosis quickly results,[14, 15] especially in those patients whose airways are already likely compromised and who are therefore candidates for this procedure.

INDICATIONS AND CONTRAINDICATIONS

Manual TLJV should be considered a legitimate form of emergency airway control that can be life-saving in some patients. It can give some assurance to the clinician who, for whatever reason, cannot readily oxygenate, ventilate, or protect the airway of an unconscious, seriously ill, or injured patient. Those patients in whom direct visualization of the airway is difficult or impossible, those whose anatomy is distorted due to injury, or those with suspected or actual cervical spine injury should be considered candidates for this technique.

A relative contraindication to the technique is an inability to locate the cricothyroid membrane. However, in dire circumstances, insertion of the cannula into the trachea at the sternal notch could be considered an acceptable alternative, considering the consequences of an uncontrolled airway. The only absolute contraindication to this procedure is total obstruction of the airway at or above the cords. The inability of the high volume oxygen to escape through the proximal airway could create very high intrapulmonary pressures, possibly resulting in life-threatening barotrauma.[14] Fortunately, complete *expiratory* upper airway obstruction is rare, and this is seldom a consideration in emergency patients.

The greatest problem with this technique is perhaps that it is underused by clinicians. It is often considered a last resort, and it is not yet thought of as an integral part of emergency airway procedure. It is *not* a technique that can be highly recommended for the novice. Neither the equipment nor details of the technique itself can be safely improvised in a crash situation. The safe performance of manual TLJV requires knowledge of upper airway anatomy, the right equipment, and the right patient.

COMPLICATIONS

Complications of this airway technique should be low, but the actual incidence of major complications is unknown. Problems related to the actual cricothyroid membrane puncture may include bleeding at the site with hematoma formation, damage to the cartilage or vocal cords with a misdirected cannula, and a later complication, infection. Most serious is puncture of the posterior tracheal wall or misplacement of the cannula into the soft tissues. Such a complication would result in life-threatening barotrauma to the soft tissues and mediastinum, but careful attention to the technique of cannula insertion—with easy and consistent aspiration of air—make this complication unlikely. Slight subcutaneous emphysema commonly results around the puncture site of the cannula. This need not be troublesome, and can be prevented or lessened by keeping the hub of the cannula firmly applied against the puncture site.

Damage to the tracheal wall has been reported in experimental animals undergoing manual TLJV.[15] Although such damage has not been reported in patients in whom cannulas with side holes were used,[17] it should be recognized that insufflation of dry oxygen under high pressure would likely cause some tracheal wall changes or perhaps damage in most patients.

EQUIPMENT

Manual TLJV requires a translaryngeal cannula, a high pressure oxygen source, tubing, and a method of interrupting the oxygen flow to allow exhalation. The cannula should be at least a 14-gauge overneedle cannula, preferably with side holes. The side holes reduce resistance to flow and will "blow" the cannula away from the tracheal wall should it be resting against it. This likely lessens the risk of tracheal wall rupture or damage. A 13-gauge cannula designed especially for translaryngeal ventilation is now commercially available, and is recommended.[17] (Actronics Corp., Zurich, Switzerland, and Pittsburgh, Pa.). This cannula has the advantage of side holes, a flange for securing the cannula to the neck, a Luer-Lok connector, and a curved design. Unfortunately, a 15-mm blue adaptor is included in this design, and this would suggest attaching a bag-valve resuscitator bag for ventilation, even though the report that studied the cannula demonstrated a dangerous inability to maintain normocapnia.[17]

The high pressure oxygen source (50 psi) required for ventilation can be obtained from any standard oxygen cylinder or hospital wall outlet, *provided there is no flow regulator interposed between the oxygen source and the TLJV tubing.* Liter flow regulators reduce the pressure of the oxygen and regulate the flow to a maximum of 15 to 17 L/min at the regulator. This will not be sufficient to provide adequate

ventilation to the patient. The flush valve on most anesthesia machines will provide sufficient pressure to provide adequate delivered volumes, but these are less than those obtained by connecting directly into the wall outlet or oxygen cylinder.[15]

Oxygen should be carried to the translaryngeal cannula in high pressure tubing, with some type of valve or "interrupter" placed between the oxygen source and the cannula. This is essential to allow the patient to exhale in the same way as conventional positive pressure ventilation. This can be very simple, e.g., a hole cut in the tubing. Commercial valves are available (Instrumentation Industries, Bethel Park, Pa.) that activate the flow of high pressure oxygen through a button mechanism. The tubing attachments should be reinforced with plastic tie-backs available from any hardware store.

The equipment should be assembled, packaged, and available on the "crash-cart," in the operating room, in the ambulance, or with the airway cart or kit in the emergency department. All personnel should be thoroughly familiar with the use of the equipment and with the principles of manual TLJV. The equipment should be subjected to regular maintenance, checks, and testing, and personnel should undergo periodic crash airway drills that should include manual TLJV.

TECHNIQUE

The technique of manual TLJV can be instituted quickly in any suitable patient. It may be lifesaving. Its success will depend upon the availability of the equipment, the correct placement of the cannula, and the correct technique of ventilation.[18] The patient must have a partially or completely open proximal airway. Otherwise, dangerously high intrapulmonary pressures and barotrauma may result.

The translaryngeal cannula is attached to a 5- or 10-mL syringe. If time permits, it is filled with 1 or 2 mL of 2% to 4% lidocaine, so that any tissue plugs that might block the cannula after puncture of the membrane can be forced out. It will also provide some anesthesia to the larynx and tracheal wall and reduce subsequent coughing in the patient whose reflexes may be intact.

The cricothyroid membrane should be palpated first. This is best done by feeling the sternal notch, and working the examining finger up the midline. The first prominent cartilage felt is the cricoid cartilage. Above this is the cricothyroid membrane, which is connected to the prominent thyroid cartilage above. If time permits, the area can be infiltrated with local anesthetic in the conscious patient, and a small puncture of the skin over the membrane with the tip of a no. 11 scalpel blade will make insertion of the cannula easier.

The cannula with syringe attached is inserted at about a 45-degree angle through the membrane while the thumb and index fingers of the dominant hand steady the cricoid cartilage and stretch the skin over the membrane (Fig 15–1). The cannula is advanced with continuous aspiration on the syringe. Entry to the larynx is indicated by easy and consistent aspiration of air into the syringe. If the syringe is filled with anesthetic solution, this can now be injected. The outer plastic cannula is advanced off the inner needle until the hub or flange lies firmly against the skin. Air should be continuously aspirated in order to confirm intratracheal placement of the tip of the cannula. The oxygen tubing can then be connected and ventilation begun, (Fig 15–2) using very gentle, short bursts of oxygen at first and observing the patient carefully for untoward effects, particularly subcutaneous emphysema. Oxygen should be heard and seen escaping from the mouth and nose of the patient. An assistant can anchor the flange, if there is one, around the neck. It is good practice to constantly hold the hub of the cannula against the puncture site while the patient is being ventilated. Displacement of the cannula has been reported, with resultant serious emphysema.[17]

The ventilatory rate should be from 12 to 20/min, insufflation time being about 1 second. An inspiratory-expiratory ratio of 1:2 (20 breaths/min) will usually result in a slight respiratory alkalosis,

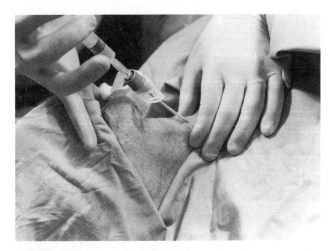

FIG 15–1.
Puncture of the cricothyroid membrane with translaryngeal jet ventilation cannula. Note aspiration of air on entry to the larynx, and the angle of the cannula.

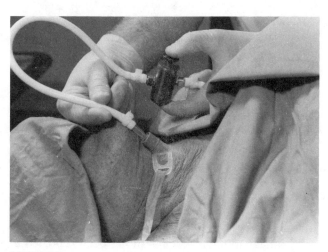

FIG 15–2.
Translaryngeal jet ventilation set up in place. The tubing is reinforced with plastic tiebacks, and the cannula is held firmly in place by a flange and tie around the neck. The button-activated mechanism provides an interrupted oxygen supply from the 50-psi source.

and blood gas samples should be obtained as soon as possible after institution of manual TLJV. The ventilatory rate can be adjusted accordingly after the results of blood gas analysis are known.

Clinical experience has shown that upper airway secretions, blood, or foreign material in the upper airway above the cords will be blown out of the mouth and nose during insufflation. Studies in animals have suggested that the positive airway pressure during this phase will be protective of aspiration, provided the patient is kept supine at or below 30 degrees.[13]

Using the proper equipment and technique for manual TLJV, the clinician can provide to the patient oxygenation *and* ventilation in the emergency setting. Following the establishment of definitive airway control, the patient should be observed for complications. Arterial blood gas analysis should be standard, as well as a chest radiograph to rule out mediastinal emphysema. The technique and equipment for manual translaryngeal jet ventilation should be familiar and readily accessible to all clinicians responsible for the care of the seriously ill and injured.

REFERENCES

1. Meltzer SJ, Auer J: Continuous respiration without respiratory movements. *J Exp Med* 1909; 11:622–625.
2. Reed JP, Kemph JP, Hamelberg W, et al: Studies with transtracheal artificial respiration. *Anesthesiology* 1954; 15:28–41.

3. Smith RB, Babinski M, Klain M, et al: Percutaneous transtracheal ventilation. *JACEP* 1976; 5:765–770.

4. Jorden RC, Moore EE, Marx JA: A comparison of PTV and endotracheal ventilation in an acute trauma model. *J Trauma* 1985; 25:978–983.

5. Jacoby JJ, Hemelberg W, Ziegler CH, et al: Transtracheal resuscitation. *JAMA* 1956; 162:625–628.

6. Smith RB, Schaer WB, Pfaeffle H: Percutaneous transtracheal ventilation for anaesthesia and resuscitation: A review and report of complications. *Can J Anaesth J* 1975; 22:607–612.

7. Spoerel WE, Narayanan PS, Singh NP: Transtracheal ventilation. *Br J Anaesth* 1971; 43:932–939.

8. Carlon GC, Cole R, Pierri MK, et al: High-frequency jet ventilation: Theoretical considerations and clinical observations. *Chest* 1982; 81:350–354.

9. Yealy DM, Stewart RD, Kaplan RM: Myths and pitfalls in emergency translaryngeal ventilation: Correcting misimpressions. *Ann Emerg Med* 1988; 17:690–692.

10. Little CM, Parker MG, Tarnopolsky R: The incidence of vasculature at risk during cricothyroidostomy. *Ann Emerg Med* 1986; 15:805–807.

11. McGill J, Clinton JE, Ruiz E: Cricothyrotomy in the emergency department. *Ann Emerg Med* 1982; 11:361–364.

12. Jacobs HB: Emergency percutaneous transtracheal catheter and ventilator. *J Trauma* 1972; 12:50–55.

13. Yealy DM, Plewa MC, Reed JJ, et al: Manual translaryngeal jet ventilation and the risk of aspiration in a canine model. *Ann Emerg Med* 1990; 19:1238–1241.

14. Neff CC, Pfister RC, van Sonnenberg E: Percutaneous transtracheal ventilation: Experimental and practical aspects. *J Trauma* 1983; 23:84–90.

15. Zornow MH, Thomas TC, Scheller MS: The efficacy of three different methods of transtracheal ventilation. *Can J Anaesth* 1989; 36:624–628.

16. Stinson TW: A simple connector for transtracheal ventilation (letter). *Anesthesiology* 1977; 47:232.

17. Ravussin P, Freeman J: A new transtracheal catheter for ventilation and resuscitation. *Can J Anaesth* 1985; 32:60–64.

18. Stewart RD: Manual translaryngeal jet ventilation. *Emerg Med Clin North Am* 1989; 7:155–164.

Cricothyrotomy and Tracheotomy

Cheryl Melick, M.D.

Peter Rosen, M.D.

There are few situations in emergency medicine that inspire more concern than the airway that needs to be managed surgically. The incidence is low and the acquisition of the necessary skills difficult. Therefore, even when the clinical situation mandates a surgical airway, there is often a psychological reluctance to attempt the procedure. This tends to make the procedure even more difficult since delay only places greater time constraints upon the emergency physician to achieve a successful airway.

The only mandatory indication for a surgical airway is total upper airway obstruction, which is a very rare condition. The most common reason is failure to achieve intubation by nonsurgical means. The emergency physician, usually more familiar and comfortable with alternative forms of airway management, often persists in attempts to achieve oral or nasal intubation when, in fact, the patient needs a surgical airway.

CRICOTHYROTOMY

History

Tracing the history of cricothyrotomy is difficult owing to the interchangeable usage of the terms *tracheotomy, laryngotomy,* and *high tracheotomy.* These terms described various incisions located anywhere in the neck, including the cricothyroid membrane. Some descriptions clearly describe the division of the tracheal rings, but in most writings, the anatomic location of the airway is not clear. The earliest reference to laryngotomy appears in the writings of the 7th-century surgeon Paulus Aegineta.[1, 2] From its

first description until the 19th century the procedure was widely condemned and rarely performed.

Renewed interest in tracheotomy occurred in 1833 when during the diphtheria epidemic, Bretonneau and Trousseau published a 25% success rate using the procedure in over 200 patients.[2, 3] Following this a new era of enthusiasm began with the "high tracheotomy" becoming the favored approach owing to speed and ease of performance. The procedure was actually an incision placed above the thyroid isthmus and included a division of the cricoid cartilage.

The first description of cricothyrotomy was Upham's case report in 1852 describing a suicidal patient who performed cricothyrotomy upon herself. She ultimately succumbed to a tracheal stricture and stenosis.[4, 5] In 1869, Erichsen, in his book *The Science and Art of Surgery,* stated that a tracheotomy should be performed in a child but a laryngotomy should be used in the adult.[2]

In 1909 Jackson described the surgical techniques of a safe tracheotomy.[6] At this time, confusion between procedures was rampant; authors were careless in their use of terminology and often failed to distinguish between cricothyrotomy, division of the cricoid cartilage (high tracheostomy), and tracheostomy. Jackson treated many patients who could not be successfully decannulated after tracheostomy. In 1921, he reported on 200 patients with chronic subglottic stenosis.[7] Of these, 158 had high tracheotomies performed; however, only 32 of these were true cricothyrotomies placed through the cricothyroid membrane and thyroid cartilage regions. From his limited study, Jackson concluded that the most common cause of chronic subglottic stenosis was high tracheotomy and he decreed that cricothyrotomy "should never be taught even in a life threatening situation." With this statement, cricothyrotomy was labeled as a procedure that should never be performed.

This doctrine was followed until one of Jackson's former pupils, John Grow Sr., questioned the teachings and began performing cricothyrotomies in his postoperative cardiac surgery patients.

Much later, in 1976, Brantigan and Grow published their results of cricothyrotomy on 655 patients.[8] They had a complication rate of only 6.1% and a zero incidence of chronic subglottic stenosis. Subsequent studies have confirmed the safety of cricothyrotomy.[9-15] While there is at present no longer any disagreement over the use of cricothyrotomy for the attainment of an emergency surgical airway, controversy remains over its use for elective airway management and whether it must always be converted to a tracheostomy if more than emergency airway management is needed.[1, 16-20]

Advantages

Cricothyrotomy became established as the preferred method of surgical emergency management during the 1970s and early 1980s. It is an easier procedure to learn since the anatomy is less complicated and there is less tendency to stray from the midline. This makes it quicker to perform and a safer procedure for the emergency physician who performs only infrequent surgical airways.[8, 9, 10, 16, 21] It is performed with the neck in neutral, the position necessary for a successful tracheotomy. Extension of the neck, especially in the context of facial injury, which is the primary indication for a surgical airway, is contraindicated during the initial management of the multiple trauma patient where the status of the cervical spine is either unstable or unknown. Cricothyrotomy is less likely to impinge upon the mediastinum producing pneumothorax, hemorrhage from an enlarged thyroid gland, injury to parathyroid glands, and damage to major vessels, or to the recurrent laryngeal nerve.[13, 16, 22] The advantages of cricothyrotomy over tracheostomy are summarized in Table 16-1.

There are situations that mandate tracheotomy over cricothyrotomy. These are principally during childhood. There is no absolute age at which cricothyrotomy becomes possible to perform. The emergency physician must gauge the size of the child, but also must be guided by the availability of pediatric

TABLE 16-1.

Advantages of Cricothyrotomy Over Tracheostomy

Faster than tracheotomy
Easier to perform for the infrequent operator
Safer; fewer surgical errors
Less encroachment upon the mediastinum
Does not require extension of the neck

equipment as well as familiarity with surgical procedures in children. The anatomic considerations are similar, but pediatric tissues do handle differently from adult tissues and this also contributes to the difficulties of surgical airway management in children.

Indications

Cricothyrotomy has many indications (Table 16-2). Intubation for the traumatized patient is often harder than for the nontraumatic, since one must be concerned about the integrity of the spinal cord. While there are no good data to teach us what is the safest method of intubation, there has been a gradual change in our thinking. For 20 years we have operated under the hypothesis that oral intubation in the multiple trauma patient is unsafe in the presence of cervical spine fracture or when the status of the cervical spine is unknown. There now appear to be data to support a new hypothesis: specifically, that oral intubation is safe so long as hyperflexion, hyperextension, and hyperdistraction at any potential fracture site are avoided.[23-25] In the past, we have recommended that in the face of cervical spine fracture or if the status is unknown, the active form of intubation chosen should be nasotracheal. If this route is unsuccessful, or not possible due to facial injuries, with loss of bony structure and support or massive hemorrhage, then one must perform a cricothyrotomy.[21, 23, 26, 27] It is increasingly less frequent that suspected cervical spine fracture is recognized as an indication for cricothyrotomy.

In most trauma centers, obstruction of the airway is a more frequently recognized indication for cricothyrotomy. The patient with massive facial injuries or with anatomic distortion of the lower airway, such as with penetrating injuries of zone I or lower zone II, will preferentially be managed with cricothyrotomy. A helpful rule is: *All patients should have a cricothyrotomy in whom it will be dangerous to remove spontaneous respirations by paralysis and in whom nasal or oral intubation is impossible or contraindicated.*[21, 25]

In addition to the trauma patient with a need for

TABLE 16–2.

Indications for Cricothyrotomy

Cervical spine injuries or suspected injury
Maxillofacial trauma
Oropharyngeal obstruction
   Edema
      Infection (Ludwig's angina, epiglottitis)
      Caustic ingestion
      Anaphylaxis (allergic reaction)
      Inhalation injuries
      Thermal injuries
      Angioneurotic edema
   Foreign body
   Mass lesion
   Cancer
Oral or nasal tracheal intubation technically difficult
   Anatomic variants, congenital or acquired
   Massive hemorrhage
   Massive aspiration, regurgitation
   Laryngospasm
Unable to obtain an airway after multiple attempts

immediate airway management, cricothyrotomy is indicated in any other disease state that produces upper airway obstruction. Edema of the airway resulting from infections, such as Ludwig's angina, retropharyngeal abscess, and epiglottitis, may occur at the same time as an anatomic deformity or inability to open the mouth, e.g., trismus that may accompany an intraoral abscess. In this case cricothyrotomy may be the only way to achieve airway management. In the child, who frequently develops total obstruction from epiglottitis, the small size of the airway may preclude cricothyrotomy.

Acute anaphylaxis, allergic reactions, and angioneurotic edema may produce such profound and rapidly progressive edema that there may be no time for any form of airway management other than cricothyrotomy.

Thermal, chemical, and inhalation burns of the face and upper airway can also cause massive upper airway edema. Caustic ingestion of acid rarely produces upper airway obstruction but alkali ingestion may be productive of massive swelling and obstruction. Smoke inhalation may complicate oropharyngeal burns compounding the necessity to control the airway. In the above situations oral intubation is always preferable, but may not be possible. In these instances cricothyrotomy should be performed.

Another common cause of obstruction are foreign bodies that obstruct the larynx and may not be removable by the Heimlich maneuver while remaining out of reach of fingers.[28] A majority of foreign bodies are seen in the intoxicated adult who does not properly chew his food or the small child who

chokes on a hot dog or a small part from a toy. If an immediate cricothyrotomy is not performed, the patient will not survive.

Mass lesions of the tongue, tonsil, and upper pharynx may sometimes enlarge precipitously via hemorrhage or posttreatment edema and therefore require lifesaving cricothyrotomy. Tumors of the larynx may also obstruct the airway but they preclude cricothyrotomy owing to their location. In this instance fiberoptic-assisted oral intubation or tracheotomy should be performed.

Finally, some patients require a cricothyrotomy because the oral or nasal route is technically difficult. This may be the result of an anatomic deformity due to congenital malformation or one acquired from prior intubation.[29] Massive hemorrhage or aspiration that cannot be suctioned may contribute to the difficulty of the procedure. In rare patients, laryngospasm may occur after administration of sedating drugs such as fentanyl, or masseter spasm may follow the administration of paralyzing drugs such as succinylcholine.[26, 30]

The most difficult indication for the emergency physician to recognize is the patient for whom oral and nasal routes are not contraindicated, but in whom intubation is unsuccessful. Each patient must be managed individually, but there is a limit beyond which surgical airway management must be chosen. **The hardest technical part of cricothyrotomy performance is the decision to pick up the knife![31]**

Contraindications

In the emergency situation, few contraindications exist for cricothyrotomy (Table 16–3). Most authors agree that poor landmarks and the small size of the cricothyroid space are contraindications to cricothyrotomy in the pediatric patient.[15, 26, 32] The exact age at which a cricothyrotomy becomes safe has not been determined. Many authors arbitrarily use age 10 to 12 as their cutoff[21, 25, 26, 33, 34] while some go as low as age 5.[31, 35–37]

TABLE 16–3.

Contraindications to Cricothyrotomy

Age <10–12 yr
Crush injury to larynx
Preexisting laryngeal pathologic condition (e.g., tumor or stricture)
Tracheal transection
Subglottic stenosis
Expanding upper zone II or III hematoma
Coagulopathy

When direct trauma to the larynx has occurred, there is a potential for tracheal separation. The transected airway may be tenuously held together by the cervical fascia. When an incision divides the fascia, the distal stump of the trachea may retract into the mediastinum with disastrous consequences for the patient. If an endotracheal (ET) tube cannot be passed across the separation to act as a stent, a tracheostomy is the preferred surgical approach.[23, 38–40]

Penetrating trauma to the neck in either high zone II or zone III associated with an expanding hematoma is a definite contraindication.[41] An attempt at cricothyrotomy may produce an exsanguinating hemorrhage. Likewise, patients with known coagulopathy may also develop uncontrollable hemorrhage resulting in aspiration, exsanguination, or inability to complete the procedure because of inability to identify landmarks. Whenever possible the coagulopathy should be corrected with appropriate clotting factors prior to surgical intervention.[31]

A larynx with an underlying abnormality from tumor, trauma, or previous intubation with resultant stenosis or scarring is a contraindication for a cricothyrotomy as the long-term complications, including the development of subglottic stenosis, are significantly increased.[9, 10, 19, 20, 29, 31, 42, 43]

Anatomy

The surface anatomy of the neck is usually easily identified. The hyoid bone lies midway between the mental protuberance of the mandible anteriorly and C3 posteriorly. It is inferior to the base of the tongue and superior to the thyroid cartilage. The hyoid bone is suspended from the base of the skull and mandible by several strong musculotendinous structures and serves as an anchor for the trachea and larynx. The midpoint of the hyoid separates the strap muscles of the neck arising from opposite sides. This provides an excellent landmark for locating the midline of the neck. The hyoid bone is rarely injured in major trauma and in the presence of major swelling and distortion of the neck it may be the only identifiable structure by which to locate the midline.[41, 44] The hyoid bone is differentiated from the thyroid cartilage by the smoothness of its anterior surface. Nevertheless, the hyoid bone is often hard to palpate in the face of induration, cellulitis, hemorrhage, or edema, especially in the short-necked or obese patient.

The thyroid cartilage lies inferior to the mandible and hyoid bone and normally is located in the midline. It is a shieldlike structure consisting of two quadrilateral laminae which meet in the middle and form a V-shaped notch superiorly. This structure, known popularly as the "Adam's apple," is very prominent in men and thin patients, but is much harder to palpate in children, women, obese patients, or when there is massive hemorrhage or edema. There is no other structure in the neck that has a V shape and identification of this notch is critical for successful performance of a cricothyrotomy.[5] Once the thyroid cartilage is located, the next cartilage below its inferior border, approximately 2 to 3 cm caudad, is the cricoid cartilage.[21] This is the only circumferential ring in the airway. It is a signet-ring structure with the large shield located posteriorly. The space between these two structures is the cricothyroid membrane, the desired location for a cricothyrotomy.

The cricothyroid membrane is a dense fibroelastic membrane, trapezoid in shape. It is bounded laterally by the cricothyroid muscles. The usable width of the membrane is 2.7 to 3.2 cm with a mean of 3.0 cm.[45] In 1957, a study by Caparosa and Zavatsky on 50 cadavers found its height to be 0.5 to 1.2 cm from the inferior border of the thyroid cartilage to the superior aspect to the cricoid cartilage, with an average of 0.9 cm.[45] A similar study by Carter and Meyers found the average height in males and females to be 0.81 cm and 0.69 cm, respectively.[46]

The soft tissue space between the skin and larynx contains no important structures. It does not calcify with age. There are no overlying muscles. Superficial veins are encountered that arise from the anterior jugular and superior and inferior thyroid systems. The right and left cricothyroid arteries, branches of the right and left superior thyroid arteries, anastomose across the superior portion of the cricothyroid membrane. The vocal cords, protected by the thyroid cartilage, lie 1.0 to 1.3 cm superior and posterior to the cricothyroid membrane.[11, 45] The vascular thyroid gland and its isthmus lie anterior to the tracheal rings that commence caudal to the cricoid cartilage. The esophagus lies posterior to the cricoid cartilage and is protected by it. The carotid arteries, jugular veins, and superior and recurrent laryngeal nerves run lateral to the respiratory apparatus and are therefore unlikely to be injured by surgery confined to the midline.[5, 26, 31, 47–49]

In children the landmarks are different. The larynx is much higher, lying at about the C2–3 level as opposed to the C5–6 level in adults. The thyroid cartilage consists of two quadrilateral laminae of hyaline cartilage that do not fuse anteriorly to form a prominent thyroid notch or V until adolescence. Because of this, in infants and young children, the hyoid bone and cricoid cartilage are the prominent structures in the anterior neck, making identification of the cricothyroid membrane difficult.[21, 50] The membrane in a term infant is 3 mm wide, too small to admit an ET tube of even 2.5 mm inside diameter.[33, 50] The cricoid cartilage is the narrowest part of the pediatric airway.[32, 36]

Equipment

The equipment is identical for both cricothyrotomy and tracheotomy (Tables 16–4 and 16–5). Most trays that are preset for these procedures contain far too many instruments. The most critical instruments, in addition to a scalpel, are a tracheostomy hook and dilator. The hook is necessary to stabilize the larynx and trachea. This is particularly critical during the performance of a tracheotomy when the neck cannot be hyperextended. Once the cervical fascia is incised, the trachea and larynx tend to fall posteriorly. This makes them hard to control and it is easy for the operator to stray from the midline where complications become frequent and serious.

Procedure

The patient is oxygenated with 100% oxygen while materials are being assembled for the procedure. Frequently the performance of a simple chin lift and jaw thrust maneuver is overlooked in the excitement of the moment, but this may buy extra time.

A midline vertical skin incision (Fig 16–1) is used to assist the operator in staying within the midline.[31, 47, 51] While a transverse skin incision is pref-

TABLE 16–4.

Equipment for Cricothyrotomy and Tracheotomy

Tracheostomy tube, no. 4 Shiley*
Scalpel, no. 11 blade
Trousseau dilator
Tracheostomy skin hook
Curved hemostats (2)
Curved Mayo scissors
25-gauge needle
10-mL syringe
2% lidocaine with epinephrine
Povidone-iodine (Betadine) scrub solution
Gauze pads, 4 × 4 in.
Suction apparatus and tubing
Twill (umbilical) tape

*See Table 16–5.

TABLE 16–5.

Shiley Tracheostomy Tube Sizes

Tube Size	Inside Diameter (mm)	Outside Diameter (mm)
3	4.8	7.0
4	5.0	8.5
6	7.0	10.0
8	8.5	12.0

erable for improved skin cosmesis, the final appearance of the scar is not a consideration when performing a lifesaving procedure. It has been shown by McGill et al. that there are fewer complications when a vertical rather than a transverse incision is used.[30] Before making the incision, the thyroid cartilage is identified by palpation of the superior V notch. The cricothyroid membrane is then identified just inferior. Many authors recommend identifying the three major landmarks, the hyoid bone, thyroid cartilage, and cricoid cartilage, to ensure proper location, as the V notch is not always readily identified in all patients.[31] The skin incision is preferably made with a no. 15 blade, but most kits carry a single blade for the sake of convenience. In this circumstance, a no. 11 blade is useful for both the skin incision and the subsequent incision into the cricothyroid membrane (Fig 16–2).

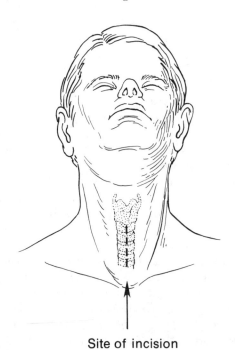

Site of incision

FIG 16–1.
Midline vertical skin incision. (From Rosen P, Barkin RM, Sternbach GL: *Essentials of Emergency Medicine.* St Louis, Mosby–Year Book, 1990. Used by permission).

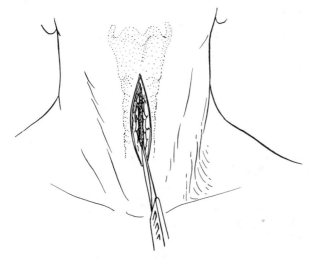

FIG 16–2.
Incising the skin and cricothyroid membrane. (From Rosen P, Barkin RM, Sternbach GL: *Essentials of Emergency Medicine.* St Louis, Mosby–Year Book, 1990. Used by permission).

Bleeding is often profuse, even from small capillary vessels in the anterior neck and soft tissue, when there is any obstruction to the airway, but these can be ignored until an airway is established. This bleeding will usually subside once the patient is less hypoxic and air-hungry. A right-handed operator should operate from the patient's left side and a left-handed operator from the left side. It is possible to operate from the left side if this is necessary in the field. In this case, the incision should be made from the chest cephalad, rather than from the thyroid caudad.

Before the incision is made, the larynx should be grasped with the nonoperating hand. It must be stabilized until the tracheostomy hook can be inserted. A vertical incision is made extending from the superior aspect of the thyroid cartilage caudad to the sternal notch. Do not attempt either procedure through a tiny incision. It will only increase the risk of straying from the midline, with disastrous consequences. The incision should be carried down to the larynx without any effort to identify the individual strap muscles. As soon as the larynx is reached, the tracheostomy hook is inserted through the cricothyroid membrane and the inferior border of the thyroid cartilage is grasped. At this time, the larynx can be released by the nonoperating hand and this hand is now used to stabilize the larynx by holding the hook until an incision can be made into the trachea and an airway established. By constant stabilization of the larynx, it is possible to avoid a very common error of cricothyrotomy, i.e., making the incision

into a location other than the cricothyroid membrane. No harm is done if a tracheotomy is thus inadvertently performed, but if the incision is made superior to the thyroid cartilage, grave injury to the vocal cords may occur. The tip of a no. 11 blade is inserted through the membrane horizontally and caudad to avoid damage to the vocal cords that lie 1 cm cephalad. The incision should be made only with the tip of the scalpel blade to avoid damage to posterior structures such as the esophagus. If possible, the incision should be placed in the inferior aspect of the membrane to avoid the arterial cascade that crosses superiorly. As the airway is entered a rush of air or bubbling is usually noted.

The Trousseau dilator is now inserted and spread vertically to enlarge the diameter of the cricothyroid space. A common error is to spread transversely, which makes it harder to insert the tracheostomy tube. If needed, Mayo scissors may be used to help enlarge the space in the transverse direction. Once the dilator is in place, the tracheostomy hook should be removed so that it will not puncture the balloon of the tracheostomy tube. It is important not to release the dilator before the tracheostomy tube is in place since it would then become very difficult to insert the tube properly.

A critical error is to slide the tube into the anterior mediastinum thinking that the tube is entering the trachea. If a Shiley tracheostomy tube is not available, a cutdown ET tube may be used. This is not ideal because it has the wrong curvature and no inner cannula, which makes insertion into the trachea more difficult. Moreover, if the tube has not been precut and a standard-length ET tube is used, it is very easy to insert the tube into the right mainstem bronchus. Even if this is avoided, it is often difficult to ventilate the patient without kinking the long flexible tube.

The average cricothyroid space in the male will accept a no. 6 Shiley tube but it is too large for the average space in the female. If a tube that is too large is forced into the trachea, it may fracture the cricoid or thyroid cartilages with subsequent permanent injury. It is safest to use a no. 4 Shiley tube that has an inside diameter of 5.0 mm and an outside diameter of 8.5 mm.[26, 30, 51] Once the tube has been inserted, the stylet is removed and the inner cannula is inserted. This step is often forgotten, but the connector to the Ambu bag or ventilator will only fit the inner cannula. The balloon is inflated and the tube position is checked by auscultating for breath sounds.

Bleeding that is persistent can now be identified

TABLE 16–6.

Cricothyrotomy Procedure

1. The patient is oxygenated with 100% oxygen while materials are assembled.
2. If there is no contraindication to cervical extension, place a rolled towel beneath the patient's shoulders. If the status of the cervical spine is in question, maintain neutrality of the cervical spine.
3. If time permits, prepare and drape the anterior neck and raise a vertical wheal with 2% lidocaine with epinephrine.
4. Identify the **V** notch of the superior border of the thyroid cartilage. Stabilize the larynx with the nonoperating hand. Make a vertical incision from the superior border of the thyroid cartilage caudad to the suprasternal notch.
5. Carry the incision down through the strap muscles and the cervical fascia to the larynx.
6. Insert the tracheostomy hook into the cricothyroid space and retract the inferior portion of the thyroid cartilage.
7. Make a transverse incision the width of the cricothyroid space.
8. Insert the Trousseau dilator and spread vertically.
9. Remove the tracheostomy hook and insert a no. 4 Shiley tracheostomy tube.
10. Remove the stylet, insert the inner cannula, and inflate the balloon.
11. Remove the dilator and check the position of the tracheostomy tube. If correct, tie the tube to the patient's neck with twill (umbilical) tape.
12. Obtain a chest film.

and controlled. Be aware that blind clamping lateral to the trachea or larynx may damage important structures, nerves, or vessels. A chest film should always be obtained, not only to insure proper positioning of the tracheostomy tube but to ensure that a pneumothorax has not occurred. This complication is more common following tracheotomy, especially in the infant, but may occur with cricothyrotomy. With positive pressure ventilation, it is all too possible to convert a simple pneumothorax into a tension pneumothorax.

If time and the patient's condition permit, it is useful to place a stay suture on either side of the lateral wall of the larynx. This may be done with 3-0 nylon. The suture is tied to itself and left in place. It serves as a substitute tracheostomy hook should the tracheostomy tube become dislodged and require reinsertion on an emergency basis. The tube should be secured with twill (umbilical) tape and tied around the patient's neck.[5, 8, 21, 26, 30, 31, 47, 52]

The most common error to avoid is taking too much time to decide to pick up the knife and perform the surgical airway and then spending too much time performing the procedure. This delay can lead to irreversible brain hypoxia.

The cricothyrotomy procedure is summarized in Table 16–6.

Complications

Cricothyrotomy compared to tracheotomy has fewer serious acute complications (Table 16–7).

This is due primarily to the superficial location of the cricothyroid membrane and the resulting absence of any important structures overlying the region. Most studies of cricothyrotomy have been performed in the semielective situation with the airway previously controlled. Few studies address complications from cricothyrotomies performed in the emergency situation. In these studies a complication rate of 28% to 32% was found.[19, 28, 30] This compares with a 6% to 8% rate in the elective situation.[8, 9, 11, 15, 27]

The common technical errors of performance have been discussed under Procedure. The two most important errors to avoid are too much time spent in performing the procedure, i.e., greater than 3 min-

TABLE 16–7.

Complications of Cricothyrotomy

Acute	Chronic
Incorrect tube placement	Infection
Long execution time (>3 min)	Hemorrhage
Hemorrhage	Plugging with secretions
False passage	Persistent stoma
Subcutaneous emphysema	Dysphonia, hoarseness
Plugging with secretions	Subglottic stenosis
Pneumomediastinum	Laryngeal stenosis
Self-extubation	Vocal cord paralysis
Aspiration	Tracheomalacia
Asphyxia	Aerophagia
Thyroid gland damage	Aspiration
Esophagus damage	
Cartilage fracture	
Recurrent laryngeal nerve damage	
Cardiac arrest	

utes, (28%), and incorrect site of tube placement (36%).[9, 30] This can lead to irreversible damage from hypoxia.

In the immediate postoperative period, the patient may have obstruction from secretions, hemorrhage, or kinking of the tube. The airway must therefore be observed carefully and suctioned as necessary. Cardiac dysrhythmias are common during suctioning, as is marked oxygen desaturation. This can be guarded against by the use of atropine, quick suctioning, and intravenous lidocaine. Bucking on the tube may require paralysis or sedation of the patient to prevent accidental dislodgment. Proper securing of the tube and patient is needed to prevent extubation. If the patient self-extubates, it may be very difficult to reintubate, especially if stay sutures have not been placed.

Leakage or breakage of the Shiley tube balloon is common. This may make it difficult to provide adequate ventilation. The risk of balloon damage is lower if the tracheostomy hook is removed prior to tube insertion and if the dilator is removed carefully.

Subcutaneous emphysema and pneumomediastinum are common and may be profound if the incision has been closed too tightly.[53, 54] This can produce a tension pneumothorax or a tension pneumomediastinum that behaves like a pericardial tamponade. In hurried situations, if the blade is not directed in precisely, damage to the vocal cords, esophagus, thyroid gland, and recurrent laryngeal nerve may result.

Chronic complications of cricothyrotomy are related to the surgical technique as well as to how long the surgical airway is maintained. Most commonly, minor problems, such as dysphonia or hoarseness, are noted in up to 40% of patients.[10, 11, 15] The dreaded complication, chronic subglottic stenosis, is seen in about 2% of patients.[9, 10, 15, 19] This rate is not higher than that seen with long-term endotracheal intubation, but it is not seen with tracheotomy.[18, 42, 55–58]

More commonly, infection at the site, including cellulitis, abscess formation, and perichondritis, develops if proper postoperative wound care is not maintained. Tracheomalacia may result from cartilage damage or serious infection. Once injured, cartilage does not have the ability to regenerate. Late bleeding may develop from erosion or improperly ligated vessels. Plugging of the tube with secretions, if not properly humidified and sectioned routinely, will develop and may result in death if not recognized. A persistent stoma or inability to decannulate due to laryngeal stenosis or vocal cord paralysis may

occur. Some patients have the persistent feeling of a "lump" in their throat and will continuously swallow air (aerophagia) or have trouble with deglutition as a result. With proper postoperative care and close follow-up by an otolaryngologist, many of these complications may be avoided.

TRACHEOTOMY

History

The writings of Galen and Aretaeus of Cappadocia around the 2nd century A.D. ascribe the first elective tracheotomy to Asclepiades of Bithynia near the end of the 1st century B.C.[3] Since its first description until the 19th century, when it became popularized, tracheotomy was widely condemned as a futile and dangerous procedure. The first successful tracheotomy on a human was done in 1546 by Musa Brassarolo who performed it to relieve an abscess in the windpipe.[59, 60] The first technical descriptions are found in the writings of Fabricius and Habicot, in 1617 and 1620 respectively.[60] Widespread use and popularity for the procedure developed following the publication in 1833 by Bretonneau and Trousseau on its successful performance in children with airway obstruction resulting from the croup and diphtheria epidemic sweeping France at the time.[2, 3] The remainder of the century brought an explosion of literature detailing the performance, complications, and controversies of the procedure.[61]

In 1909 the definitive paper on appropriate surgical technique was published by Chevalier Jackson.[6] In 1921 Jackson published a landmark paper condemning high tracheostomies and more clearly defining surgical airway management to a standard tracheostomy.[7] Until the 1940s, performance of a tracheotomy was only indicated for relief of an obstruction of the upper airway from such causes as croup, diphtheria, foreign bodies, and trauma. In 1943, during the polio epidemic, Galloway demonstrated the usefulness of the procedure in helping to manage secretions in polio patients.[62] Following this, multiple indications for the procedure developed, including management of severe chest and head injuries along with the management of chronic obstructive pulmonary disease (COPD) due to the decrease in dead space which results. With the advent of endotracheal intubation, first performed in 1878 by Macewen, and popularized in 1907 by Bartholomy for anesthesia, one of the main dramatic uses for tracheotomy was removed.[2] With the realization

TABLE 16–8.

Indications for Tracheotomy

Pediatric patients
Laryngeal fracture
Tracheal transection
Expanding high zone II or III hematoma
Laryngeal foreign body or tumor
Subglottic stenosis

of the safety, speed, and relative ease of endotracheal airway control for many situations, a more limited and rational approach to the use of tracheostomy has developed in the past 30 years.

Indications

In most emergency situations, cricothyrotomy is the procedure of choice, as tracheotomies are more difficult and time-consuming with more serious potential complications.[10, 16, 19, 33, 52] There are, however, situations when a tracheotomy is the surgical airway of choice (Table 16–8).

In the pediatric patient, owing to a very small cricothyroid membrane (3 mm wide),[50, 33] and poorly defined landmarks, a cricothyrotomy is an anatomically impossible procedure.[63] The smallest ET tube of 2.5 mm has an outside diameter of 3.5 mm, and forcing a tube through an opening that is too small carries significant long-term morbidity should the patient survive. The age up to which a tracheotomy should be performed is not known, and depends largely on the size of the child. Some authors recommend age 5 years[31, 35, 36, 37] as the cut-off, but more commonly age 10 to 12[21, 25, 26, 33, 34] is the age above which most feel a cricothyrotomy may be safely performed.

The most common indication for an emergent tracheotomy is laryngeal fracture or destruction.[64–66] Performance of a cricothyrotomy through a badly deformed larynx presents multiple difficulties including inability to identify landmarks with inappropriate tube placement resulting. An expanding zone III or high zone II hematoma indicates serious large-vessel injury and controlling an airway through this hematoma may result in an exsanguinating hemorrhage. A transected trachea will quickly retract into the chest out of reach if attempts at airway control other than a tracheotomy are performed.[23, 39, 40] Laryngeal foreign bodies, tumors, or stenosis from previous airway control procedures may make performance of cricothyrotomy impossible.

Contraindications

A major contraindication to performance of a tracheotomy is the situation in which a cricothyrotomy may be performed safely in its place (Table 16–9). Doing a tracheotomy simply because it is felt at the time that a long-term airway may be needed is not relevant to the emergent situation. Cricothyrotomy for surgical access is by far quicker and safer in an emergency. It may be converted to a standard tracheotomy under more controlled and safer conditions at a later date. An expanding zone I or low zone II hematoma, besides making a technically difficult procedure more difficult by obscuring the field with blood, may cause rapid exsanguination once the tamponade is violated. Lastly, a relative contraindication, as in any surgical procedure, is the presence of a coagulopathy. If at all possible, this should be corrected prior to performance of a surgical airway.

Anatomy

The trachea is composed of 16 to 20 hyaline cartilage U-shaped structures connected posteriorly by fibroelastic tissue. The trachea begins at the inferior border of the cricoid cartilage at the level of C6 in the adult. It extends 10 to 11 cm caudad (4–5 cm in the newborn), ending at the carina opposite the upper edge of T5. Its external diameter measures 1.5 to 2.0 cm in the adult and 0.3 to 0.4 cm in the newborn.[48, 50] The trachea runs much deeper in the neck than the cricothyroid membrane and this requires more technical expertise in the performance of a tracheotomy than in cricothyrotomy.

The skin and subcutaneous tissue are anterior to the trachea. Below is the fascia that invests the anterior jugular veins which frequently anastomose across the midline. The thyroid isthmus is situated below this fascia and overlies the second through fourth tracheal rings, the optimal site for the tracheotomy incision. The thyroid isthmus is attached superiorly via a suspensory ligament to the inferior border of the cricoid cartilage. Above the isthmus, the superior thyroid arteries anastomose, while just below the isthmus, the inferior thyroid veins are

TABLE 16–9.

Contraindications to Tracheotomy

Zone I or low zone II hematoma
Cricothyrotomy possible
Coagulopathy

found along with the remnants of the thymus gland. In the adult, the inferior thyroid veins are frequently behind the manubrium and are not a source of bleeding. In the infant, however, identifying these veins is a warning that you are too low in the neck and in danger of injuring the brachiocephalic artery and left brachiocephalic vein that cross just above the manubrium near these vessels.[49, 54]

Lateral to the trachea are the sternocleidomastoid muscle and the strap muscles of the neck. These cover and protect the carotid sheath and lobes of the thyroid gland. The carotid sheath contains the carotid artery, internal jugular vein, and vagus nerve, which are especially prone to damage in the pediatric patient owing to their small size and close proximity to the trachea. The thyroid lobes lie adjacent to the trachea from its origin at the cricoid cartilage down to the fifth or sixth tracheal ring.

The posterior aspect of the trachea lacks cartilaginous support and is enclosed by fibroelastic tissue. The posterior wall is flattened and lies against the esophagus. On either side, running obliquely, lie the recurrent laryngeal nerves.

Procedure

The most critical instruments in addition to the scalpel are a tracheostomy hook and tracheal dilator. The hook is necessary to stabilize the larynx and trachea. This is particularly critical during the performance of a tracheotomy when the neck cannot be hyperextended. Once the fascia is incised, the trachea and larynx fall posteriorly. This makes the trachea, which already tends to run posteriorly, hard to control, making it easy for the operator to stray from the midline where complications are frequent and serious.

The patient is oxygenated with 100% oxygen while the materials are assembled. In a routine tracheotomy the neck is hyperextended by placing a folded towel below the shoulders to bring the trachea more into the field of view (Fig 16–3). If a cervical spine fracture is not a concern and if the neck can be hyperextended, care should be taken to not overextend the neck, especially in short and thick-necked patients, because the trachea is so deep that accidental decannulation may occur when the neck is flexed postoperatively and the stoma recedes away from the surface.[22, 67, 68]

A vertical midline incision is used to assist the operator in staying within the midline. Disastrous hemorrhage can occur from injury to major vessels if a transverse incision is used.[54, 68–70] While a transverse skin incision may be preferred for improved

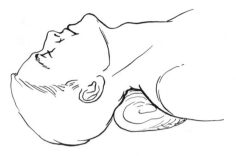

FIG 16–3.
A folded towel placed below the shoulders for routine tracheotomy. (From Rosen P, Barkin RM, Sternbach GL: *Essentials of Emergency Medicine*. St Louis, Mosby–Year Book, 1990. Used by permission).

skin cosmesis, the final appearance of the scar is not a consideration when performing a lifesaving procedure. Before making the incision, landmarks are identified by palpation (see Anatomy). The superior V notch of the thyroid cartilage is the most easily recognized landmark, except in the infant. Immediately inferior is the cricoid cartilage, and then the tracheal rings. The skin incision is preferably made with a no. 15 blade, but most kits carry a single blade for convenience. In this circumstance a no. 11 blade is useful for both the skin incision and subsequent entry into the trachea.

Prior to making the incision, the larynx should be stabilized with the nonoperating hand. This is facilitated by the right-handed operator standing at the patient's right side. The larynx must be held until the tracheostomy hook is inserted. This helps to maintain the midline and prevent complications. A vertical incision is made from the cricoid cartilage caudad to the sternal notch. Do not attempt the procedure through a small incision; it will only increase the risk of straying from the midline.

In carrying the incision through the investing fascia, branches of the anterior jugular veins are encountered. If identified, these veins are clamped and ligated to prevent major hemorrhage (Fig 16–4). These vessels achieve prominent size, especially in the struggling and hypoxic patient. Incising the investing fascia reveals the thyroid isthmus (Fig 16–5). It overlies the second through fourth tracheal rings, the site for performance of the tracheotomy. If the thyroid isthmus cannot be easily retracted out of the field, then it must be clamped and ligated. It may be mobilized by cutting its suspensory ligament at the inferior border of the cricoid cartilage. Using a blunt clamp or hemostat, dissect beneath the isthmus along the tracheal wall to free it. Clamps are then

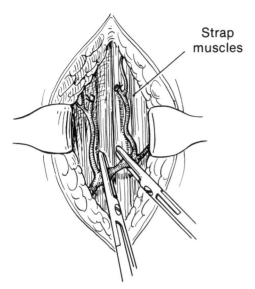

FIG 16–4.
Clamping branches of the anterior jugular veins. (From Rosen P, Barkin RM, Sternbach GL: *Essentials of Emergency Medicine.* St Louis, Mosby–Year Book, 1990. Used by permission).

placed on either side of the midline and the isthmus is cut. Suture ligation with a 2-0 silk may be performed later.

Identification of the second tracheal ring is now possible. Place the tracheostomy hook between the first and second rings and use gentle upward traction to better elevate the trachea into the surgical field. The trachea is incised transversely between the second and third ring interspace using a no. 11

too far laterally, which will transect the trachea, or too far posteriorly, which will damage the esophagus. When performing this procedure in the newborn it should be remembered that the structures are anatomically small and the carotid artery lies next to the trachea. If in doubt about the appropriate structure being entered, prior needle aspiration may avert serious consequences. The anterior portion of the third ring is then cut on each side using the no. 11 blade. Occasionally, owing to calcification of the tracheal cartilage, heavy scissors are required. The anterior portion of the third cartilage is removed (Fig 16–7). A Trousseau dilator is inserted and spread vertically. Once the dilator is in place, the tracheostomy hook may be removed to prevent puncture of the balloon. A no. 7 Shiley tube is the appropriate size for most male tracheas and a no. 6 Shiley tube is used for the female patient. An ET tube is best avoided because it has the wrong curvature, is too long and thus risks entering the right mainstem bronchus, and is too flexible, which causes kinking.

Once the tracheostomy tube has been inserted, proper placement is checked by auscultating over the lung fields and watching for chest movement. Suctioning of blood and debris is necessary to prevent tube expulsion from coughing. Control of any persistent bleeding should now be performed. A chest film should be obtained to evaluate tube placement as well as search for a pneumothorax. Pneumothorax is a common complication in tracheoto-

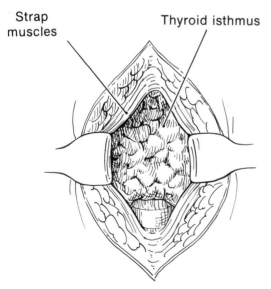

FIG 16–5.
The thyroid isthmus. (From Rosen P, Barkin RM, Sternbach GL: *Essentials of Emergency Medicine.* St Louis, Mosby–Year Book, 1990. Used by permission).

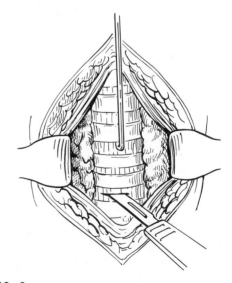

FIG 16–6.
Transverse incision in the trachea. Note position of the tracheostomy hook. (From Rosen P, Barkin RM, Sternbach GL: *Essentials of Emergency Medicine.* St Louis, Mosby–Year Book, 1990. Used by permission).

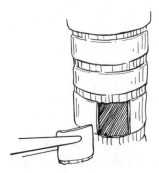

FIG 16–7.
Removal of the anterior portion of the third cartilage. (From Rosen P, Barkin RM, Sternbach GL: *Essentials of Emergency Medicine.* St Louis, Mosby–Year Book, 1990. Used by permission).

mies, especially those performed in the pediatric population.[67, 70–72]

If time and the patient's condition permit, it is useful to place a stay suture on either side of the lateral wall of the trachea. This may be done with 3-0 nylon. The suture is tied to itself and left in place. It serves as a substitute tracheostomy hook should the tracheostomy tube become dislodged and require reinsertion on an emergent basis prior to development of an epithelialized tract, which normally requires 7 to 10 days. The tube should be secured with twill (umbilical) tape and tied around the patient's neck. The skin incision should be closed loosely or left open. A skin closure that is too tight will prevent escape of air during forced expiration, causing subcutaneous emphysema.[33, 39, 50, 52, 53, 54, 68, 73, 74]

The tracheotomy procedure is summarized in Table 16–10.

Complications

Most complications following tracheotomy are similar to those encountered in the performance of a cricothyrotomy (Table 16–11). Acute complications that are common to both procedures include subcutaneous emphysema, pneumomediastinum, aspiration, false passageway, cardiac arrest due to asphyxia or increased vagal stimulation, plugging of the tube with secretions, and self-extubation.

Acutely, hemorrhage is the most commonly encountered problem during a tracheotomy, occurring in about 5% of cases.[8, 39, 68, 75] This area is rich in vasculature. The branches of the anterior jugular vein cross the investing fascia in the midline at the site of the incision, while the superior thyroid arteries cross the superior aspect of the thyroid isthmus. The carotid sheath containing the common carotid artery and jugular vein are just lateral to the trachea, a significant relationship in the newborn. Lastly, in some patients the innominate artery crosses just superior to the manubrium and is easily nicked with a scalpel as the incision is extended inferiorly, especially in a struggling patient.[54, 76]

Pneumothorax is much more frequent than after cricothyrotomy. In patients with COPD and in infants, the pleural domes extend out of the chest into the lower neck in the region of the tracheotomy. This complication is seen in 5% to 7% of pediatric patients and the consequences are disastrous if not immediately recognized.[33, 53, 67, 70, 72, 77] Owing to the multitude of large vessels in the region, air embolism is a rare but potentially serious complication.

TABLE 16–10.

Tracheotomy Procedure

1. The patient is oxygenated with 100% oxygen while materials are assembled.
2. If there is no contraindication to cervical extension, place a rolled towel beneath the patient's shoulders. If the status of the cervical spine is in question, maintain neutrality of the cervical spine.
3. If time permits, prepare and drape the anterior neck and raise a vertical wheal with 2% lidocaine with epinephrine.
4. Once the larynx is identified, stabilize it with the nonoperating hand. Make an incision from the inferior border of the thyroid cartilage down to the suprasternal notch.
5. Carry the incision down through the cervical fascia to the trachea.
6. Insert the tracheostomy hook into the third tracheal interspace.
7. Make a transverse incision above and below the third tracheal cartilage.
8. Remove the anterior portion of the third cartilage.
9. Insert the Trousseau dilator and spread vertically.
10. Insert an appropriate-sized Shiley tracheostomy tube.
11. Remove the stylet, insert the inner cannula, and inflate the balloon.
12. Remove the dilator and check the position of the tube. Tie the tube to the patient's neck with twill (umbilical) tape.
13. Obtain a chest film.

TABLE 16–11.

Complications of Tracheotomy

Acute	Chronic
Hemorrhage	Infection
Pneumothorax	Plugging with secretions
Subcutaneous emphysema	Hemorrhage
Pneumomediastinum	Tracheal stenosis
Aspiration	Tracheoesophageal fistula
False passage	Innominate artery erosion
Cardiac arrest	Aspiration
Plugging with secretions	Aerophagia
Air emboli	Persistent stoma
Thyroid gland damage	Vocal cord paralysis
Esophagus damage	Tracheomalacia
Self-extubation	Mediastinitis

Damage to the thyroid gland that is more extensive with increased bleeding may occur with suture ligation of the thyroid isthmus occurs during a tracheotomy. Esophageal damage during incision into the trachea is more readily caused as there is no posterior support structure to protect the thin-walled tracheoesophageal interface. During a cricothyrotomy, the large signet-ring shape of the posterior cricoid cartilage protects the esophagus against inadvertent entry or damage.

Chronic complications, which are the same for cricothyrotomy and tracheotomy, include infection at the surgical site; plugging of the tube with secretions; aspiration; aerophagia; and a persistent stoma.

Tracheal stenosis is seen in over 65% of autopsy studies[57] but is only clinically significant in 2% to 4% of patients.[77–79] Tracheoesophageal fistula and innominate artery hemorrhage are two devastating complications resulting from erosion and constant pressure of a poorly fitting tracheostomy tube.[53, 80] In some situations smaller bleeds herald the exsanguinating hemorrhage from the innominate artery erosion. Another common complication, tracheomalacia, may develop from a low-grade infection. A more severe and devastating complication is mediastinitis that may occur due to extension of infection from the surgical site to the chest. Lastly, vocal cord paralysis, which frequently is caused by damage to the recurrent laryngeal nerve at the time of performance of the surgical airway, is only noticed at a later date when attempts at decannulation are unsuccessful.

Mortality from the tracheotomy procedure itself is usually reported at less than 5%,[57, 67, 78–80] but most studies have been performed in the semielective situation with the airway already controlled by other methods. It is believed that mortality for emergent tracheotomy is in the vicinity of 30%,[40, 79] with this figure being much higher in the infant than in the adult.[77, 80–82] While this probably represents death from the underlying condition that necessitated the tracheotomy, the emergent procedure is difficult and technical errors are common.

Postoperative Care

Following surgical airway management, patients are admitted to the intensive care unit (ICU) for proper postoperative wound care and monitoring. Immediately postoperation, sudden tube occlusion from crusting and plugging of secretions may occur with disastrous consequences if it is not immediately recognized and corrected. To minimize this possibility, aggressive humidification of inspired oxygen in conjunction with frequent suctioning and good pulmonary toilet must be carried out.

Head positioning is very important. Multiple skin folds or a short neck can easily cause tube occlusion. In neonates and small children, owing to the small size of the trachea, the length of the tube will be only a few centimeters. In this situation slight hyperextension of the neck may cause extubation that can remain undetected until serious hypoxia has occurred.

Replacement of an extubated tracheostomy tube is extremely difficult in the first 7 to 10 days before an epithelialized tract has developed. During the development of this fistula, patients should be monitored in the ICU with a spare tracheostomy tube at the bedside. When extubated, the ends of the trachea frequently retract, making replacement of the tube difficult. It is common for a displaced tube to be replaced into a false passageway between soft tissue planes. If stay sutures have been left in place, traction on them will allow the ends of the trachea to be pulled into view so that appropriate tube replacement may be done.

Chronic complications of stenosis, granuloma formation, and innominate artery erosion may occur due to pressure from the tube. A cuff pressure that is too high can cause damage that may lead to chronic problems. Tracheomalacia, from chronic or low-grade infection of the cartilage, is another devastating long-term complication. Once damaged from infection, cartilage will not regenerate. This is an important reason to maintain proper aseptic technique during all suctioning and care of the surgical site as well as to prevent nosocomial infections of the neck and lung.[5, 12, 22, 53, 54, 59, 67, 69, 70, 76, 77, 82]

The postoperative complications of surgical airways are summarized in Table 16–12.

TABLE 16–12.
Postoperative Care of Surgical Airways

Complications	Care and Prevention
Tube occlusion	Humidification
	Frequent suctioning/pulmonary toilet
	Correct head positioning
Premature decannulation	Spare tracheostomy tube at bedside
	Stay sutures in place
Infection	Aseptic technique
Tracheal stenosis	Cuff pressure monitoring
	Proper tube size
	Correct head positioning

SUMMARY

The ability to perform a surgical airway is an important skill for the emergency physician to possess. Technical competency comes only with practice and clinical wisdom only with experience. The emergency physician must have a psychological readiness for these difficult procedures so that the ability will exist to carry them out in those patients for whom it will be lifesaving.

REFERENCES

1. Gleeson MJ: Cricothyroidotomy: A satisfactory alternative to tracheostomy? (Editorial). *Clin Otolaryngol* 1984; 9:1–2.
2. Frost EA: Tracing the tracheostomy. *Ann Otol* 1976; 85:618–624.
3. Goodall EW: The story of tracheotomy. *Br J Child Dis* 1934; 31:167–176, 253–272.
4. Upham JB: Report of a case of incised wound of the throat resulting in closure of the larynx by cicatrix. *New Hampshire J Med* 1852; 2:206.
5. Brantigan CO: Emergency cricothyroidotomy, in Roberts JR, Hedges JR (eds): *Clinical Procedures in Emergency Medicine*. Philadelphia, WB Saunders Co, 1985.
6. Jackson C: Tracheotomy. *Laryngoscope* 1909; 18:285–290.
7. Jackson C: High tracheotomy and other errors: The chief causes of chronic laryngeal stenosis. *Surg Gynecol Obstet* 1921; 32:392–395.
8. Brantigan CO, Grow JB: Cricothyroidotomy: Elective use in respiratory problems requiring tracheotomy. *J Thorac Cardiovasc Surg* 1976; 71:72–81.
9. Boyd AD, Romita MC, Conlan AA, et al: A clinical evaluation of cricothyroidotomy. *Surg Gynecol Obstet* 1979; 149:365–368.
10. Cole RR, Aguilar EA: Cricothyroidotomy versus tracheotomy: An otolaryngologist's perspective. *Laryngoscope*. 1988; 98:131–135.
11. Greisz H, Qvarnstrom O, Willen R: Elective cricothyroidotomy: A clinical and histopathological study. *Crit Care Med* 1982; 10:387–389.
12. McDowell DE: Cricothyroidostomy for airway access. *South Med J* 1982; 75:282–284.
13. Morain WD: Cricothroidostomy in head and neck surgery. *Plast Reconstr Surg* 1980; 65:424–428.
14. Romita MC, Colvin DB, Boyd AD: Cricothyroidotomy. *Surg Forum* 1977; 28:174.
15. Sise MJ, Shackford SR, Cruickshank JC, et al: Cricothyroidotomy for long-term tracheal access. *Ann Surg* 1984; 200:13–17.
16. Booth RP, Brown J, Jones K: Cricothyroidotomy, a useful alternative to tracheostomy in maxillofacial surgery. *Int J Oral Maxillofac Surg* 1989; 18:24–26.
17. Kennedy TL: Epiglottic reconstruction of laryngeal stenosis secondary to cricothyroidostomy. *Laryngoscope* 1980; 90:1130–1136.
18. Brantigan CO, Grow JB. Cricothyroidotomy revisited again. *Ear Nose Throat J* 1980; 59:26–38.
19. Esses BA, Jafek BW: Cricothyroidotomy: A decade of experience in denver. *Ann Otol Rhinol Laryngol* 1987; 96:519–524.
20. Kuriloff DB, Setzen M, Portnoy W, et al: Laryngotracheal injury following cricothyroidotomy. *Laryngoscope* 1989; 99:125–130.
21. Kress TD, Balasubramaniam S: Cricothyroidotomy. *Ann Emerg Med* 1982; 11:197–201.
22. Kenan PD: Complications associated with tracheostomy: Prevention and treatment. *Otolaryngol Clin North Am* 1979; 12:807–815.
23. Jordan R: Airway management. *Emerg Med Clin North Am* 1988; 6:678–685.
24. Apple JS, Kirks DR, Merten DF, et al: Cervical spine fractures and dislocations in children. *Pediatr Radiol* 1987; 17:45–49.
25. American College of Surgeons, Committee on Trauma: *ATLS Instructor Manual*. American College of Surgeons, 1989, pp 35–37.
26. Mace SE: Cricothyrotomy. *J Emerg Med* 1988; 6:309–319.
27. Kastendieck J: Airway management, in Rosen P, Baker FJ, Barkin RM, et al (eds): *Emergency Medicine: Concepts and Clinical Practice*, ed 2. St Louis, Mosby–Year Book, Inc, 1988 pp 41–68.
28. Spaite DW, Joseph M: Prehospital cricothyrotomy: An investigation of indications, technique, complications and patient outcome. *Ann Emerg Med* 1990; 19:279–285.
29. Whited RE: A prospective study of laryngotracheal sequelae in long-term intubation. *Laryngoscope* 1984; 94:367–377.
30. McGill J, Clinton JE, Ruiz E: Cricothyrotomy in the emergency department. *Ann Emerg Med* 1982; 11:361–364.

31. Walls RM: Cricothyroidotomy. *Emerg Med Clin North Am* 1988; 6:725–736.
32. American Heart Association: *Textbook of Pediatric Advanced Life Support*. Dallas, American Heart Association, 1988.
33. Piotrowski JJ, Moore EE: Emergency department tracheostomy. *Emerg Clin North Am* 1988; 6:737–744.
34. Linscott MS, Horton WC: Management of upper airway obstruction. *Otolaryngol Clin North Am* 1979; 12:351–373.
35. Barkin RM, Rosen P: *Emergency Pediatrics*, ed 2. St Louis, Mosby–Year Book, Inc, 1986, p 13.
36. Barkin RM: Pediatric airway management. *Emerg Med Clin North Am* 1988; 6:687–692.
37. Rosen P, Barkin R: Pediatric respiratory distress. *J Emerg Med* 1983; 1:81–82.
38. Mace SE: Blunt laryngotracheal trauma. *Ann Emerg Med* 1986; 15:836–842.
39. Orringer MB: Endotracheal intubation and tracheotomy. Surg Clin *North Am* 1980; 60:1447–1464.
40. Price HC, Postma DS: Tracheostomy. *Ear Nose Throat J* 1983; 62:474–483.
41. Simon RR, Brenner BE, Rosen MA: Emergency cricothyroidotomy in the patient with massive neck swelling. Part 2: Clinical aspects. *Crit Care Med* 1983; 11:119–123.
42. Brantigan CO, Grow JB: Subglottic stenosis after cricothroidotomy. *Surgery* 1982; 91:217–221.
43. Weymuller EA, Cummings CW: Cricothyroidotomy: The impact of antecedent endotracheal intubation. *Ann Oto Rhinol Laryngol* 1982; 91:437–439.
44. Simon RR, Brenner BE: Emergency cricothroidotomy in the patient with massive neck swelling: Part 1: Anatomical aspects. *Crit Care Med* 1983; 11:114–118.
45. Caparosa RJ, Zavatsky AR: Practical aspects of the cricothyroid space. *Laryngoscope* 1957; 67:577–591.
46. Carter DR, Meyers AD: The anatomy of the subglottic larynx. *Otolaryngology* 1978; 86:279.
47. Narrod JA, Moore EE, Rosen P: Emergency cricothyrotomy: Technique and anatomical considerations. *J Emerg Med* 1985; 2:443–446.
48. Morris IR: Functional anatomy or the upper airway. *Emerg Med Clin North Am* 1988; 6:659–669.
49. Williams Warwick: The Larynx, in *Gray's Anatomy*, ed 36. Philadelphia, WB Saunders Co, 1980, pp 1229–1241.
50. Tucker JA: Obstruction of the major pediatric airway. *Otolaryngol Clin North Am* 1979; 12:329–341.
51. Clinton JE, Ruiz E: Emergency airway management: Methods to meet the challenge. *Top Emerg Med* 1988; 10:31–41.
52. Simon RR, Brenner BE: *Procedures and Techniques in Emergency Medicine*. Baltimore, Williams & Wilkins Co, 1982.
53. Scholl PD, Pashley NR: Tracheotomy, in Balkany TJ (ed): *Clinical Pediatric Otolaryngology*. St Louis, Mosby–Year Book, Inc, 1986.
54. Kirchner JA: Tracheotomy and its problems. *Surg Clin North Am* 1980; 60:1093–1104.
55. Gaynor EB, Greenberg SB: Untoward sequelae of prolonged intubation. *Laryngoscope* 1985; 95:1461–1467.
56. Mackenzie CF: Compromises in the choice of orotracheal or nasotracheal intubation and tracheostomy. *Heart Lung* 1983; 12:485–492.
57. Stauffer JL, Olson DE, Petty TL: Complications and consequences of endotracheal intubation and tracheotomy. *Am J Med* 1981; 70:65–76.
58. Marshak G, Grundfast KM: Subglottic Stenosis. *Pediatr Clin North Am* 1981; 28:941–948.
59. Koopmann CF, Feld RA, Coulthard SW: The effects of cricoid cartilage injury and antibiotics in cricothyroidotomy. *Am J Otol* 1981; 2:123–128.
60. Borman J, Davidson JT: A history of tracheostomy. *Br J Anaesth* 1963; 35:388–390.
61. Colles CJ: On stenosis of the trachea after tracheotomy for croup and diphtheria. *Ann Surg* 1886; 3:499–507.
62. Galloway TC: Tracheotomy in bulbar poliomyelitis. *JAMA* 1943; 123:1096.
63. Kinnerfors A, Olofsson J: Acute epiglottitis in children: Experiences with tracheotomy and intubation. *Clin Otolaryngol* 1983; 8:25–30.
64. Whited RE: Laryngeal fracture in the multiple trauma patient. *Am J Surg* 1978; 136:354–355.
65. Schaefer SD: Primary management of laryngeal trauma. *Ann Otol Rhinol Laryngol* 1982; 91:399–402.
66. Trone TH, Schaefer SD, Carder HM: Blunt and penetrating laryngeal trauma: A 13-year review. *Otolaryngol Head Neck Surg* 1980; 88:257–261.
67. Rodgers BM, Rooks JJ, Talbert JL: Pediatric tracheostomy: Long-term evaluation. *J Pediatr Surg* 1979; 14:258–263.
68. Tepas JJ, Heroy JH, Shermeta DW, et al: Tracheostomy in neonates and small infants: Problems and pitfalls. 1981; 89:635–639.
69. Carter P, Benjamin B: Ten-year review of pediatric tracheotomy. *Ann Otol Rhinol Laryngol* 1983; 92:398–400.
70. Gerson CR, Tucker GF: Infant tracheotomy. *Ann Otol Rhinol Laryngol* 1982; 91:413–416.
71. Johnson DG, Jones R: Surgical aspects of airway management in infants and children. *Surg Clin North Am* 1976; 56:263–279.
72. Perrotta RJ, Schley WS: Pediatric tracheotomy. *Arch Otolaryngol* 1978; 104:318–321.
73. McLaughlin J, Iserson KV: Emergency pediatric tracheostomy: A usable technique and model for instruction. *Ann Emerg Med* 1986; 15:463–465.
74. McKelvie P: How to do an emergency tracheostomy. *Br J Hosp Med* 1981; 25:640–641.
75. James OF, Moore PG: Tracheostomy in the management of chest injuries: Its use and complications. *Aust N Z J Surg* 1981; 51:598–602.

76. Stemmer EA, Oliver C, Carney JP, et al: Fatal complications of tracheostomy. *Am J Surg* 1976; 131:288–240.

77. Gilmore BB, Mickelson SA: Pediatric tracheotomy. *Otol Clin North Am* 1986; 19:141–151.

78. Schusterman M, Faires RA, Brown D, et al: Local complications and mortality of adult tracheostomy. *J Ky Med Assoc.* 1983; 81:885–888.

79. Head JM: Tracheostomy in the management of respiratory problems. *N Engl J Med* 1961; 264:587–591.

80. Wetmore RF, Handler SD, Potsic WP: Pediatric tracheostomy experience during the past decade. *Ann Otol Rhinol Laryngol* 1982; 91:628–632.

81. Okafor BC: Tracheostomy in the management of pediatric airway problems. *Ear Nose Throat J* 1983; 62:28–33.

82. Hawkins DB, Williams EH: Tracheostomy in infants and young children. *Laryngoscope* 1976; 86:331–340.

17

Cricotomes

Steven Hulsey, M.D.

HISTORY

Currently, surgical cricothyrotomy is the accepted alternative emergency procedure when translaryngeal intubation is impossible. However, cricothyrotomy has potential for major hemorrhage, infection, pneumothorax, and damage to surrounding structures. Also, it requires greater surgical experience than most emergency physicians have acquired, and ideally an assistant as well. Most important, this procedure may be too time-consuming in a critical situation.

Cricotomes are percutaneous devices designed to overcome these problems. The underlying concept of the cricotome is the insertion of a needle or stylet into the airway and subsequent dilation of the tract to allow placement of a functional airway. They have been developed to improve speed and safety, allow for lesser surgical skills in the operator, expand their use to children, and provide more effective ventilation and oxygenation than found with percutaneous transtracheal ventilation (PTTV) devices. Operative lighting is unnecessary. The small entrance hole minimizes bleeding by pressure against surrounding tissues, and may reduce the chance of infection. After removal, the cricotome leaves a more satisfying cosmetic result. Whether these objectives have been met or are indeed attainable is open to question since these devices are rarely used and there exists almost no literature on the subject. Available reports are primarily from the cricotome developers themselves, and there are no clinical comparisons with standard surgical tracheostomy, cricothyrotomy, or PTTV. This chapter discusses the currently marketed cricotomes.

INDICATIONS AND CONTRAINDICATIONS

Indications for cricotome use are the same as those for standard cricothyrotomy and tracheostomy (see Chapter 16). An acute laryngeal pathologic condition is considered a relative contraindication because of the high rate of subglottic stenosis.[1]

EQUIPMENT, PROCEDURE, AND COMPLICATIONS

Pertrach

The Pertrach (Fig 17–1) was first described in 1969 by Toye and Weinstein,[2] neurosurgeons. It was developed with the goal of achieving the equivalent of a surgical airway faster and safer than with standard surgical technique. Although intended for emergency as well as chronic use, the authors subsequently reported only six insertions in emergency situations.[3] The device has evolved considerably to its present form, which is an adult size cuffed tracheostomy tube with an inner diameter (ID) of 6 mm. It is introduced by Seldinger technique with a dilator inserted over a Teflon-coated wire through a split-away needle. The procedure for insertion of the Pertrach (Fig 17–2) is as follows:

1. Insert the Teflon guide into the tracheostomy tube and test the balloon. Deflate. Check the needle-syringe unit for air leaks prior to insertion by placing a finger over the end of the needle and confirming a vacuum.

2. Extend the patient's neck prior to the proce-

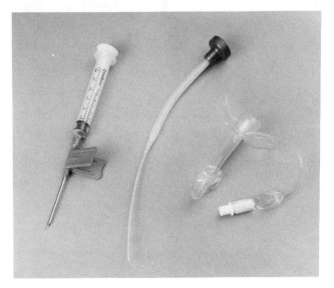

FIG 17–1.
Adult Pertrach kit. (Courtesy of Pertrach Inc., Clarksburg, W. Va.)

dure to improve access to the area; if this is not advisable, use cephalad traction applied at the mandibular angles by an assistant.

3. For cricothyrotomy, locate the notch on the superior aspect of the thyroid cartilage; follow caudally to the soft cricothyroid membrane between the thyroid and cricoid cartilages. For tracheotomy, locate the space between the second or third tracheal ring. In the conscious patient infiltrate local anesthetic into the tissue and trachea.

4. Make a vertical skin incision of 1 to 2 cm over the trachea or cricothyroid membrane in the midline.

5. With the syringe attached, insert the splitting needle into the airway perpendicular to the skin and advance it until you are able to aspirate air easily.

6. Redirect the needle inferiorly.

7. Remove the syringe and fully insert the guide wire portion of the dilator and tracheostomy tube unit into the needle, and then split and remove the needle.

8. Exert pressure with the thumb and force the lubricated dilator-tube unit into the airway until the faceplate touches the skin. Easy passage and patient cough suggest proper placement.

9. Remove the dilator, inflate the cuff (1–8 mL) and begin ventilation. Secure the tube using the tie strap.

The only reported studies of the Pertrach are those by Toye and Weinstein.[2, 3] Their largest series is 100 insertions, 94 tracheostomies, and 6 cricothyrotomies over a 17-year period. None of the inser-

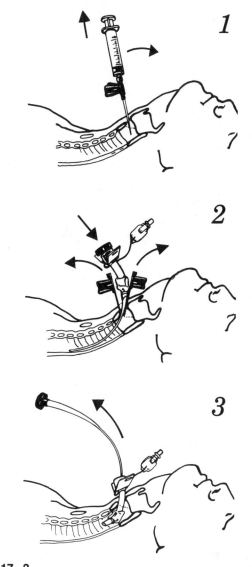

FIG 17–2.
Insertion procedure for adult Pertrach. See text. (Courtesy of Pertrach Inc., Clarksburg, W. Va.)

tions was performed with the cricotome in its current form and most were done by the authors themselves. They were able to insert the Pertrach in about 30 seconds and never required more than 2 minutes.

Eleven of 100 patients had complications. In 6 patients the initial insertion was outside the tracheal lumen. There were four subcutaneous emphysemas, two pretracheal hematomas, one pretracheal cellulitis; and one bilateral pneumothorax. One death occurred in a very obese patient when the airway tube was of insufficient length to enter the trachea. Follow-up after decannulation in 19 patients showed no long-term complications.[3]

In summary, the Pertrach is a sophisticated device that functions comparably to a surgical tracheostomy or cricothyrotomy and has been used by its originators in more than 100 patients. The complication rate in emergency situations may be expected to exceed the 11% reported in elective situations. Theoretically, this cricotome appears to be suitable for emergency use, but more experience is needed in emergency situations and by multiple operators.

Nu-Trake

In 1983 Weiss introduced the Nu-Trake[4] (Fig 17–3,A–C). This device incorporates a sharp stylet within a blunt expanding needle and rigid straight metal airway tube. The instrument has changed little since its development and includes a 4.0-, 6.0-, and 7.2-mm-ID airway in each kit. For adults it is advised to enlarge the airway progressively to accommodate the 7.2-mm size after ventilation has been initially established with a smaller tube. The average vertical diameter of the adult cricothyroid membrane is 9 mm. A 6-mm-ID tube has an outer diameter (OD) of 8.2 mm; a 6.5-mm tube has an OD of almost 9 mm.[5] The procedure for insertion of the Nu-Trake is as follows:

1. Insert the stylet into the blunt needle housing unit and attach the syringe.

2. Identify the cricothyroid membrane, as described with the Pertrach, and make a 1- to 2-cm vertical skin incision in the midline. Extreme difficulty in inserting the stylet-housing unit will be encountered if the skin and subcutaneous tissue is not first incised with the scalpel.

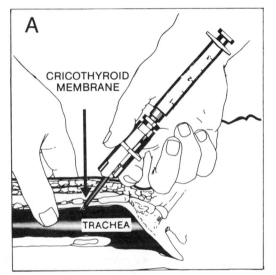

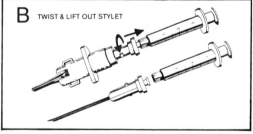

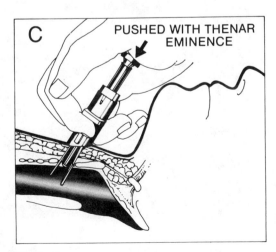

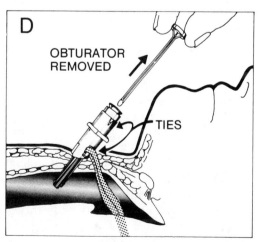

FIG 17–3.
A–D, insertion procedure for Nu-Trake. See text. (Courtesy of International Medical Devices Inc., Northridge, Calif.)

3. Puncture the cricothyroid membrane with the stylet and housing unit through the incision at approximately a 45-degree angle caudad and aspirate air from the trachea to confirm proper placement.

4. Twist and remove the stylet and syringe from the housing unit, and gently advance the housing until the base rests on the skin. A free rocking motion of the housing unit after removal of the stylet helps confirm proper placement.

5. Insert an appropriate obturator into a 4-mm airway and insert them into the housing. Hook the index and middle fingers around the phalanges of the housing and push the obturator with the thenar eminence toward the trachea to divide the blunt needle. Do not use a squeezing action when inserting the obturator-airway unit; this could pull the housing from the trachea.

6. Remove the obturator, leaving the airway and housing in the trachea. Ventilate the patient and secure the airway with umbilical tape.

In a study by Ravlo et al.,[6] following audiovisual training, physicians were able to establish a Nu-Trake airway in an average of 30 seconds, with subsequent autopsy proving that all were properly placed, whereas only 70% of Nu-Trakes were properly placed by the untrained group.

Bjoraker et al.[7] had six anesthesiologists and five residents attempt Nu-Trake placement in 11 dogs. There was difficulty inserting the stylet and blunt needle through the cricothyroid membrane; this caused slippage and two subcricoid insertions. There were also frequent air leaks from the anterior notch in the housing, and the unit's lumen had a tendency to occlude on the posterior wall of the trachea if held perpendicular to the neck. Subcutaneous emphysema occurred in 2 dogs, the cricoid cartilage was injured in 2, the cricotracheal ligament perforated in 2, the posterior tracheal wall perforated in 3 (without esophageal injury), and incidental submucosal airway hemorrhage was found in 6 dogs.[7]

There appear to be several defects in the Nu-Trake device. The 4-mm airway initially used must be dilated twice to achieve the recommended adult size. The metal airways are uncuffed, doing little to prevent aspiration, and in Bjoraker's small animal study complications were frequent and significant. It appears that the Nu-Trake needs further development or solid clinical evidence of safety and efficacy before it can be recommended for use in emergency medicine practice.

Melker Catheter

In 1985 Ciaglia et al.[8] proposed their modification of a renal dilator set, using the Seldinger technique, to perform percutaneous cricothyrotomy. With the renal set, progressively larger dilators allow a 6-mm-ID uncuffed curved plastic airway to be inserted. It has been modified by Melker for emergency cricothyrotomy by eliminating the progressive dilations, using a single 18F device (Fig 17–4). The procedure is as follows:

1. Locate the cricothyroid membrane as described for the Pertrach.
2. Make a 1- to 2-cm vertical incision in the skin over the membrane.
3. Pass the needle-catheter unit with the syringe attached through the incision and cricothyroid membrane and into the airway at a 45-degree angle caudad. Verify proper position by easy aspiration of air.
4. Remove the needle and syringe, leaving the soft catheter in place.
5. Advance the guide wire through the catheter, in the usual Seldinger technique, a few centimeters into the airway and remove the Teflon catheter, leaving only the guide wire in the trachea.
6. Slide the plastic airway over the dilator and lubricate the surface. Thread this unit over the guide wire.
7. Always visualize and control the proximal end of the wire to prevent its loss in the trachea.

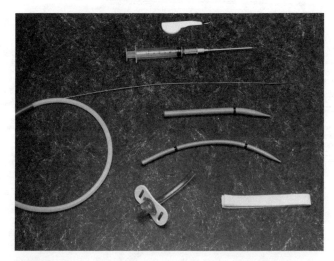

FIG 17–4.
Melker catheter kit. (Courtesy of Cook Inc., Bloomington, Ind.)

8. Advance the dilator into the trachea a few centimeters with a rotating motion. Push the airway into the trachea over the dilator.
9. Remove the guide wire and dilator simultaneously. Begin ventilation and fix the airway to the neck with a tie.

Ciaglia et al.[8] found no intraoperative or long-term complications in 26 elective tracheostomies performed with the Melker device. Holtzman[9] reported one case of self-limiting subcutaneous emphysema as the only complication in eight insertions. Hazard et al.[10] used the Melker device on 55 elective cases; they reported moderate bleeding in 2 patients with coagulation disorders, but only minimal bleeding in the 10 other coagulopathy patients in the study group. Subcutaneous emphysema occurred in 2, pneumothorax in 1, posterior tracheal wall puncture in 1, and operative site cellulitis in 1 patient. Twenty decannulated survivors (four of them long-term) had no complications.[10]

Again, there are no published data on use of the Melker device in the emergency situation, but in the elective setting it appears to be reasonably safe. The Seldinger technique is familiar to most emergency physicians, and eliminating the splitting needle of the Pertrach may make it easier for one operator to handle. A flaw in the Melker device is the potential for losing the guide wire in the airway, and the absence of a cuff permits aspiration.

PEDIATRIC PERSPECTIVE

Considerable controversy exists regarding the proper establishment of the airway from below in pediatric patients; some authors recommend only needle transtracheal ventilation, others only tracheostomy, and still others only cricothyrotomy.[11-13] Developers of cricotomes have not resolved this issue. Toye and Weinstein[3] recommend the Pertrach only for tracheostomy in children, and market a pediatric model of their device with 3.0-, 3.5-, and 4-mm-ID uncuffed plastic airways for children of ages 0 to 11 months, 1 to 4 years, and 3½ to 10 years respectively (Fig 17–5). The method of insertion is the same as for the adult model. Nu-Trake offers the Pedia-Trake for both cricothyrotomy and tracheostomy. This uses a curved stylet expanded with a plastic plier and curved, uncuffed plastic airways in sizes of 3, 4, and 5 mm ID. Pedia-Trake is not recommended in children under 1 year of age. The

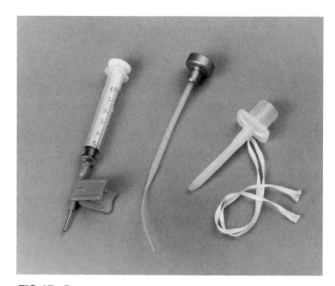

FIG 17–5.
Pediatric Pertrach kit. (Courtesy of Pertrach Inc., Clarksburg, W. Va.)

Melker catheter is not recommended for pediatric use. It is recommended that the manufacturers' instructions in their product literature be followed with regard to the use of these devices in pediatric patients.

PREHOSPITAL PERSPECTIVE

Cricothyrotomy is the accepted standard for securing the airway in the prehospital setting when oral or nasotracheal intubation is not possible. However, a surgical airway is difficult to perform in the emergency department, let alone in a moving vehicle or poorly lighted accident scene. Studies using cricotomes in the prehospital setting are needed as cricotomes are not currently available to emergency medical services providers. Conceivably, the cricotome could provide an airway maneuver that is more expedient, safer, and easier for paramedical workers to learn.

REFERENCES

1. Bratigan CO, Grow JB Sr: Subglottic stenosis after cricothyroidotomy. *Surgery* 1982; 91:217.
2. Toye FJ, Weinstein JD: A percutaneous tracheostomy device. *Surgery* 1969; 65:384–389.
3. Toye F, Weinstein J: Clinical experience with percutaneous tracheostomy and cricothyroidotomy in 100 patients. *J Trauma* 1986; 26:1034.

4. Weiss S: A new emergency cricothyroidotomy instrument. *J Trauma* 1983; 23:155–158.

5. Safar P, Penninckx J: Cricothyroid membrane puncture with a special cannula. *Anesthesiology* 1967; 28:943.

6. Ravlo O, Bach V, Lybecker H, et al: A comparison between two emergency cricothyroidotomy instruments. *Acta Anaesthesiol Scand* 1987; 31:317–319.

7. Bjoraker D, Kumar NB, Brown AC, et al: Evaluation of an emergency cricothyrotomy instrument. *Crit Care Med* 1987; 15:157.

8. Ciaglia P, Firsching R, Syniec C: Elective percutaneous dilatational tracheostomy. *Chest* 1985; 87:715.

9. Holtzman RB: Percutaneous approach to tracheostomy (letter). *Crit Care Med* 1989; 17:595.

10. Hazard PB, Garrett HE, Adams JW, et al: Bedside percutaneous tracheostomy; experience with 55 elective procedures. *Ann Thorac Surg.* 1988; 46:63–67.

11. Brantigan C: Emergency cricothyroidotomy in emergency procedures. 1985.

12. Campbell WH, Cantrill SV: Neck injuries, in Rosen P, et al (eds): *Emergency Medicine*. Mosby–Year Book, Inc, 1988, pp 423.

13. Marlowe FI: Otolaryngologic Emergencies, in Tintinalli J, et al (eds): *Emergency Medicine, a Comprehensive Study Guide*. Dallas, American College of Emergency Medicine, 1985, p. 593.

18

Respiratory Adjuncts

18A
Therapeutic

Jay A. Johannigman, M.D.*

Once a patent airway has been established, it is often necessary to increase the oxygen content of the inspired gas in order to improve or eliminate arterial hypoxemia. Despite the fact that O_2 is a widely used drug, the provision of precise, constant concentration of this therapeutic agent is rarely understood or achieved. The rational and effective administration of O_2 requires a working familiarity with the principles of O_2 delivery and the equipment used to achieve this delivery.

Oxygen therapy devices are commonly grouped into two broad categories which assist in the understanding of the capabilities and limitations of the equipment. These categories are *low-flow* or *variable-performance equipment* and *high-flow* or *fixed-performance equipment.*[1] Low-flow or variable-performance equipment provides only a portion of the total gas volume inspired by the patient. As ventilatory demands or respiratory patterns change, a variable amount of room air will dilute the O_2 flow. High-flow or fixed-performance equipment supplies all of the patient's inspired gas at a prescribed fractional concentration of oxygen in inspired gas (FiO_2). In most cases, the performance of this equipment is not significantly altered by a patient's ventilatory demand or respiratory pattern. Oxygen therapy devices, their flow rates, and FiO_2 are shown in Table 18A–1.

*The views expressed in this chapter are those of the author and do not reflect the official policy of the Department of Defense or other departments of the U.S. government.

VARIABLE-PERFORMANCE EQUIPMENT

Nasal Cannula

The nasal cannula, first introduced in 1871, remains the most commonly employed O_2 delivery device. The catheter is simple in design and consists of a soft, plastic tube with either an over-the-ear or under-the-chin adjustment. Since the nasal cannula is a low-flow device, the FiO_2 provided at a given flow rate may vary dramatically from patient to patient as well as hour to hour in a given patient.[2, 3] As the patient's ventilatory flow and pattern change, a variable portion of room air will be mixed with the O_2 provided by the cannula. An important additional consideration is the relative distribution of mouth vs. nasal breathing. With these considerations in mind, it must be recognized that studies that quote FiO_2 values obtained with the use of a nasal cannula are, at best, rough estimates. The estimated FiO_2 is subject to significant changes based upon alterations in ventilatory patterns. A reasonable estimate of the range of potential FiO_2 values with a nasal cannula is provided in Table 18A–2.[4, 5]

The ability of the nasal cannula to increase FiO_2 plateaus at approximately 6 L/min of O_2 flow.[6] Above this level, increases in O_2 flow result in only negligible increases in FiO_2. For this reason, as well as patient complaints of drying of nasal mucosa when flow rates are high, the maximal delivered flow from a nasal cannula is normally limited to 6 to 8 L/min.

199

TABLE 18A–1.

Oxygen Therapy Devices

Device	Flow (L/min)	FiO$_2$*
Nasal cannula	1–10	0.23–0.45
Simple mask	5–15	0.40–0.60
Partial rebreathing	10–15	0.60
Nonrebreathing	10–15	0.60–0.80
Anesthesia bag-valve-mask	15	0.90–1.0
Air entrainment	4–12	0.24–0.50
Aerosol	5–15	0.40–1.0

*Fractional concentration of inspired oxygen (FiO$_2$) is approximate. Value varies based on inspiratory flow (see text).

Oxygen Masks

Simple Masks

Of the various mask devices available, the simple mask is the one most commonly employed. The simple mask is a disposable, lightweight plastic device that covers the nose and mouth and is secured with an elastic strap (Fig 18A–1). The face seal of the simple mask is normally not fitted with any special system to ensure a leak-free system. The poorer the mask fit, the greater the volume of air entrainment that will occur with each breath. Even a reasonably well-fitting mask will display a great variability in FiO$_2$ based upon the patient's ventilatory pattern. Simple masks must be run at a minimum flow of 5 L/min O$_2$ to ensure adequate washout of the patient's exhaled carbon dioxide. With proper fit, adequate O$_2$ flow, and a standard ventilatory pattern, FiO$_2$ values in the range of 40% to 60% may be achieved.[7] Patients often find these masks hot and uncomfortable, and the plastic irritating to the skin. Some patients, particularly if hypoxic, complain of feeling claustrophobic. Generally speaking, simple masks are only tolerated for relatively short periods of time.

Partial Rebreathing Mask

The concept behind the partial rebreathing mask is that it uses a reservoir to provide a source of

TABLE 18A–2.

Estimated Range of FiO$_2$ Values With a Nasal Cannula

L/min	FiO$_2$
1	0.23
2	0.24–0.38
3	0.25–0.32
4	0.26–0.36
5	0.30–0.40
6	0.36–0.42
10	0.40–0.45

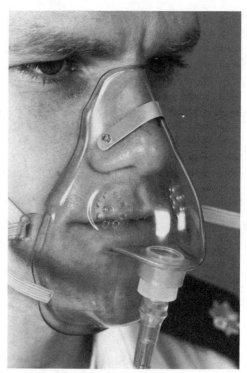

FIG 18A–1.
Simple mask. Note the open air entrainment ports.

O$_2$ to the patient during inspiration. When a patient inspires through this type of mask the O$_2$ is drawn from the mask, the reservoir bag, and the tubing. A variable degree of room air is entrained around the mask. The mask's reservoir serves as a means of meeting a portion of the inflow demands which occur during peak inspiratory flow. These devices are called partial rebreathing masks because a portion of the expired gas returns to the mask and reservoir before the remainder is vented to the ambient surrounding. Theoretically, the first portion of exhaled gas is dead space and therefore does not contain CO$_2$. If the system's flow is high enough to prevent the reservoir bag from deflating more than one-half its volume during inhalation, no CO$_2$ accumulates during exhalation. The partial rebreathing mask provides an FiO$_2$ of approximately 60% if correctly used, with a minimum flow of 8 L/min of O$_2$. With increased ventilatory effort, flows up to, or exceeding 15 L/min may be required to keep the reservoir bag adequately filled.

Nonrebreathing Mask

The nonrebreathing mask utilizes the same basic design concepts as the partial rebreathing mask but incorporates one-way flap valves between the reservoir bag and mask, and between the mask and the exhalation ports (Fig 18A–2). During optimal operation, the patient inspires O_2 from the mask, the reservoir bag, the inlet tubing, and if necessary, entrains room air around the face mask seal.[8] If the available O_2 reservoir exceeds the patient's peak inspiratory need, then an FiO_2 approaching 100% will be attained.[9] Practically speaking, this situation only occurs when a patient has a slow, shallow respiratory pattern. Oxygen flow into the system should be great enough to ensure a flushing of the mask with O_2 and complete filling of the reservoir prior to the next breath. Proper operation requires a flow of at least 10 L/min, but preferably should be maintained in excess of 15 L/min. The nonrebreathing mask provides FiO_2 values in the range of 60% to 80% when high-flow O_2 is utilized.

Anesthesia Bag-Valve-Mask Systems

The basic design of these devices is similar to the reservoir masks. The most significant difference with these devices deals with the use of more competent components. The reservoir bag consists of a 1- or 2-L anesthesia bag with a tailpiece gas inlet of variable length. The masks used with these systems possess good facial sealing characteristics and come in a number of shapes and sizes. The mask is fitted to the face and secured in order to provide a leak-free seal. Sys-

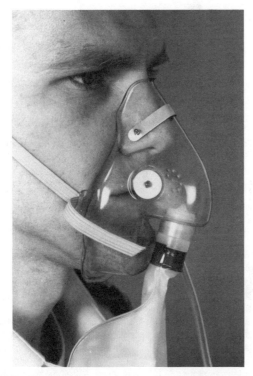

FIG 18A–2.
Nonrebreathing mask. Note the oxygen reservoir and one-way valves which prevent entrainment of room air.

tems such as these are capable of delivering 100% O_2 when inlet flow is greater than 15 L/min.

HIGH-FLOW OR FIXED-PERFORMANCE EQUIPMENT

High-flow O_2 systems provide a patient's entire inspired minute volume. There are three high-flow systems in common use: (1) *air entrainment masks;* (2) *large-volume aerosol systems,* and (3) *large-volume humidification systems.*

Air Entrainment Masks

Although often incorrectly termed *Venturi masks,* these devices employ the principle of *jet drag* to achieve their effect. Oxygen under pressure is forced through a small nozzle at the base of the mask (Fig 18A–3, A and B). The velocity of the O_2 flow is accelerated at the nozzle owing to the change in cross-sectional diameter. The increased velocity creates a jet drag or shearing effect distal to the nozzle which causes room air to be entrained or "dragged" into the mask[1, 4] (Fig 18A–4). The resultant FiO_2 is a function of the proportions of the mixture of O_2 and entrained air.[10] The proportions of mixing are determined by the size of the nozzle and the size of the entrainment ports. These characteristics allow a system to be designed with the capability of providing a specific, precise FiO_2. The basic design requires that the flow generated by the mask meet or exceed patient demands. A basic approximation of patient inspiratory flow rates is provided in Table 18A–3.[10, 11]

When O_2 flow rates recommended by manufacturers are used, the total flow provided by these systems may not be adequate for patients with rapid inspiratory flows. At levels of FiO_2 greater than 35%, the total flow of the mask system may be less than patient demand, particularly for patients with chronic obstructive pulmonary disease (COPD) or respiratory distress[12] (Tables 18A–3 and 18A–4). In this setting dilution of FiO_2 will occur as the high

TABLE 18A–3.

Basic Approximation of Inspiratory Flow Rates

Patient	Minute Ventilation (L/min)	Inspiratory Time (sec)	Peak Inspiratory Flow (L/min)
Normal	7.0	2.00	28
COPD	6.5	1.43	39
Respiratory distress	10.0	0.71	73

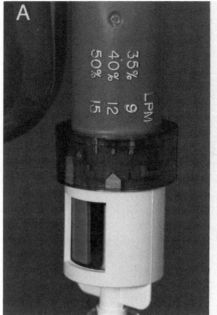
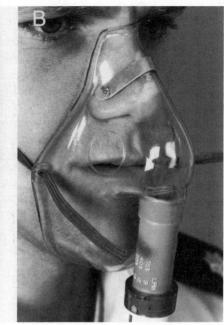

FIG 18A–3.
A, base unit of air entrainment mask. Note air entrainment port which is variably adjustable. **B,** air entrainment mask.

inspiratory flow results in the entrainment of additional room air around the mask seal.

Air entrainment masks are particularly suited for patients whose hypoxemia cannot be controlled on lower FiO_2 devices such as the nasal cannula. Patients with COPD who tend to hypoventilate at moderate levels of FiO_2 are candidates for an air entrainment mask because it allows for more precise FiO_2 delivery. The air entrainment mask works well in patients with severe asthma or patients who are hyperventilating because of its ability to provide relatively high flows without the use of particulate aerosols which may induce bronchospasm.

Large-Volume Aerosol Systems

These systems utilize a variable FiO_2 delivery capability via gas entrainment, as described above. In addition, they incorporate either a disposable or nondisposable large-volume aerosol nebulizer in conjunction with an increased delivered gas volume.

TABLE 18A–4.

Input Flow and Total Flow for Representative Air Entrainment System

FiO_2	Input Flow (L/min)	Total Flow (L/min)
0.24	4	97
0.28	6	68
0.30	6	54
0.35	8	45
0.40	12	50
0.50	12	33

Both the disposable and permanent nebulizers have an adjustable dilution setting which varies the size of the entrainment ports to produce the desired FiO_2. The FiO_2 may be set at fixed points (40%, 60%, or 100%) or be continuously adjustable from 30% to

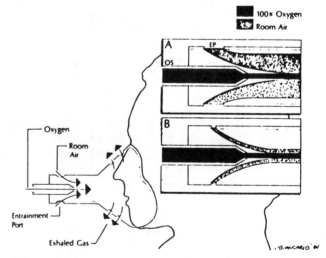

FIG 18A–4.
Principle of an air entrainment device. Pressurized oxygen is forced through a nozzle (constricted orifice); the increased gas velocity distal to the orifice creates a jet drag or shearing effect that causes room air to be entrained through the entrainment ports. The high flow of gas fills the mask, which has holes, allowing both exhaled and delivered gas to escape. *A* and *B* illustrate that the size of the entrainment ports *(EP)* determines the amount of room air to be entrained. *OS* = oxygen source. *A* illustrates large ports, resulting in relatively higher FiO_2. For any size entrainment port, the FiO_2 is stable; however, the total gas flow will vary with the pressurized oxygen flow. (From Kacmarek RM: *Probl Respir Care* 1990; 3:568. Used by permission.)

100%. As with air entrainment masks, as FiO_2 increases, total delivered flow decreases. To produce an FiO_2 of 100%, total flow is limited to 15 L/min.[13] If a patient is dyspneic or displays an increased respiratory drive, peak flows may exceed the delivery capability of the system and entrainment of room air around the mask will occur.

Nebulizers may be applied to the patient via many different routes. The aerosol mask, tracheostomy collar, face tent, and T-piece (Briggs adaptor) may all be utilized by attaching large-bore tubing to the nebulizer. These devices use an open system that freely vents inspiratory and expiratory gases. Because of this feature these devices also allow the patient to readily entrain surrounding room air, and therefore the FiO_2 is often quite variable.

The T-piece is one specific form of an aerosol system that is commonly used with an intubated patient. It may be attached to an endotracheal tube to provide a reasonably constant FiO_2. It is common practice to use either a reservoir bag before the T, or a reservoir tube on the distal side of the T to provide a large reservoir volume to meet inspiratory flow demands. The long-term use (>2 hours) of a T-piece in the intubated patient may promote atelectasis and loss of functional residual capacity since this system fails to provide physiologic levels of positive end-expiratory pressure (PEEP).

The primary concern in evaluating the performance of large-volume aerosol systems is to ensure that the system is providing sufficient flow to meet patient demands. The mist generated by the system may be employed as a tracer to evaluate the adequacy of flow. If the visible mist exiting the distal port of the T-piece obviously disappears during inspiration, the flow should be increased in order to provide adequate flow without entrainment of room air.

Large-Volume Humidifier Systems

The most accurate and precise method of delivering O_2, other than a ventilator or continuous positive airway pressure (CPAP) system, is through the use of a large-volume humidification system. These systems utilize a blender to mix pressurized oxygen and air to provide any desired FiO_2 at flow rates up to 150 L/min.[12] The flow is routed through a large-volume humidifier and delivered to the patient via large-bore aerosol tubing. The flow is interfaced to the patient by an artificial airway (endotracheal tube) or face mask. The major drawback of these systems is the noise created as gas flows of greater than 80 to 100 L/min move through the system. In addition to

their adult applications, these are the systems most commonly used in infant oxygen hoods, incubators, and oxygen tents.

CLINICAL APPLICATIONS

When a clinician is faced with a decision regarding which O_2 therapy device to use, he or she must consider the following questions: What FiO_2 is required? Is consistency and accuracy of FiO_2 important? Does the patient require humidification? Is the patient intubated or does he or she have a tracheostomy? Is patient compliance a problem?

Patient compliance is an important consideration since O_2 delivery devices are of little use if they are not worn by the patient. Patient compliance and tolerance of high-flow systems is normally quite low unless constantly monitored. Face masks are often poorly tolerated because they engender a sense of claustrophobia in the hypoxic patient and the mask must be removed for eating, oral hygiene, and conversation. As a result of these considerations, the nasal cannula remains the most commonly employed O_2 therapy device. The majority of patients that require supplemental O_2 are easily maintained on a nasal cannula and normally tolerate this modality well. In the setting of trauma, field resuscitation, or during the initial emergency room evaluation, a simple O_2 mask or a partial rebreathing mask serves as a readily available means of providing an FiO_2 unobtainable with a cannula. Patients who require supplemental O_2 for a prolonged period should be considered for an entrainment or aerosol system that provides a source of humidification. The provision of humidification will eliminate the difficulties of nasal drying or the thickening of secretions which can occur with chronic use of an unhumidified source. All patients that have been placed on O_2 therapy to reverse hypoxemia should undergo evaluation of their arterial oxygen partial pressure (PaO_2), either directly by arterial blood gas measurements or indirectly by O_2 saturation monitoring.

In the intubated patient only high-flow systems are suitable since the system must meet or exceed the patient's peak inspiratory flow. If an endotracheal tube is in place, O_2 enrichment is most effectively accomplished via a large-volume aerosol system and T-piece until definitive mechanical ventilation is instituted or extubation accomplished. As mentioned previously, long-term use of the T-piece should be avoided since it fails to provide physiologic levels of PEEP and therefore may promote distal airway collapse and atelectasis. Patients with tracheostomy tubes are managed with either a T-piece (short term) or a tracheostomy mask (long term). In the majority of patients with chronic tracheostomies, the primary concern is for consistent humidification rather than precise FiO_2 delivery. For this reason a heated aerosol system or a high-flow humidification system is most appropriate for the patient with a chronic tracheostomy. An aerosol system offers the advantages of simplicity and ease of maintenance but is limited in its FiO_2 delivery. If an FiO_2 greater than 40% is required, a high-flow humidifier system should be employed because of its accuracy, versatility, and high-flow–high FiO_2 capability.

Despite concern regarding O_2 toxicity, absorption atelectasis, and O_2-induced hypoventilation, 100% O_2 is indicated when there is concern for tissue hypoxia. The use of 100% O_2 is proper during cardiac arrest, acute cardiopulmonary instability, carbon monoxide poisoning, or trauma with systemic hypotension. Once stabilization is achieved, the FiO_2 should be reduced to the lowest level which maintains a PaO_2 greater than 60 mm Hg (saturation >90%).

Suctioning

Normal bronchial clearance is accomplished by the mucociliary escalator in conjunction with the cough mechanism which clears the upper airway. Tracheobronchial suctioning is indicated when these normal protective mechanisms are not effective in clearing the airway. Although usually viewed as a routine part of care of the airway, it must be recognized that suctioning poses a number of potential hazards which include mucosal bleeding, abrupt and significant drops in PaO_2, excessive vagal stimulation, bradycardia, and patient discomfort.[12] The majority of these adverse effects can be avoided by adequate preoxygenation and limiting the duration of suctioning procedures.

In the unintubated patient nasotracheal suctioning provides the most adequate means of clearing secretions from the oropharynx and trachea. This technique is also of value because of its ability to stimulate a vigorous coughing response. This coughing response may be the primary advantage of nasotracheal suctioning. The placement of a nasopharyngeal airway (nasal trumpet) will facilitate suctioning and is more readily tolerated than an oral airway in the alert or semiconscious patient. The nasal trumpet is designed to follow the curvature of the nasopharynx so that the terminal portion is located at the base of the tongue just above the epi-

glottis. This serves to provide an open airway as well as a path for passage of a suction catheter directly into the upper trachea. Suctioning should be limited to 10- to 15-second intervals with intervening oxygenation with 100% FiO_2. A useful guideline is for the therapist to hold his or her breath during suctioning as a indication of the duration of the procedure.

Endotracheal or tracheostomy suctioning employs the same basic techniques used for nasotracheal suctioning. The use of artificial airways often impairs the efficacy of normal mucociliary clearance and therefore frequent and effective suctioning is absolutely essential to adequate pulmonary toilet. Endotracheal intubation circumvents the normal humidification of inhaled gases by the upper airway and tracheobronchial secretions may become thick and tenacious as a result. The instillation of 1 to 2 mL of normal saline directly into the endotracheal tube immediately prior to suctioning often facilitates the mobilization of secretions.

Humidification

Humidity therapy is the process of providing increased levels of humidity in an inspired gas. Medical gases such as O_2 are supplied from tanks or central piping systems that are completely free of humidity. If such gas is mixed with ambient air, the net result can be irritation of the nasal and oropharyngeal mucosa as well as thickening of secretions in the tracheobronchial tree. With the use of low-flow devices such as nasal cannulas or simple face masks, a relatively large proportion of humidified room air is entrained with each breath. The requirements for additional humidification in this setting are minimal and are readily satisfied through the addition of a bubble humidifier. In situations in which O_2 flow is limited to 1 to 4 L/min, additional humidification is usually not necessary.

High-flow or fixed-performance devices deliver a substantially larger volume of medical gas and therefore the humidification system used must be capable of a greater volume of delivery. For the intubated patient it is preferable to use a large-volume humidifier or an artificial nose to provide humidification. The artificial nose is a device that is inserted in line with the delivery system. It consists of a tightly packaged membrane surface which functions as a countercurrent heat and moisture exchanger. In the intubated patient humidification (the creation of water vapor) is preferred to aerosolization or nebulization (particulate water) sources because of the tendency of particulate water to transport bacteria and irritate the upper airway.[13] Aerosol therapy is usually reserved for the therapeutic deposition of bronchoactive medications, for sputum induction, or for short-term use in high-flow devices such as T-pieces or face shields.

Tracheostomy Tubes

The tracheostomy tube is utilized as an artificial airway when there is an anticipated need for long-term ventilatory support or pulmonary toilet. A tracheostomy is also commonly employed in the setting of facial or neck trauma where endotracheal intubation is precluded due to injury, edema of the upper airway, or the need for surgical repair. The tracheostomy tube is surgically inserted into the trachea, usually at the level of the third tracheal ring at a level below the vocal cords.

The important components of tracheostomy care are to maintain patency of the airway, proper wound care, and regular assessment of ventilatory needs. Until a well-formed tract is established (5–7 days postoperatively) the inadvertent dislodgment of a tracheostomy tube may prove disastrous. Care should be exercised in the perioperative period to maintain the security of the airway and an additional tracheostomy tube of the same size should be kept at the patient's bedside. The tracheostomy tape or fixation sutures which hold the tracheostomy in position during the immediate postoperative period should be visually inspected and adjusted as the patient's condition dictates.

Because tracheostomy tubes are commonly used in chronic situations, a number of design innovations have been incorporated to prevent accumulation of secretions and subsequent airway obstruction. The metal (Jackson) tracheostomy tube as well as the plastic Shiley tube have an inner cannula that may be removed in order to clear accumulated secretions. An airway seal is usually maintained via an air-filled balloon cuff, but alternative methods such as a foam cuff (Bivona) or concentric silicone rings (Dow Corning) may also be employed.

Since a tracheostomy tube bypasses the upper airway, the normal mechanism for heating and humidification of inspired gases is eliminated. It is necessary to provide a source of heated, humidified gas in order to ensure patient comfort as well as to eliminate thickening of pulmonary secretions. A tracheostomy also circumvents glottic closure, and therefore decreases the effectiveness of the normal cough mechanism for the clearing of secretions. Adequate humidification of inspired gases as well as careful attention to the patient's hydration status will aid in the thinning of secretions and promote their mobilization. The provision of humidification is most easily accomplished through the use of an aerosol system (short term) or a heated humidifier (long term) in conjunction with a tracheostomy mask.

The fenestrated tracheostomy tube is a device that is useful in assessing the patient's ability to be extubated or to allow the patient to speak while a tracheostomy is in place. The fenestrated tracheostomy tube utilizes an opening in the tube above the cuff. If the inner cannula is inserted and the cuff inflated, the system functions as a normal tracheostomy tube. When the inner cannula is removed, the cuff deflated, and the normal inlet occluded with a cap, the patient can inhale and exhale through the fenestration and into the native upper airway.

Mask Continuous Positive Airway Pressure

The first report of the application of positive pressure by face mask was by Sterling Bunnell in 1912.[14] In his report Bunnell described the use of a "slider and spring device" which was adapted to a standard anesthesia face mask to maintain lung expansion during thoracic surgery. Episodic reports over the next 30 years documented the use of positive pressure in the treatment of pneumonia,[15] asthma,[16] and pulmonary edema.[17, 18] During the 1940s the science of positive pressure breathing was advanced by the military medical corps, who used it to treat "traumatic wet lung"[19] and for improving the altitude tolerance of pilots.[20] In 1946 and 1947 Barach and colleagues published voluminous reports on the effects of positive pressure breathing on respiration, circulation, and arterial blood gases from sea level to 45,000 ft.[21–24] Barach and co-workers were the first to elucidate the relationship between the work of breathing and the efficiency of the CPAP system. They also noted a decrease in the cardiac silhouette at a pressure of 20 cm H_2O and were therefore the first to describe the hemodynamic consequences of positive pressure. The term *continuous positive airway pressure* was introduced by Gregory et al.[25] who reported its use as a treatment for spontaneously breathing neonates with hyaline membrane disease. In recent years an increasing number of reports have focused on the use of mask CPAP in the adult population as a treatment modality to relieve hypoxemia in the setting of acute respiratory failure (ARF), pulmonary contusion and flail chest, cardiogenic pulmonary edema, COPD, and postoperative atelectasis.[26-31]

CPAP systems provide gas by a continuous-flow or demand-valve system. A typical system is depicted in Figure 18A–5. Gas is directed from a high-flow blender through a large-volume, low-resistance humidifier. The inspiratory limb contains a 3- to 5-L reservoir bag and connects the humidifier to the patient T-piece. The patient T-piece contains one-way valves to direct flow. The expiratory limb is routed to an expiratory pressure valve, typically a threshold resistor type. A combination manometer–low pressure alarm is interfaced at the patient T-piece to accurately measure airway pressure and detect disconnection. The flow required to maintain constant pressure in the CPAP system is approximately two to three times the patient's minute ventilation (30–90 L/min). In practical terms this requires that flow in the system be increased until a pressure drop no greater than 2 to 3 cm H_2O is observed during the patient's peak inspiration.[32] Currently, there are a limited number of commercially available systems that provide a continuous flow adequate to maintain CPAP. Of these systems, the Downs adjustable flow generator has the greatest applicability to the emergency department setting. The Downs adjustable FiO_2 flow generator operates from a standard 50-psi outlet and is capable of delivering an FiO_2 from 0.32 to 1.0 at a continuous flow ranging from 90 to 230 L/min.

Physiology

The physiologic goals of mask CPAP are an increase in functional residual capacity (FRC) with its accompanying increase in arterial oxygenation. In-

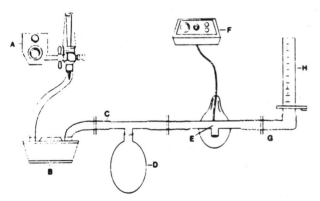

FIG 18A–5.
Continuous-flow CPAP system. *A,* high-flow blender. *B,* large-volume, low-resistance humidifier. *C,* inspiratory limb. *D,* reservoir bag (3–5 L). *E,* patient T-piece. *F,* high-low pressure alarm and manometer. *G,* expiratory limb. *H,* threshold resistor.

creasing FRC recruits collapsed alveoli, improves lung compliance, and therefore decreases the work of breathing.[33-35] Additionally, reversal of alveolar collapse decreases intrapulmonary shunt (Qs/Qt), thereby improving oxygenation.[36, 37] The goal of mask CPAP (vs. conventional CPAP delivered via endotracheal tube) is to avoid endotracheal intubation and mechanical ventilation with its complications. Mask CPAP is particularly appealing for the patient who presents with hypoxemia from a potentially readily reversible cause such as pulmonary edema, mild pulmonary contusion, or postoperative atelectasis. In this setting the clinician is often forced to intubate the patient during the time lag between the initiation of medical therapy and the subsequent clinical improvement in the patient's pulmonary function. Mask CPAP can effect a rapid and significant improvement in oxygenation but should not be considered a replacement for controlled intubation and mechanical ventilation. The technique of mask CPAP is most appropriately applied when there is a reasonable expectation of significant improvement in pulmonary dysfunction once therapy is instituted or a short-term condition resolves.

A number of studies have examined the use of mask CPAP in treating pulmonary edema. In 1985 Rasanen et al.[38] reported on a series of 40 patients who presented with clinical and radiographic evidence of pulmonary edema as well as a respiratory rate greater than 25 breaths per minute, and a PaO_2/FiO_2 ratio of less than 200. The control group was treated with face mask O_2 while the study group received 10 cm CPAP; both groups were set at an FiO_2 of 0.35. Ten minutes after the institution of therapy the study group displayed a significant increase in PaO_2 and a significant decrease in heart rate and respiratory rate. At the end of the 3 hours of therapy, 62% of the control group required intubation compared with only 27% of the study group. In a second study utilizing a prospective randomized trial of increasing FiO_2 vs. mask CPAP, Vaisan and Rasanen[39] demonstrated that the use of mask CPAP was associated with a statistically significant fall in respiratory rate, blood pressure, and the need for intubation. Two other studies, by Perel et al.[40] and O'Halloren and Kalter[41] also document the efficacy of mask CPAP in treating pulmonary edema with associated hypercarbia. The supposition is that mask CPAP improves lung compliance, decreases shunt, and improves oxygenation and the work of breathing. A significant added benefit of mask CPAP in the treatment of cardiogenic pulmonary edema is that it increases airway and intrathoracic pressure which in turn favorably decreases venous return, ventricular filing pressure, and preload.[38]

A patient who presents to the emergency department with hypoxemia from a potentially readily reversible cause may be considered a candidate for mask CPAP. For hypoxemia secondary to cardiogenic pulmonary edema, mask CPAP with pressure of 10 cm H_2O is appropriate. Continual oximetric monitoring should be undertaken as well as intermittent arterial blood gas determinations of acid-base status and monitoring for the possible development of hypercarbia. The most reliable indicators of a favorable response are a decrease in respiratory and heart rate accompanied by an arterial O_2 saturation greater than 93%.[28, 39] The most common indications for abandonment of mask CPAP (with subsequent intubation of the patient) are hypercarbia and hypoventilation, inability to clear or protect the airway, and inability of the patient to tolerate the tight fit of the mask.

The initial FiO_2 should be 1.0 to relieve hypoxemia as rapidly as possible. The FiO_2 may be subsequently weaned using oximetric or arterial blood gas determination. If necessary, the mask CPAP pressure may be elevated to 15 cm H_2O. At pressures equal to or greater than 15 cm H_2O, attention must be paid to signs of CO_2 retention, obtundation, and hypotension (due to decreased venous return). Consideration should be given to the placement of a nasogastric (NG) tube to prevent aerophagia and potential aspiration. The level of airway pressure at which gastric insufflation occurs has not been established but is easily prevented by the placement of an NG tube.

The length of therapy of mask CPAP is variable and is primarily determined by the degree of underlying pulmonary dysfunction. Patients may be weaned from mask CPAP within several hours or may require several days before therapy can be discontinued. The clinician must be constantly prepared to intubate the patient if there is evidence of deterioration such as lethargy, obtundation, or rising arterial carbon dioxide partial pressure ($PaCO_2$).

The presence of facial fractures, extensive facial lacerations, laryngeal trauma, or a basilar skull fracture should be considered a contraindication to the use of mask CPAP. Patients at risk for vomiting or aspiration (gastrointestinal bleeding, esophageal varices, ileus) may also need to be excluded. The CPAP mask employed in the system should be composed of clear material to facilitate observation and early detection of potential airway compromise.

The largest published series of the use of mask

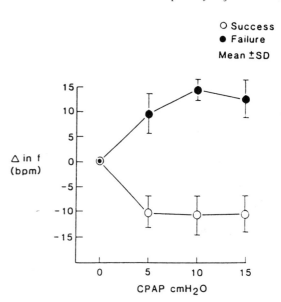

FIG 18A–6.
Changes in respiratory rate *(bpm)* in response to mask continuous positive airway pressure *(CPAP)*. *Open circles* denote mask CPAP "successes" (125/135) and *closed circles* denote "failures" (i.e., those that were subsequently intubated and mechanically ventilated). (From Branson RD: *Respir Care* 1988; 33:598–610. Used by permission.)

CPAP is that of Branson et al.[42] who described the use of this technique in 135 patients with a variety of disorders that resulted in acute respiratory failure. Their overall success rate was 93% and in their experience success or failure could be predicted by monitoring the respiratory rate. Those patients who responded favorably to CPAP showed a fall in respiratory rate while those who failed displayed no change or an increase (Fig 18A–6).

The reader is referred to a number of excellent reviews and articles regarding the use of mask CPAP, notably those of Barach et al.[16, 17] and Branson and colleagues,[32, 42] for further details regarding this technique.

The goal of O_2 therapy is to provide this therapeutic agent in such a way that hypoxemia is eliminated without imposing undue toxicity. With a careful consideration of patient needs as well as a recognition of the fundamental properties of the various delivery systems, this goal may be readily met in most patients.

REFERENCES

1. Shapiro BA, Harrison RA, Kacmarek RM, et al: *Clinical Application of Respiratory Care*, ed 3. St Louis, Mosby–Year Book, Inc, 1985.
2. Schacter EN, Littner MR, Luddy P, et al: Monitoring

of oxygen delivery systems in clinical practive. *Crit Care Med* 1980; 8:405–409.

3. Kory RD, Bergmann JC, Sweet RO, et al: Comparative evaluation of oxygen therapy techniques. *JAMA* 1962; 179:123–128.

4. Kacmarek RM: Oxygen therapy techniques, in *Current Respiratory Care.* Toronto, BC Decker Co, 1988.

5. Redding JS, McAfee DD, Parkam AM: Oxygen concentrations received from commonly used delivery systems. *South Med J* 1978; 71:169.

6. Kacmarek RM: Methods for oxygen delivery in the hospital. *Probl Respir Care* 1990; 3:563–574.

7. Hill AL, Barnes PK, Holloway T, et al: Fixed performance oxygen masks: An evaluation. *Br Med J* 1984; 288:1261–1263.

8. Leigh JM: Variation in performance of oxygen therapy devices. *Ann R Coll Surg Engl* 1973; 52:234–253.

9. Hedley-White J, Winter PM: Oxygen therapy. *Clin Pharmacol Ther* 1968; 8:696–737.

10. Spearman CB, et al: Effects of changing jet flows on O_2 concentrations in adjustable air entrainment masks. *Respir Care* 1980; 25:1266.

11. Friedman SA, Weber B, Briscoe WA, et al: Oxygen therapy—evaluation of various air-entraining masks. *JAMA* 1974; 228:474.

12. Barnes TA: *Respiratory Care Practice.* St Louis, Mosby–Year Book, Inc, 1988.

13. McPherson SP: *Respiratory Therapy Equipment,* ed 3. St Louis, Mosby–Year Book, Inc, 1985.

14. Bunnell S: The use of nitrous oxide and oxygen to maintain anesthesia and positive pressure for thoracic surgery. *JAMA* 1912; 58:835–838.

15. Bullowa JGM: *The Management of Pneumonias.* New York, Oxford University Press, 1936, pp 192–195.

16. Barach AL, Martin J, Eckman L: Effect of breathing gases under positive pressure on lumens of small and medium sized bronchi. *Arch Intern Med* 1939; 63:946–948.

17. Barach AL, Martin J, Eckman M: Positive pressure respiration and its application to the treatment of acute pulmonary edema. *Arch Intern Med* 1938; 12:754–793.

18. Poulton EP, Oxon DM: Left-sided heart failure with pulmonary edema: Its treatment with the "pulmonary plus pressure machine." *Lancet* 1936; 231:981–983.

19. Brewer LA III, Samson PC, Burbank B, et al: The wet lung in war casualties. *Ann Surg* 1946; 123:343–361.

20. Gagge AP, Allen SC, Marbager JP: Pressure breathing. *J Aviat Med* 1945; 17:290–380.

21. Barach AL, Eckman M, Ginsburg E, et al: Studies on positive pressure respiration: (I.) General aspects of pressure breathing. (II.) Effects on respiration and circulation at sea level. *J Aviat Med* 1946; 17:290–380.

22. Barach AL, Eckman M, Eckman I, et al: Effect of continuous positive pressure breathing on arterial blood gases at high altitude. *J Aviat Med* 1947; 18:139–148.

23. Barach AL, Eckman M, Bloom WL, et al: IV. Subjective clinical and psychological effects of continuous positive pressure breathing at high altitudes. *J Aviat Med* 1947; 18:252–305.

24. Barach AL, Ferns EB, Schmidt CF: The physiology of pressure breathing. A brief review of its present status. *J Aviat Med* 1947; 18:73–87.

25. Gregory GA, Kitterman, JA, Phibbs RH, et al: Treatment of the idiopathic respiratory distress syndrome with continuous positive airway pressure. *N Engl J Med* 1971; 284:1333–1340.

26. Hoff BH, Flemming DC, Sasse F: Use of positive airway pressure without endotracheal intubation. *Crit Care Med* 1979; 7:559–561.

27. Smith RA, Kirby RR, Gooding JM, et al: Continuous positive airway pressure by face mask. *Crit Care Med* 1980; 8:483–495.

28. Suter PM, Kobel N: Treatment of acute pulmonary failure by CPAP via face mask. When can intubation be avoided? *Klin Wochenschr* 1981; 59:613–616.

29. Linton DM, Potgieter PD: Conservative management of blunt chest trauma. *S Afr Med J* 1982; 61:917–919.

30. Hurst JM, DeHaven CB, Branson RD: Sole use of mask CPAP in respiratory insufficiency. *J Trauma* 1985; 25:1065–1068.

31. Covelli HD, Weled BJ, Beckman JF: Efficacy of continuous positive airway pressure administered by face mask. *Chest* 1982; 81:147–150.

32. Branson RD: PEEP without endotracheal intubation. *Respir Care* 1988; 33:598–610.

33. Powers SR, Mannal R, Naclerio M, et al: Physiologic consequences of positive end-expiratory pressure (PEEP) ventilation. *Ann Surg* 1973; 178:265–272.

34. Vuori A, Jalonen J, Laaksonen V: Continuous positive airway pressure during mechanical spontaneous ventilation: Effects on central hemodynamics and oxygen transport. *Acta Anaesth Scand* 1979; 23:453–461.

35. Gherini S, Peters RM, Virgilio RW: Mechanical work on the lungs and work of breathing with positive end-expiratory pressure and continuous positive airway pressure. *Chest* 1979; 76:251–256.

36. Matthay MA, Hopewell PC: Critical care for acute respiratory failure, in Baum GL, Wolinsky E (eds): *Textbook of Pulmonary Diseases.* Boston, Little, Brown & Co, 1989, pp 1055–1101.

37. Weisman IM, Rinaldo JE, Rogers RM: Positive end-expiratory pressure in adult respiratory failure. *N Engl J Med* 1982; 307:1381–1384.

38. Rasanen J, Heikkila J, Nikki P, et al: Continuous positive airway pressure by face mask in acute cardiogenic pulmonary edema. A randomized study. *Am J Cardiol* 1985; 55:296–300.

39. Vaisanen IT, Rasanen J: Continuous positive airway pressure and supplemental oxygen in the treatment

of cardiogenic pulmonary edema. *Chest* 1987; 92:481–485.

40. Perel A, Williamson DC, Modell JH: Effectiveness of CPAP via face mask for pulmonary edema associated with hypercarbia. *Intensive Care Medicine* 1983; 9:17–19.

41. O'Halloren K, Kalter C: Acute pulmonary edema with hypercarbia. An alternative approach. *Respir Tract* 1984; 10:1–6.

42. Branson RD, Hurst JM, DeHaven CB: Mask CPAP: State of the art. *Respir Care* 1985; 30:846–857.

18B
Diagnostic

Robert H. Dailey, M.D.

OXIMETRY AND CAPNOGRAPHY

The bedside assessment of ventilation and oxygenation is notoriously unreliable and poses major problems for the emergency physician. Traditionally, the arterial blood gas determination (ABG) has bridged the gap, and because of its accuracy it remains the gold standard for pH, PaO_2, and $PaCO_2$. However, this test requires an arterial puncture (it is always painful and often produces hematomas); it requires laboratory analysis (and is therefore not real time); it is costly; and continuous sampling requires arterial catheter placement. Therefore, means have been sought to obviate these problems through indirect measurements of PaO_2 and $PaCO_2$. In the past 10 years, giant technological strides have been made in this regard; it is now quite easy to efficiently monitor O_2 saturation, and practical ventilation monitoring may not be far behind. Two recent excellent reviews provide information appropriate to the emergency physician.[1, 2]

Oximetry refers to the process of noninvasive bedside monitoring of arterial O_2 saturation (SaO_2). Capnography refers to the bedside estimation of $PaCO_2$ by graphic waveform display of end-tidal PCO_2 ($PetCO_2$). Capnometry refers to a numerical display.

Oximetry

Technology and Equipment

The development of oximetry has spanned five decades. Two technologies have been developed. One, transcutaneous oximetry, is probably now becoming obsolete.[3] It depends on the polarographic measurement of O_2 diffusing from the capillary bed through the dermis of the skin. It requires skin preparation and, to provide vasodilatation, heating of the monitoring site to 43° C (burns sometimes result). Initial and subsequent calibrations are necessary. There is about a 15 second delay in readings. Pigmented, thick, or edematous skin incur errors, as do low-flow states. Preferred sites for transcutaneous oximetry are fingers, earlobes, and conjunctivae. A conjuntival site necessitates use of local anesthetic, and because blinking cannot occur, corneal ulcerations are a real danger with prolonged usage.[4]

Pulse oximetry has become the ascendant technology. It is based on the physical principles of (1) differential absorbtion of red and infrared light by oxyhemoglobin and reduced hemoglobin, and (2) arterial pulsation. A sturdy, lightweight, and inexpensive light-emitting diode is incorporated into the probe, and a simple microchip processor reliably interprets the signal. In addition to SaO_2, a visual pulse rate is displayed (and is audible). Technically, these instruments do not require calibration; they provide real-time data; need no site preparation or heating; are unaffected by thick, pigmented, or edematous skin; and are painless and noninvasive. Physically, they are compact, lightweight, and portable; they have no moving parts; and they are sturdy and relatively affordable. These devices have now reached a high degree of sophistication and reliability (i.e., they are fully evolved).

However, pulse oximeters have some technical limitations. Strong room lights, particularly those that flicker (fluorescent), can interfere with the probe's internal monochromatic light source; covering the probe or dimming the room lights easily rectifies this problem. Finger and hand motion may simulate a pulse to the sensor; this should not be a significant problem unless there is a continuous severe hand tremor, in which case the probe can be attached to a toe.

Interpretation

Pulse oximeters do *not* measure O_2 tension (pO_2). The oxyhemoglobin dissociation curve is needed to translate exactly the O_2 saturation reading into PaO_2 (Fig 18B–1). Fortunately, for our clinical purposes, the following obtain: (1) this translation has been shown to be very accurate; (2) within the range of clinically pertinent O_2 saturation values, the relationship of SaO_2 to PaO_2 is nearly linear (on the straight midportion of the curve); and (3) we can use two "shorthands" that obviate the need to reference the curve at all: *(a)* over the extremes of the useful SaO_2 range, 90% correlates roughly with a PaO_2 of 60 mm Hg, and 75% with a PaO_2 of 40 mm Hg (see inset of Fig 18B–1); and *(b)* within this "clinical" range, $PaO_2 = SaO_2 \simeq 30$.

Pulse oximetry is a relatively insensitive indicator of PaO_2 in the higher SaO_2 ranges (94% to 96%): subtle decrements in SaO_2 mask relatively large falls in PaO_2 (the flat end of the curve). Therefore, a reading in this range might or might not be associated with an abnormal PaO_2. Also, in the lower ranges (below 55%), the pulse oximeter becomes progressively inaccurate, overestimating the true SaO_2.

Certain clinical states provide problems in interpretation. Severe anemia has been cited, though pulse oximetry has been found accurate with hematocrit readings as low as 20%.[5] The presence of carbon monoxide or large amounts of methemoglobin will give erroneous readings.[1] But the most important problem is low-flow states (e.g., hypotension, increased peripheral vascular resistance, hypothermia, peripheral vascular disease, and vasoconstrictive pressors). The increased peripheral O_2 consumption associated with these low-flow states is associated with spuriously low readings. Practically, however, low-flow states must be severe for pulse oximeters to be in error, and the microprocessors have been programmed internally to automatically cease functioning at critical levels. Also, one can warm the monitored extemity and/or smear nitroglycerin on the monitored finger.[6]

Emergency Department Use

Pulse oximetry has added immeasurably to the clinical assessment of the dyspneic patient, to both identify and quantify significant hypoxemia (Table 18B–1). It is wise to get an initial room air reading as a baseline, both for diagnostic and therapeutic considerations. Of course, this won't be possible for the many patients who are transported by ambulance and in whom O_2 delivery has already begun. The use of pulse oximetry has already ben shown to uncover otherwise unsuspected severe hypoxemia (<85% SaO_2).[7] For the same reason this instrument will find a place in emergency department (ED) nurse triage.

One of the best usages of oximetry is for following the progress and/or deterioration of acutely ill patients with cardiac or respiratory disease.[5] However, to monitor *change,* one must keep the inspired O_2 concentration (FiO_2) constant. *Each increase/decrease in FiO_2 forms a new baseline for interpretation!* And simply increasing the FiO_2 in response to a falling SaO_2 does not mean that clinical improvement is necessarily occurring. Then too, *oximetry cannot give information about alveolar ventilation!* There is a real danger of the clinician accepting adequate SaO_2 values while neglecting gross hypoventilation.

In the patient with acute respiratory distress, pulse oximetry can *help* in the decision to intubate. It cannot be used in isolation to make that decision; other clinical factors such as mental alertness, adequacy of respiratory muscular effort, and severity and tempo of deterioration of the underlying pathological process also come into play. The SaO_2 is important to monitor during intubation as well; when attempts are prolonged or fail, oximetry has been shown to provide early detection of severe hypoxic episodes.[8]

A very different potential use of pulse oximetry

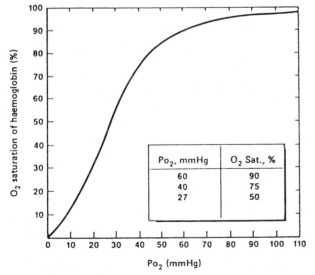

FIG 18B–1.
Adult hemoglobin-oxygen dissociation curve; arterial saturation plotted against oxygen tension (pO₂). (From Moore FA, Haenel JB: *Med Instrumentation* 1988; 22:138. Used with permission.)

TABLE 18B–1.

Indications for Oximetry Use in Emergency Medicine*

1. Early identification of significant hypoxemia by EMTs and for triage into ED
2. Aid in monitoring clinical improvement or deterioration in acutely dyspneic patients
3. Aid in determining when to intubate patients
4. Aid during intubation or other airway manipulations
5. Cost savings: to avoid ABGs when deemed unnecessary

*ED = emergency department; EMTs = emergency medical technicians; ABGs = arterial blood gas analyses.

1. The PaO_2 is likely to be out of the sensitive range of the oximeter (and clinically relevant)
2. The accuracy of the oximeter is in doubt
3. Hypercarbia is a real possibility

has recently been suggested: to determine systolic blood pressure in circumstances in which it is otherwise difficult. The oximeter was placed on the same arm as the cuff, and the appearance and disappearance of the pulse wave observed in conjunction with the blood pressure reading. Excellent correlation was found with Doppler readings in the range of 85 to 250 mm Hg.[9] This technique might prove very useful indeed if there were good correlations in patients in severe shock.

Finally, the cost savings potential of oximetry should be considered. Pulse oximetry should be performed immediately in patients with respiratory problems. ABGs should be considered only if (1) the PaO_2 is likely to be out of the range or in the insensitive area (95% to 96%) of the oximeter (and relevant!); (2) the accuracy of the oximeter is in doubt; (3) hypercarbia is a possibility (requiring $PaCO_2$ assessment); or (4) the arterial pH is needed (Table 18B–2). One should always ask, "Will an ABG give me additional necessary information?" Although pulse oximetry holds the potential for significant savings,[10] a recent study in a tertiary care teaching hospital ED showed no decrease in ABG usage following introduction of oximetry.[11]

Capnography

Technology and Equipment

The arterial carbon dioxide tension ($PaCO_2$) is the clinical standard for measurement of alveolar ventilation. It is affected by both production and elimination of carbon dioxide. But in 99% of clinical situations it is only the elimination (through ventilation) of CO_2 that is quantitatively significant. Thus, for practical purposes, the $PaCO_2$ solely measures ventilation. Normal values range from 37 to 43 mm Hg.

There are several means by which $PaCO_2$ can be measured without performing ABGs. Miniaturized intra-arterial electrodes have been devised that can directly measure $PaCO_2$ values continuously; but these are invasive and, as yet, experimental.[12]

There are two indirect measurement techniques: (1) sampling end-tidal air and analyzing for P_{CO_2}

($PetCO_2$) by infrared light absorption, and (2) performing transcutaneous polarographic measurement of P_{CO_2} ($PtcCO_2$) in either fingers or conjuntivae. Currently, $PetCO_2$ is being utilized clinically more than $PtcCO_2$, since the many technical drawbacks of $PtcCO_2$ are identical to those of $PtCO_2$ (see above). Several analyzers are commercially available, and have been recently tested and compared.[13] They are not inexpensive ($8,000 to $15,000 in the United States). Analysis of infrared light absorbtion of CO_2 by a digital diode, analogous to the pulse oximeter, has not been developed. Recently, two devices have been developed for use primarily in assessing correct positioning of endotracheal tubes following intubation (see following discussion).

Although sampling of respiratory gases can be performed in both intubated and nonintubated patients, most of the literature deals with the former, since it has been generated in ICUs. With the patient on a ventilator, air sampling can be either "mainstream" (in-line) or "sidestream" (Fig 18B–2). *Mainstream* means that the detector is located next to the endotracheal tube; this adds considerable bulk to the airway apparatus, necessitating a separate mount and posing the threat of system disconnections! *Sidestream* sampling, on the other hand, is prone to interference by secretions and water vapor. The mainstream devices tend to yield more accurate values. A modified nasal cannula for use in nonintubated patients has been recently devised, but no data have yet been published.[1]

Physiology

In persons with normal cardiopulmonary function there is virtually complete equilibration of CO_2 at the alveolar-capillary interface during the end of expiration; thus, the blood (which is then delivered to the arterial circulation) and the end-tidal air will normally both have a P_{CO_2} of about 40 mm Hg. One can measure $PetCO_2$ continuously and obtain a nearly real-time graphic display, so-called capnography (Fig 18B–3). Note the four distinct segments: end inspiration *(A to B),* rapid (beginning) expiration *(B to C),* slow (end) expiration *(C to D),* and rapid inspiration *(D to E).* In the figure, it is the peak of the plateau of expiration *(point D)* that represents end-tidal P_{CO_2}. However, abnormalities of either ventilation or perfusion, whether related to equipment or pathophysiology, will cause the $PetCO_2$ to be no longer a fair approximation of the $PaCO_2$ (producing a $PetCO_2/PaCO_2$ gradient).

Central perfusion (cardiac output) also can markedly alter the gradient between $PetCO_2$ and

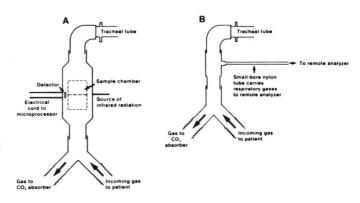

FIG 18B–2.
A, mainstream CO_2 analyzer. The sample chamber resides within the breathing circuit as close to the patient's airway as possible. Only infrared mainstream CO_2 analyzers are currently available. **B,** sidestream CO_2 analyzer. The small-bore tube carries the sample from the airway to a distant sample chamber. All mass spectrometry and some infrared analyzers are of this variety. (From Carlon GC, Ray C, Miodownik S, et al: *Crit Care Med* 1988; 16:550–556. Used with permission.)

$PaCO_2$. Markedly diminished cardiac output (CO) results in very little blood being presented to the lung for gas exchange. Therefore, little carbon dioxide is extracted, and accordingly the $PetCO_2$ is quite low and the $PaCO_2$ high—a large gradient.

The two types of ventilation abnormalities are (1) air that does not participate in gas exchange (dead space), and (2) pulmonary blood flow that perfuses unventilated alveoli (shunting); shunting accounts for very little alteration under most clinical circumstances. Dead space is of three types: (1) equipment-related (ventilator), (2) anatomically related (airways), and (3) physiologic, due to pulmonary disease.

It is unfortunate for the clinician that the above mentioned pathophysiologic alterations produce gradients, since it is during disease states that we most desire a close correlation between the two values! However, analysis of capnography waveforms can still give extremely useful information about both ventilatory equipment function and patient pathophysiology[14, 15] (Table 18B–3).

Emergency Department Use

As yet capnography/capnometry has had limited utility in the ED. Most experience has been with two

devices that help confirm tracheal placement of endotracheal tubes following intubation. The FEF endtidal CO_2 detector (Fenem, Inc., New York, NY, 10038; approximately $25) is a disposable device that is applied to the end of the endotracheal tube following intubation (Fig 18B–4). Its face changes color continuously, from inspiration to expiration, in response to changing carbon dioxide concentrations. It is purple on inspiration (i.e., absent or very low CO_2 concentrations: 0.03% to <0.5%, = 0.23 to <3.8 mm Hg) and yellow on expiration (i.e., relatively high CO_2 concentrations: 2% to 5%, = 15 to 38 mm Hg). Intermediate readings give a tan hue. Thus, incorrect esophageal placement would give a purple color. Several sources of error are possible. If

TABLE 18B–3.
Clinical Conditions Associated With Alterations in $PetCO_2$*

Increases in $PetCO_2$
  Sudden
    Sudden increase in cardiac output
    Sudden release of a tourniquet
    Injection of sodium bicarbonate
  Gradual
    Hypoventilation
    Increase in CO_2 production
Decreases in $PetCO_2$
  Sudden
    Sudden hyperventilation
    Sudden decrease in cardiac output
    Massive pulmonary embolism
    Air embolism
    Disconnection of the ventilator
    Obstruction of the endotracheal tube
    Leakage in the circuit
  Gradual
    Hyperventilation
    Decrease in oxygen consumption
    Decreased pulmonary perfusion
Absent $PetCO_2$
  Esophageal intubation

*From Bongard F, Sue D: *West J Med* 1992; 156:57–64. Used by permission.

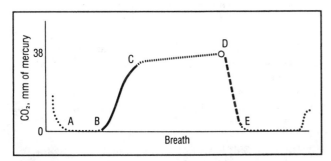

FIG 18B–3.
A normal capnograph consists of four distinct segments, beginning at the zero baseline. See text for explanation. (From Bongard F, Sue D: *West J Med* 1992; 156:61. Used with permission.)

a carbonated beverage has just been ingested, gastric air can contain enough CO_2 to give a false yellow reading; however, in a dog model it was found that over the space of seven ventilations, the CO_2 fell to the intermediate tan range.[16] A second and more probable source of error is circulatory collapse. Since patients in shock or cardiopulmonary arrest constitute a great portion of those undergoing emergency intubation, this source of error looms large. Indeed, under these circumstances paramedical physical examination was found in one study to be just as accurate as the FEF end-tidal CO_2 detector (about 15% error by each).[17]

A second device to assess endotracheal tube placement is the Minicap III (Mine Safety Appliances, Co., Pittsburg, PA; approximately $1,000). (Fig 18B–5) This is a sturdy, belt-portable device with its mainstream CO_2 detector set in an "on/off" position at 0.5% vol% (3.8 mm Hg). Its sensor (cost, approximately $5) is disposable but also reusable after cleansing. In a recent study, this device was used 100 times (21 cardiac arrests) in 88 consecutive patients. Tube placement was confirmed by either direct visualization or x-ray. The sensitivity and specificity for correct intubation was 100%.[18]

$PetCO_2$ has been studied in CPR. The delivery of CO_2 to the lungs decreases logarithmically with decreased cardiac output.[19] The $PetCO_2$ has been found to correlate, albeit roughly, with return of circulation[20] and survival outcomes.[21] Correlation in animals between $PaCO_2$ and $PetCO_2$ during cardiac arrest has not been confirmed in humans.[22]

The FEF end-tidal CO_2 detector has been described as an aid in blind nasotracheal intubation.[23] Instead of using airstream intensity to guide the tube, one observes the colorimetric change of the device while slowly advancing the tube. (No results were offered in the report.)

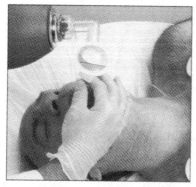

FIG 18B–4.
FEF end-tidal CO2 detector connected to endotracheal tube.

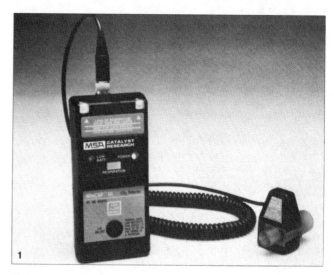

FIG 18B–5.
Minicap III CO_2 detector.

Finally, one would hope that a device might be developed that could reliably detect and monitor hypercarbia in nonintubated ED patients with respiratory distress. Given that it is precisely these patients in whom (1) there is a large gradient between the $PaCO_2$ and the $PetCO_2$,[24] and (2) air sampling has not been perfected, this hope is not likely to be realized until a finger monitor analogous to the pulse oximeter becomes available.

REFERENCES

1. Bongard F, Sue D: Pulse oximetry and capnography in intensive and transitional care units. *West J Med* 1992; 156:57–64.
2. Tobin MJ: Respiratory monitoring. *JAMA* 1990; 264:244–251.
3. Brown M, Vender JS: Noninvasive oxygen monitoring. *Crit Care Clin* 1988; 4:493–509.
4. Abraham E, Fink S: Conjunctival oxygen tension monitoring in ED patients. *Am J Emerg Med* 1988; 6:549–554.
5. Jones J, Heiselman D, Cannon L, et al: Continuous ED monitoring of arterial oxygen saturation in adult patients with respiratory distress. *Ann Emerg Med* 1988; 17:463–468.
6. McGough EK, Boysen PG: Benefits and limitations of pulse oximetry in the ICU. *J Crit Illness* 1989; 4:23–31.
7. Dunmire SM, Paris PM, Menegazzi JJ, et al: Value of pulse oximetry in prehospital care (abstract) *Ann Emerg Med* 1991; 20:492.
8. Mateer JR, Stueven HA, Aufderheide TP: Continu-

ous pulse oximetry during emergency endotracheal intubation (abstract). *Ann Emerg Med* 1991; 20:493.

9. Carlin D, Althoff M, Rancatore E, et al: Use of the pulse oximeter wave display to determine systolic blood pressure in the ED (abstract). *Ann Emerg Med* 1991; 20:493.

10. Joseph S, Kellermann AL, Cofer CA, et al: Impact of portable pulse oximetry on arterial blood gas analysis in an urban emergency department (abstract). *Ann Emerg Med* 1989; 18:232.

11. Singer A, Jouriles NJ, Rutherford WF, et al: Impact of bedside pulse oximetry on the utilization of arterial blood gas measurements in the ED (abstract). *Ann Emerg Med* 1991; 20:493.

12. Tobin MJ: Respiratory monitoring in the ICU. *Am Rev Respir Dis* 1988; 138:1625–1642.

13. Selby DG, Ilsley AH, Runciman WB: An evaluation of five carbon dioxide analysers for use in the operating theatre and ICU. *Anaesth Int Care* 1987; 15:212–216.

14. Stock CM: Capnography. *Intensive Care Mon* 1988; 4:511–527.

15. Carlon GC, Ray C, Miodownik S, et al: Capnography in mechanically ventilated patients. *Crit Care Med* 1988; 16:550–556.

16. Garnett AR, Gervin CA, Gervin AS: Capnographic waveforms in esophageal intubation: Effect of carbonated beverages. *Ann Emerg Med* 1989; 18:387–390.

17. Braun RU, Londeree RD: Paramedic physical examination skills compared with a disposable end-tidal CO_2 monitor for confirmation of endotracheal tube placement. *Ann Emerg Med* 1991; 20:487.

18. Yukmir RB, Heller MB, Stein KL: Confirmation of endotracheal tube placement: A miniaturized infrared qualitative CO_2 monitor. *Ann Emerg Med* 1991; 20:726–729.

19. Ornato JP, Garnett AR, Glauser FL: Relationship between cardiac output and the end-tidal carbon dioxide tension. *Ann Emerg Med* 1990; 19:1104–1106.

20. Garnett AR, Ornato JP, Gonzalez ER, et al: End-tidal carbon dioxide monitoring during cardiopulmonary resuscitation. *JAMA* 1987; 257:512–515.

21. Sanders AB, Kern KB, Otto CW, et al: End-tidal carbon dioxide monitoring during cardfiopulmonary resuscitation. *JAMA* 1989; 262:1347–1351.

22. Barton C, Callahan M: Lack of correlation between end-tidal carbon dioxide concentrations and $PaCO_2$ in cardiac arrest. *Crit Care Med* 1991; 19:108–110.

23. King HK, Wooten DJ: Blind nasal intubation by monitoring end-tidal CO_2 (letter to editor). *Anesth Analg* 1989; 69:412–413.

24. Heinoff J, DelGuercio C, LaMorte W, et al: Efficacy of pulse oximetry and capnometry in postoperative ventilatory weaning. *Crit Care Med* 1988; 16:701–705.

19

Ventilators

David K. English, M.D.

Mechanical ventilators routinely allow patients to survive insults that were uniformly fatal only a few decades ago. Mechanical ventilation is used primarily to improve arterial oxygenation, to supplant inadequate spontaneous ventilation, and to relieve the ill patient from the work of breathing. Ventilation should be considered for every emergency department patient that requires endotracheal intubation, and for actual or potential respiratory insufficiency complicating any illness. The ventilator may also be a useful adjunct in many situations other than primary respiratory failure.[1] Patients with elevated intracranial pressure benefit from controlled hyperventilation. Patients with marginal cardiac output may benefit from the reduced energy cost of breathing.

New ventilators, new monitors, and new modes of ventilation are being introduced constantly.[2-6] The literature is replete with arguments for and against these innovations. Fortunately, the basics of ventilation needed for acute management are easily grasped. They are the focus of this chapter.

TYPES OF VENTILATORS AND MODES OF VENTILATION

The major classes of ventilator in current use are *pressure-cycled* and *volume-cycled*. Pressure-cycled ventilators are used almost exclusively in pediatrics (Fig 19–1). They deliver gas to the patient until a preset pressure is reached. The clinician cannot directly control the volume delivered. Most adult ventilators deliver a preset volume of gas, regardless of the pressure necessary (within limits) (Fig 19–2,A and B). This discussion focuses on volume-cycled ventilators, since they are most often used by emergency physicians.

There is a plethora of ventilator modes and settings, resulting in endless confusion for any physician who does not use them regularly. Fortunately, in the emergency department, only a few settings are truly necessary for acute patient management (Table 19–1).

The first and most easily understood mode of ventilation is *controlled mechanical ventilation* (CMV). The ventilator delivers the set amount of gas at the set frequency, and the patient's efforts, if any, do not contribute to ventilation in any way. This is ideal for the paralyzed patient or the patient under general anesthesia, but is not tolerated by awake patients. *Assist-control* (AC) has almost completely replaced CMV. If the patient on AC initiates a breath, the ventilator will provide a full breath at the preset volume. If the patient does not make an inspiratory effort within a certain time, then a full breath is delivered, just as in CMV. The patient's respiratory effort may cause ventilation to exceed the set parameters, but ventilation cannot fall below the set level.

Intermittent mandatory ventilation (IMV) is another popular mode of ventilation.[7] Breaths are delivered by the machine at a set rate and volume. Between machine breaths, a fresh gas supply is available for the patient's spontaneous breaths, but the machine does not assist spontaneous breaths. Because a machine breath may be delivered at an uncomfortable moment (such as at end-inhalation), IMV has been largely replaced with *synchronized intermittent mandatory ventilation* (SIMV). Within limits, the patient's efforts are used to trigger the machine breaths. If the patient makes no effort, the preset breaths are given; if the patient breathes faster than the ventilator, the extra breaths are not assisted. By contrast, in AC mode every breath is fully assisted. Figure 19–3 graphically illustrates the changes in airway pressure with each mode.

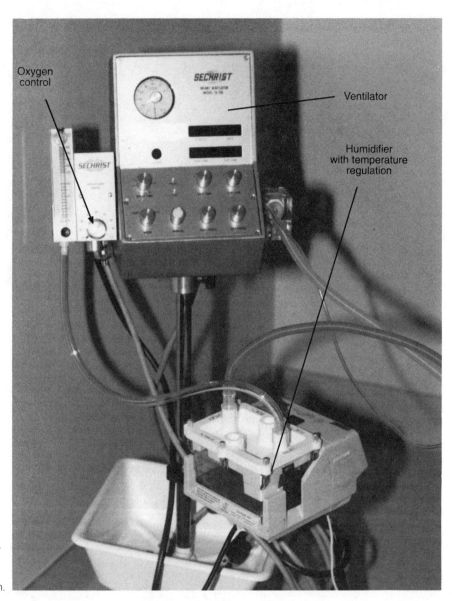

FIG 19–1.
The Sechrist IV-100 ventilator, a pressure-cycled infant ventilator. *Left, above:* oxygen control. *Right, above:* ventilator. *Below:* humidifier with temperature regulation.

For acute management in the emergency department, there is no important difference between AC and SIMV. The clinician should choose one and use it consistently, unless there is a compelling reason to change it for a particular patient. Often the institutional bias is the most important criterion. Either mode provides full ventilatory support if the set parameters exceed the patient's needs or if the patient is unable to initiate a breath. The work of breathing is similar in either mode for the awake patient.[8]

TABLE 19–1.

Comparison of Ventilator Modes

| Mode* | Response to Apnea | Response to Spontaneous Breaths | | Full Machine Breaths Delivered |
		Rate	Volume	
AC	Set rate and volume delivered	Set by patient	Always full	Always
SIMV	Set rate and volume delivered	Set by patient	Set by patient	Sometimes
PS	No breath	Set by patient	Set by patient	Never

*AC = assist-control; SIMV = synchronized intermittent mandatory ventilation; PS = pressure support.

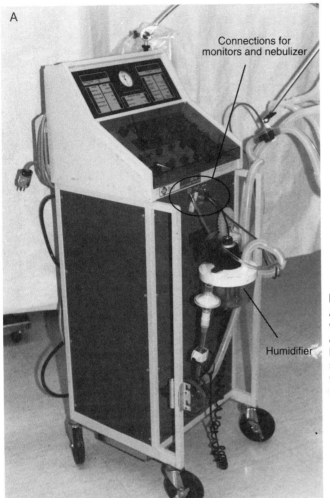

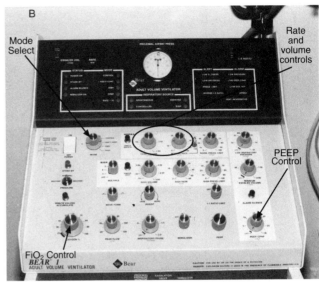

FIG 19–2.
A, the Bear ventilator by Intermed. A common adult volume-cycled ventilator. Controls are easily accessible on the top panel. *Right, above:* connections for monitors and nebulizer. *Right, below:* humidifier. **B,** control panel of the Bear ventilator. *Left, above:* mode select. *Left, below:* inspired oxygen control. *Right, above:* rate and volume controls. *Right, below:* positive end-expiratory pressure (PEEP) control.

(This last may seem counterintuitive, but the contraction of the respiratory muscles does not stop when the ventilator delivers a breath.[9]) There are theoretical advantages favoring one mode over the other, but controlled clinical trials do not show an important difference. Advocates of SIMV claim that it lowers mean intrathoracic pressure and has less tendency to produce respiratory alkalosis, but this has not been proved in trials.[10, 11]

Occasionally a patient requires intubation for an airway problem but is able to generate adequate ventilation once the airway is secure. This patient can be connected to a *T-piece,* which vents fresh gas past the end of the endotracheal tube while the patient breathes as much or as little as desired. Unfortunately, neither the rate nor tidal volume can be readily measured, the oxygen concentration may vary, and the airway pressure is the same as ambient room pressure. The preferred alternative is a mode called *pressure support* (PS), which is available on many modern ventilators. In PS the patient's inspira-

tory effort triggers a demand valve, which delivers fresh gas at a preset pressure. Gas flow continues until the inspiratory flow falls below a set threshold. The patient determines both the rate and the volume, while the pressure helps overcome resistance in the breathing circuit. Although rate and volume are not controlled, they can be monitored easily since the circuit is closed. All of the alarms and monitors provided by the ventilator are available. This mode is usually very well tolerated, unless the demand valve requires an excessive effort to initiate gas flow.[12–14] Pressure support can also be added to SIMV mode to reduce the work of the patient's spontaneous breaths.

ADJUNCTS TO VENTILATION

Most patients placed on mechanical ventilation have some pulmonary pathologic condition and require supplemental oxygen. All modern ventilators

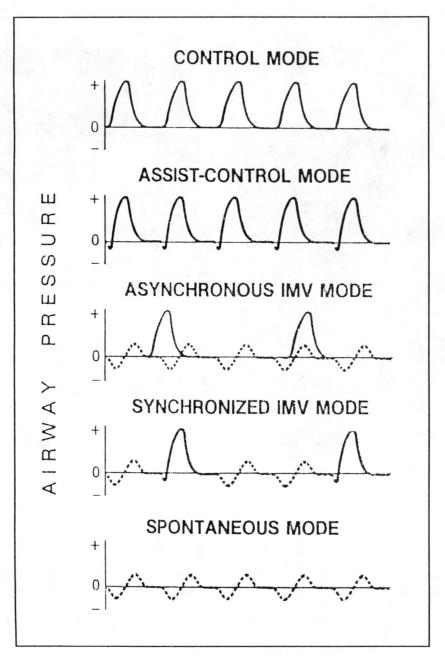

FIG 19-3.
Airway pressures in various modes of ventilation. *Broken lines* represent spontaneous breaths; *IMV* = intermittent mandatory ventilation. (Modified from Otto CW: *Emerg Med Clin North Am* 1986; 4:635-654.)

provide a straightforward method of selecting the inspired concentration of oxygen (FiO$_2$), usually by a simple dial adjustment. Although prolonged exposure to high levels of oxygen is toxic to the lung, hypoxemia is far more injurious in the short term. Supplemental oxygen should never be withheld once the decision to start mechanical ventilation is reached. Some patients with collapse or flooding of alveoli cannot be adequately oxygenated even at

100% FiO$_2$; they may require *positive end-expiratory pressure* (PEEP). PEEP maintains the airway pressure above ambient pressure, which has the beneficial effect of increasing the lung volume and holding the alveoli open. This will improve oxygenation of the blood through improvement in ventilation-perfusion matching at the alveoli. It may or may not improve oxygen delivery to peripheral tissues, because higher levels of PEEP can decrease cardiac output. The elevation of mean intrathoracic pressure also increases the risk of barotrauma.

All ventilators are supplied with a humidifier for the fresh gas. The emergency physician can usually ignore humidification, but in a few instances it is important. In case of hypothermia, the humidifier can deliver a significant amount of heat to the patient. Some humidifiers markedly increase the work of breathing, and all cause condensation which may obstruct alarm sensors or even the entire breathing circuit. Contaminated humidifiers have also resulted in iatrogenic pneumonia.

Medication nebulizers can be added easily to the breathing circuit (Fig 19–4). In principle they are no different from the hand-held nebulizers used for the nonintubated asthmatic patient. The nebulizer is placed directly in the inspiratory side of the breathing circuit, often at the attachment to the endotracheal tube. A separate supply of fresh compressed gas is attached to the nebulizer; it is usually provided by the ventilator and has the same FiO_2 as the patient gas supply. The medication is continuously aerosolized into the circuit, but the nebulizer does not interfere with ventilation of the patient. This is an extremely effective route of drug delivery because every breath will reliably contain medication, the full dose will be delivered, and access to the lower airway is assured. The asthmatic patient's β-agonist inhalation treatments can be resumed within minutes after ventilation is started, and can be provided continuously if needed.

A host of other ventilator parameters can be specified, including varied inspiratory waveforms and flows, pauses, and sighs (see Fig 19–2,B). Occasionally the emergency physician will need to modify the inspiratory flow rate, as discussed later, but the respiratory therapist will generally choose a rate that is suitable for the patient's clinical situation and response to the ventilator. The emergency physician can safely ignore waveforms, pauses, and sighs. Altered inspiratory waveforms and inspiratory pauses are sometimes used by pulmonary specialists in management of patients at special risk from barotrauma, or those with markedly abnormal airway dynamics or ventilation-perfusion relationships. They are well beyond the scope of this chapter. Sighs are extralarge breaths delivered intermittently to prevent atelectasis. Sighs are not usually necessary with current techniques of large volume ventilation, but they may be in vogue at individual institutions.

ORDERS

Every patient receiving mechanical ventilation must have orders for the mode, the rate, the tidal volume, and the concentration of oxygen (Table 19–2). As noted earlier, the physician can safely choose either AC or SIMV mode for all patients, and ignore the theoretical concerns which favor one or the other. Tidal volumes of 10 to 12 mL/kg, or 700 to 850 mL for the usual 70-kg adult, are almost always satisfactory. Smaller tidal volumes increase the risk of atelectasis, but are sometimes necessary if airway pressures are excessive at the usual volume. Larger volumes increase the risk of barotrauma without any benefit to the patient. A rate of 10 to 12 breaths per minute at these large volumes will provide complete ventilatory support for the patient with average metabolic needs. If hyperventilation is clinically indicated, for example in head trauma or severe metabolic acidosis, then a relatively small increase in rate to 14 to 16 breaths per minute will produce a large increase in ventilation.

Almost every patient should start with 100% FiO_2. It is better to err on the side of overoxygenating the patient in the first few minutes of ventilation. Usually

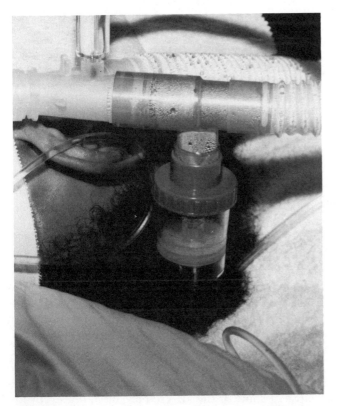

FIG 19–4.
Medication nebulizer in the inspiratory arm of the ventilator circuit. Compressed gas supply from the ventilator is attached at the bottom of the nebulizer.

TABLE 19–2.

Initial Ventilator Settings*

Patient	Mode	Rate (breaths/min)	Volume (mL/kg)	Pressure (cm H_2O)	FiO_2	Comment
Adult	AC or SIMV	10–12	10–12	NA	100%	Pressure <50 cm H_2O results in less barotrauma
Child	AC or SIMV	14–24	10–15	Alarm ≈20	100%	Pressure usually not set directly
Infant	SIMV	20–40	NA	12–20	100%	Titrate FiO_2 rapidly to avoid O_2 toxicity

*FiO_2 = fractional concentration of oxygen in inspired gas; AC = assist-control; SIMV = sychronized intermittent mandatory ventilation; NA = not available.

the clinician does not know the state of the patient's oxygenation precisely, and mechanical ventilation will slightly worsen the ventilation-perfusion relationships in the lung. Although high levels of oxygen have real risks for the patient in the long term, hypoxia is a much more serious immediate threat. The FiO_2 can be adjusted downward after the first arterial blood gas sample is measured.

The inspiratory flow rate is set by the respiratory therapist and usually need not be specified. However, patients with expiratory airflow obstruction sometimes benefit from a setting that is higher than normal, since the shorter inhalation allows more time to complete exhalation. Some patients with subjective "air hunger" will also improve with inspiratory flow that is higher than normal. The peak airway pressure alarm limit can also be specified, but it is normally set at 15 to 20 cm H_2O above the patient's usual peak pressure.

Every intubated patient needs frequent and thorough suctioning of the airway, because the endotracheal tube prevents an effective cough. In the emergency department, this can be done on an as-needed basis. If the patient is to remain under the emergency physician's care for a prolonged period, then a standing order for suctioning at intervals of every 2 hours is appropriate. Similarly, patients detained in the emergency department may benefit from routine chest physiotherapy (percussion and postural drainage) several times a day.

CLINICAL SITUATIONS

Only a few common problems are discussed here. For further details, consult the appropriate chapter in Part III for the patient's specific condition.

Many patients in status asthmaticus require mechanical ventilation. The main indications are hyper-

carbia and hypoxia, with a deteriorating mental status, inability to phonate, and inaudible breath sounds prompting emergent intubation. These patients require inordinately high airway pressures to obtain the usual tidal volumes, and they are at high risk of barotrauma. Because the obstruction to exhalation is greater than the obstruction to inhalation, high flow rates are often chosen. This allows more time for exhalation and prevents air trapping in the lungs but may raise peak airway pressures even further. Since barotrauma accounts for more morbidity than respiratory acidosis, some authors have advocated intentional hypoventilation.[15] In trials, the ventilator was adjusted to avoid pressures beyond a predetermined limit; hypercapnia and mild acidosis were disregarded. Severe acidosis was unusual and was treated with intravenous bicarbonate. When effective bronchodilation was accomplished, the carbon dioxide partial pressure (PCO_2) fell and a more normal pattern of ventilation was resumed. The incidence of barotrauma was markedly reduced. Of course, aggressive bronchodilation with in-line aerosols, intravenous steroids, hydration, and other standard measures is required. For the truly refractory patient, inhalation anesthetics such as halothane are occasionally required.

Patients with wet or "white-out" lungs, from causes such as congestive heart failure or adult respiratory distress syndrome, have in common the pathologic features of flooding and collapse of the terminal alveoli. This makes the lungs very stiff (low compliance), and impairs oxygenation far more than it affects CO_2 exchange. In addition to ongoing efforts to correct the underlying process, these patients will often benefit from PEEP. PEEP acts to hold the lung at a higher volume, preventing collapse of some of the affected alveoli and thereby improving the match between ventilation and perfusion. It does not change the underlying lung condition, nor does it force water out of the lung. It does increase the mean airway pressure and intracranial pressure, and it may decrease cardiac output, but it may permit adequate oxygenation of a patient with otherwise refractory hypoxemia. PEEP levels above 8 to 10 cm H_2O often necessitate invasive hemodynamic monitoring to determine the ultimate effect on tissue oxygen delivery.[16]

Patients with head trauma or central nervous system (CNS) infection benefit from lowering of intracranial pressure through controlled hyperventilation. The maximal benefit is obtained by lowering the PCO_2 to 25 to 30 mm Hg; below this range there are increasing complications from the severe systemic alkalosis and no further benefits to the brain.[17] Hyperventilation to PCO_2 levels below 20 mm Hg results in cerebrospinal fluid (CSF) lactic acidosis, apparently from cerebral hypoxia resulting from inadequate cerebral blood flow. If hyperventilation is initiated, it must never be stopped abruptly or intracranial pressure will rise precipitously, as the vessels dilate within minutes.

REASSESSMENT

All patients should be checked frequently in the first few minutes after connection to the ventilator. The lungs must be auscultated to assess adequacy and uniformity of ventilation. The endotracheal tube is often dislodged during the rapid manipulation of the patient, and a previously unsuspected pneumothorax may become rapidly apparent with positive pressure ventilation. A stat. chest radiograph should be obtained in this initial period to help rule out these complications, and to assess the underlying lung pathologic condition. The lungs are often much better seen in the postintubation films because adequate inflation is more easily assured.

The vital signs should be rechecked frequently in the first few minutes. Positive pressure ventilation reduces venous return to the heart, and may reduce cardiac output significantly if the patient is already relatively hypovolemic or has impaired autonomic reflexes. This hypotension will respond to intravenous crystalloid infusion if fluid is not otherwise contraindicated.

After 15 to 20 minutes of ventilation, arterial blood gases must be measured to assess oxygenation and ventilation. Shorter intervals do not allow the pH and PCO_2 to equilibrate, whereas longer intervals increase the patient's risk unnecessarily.

Hyper- or hypocapnia must be corrected promptly by adjustment of the ventilator rate. If the patient is breathing faster than the ventilator rate, then sedation may be necessary to correct the alkalosis. If the PCO_2 is low but the pH is normal or low, then hyperventilation is compensating for a metabolic acidosis, and ventilation should not be decreased until the metabolic problem is corrected. If the patient is hypercapnic with a normal pH, then it is likely that the patient chronically hypoventilates. In such a case it is better to aim for a normal pH than a normal PCO_2 or else the eventual weaning will be unnecessarily prolonged and difficult.

The oxygen tension (PO_2) should be maintained at a level that assures near-complete hemoglobin saturation, approximately 80 to 100 mm Hg. Once ventilation is started, concern about the hypoxic drive of the patient with chronic obstructive pulmonary disease (COPD) is irrelevant. If the initial PO_2 is very high, in the range of 400 to 600 mm Hg, then the FiO_2 can be reduced in one step to 50% to 60%, and further reductions left to the admitting physician. If the PO_2 is lower than 400 mm Hg on 100% FiO_2, then there is a significant impairment to oxygenation and decreases should be done more gradually. If the PO_2 is low, less than 80 mm Hg, then the oxygen supply and the ventilator settings should be immediately rechecked. Do not assume that the blood gas measurement is in error. If hypoxia is present despite a confirmed FiO_2 of 100%, then PEEP should be added in small increments, initially 3 to 5 cm H_2O and then by 2- to 3-cm increments. The lowest level that permits adequate oxygenation should be chosen. PEEP of 3 to 5 cm H_2O is well tolerated, but higher levels above 8 to 10 cm H_2O should be avoided without help from the consultant.

After the patient has been adequately stabilized, with the ventilator adjusted to desired levels of support and adequate oxygenation assured, the maintenance phase begins. The goal here is to prevent complications, while efficiently reversing the underlying pathophysiology which made ventilation necessary. Appropriate therapy might include aggressive bronchodilation for the asthmatic patient, diuresis for the patient in congestive heart failure, and antibiotics for the septic patient.

CRISIS MANAGEMENT

The emergency physician must recognize and treat the few common complications rapidly. Perhaps the most common problem is hypotension, which may be due to decreased venous return. Hypotension may also result from the underlying pathologic condition, sedative medications, or another, unsuspected complication such as tension pneumothorax or severe acid-base derangement. If due solely to decreased return, hypotension should respond easily to intravenous fluid. Some patients with impaired autonomic reflexes will need low doses of vasoconstrictive drugs. Hypotension should always lead to a thorough reassessment of the patient, searching for other more serious causes.

Pulmonary barotrauma is a common complication in patients requiring high inspiratory pressures. It may present at any time in the course of ventilation. Overdistended alveoli rupture and air dissects into the pleural space, mediastinum, pericardium, and other sites.[18] Every ventilated patient with a pneumothorax from any cause needs a chest tube. Under the positive pressure of the ventilator, a small pneumothorax can become a tension pneumothorax in only a few breaths. The usual signs of tension will be present, including asymmetric breath sounds, tympany, and ultimately hypotension. However, tension pneumothorax in a ventilated patient may present first as a rapid rise in peak airway pressure as the thorax becomes more difficult to inflate. Needle thoracostomy and chest tube placement must be done without delay.

Most awake patients will "fight" the ventilator for the first few minutes. The patient is likely to be in pain, frightened, experiencing multiple procedures, and will be receiving a pattern of ventilation different from what he or she would choose spontaneously. These initial problems of adaptation will usually resolve within a few minutes; if not, other causes should be sought. Sedation and paralysis are sometimes necessary to permit satisfactory ventilation, but they should never take the place of correcting underlying problems. Because agitation and respiratory asynchrony are self-perpetuating, the patient should be disconnected from the ventilator and manually ventilated with 100% oxygen for a few minutes. The position and integrity of the endotracheal tube should be checked, and the tube should be suctioned after preoxygenation. Mucous plugs may markedly increase airway resistance, while a leaking cuff can decrease the volume delivered to the patient. A malpositioned tube can stimulate forceful coughing, a sense of dyspnea, or air hunger.

After manual ventilation and assessment of the patient and the tube, the ventilator should be quickly checked for integrity of the circuit. The settings should be rechecked for any inadvertent change. If no problems are found, the patient should be reconnected to the ventilator briefly under close observation. If there is a large difference between delivered and expired volumes, then a leak in the circuit is likely. The respiratory therapist should perform detailed checks and possibly provide a different ventilator. If all seems well but the patient continues to fight, sedation is appropriate. Opiates such as morphine are ideal because of their combination of analgesia, suppression of respiratory drive, and rapid reversal with a specific antidote.

Modern ventilators have a host of alarms[19]; their cacophony often overwhelms the less experienced clinician. The low-pressure or low-exhaled-volume alarms may indicate disconnection or leaks in the breathing circuit. They deserve prompt attention.[20] The high-pressure alarm is frequently triggered by a cough or movement of the patient. If it is transient, it can be ignored. If it is part of an upward trend in pressure, the patient must be assessed for bronchospasm, obstruction, or pneumothorax, and appropriate treatment undertaken. Oxygen analyzers are usually entirely separate devices linked to the ventilator only by their sensors. If they indicate a low FiO_2, the patient should be manually ventilated with 100% oxygen from a separate source until the ventilator and its gas supply can be checked. Hospital gas mains (as well as equipment and its operators) can and do fail, and the connections to the lines are even more prone to trouble. In any case where equipment failure is suspected, the default mode of manual ventilation with a self-inflating bag attached to a known source of 100% oxygen should be started immediately.[21]

It is likely that future systems will incorporate still more monitoring devices. Computerized monitoring systems developed for the space program may not only detect but also diagnose a variety of mishaps.[22] Capnometers and mass spectrometers provide continuous visual display of the patient's exhaled CO_2 concentration.[23] They can detect alterations of ventilation, perfusion, and equipment function before most other types of monitors,[24] but require significant training for proper interpretation. Capnometers are gradually moving from the operating room to the emergency department.

PEDIATRIC PERSPECTIVES

Pediatric ventilation is guided by the same general principles as apply to adult patients, though the anxiety of the clinician is likely to be much greater. Because of mechanical and developmental differences, children have much more compliant chests (there is a greater change in volume for a given change in pressure), and their alveoli fill and empty in a much shorter interval. Pressure-cycled ventilators are used routinely for infants (see Fig 20–1); older children can be ventilated with the more familiar volume-cycled ventilators. For children, a tidal volume of 10 to 15 mL/kg is appropriate, with initial rates varying between 14 and 24 breaths per minute, depending on age. Because younger children are ordinarily intubated with an uncuffed endotracheal tube, some leakage of gas from the system is expected.[25] The exhaled volume will be less than the set volume, and the volume delivered to the patient will be still less because of expansion and contraction of the tubing. The blood gases and clinical assessment of the patient are far more helpful than the specific numbers on the ventilator dial. Since infants are ventilated with pressure-cycled machines, no specific tidal volume can be set. Instead, the *peak inspiratory pressure* (PIP) is set in the range from 12 to 20 cm H_2O with a rate from 20 to 40 breaths per minute.[26] Depending on the ventilator, either the flow rates or the inspiratory-expiratory ratio are set directly, to provide an expiratory time of 0.3 to 0.6 second. Too little expiratory time results in air trapping and barotrauma.[27] Because of the uncuffed endotracheal tube, an increase in PIP may not result in a corresponding increase in ventilation, and blood gases and clinical evaluation are essential. Because infant endotracheal tubes are very small, even small mucous plugs may cause sudden and severe deterioration in ventilation.

REFERENCES

1. Otto CW: Ventilatory management in the critically ill. *Emerg Med Clin North Am* 1986; 4:635–654.
2. Froese AB, Bryan AC: High frequency ventilation. *Am Rev Respir Dis* 1987; 135:1363–1374.
3. Hayes B: Ventilation and ventilators—an update. *J Med Eng Technol* 1988; 12:197–218.
4. Hayes B: Ventilation and ventilators. *J Med Eng Technol* 1982; 6:177–192.
5. Slutsky AS: Nonconventional methods of ventilation. *Am Rev Respir Dis* 1988; 138:175–183.
6. Petty TL: The modern evolution of mechanical ventilation. *Clin Chest Med* 1988; 9:1–10.
7. Weisman IM, Rinaldo JE, Rogers RM, et al: Intermittent mandatory ventilation. *Am Rev Respir Dis* 1983; 127:641–647.
8. Groeger JS, Levinson MR, Carlon GC: Assist control versus synchronized intermittent mandatory ventilation during acute respiratory failure. *Crit Care Med* 1989; 17:607–612.
9. Marini JJ, Smith TC, Lamb VJ: External work output and force generation during synchronized intermittent mechanical ventilation. Effect of machine assistance on breathing effort. *Am Rev Respir Dis* 1988; 138:1169–1179.
10. Culpepper JA, Rinaldo JE, Rogers RM: Effect of mechanical ventilator mode on tendency towards respiratory alkalosis. *Am Rev Respir Dis* 1985; 132:1075–1077.
11. Hudson LD, Hurlow RS, Craig KC, et al: Does intermittent mandatory ventilation correct respiratory alkalosis in patients receiving assisted mechanical ventilation? *Am Rev Respir Dis* 1985; 132:1071–1074.
12. Fiastro JF, Habib MP, Quan SF: Pressure support compensation for inspiratory work due to endotracheal tubes and demand continuous positive airway pressure. *Chest* 1988; 93:499–505.
13. MacIntyre NR: Respiratory function during pressure support ventilation. *Chest* 1986; 89:677–683.
14. Brochard L, Pluskwa F, Lemaire F: Improved efficacy of spontaneous breathing with inspiratory pressure support. *Am Rev Respir Dis* 1987; 136:411–415.
15. Darioli R, Perret C: Mechanical controlled hypoventilation in status asthmaticus. *Am Rev Respir Dis* 1984; 129:385–387.
16. Luce JM: The cardiovascular effects of mechanical ventilation and positive end-expiratory pressure. *JAMA* 1984; 252:807–811.
17. Heffner JE, Sahn SA: Controlled hyperventilation in patients with intracranial hypertension. Application and management. *Arch Intern Med* 1983; 143:765–769.
18. Strieter RM, Lynch JP III: Complications in the ventilated patient. *Clin Chest Med* 1988; 9:127–139.
19. Klein MT, Moyes DG: Ventilation monitors and alarms. *S Afr Med J* 1985; 67:410–413.
20. Raphael DT, Weller RS, Doran DJ: A response algorithm for the low-pressure alarm condition. *Anesth Analg* 1988; 67:876–883.
21. Glauser FL, Polatty RC, Sessler CN: Worsening oxygenation in the mechanically ventilated patient. Causes, mechanisms, and early detection. *Am Rev Respir Dis* 1988; 138:458–465.
22. Brunner JX, Westenskow DR, Zelenkov P: Prototype ventilator and alarm algorithm for the NASA space station. *J Clin Monit* 1989; 5:90–99.
23. Carlon GC, Ray C Jr, Miodownik S, et al: Capnography in mechanically ventilated patients. *Crit Care Med* 1988; 16:550–556.
24. Weingarten M: Anesthetic and ventilator mishaps: Prevention and detection (editorial). *Crit Care Med* 1986; 14:1084–1086.
25. McWilliams BC: Mechanical ventilation in pediatric patients. *Clin Chest Med* 1987; 8:597–609.
26. Carlo WA, Martin RJ: Principles of neonatal assisted ventilation. *Pediatr Clin North Am* 1986; 33:221–237.
27. Ramsden CA, Reynolds EO: Ventilator settings for newborn infants. *Arch Dis Child* 1987; 62:529–538.

ADDITIONAL READINGS

Braman SS, Dunn SM, Amico CA, et al: Complications of intrahospital transport in critically ill patients. *Ann Intern Med* 1987; 107:469–473.

Gervais HW, Eberle B, Konietzke D, et al: Comparison of blood gases of ventilated patients during transport. *Crit Care Med* 1987; 15:761–763.

Hudson LD: Survival data in patients with acute and chronic lung disease requiring mechanical ventilation. *Am Rev Respir Dis* 1989; 140:S19–24.

Knaus WA: Prognosis with mechanical ventilation: The influence of disease, severity of disease, age, and chronic health status on survival from an acute illness. *Am Rev Respir Dis* 1989; 140:pS8–13.

PART III

Special Emergency Clinical Situations

20

Ethical Issues in Airway Management

Terri A. Schmidt, M.D.

Susan W. Tolle, M.D.

With prompt medical care a vast majority of emergency calls result in the patient arriving alive at the emergency department. With the advent of modern cardiopulmonary resuscitation (CPR) techniques in the 1960s, even patients in full cardiopulmonary arrest are being saved. Up to 1,000 cardiac arrests occur in the United States every day.[1] Survival rates vary from 2.9% for patients presenting in asystole to 30% for those patients presenting in ventricular fibrillation or tachycardia.[2] In the subset of patients with advanced age, sepsis, or cancer, the survival rates approach zero.[3, 4] As we become increasingly skillful in the swift application of emergency medical support, among our most challenging tasks is its wise application.

Cardiopulmonary resuscitation was first developed as part of the treatment for sudden cardiac death associated with coronary artery disease. Initially, it was assumed that, as with other medical treatment, it was indicated in some situations and not in others. However, since rapid initiation of CPR is required if efforts are to be successful, CPR began to be performed in any cardiac arrest situation with little thought given to the risks vs. benefits. Soon the indications for its use became more broad and it was attempted on most patients who sustained a cardiac arrest regardless of the underlying medical condition. Beginning CPR became so automatic that withholding it seems tantamount to an interference with patients' rights.[1] CPR and, in some states, tube feedings are the only health care technologies which are given unless specifically refused. In other invasive procedures informed consent is generally obtained prior to treatment.

Despite our difficulty in deciding whether to withhold intubation in a particular patient, there is national consensus that at times withholding treatment is appropriate. The courts and medical ethicists agree that, in general, competent patients have the right to refuse *any* medical treatment. The right to refuse treatment rests on our strong support for the ethical principle of autonomy. This principle is legally protected by the common-law right of self-determination.[5]

In selected circumstances, patients can exercise their right to refuse intubation by completing an advance directive (living will or durable power of attorney). As of Dec 1, 1991, the Patient Self-Determination Act mandates that all hospitals and long-term care facilities provide adults an opportunity to complete an advance directive during the process of admission. These documents (when criteria have been met) compel health care providers to withhold treatment and provide legal protection for those who do so. Forty-nine states have laws authorizing some form of living will.[6] State statutes regarding advance directives vary, but they all share several major limitations.[7]

First, only about 7% of the adult population has a written form of advance directive.[8] Where does that leave those terminally ill patients who have orally expressed their strong desire to refuse intubation? Must we intubate them because we lack written documentation of their refusal? The United States Supreme Court clarified the right of patients to refuse medical treatment in the 1990 *Cruzan* decision. Written documentation is not required. However, it may be difficult to verify the patient's orally expressed wishes, particularly if there is a dispute among family members.

Second, many advance directives contain the words "imminent" and "terminal." While definitions of imminent death and terminal illness vary, these terms strongly suggest that the patient will die within weeks to months with or without medical intervention. Does that mean that we must intubate those patients who have signed an advance directive but are not terminally ill? A bedridden stroke patient in a nursing home may not be considered to have a progressive medical condition and may not fit some states' definition of terminal illness. Thus, though the patient has a living will and strongly expressed preferences about withholding all forms of life-sustaining treatment, health care providers may feel ethically bound to respect the patient's wishes and yet be concerned about their legal protection.

Third, even if the first two criteria are met (the patient has completed an advance directive and is terminally ill) special challenges still face emergency health care providers. Often the document is not readily available for the responding personnel to read, leaving care providers with questions about the existence of the document and its precise intent. Questions arise about what treatment the patient would want to receive and what should be withheld. For example, it may seem clear that the patient does not desire intubation and mechanical ventilation, but does that mean no intravenous lines should be started, no medications given, no oxygen administered?

In this area a durable power of attorney differs from a do not resuscitate (DNR) order. DNR orders are only meant to apply if a person has sustained a cardiac arrest. They do not restrict or direct treatment for other medical problems prior to the moment of arrest. A durable power of attorney allows patients greater flexibility. This document permits patients to direct and limit all forms of medical treatment through their surrogate at the point when the patient is unable to express his or her wishes.

In general, quality health care is supported both by the ethics of the health care professions and by the courts. However, the courts often do not provide precise guidelines in a specific case and decision making rests on ethical guidelines. In this chapter we will further explore decision making using a structured model to approach ethical issues in patient management. This model was developed by Jonsen et al.[9] and utilizes the evaluation of information in four specific areas to guide decision making (Table 20–1). The four areas are: (1) medical indications, (2) patient preferences and values, (3) quality of life, and (4) external factors. We briefly de-

TABLE 20–1.
Ethical Model for Decision Making Regarding Health Care Treatment

1. Medical indications (risks and benefits)
2. Patient preferences and values (autonomy)
3. Quality of life
4. External factors (cost, the wishes of family, professional standards, institutional policy, legal boundaries)

scribe our process of decision making in evaluating each of these areas before applying the model to three case scenarios.

The first factor in considering an ethical issue is to review the medical indications. What are the potential risks and benefits of a proposed treatment? The ethical principles at issue are beneficence (doing good and acting in the best interest of the patient) while acting with nonmaleficence (do no harm). When considering the medical indications for a patient in need of urgent intubation, the alternative is almost certain death without intubation and a varying probability (depending on the clinical situation) of extending life with intubation. At times the likelihood of resuscitating the patient with intubation is remote and the question of futility is considered. Unless treatment is clearly futile, the medical indications analysis, when considered alone, usually favors intubation.

The second factor for careful consideration is information about the patient's values and preferences. In an emergency situation, time and the patient being in extremis often prevent dialogue with the patient to clarify his or her preferences regarding intubation. At times, patients have clearly expressed a prior wish not to be resuscitated. In general, informed and otherwise competent patients can refuse medical treatment and their wishes should be respected. Emergency personnel face several unique challenges as they attempt to respect the patient's autonomy with regard to a wish to limit treatment. Among the issues confronting emergency personnel are (1) obtaining evidence of the patient's prior wishes in a timely manner, (2) assessing the applicability of the prior wishes to the current medical problem, and (3) clarifying which treatments are to be given and which withheld.

The third factor to be evaluated is quality of life. This factor requires time to consider, more time than is usually available when a patient requires emergency intubation. Quality of life may be assessed differently by the patient, the family, and the physician. Patients who have prepared advance directives (living will and durable power of attorney) have usually incorporated an assessment of their quality of life in their decision to limit treatment. In the emergency situation, unless the patient has previously made an assessment that his or her current quality of life is such that he or she does not wish to be intubated, intubation should be done. Further evaluation of the patient's quality of life should be subsequently undertaken at the hospital and the indications for continued treatment reevaluated.

The fourth and final consideration is the evaluation of all of the external factors of the case that do not relate directly to the health care provider–patient relationship but which, directly or indirectly, influence the decision-making process. These factors vary in importance from case to case but often include: (1) state statutory precedent, if one exists; (2) family needs and conflicts; (3) the policy of the institution; (4) cost; and (5) professional standards.

The importance of a particular factor is affected by the clinical situation. The following three case scenarios are presented to illustrate a systematic process which can be used to approach decisions about withholding emergency intubation.

Scenario 1

Mr. Johnson is a 57-year-old man with lung cancer who has gone out to a park with his daughter and wife. He sits down on a park bench to enjoy the afternoon sun, while his wife and daughter walk a short distance. Suddenly, he develops chest pain and becomes extremely short of breath. A person who is jogging by notices his distress and calls an ambulance. His wife and daughter return and find the paramedical workers at the scene.

The paramedical personnel find a thin, chronically ill–appearing man in acute distress. He is grasping his chest, moaning softly, and is diaphoretic and confused. His blood pressure is 180/110 mm Hg, the heart rate is 120 beats per minute and the respiratory rate is 40 breaths per minute. His lungs have rales throughout.

The wife and daughter tell the paramedical workers that Mr. Johnson has lung cancer and that he, the family, and his physician have discussed his wishes. Although he has been feeling well in the past few weeks, he has stated that should he become ill and require any mechanical life support, he would not want this done. He has written a living will which they have at home. The family seem caring and appropriately concerned about Mr. Johnson.

Oxygen is started and Mr. Johnson is brought to the nearest hospital, which he has never visited be-fore. He is now obtunded, ashen, and in severe respiratory distress. A decision must be made about intubation. The family arrives at the emergency department along with the patient, and they reconfirm the patient's desire for no intubation or any measures to prolong his life.

DISCUSSION

Using the four factors of ethical decision making, we can discuss the decision whether or not to intubate Mr. Johnson. In this case the answer should be quite clear.

The first factor is medical indications. Mr. Johnson is in severe respiratory distress and in imminent danger of death from his acute, life-threatening decompensation unless he is quickly intubated and supported. However, even with intubation and aggressive treatment, he has an underlying terminal illness which decreases his chance of long-term survival. With metastatic lung cancer he has approximately a 90% chance of dying in the next 2 years.[10] Thus, intubation is not futile in the case of Mr. Johnson because he has a modest chance of short-term benefit, and of leaving the hospital.

The second factor of patient preference is at the heart of this decision. At the time of presentation to the emergency department Mr. Johnson is unable to express his wishes. However, we have clear, previously stated wishes to help guide our decision about treatment. A competent person is able to direct treatment he or she would want and we can use the previously expressed wishes of a competent person.

For a person to make a valid decision to accept or refuse treatment, four criteria must be met[11] (Table 20–2). The person making a decision must be able to *communicate choices*. Mr. Johnson is currently unable to communicate his choices but he was able to do so in writing and with his family in the past. Secondly, the person must be able to *understand relevant information*. The third requirement is an *appreciation of the situation and its consequences*. This involves understanding the existence of the disease, and the

TABLE 20–2.

Criteria for Valid Decision to Accept or Refuse Treatment

1. The patient is able to *communicate choices*
2. The patient is able to *understand relevant information*
3. The patient has an *appreciation of the situation and its consequences*
4. The patient is able to *rationally manipulate information*

likely consequences of refusal. Finally, the person must be able to *rationally manipulate information*. This is the ability to use logical thought processes to compare the benefits and risks of treatment or refusal.

A conversation with the family should allow the health care team to understand Mr. Johnson's wishes and his ability to make an informed choice at the time he expressed his wishes. The family can reassure the providers that Mr. Johnson made a prior choice against intubation and at the time he made that decision, that he was competent to make it.

The third factor involved in the decision to intubate this person is quality of life. Quality-of-life issues are hard to assess in the emergency setting. Plans must be made quickly and in this case there is insufficient information on which to base a decision.

Finally, there are the external factors that play a role in the ethical decision, including the legal ramifications. In this case the family states that the patient has a living will. Since Mr. Johnson has a terminal illness and death can be thought to be imminent, the living will would appear to apply. Because of the emergency situation that takes place away from home, we are unable to see the written document, and can only go by the family's report that it exists. However, seeing the document is really only corroborative since our actual decision is based on the ethical principle of autonomy and respecting the patient's right to refuse treatment.

Family wishes, rather than the family's expression of the patient's wishes, may be an external factor. In this case the family members appear to be in agreement with each other and supportive of the patient's previously expressed wishes. If the situation were different and a member of the family was unwilling to withhold life support despite the patient's known desire to have treatment withheld, it would be prudent to provide support until those issues could be further clarified with the family.

Institutional policy could also impinge on the decision to intubate this patient. Some facilities may have specific guidelines directing circumstances under which treatment may be withheld. It is worthwhile to know the policies of your institution and to ensure that those policies do not conflict with ethical reasoning.

In summary, in the case of Mr. Johnson, a strong argument is made for the decision not to intubate based on respect for autonomy. While there is medical support for intubation, a beneficial outcome is far from certain. His family reports that he has a terminal illness and his appearance of chronic illness supports the diagnosis of cancer. Although we are

unable to see written documentation of his living will, his family reports that one exists and that the patient has made it clear that he wishes nothing done to extend his life. The family members appear to be reliable, caring, and supportive. There are no external factors conflicting with the decision not to intubate.

Scenario 2

Mrs. Carr is a 75-year-old woman with breast cancer. She has had a radical mastectomy and now has metastases to the bone, which cause her pain. She is frail but mentally clear despite the use of narcotics to control her pain. She has gone out to dinner at a restaurant with her son and daughter-in-law and two friends.

While eating her seafood dinner, she first complains of feeling itchy and then develops respiratory distress. The family calls for help.

When the paramedical personnel arrive they find an elderly, chronically ill–appearing woman in acute respiratory distress, pale, diaphoretic, and unable to speak. Her blood pressure is 80/50 mm Hg, the heart rate is 120, and the respiratory rate is 44. Her lungs show minimal air movement and wheezing throughout.

The family tells them that their mother has cancer that has spread through her body and that she is often in pain. They say they have discussed her wishes regarding medical treatment with her and she wants everything possible done.

While this information is being gathered, Mrs. Carr has a respiratory arrest. The paramedical workers begin oxygen and bag-valve-mask ventilation. They call the on-line medical control to ask whether they should intubate this woman with a terminal illness.

DISCUSSION

Like the previous scenario, Mrs. Carr's treatment plan will be evaluated using the four ethical factors. We will see that although both patients have metastatic cancer, because the facts are different the outcome will change.

Mrs. Carr also has an underlying terminal illness, metastatic breast cancer, but that is not her medical problem today. Currently she appears to be experiencing an anaphylactic reaction that has led to a respiratory arrest. Intubation is medically indicated. Like our previous patient, her chronic illness may soon terminate her life. However, she has a good chance of extubation and discharge from the hospital following treatment of the anaphylactic episode.

The second factor, patient preference, is vitally important. The family reports that Mrs. Carr knows about her medical illness, understands her prognosis, and wants aggressive treatment. Once again, Mrs. Carr is currently unable to express her wishes but at the time she was able to express them, she had a definite preference in favor of treatment. Assuming she met the criteria of competence at the time of her discussion with her family, these patient wishes carry strong moral weight in the decision about current treatment.

The third factor, quality of life, must also be addressed. Again, in the emergency setting little time is available to explore this issue. However, health care providers often assume that a person with metastatic cancer who requires medication for pain control has a poor quality of life. In fact, the patient may view the situation differently. Studies of the congruence of patients' and physicians' views of quality of life showed that physicians rated quality of life more negatively than patients.[12, 13] Further, physicians are more likely to write DNR orders for patients with cancer or acquired immunodeficiency syndrome (AIDS) than for patients with other diseases with similar prognoses such as cirrhosis or severe congestive heart failure.[10, 14]

Finally, external factors must be considered. In this case the decision about intubation occurs in the prehospital setting. The American College of Emergency Physicians (ACEP) has taken the following position:

> Unless a valid "do not resuscitate" document is produced at the scene of an EMS [emergency medical services] run and/or a physician (either on-line or on the scene) takes direct responsibility for withholding resuscitation efforts, prehospital personnel should perform all necessary treatments if called to the scene of a victim of cardiopulmonary arrest (unless obvious signs of death such as rigor mortis, dependent lividity, or decapitation are found).[15]

This ACEP position admits that it will lead to initial overtreatment in some cases, but allows for later withdrawal of support when legal, ethical, and medical considerations can be more fully evaluated.

The ACEP position is becoming generally accepted.[16, 17] There is general support for withholding resuscitation when written documentation exists or a physician is available to make the determination. Otherwise prehospital personnel are not asked to make an ethical judgment with limited information and only moments to make a decision.

Using the four components of ethical decision making, in this case the decision would be to intubate Mrs. Carr. There is a strong medical indication, her prior preference favors treatment, quality of life cannot be fully addressed, and there are no institutional factors weighing against intubation.

Scenario 3

Mr. Harold is a 27-year-old man with AIDS. He is eating alone at a restaurant when he suddenly becomes short of breath. The restaurant owner calls for help.

When the paramedical personnel arrive they find a thin, chronically ill–appearing man in acute respiratory distress. He is gasping for breath and unable to speak. His blood pressure is 100/70 mm Hg, his heart rate is 160, and his respiratory rate is 44.

The restaurant owner says that he knows Mr. Harold has AIDS from discussions they have had when he comes to the restaurant. He does not know Mr. Harold very well and cannot provide any other information about his illness or his wishes for treatment.

Mr. Harold is transported to the hospital. At the hospital his respiratory distress worsens and he becomes apneic. Family members are expected soon but no one is now available. A decision about intubation must be made.

DISCUSSION

The remarkable and not uncommon emergency medicine feature of Mr. Harold's scenario is the lack of information. A life-threatening situation has developed and a decision about airway management must be made with this paucity of information. When information is not available, it is advisable to provide life-sustaining treatment until the person is stabilized, further information is gathered, and time becomes available to make a reasoned decision about continuation of treatment. From an ethical point of view, there is no difference between withholding treatment and withdrawing it. Using the model for making ethical decisions about airway management, at any time that it becomes clear that treatment should be withheld, ventilatory support can be withdrawn. Despite the lack of timely information, we can still attempt to use the four ethical factors to evaluate Mr. Harold's case. However, the treatment plan will vary depending on how the situation changes as we learn more.

The first factor is the medical indications. Mr. Harold has had a respiratory arrest and will certainly die if no ventilatory support is provided. The cause of his acute decompensation is unknown. It is unlikely to be *Pneumocystis carinii* pneumonia or another simple infectious process because the onset of dyspnea is so sudden. Perhaps he has aspirated food and has an upper airway obstruction. Currently we can only assume that he has a potentially reversible airway problem and treatment is not futile although his long-term prognosis is grim. On medical grounds alone, treatment is indicated. The second factor is patient preference. Without any knowledge of clearly expressed wishes from the patient, we must act in the patient's best interests. At this point that would require airway support for the patient. The third factor is quality of life. As in our earlier cases, this is an area where little is known. We do not know the stage of Mr. Harold's disease. We only know that

he was well enough to go out to eat alone but appeared to be chronically ill. This factor does not help us to make an acute decision.

Finally, the fourth factor of external issues must be considered. Mr. Harold is reported to have AIDS. Health care providers may be reluctant to treat a person with AIDS because of the risk of transmission. The risk of transmission is low (less than 1% with a needle stick) but the consequences are likely death.[18] Considering this risk, do health care providers have a duty to treat AIDS patients? This duty is separated into two aspects: a legal obligation and an ethical obligation. In American legal tradition there is no duty to treat a person until a doctor-patient relationship is established.[17-21] Thus a physician may not have a legal duty to take new human immunodeficiency virus (HIV)–seropositive patients into treatment, but the physician would be obligated to continue to treat anyone who is currently his or her

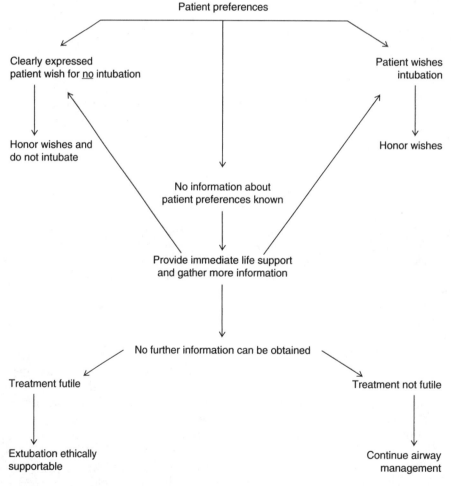

FIG 20–1.
Algorithm of ethical decisions in airway management. *In the prehospital setting, the American College of Emergency Physicians states that these wishes must be written or responsibility for withholding treatment must be taken by an on-line physician.

patient. Further, emergency physicians have a duty to treat anyone who presents for care. In some states AIDS patients are defined as handicapped and there is a legal obligation not to discriminate against classes of people, including the handicapped.[19, 22]

Physicians do have an ethical obligation to treat AIDS patients.[19, 21–25] The American Medical Association (AMA) Council on Ethical and Judicial Affairs in its position paper expressed this ethical obligation by stating a physician should not refuse to treat a patient solely because of HIV seropositivity.[22] The AMA has a long tradition favoring treatment during epidemics. During the 1800s its ethics code stated that "when pestilence prevails, it is their [physicians'] duty to face the danger, and to continue their labors for the alleviation of suffering, even at the jeopardy of their own lives."[18] ACEP has taken the position that "appropriate medical care should be provided to all patients who seek emergency care, regardless of their HIV status or risk factor."[26] Thus there is certainly an ethical obligation and likely a legal obligation to appropriately treat Mr. Harold.

In summary, in Mr. Harold's case there is no compelling factor favoring withholding treatment and hence airway support should be begun. When family, medical records, or the patient's personal physician is able to enlighten us, later decisions can then be based on the further information and treatment can be continued or stopped as appropriate.

CONCLUSIONS

In considering ethical issues in airway management we have presented four factors that deserve consideration. In patients for whom intubation offers the potential of medical benefit, the overriding ethical consideration is usually patient preference. Figure 20–1 gives a model for the decision-making process using patient wishes to guide treatment decisions.

Competent patients have the right to refuse all forms of medical therapy, including intubation, under the ethical principle of autonomy. In an emergency situation, when no information about patient preferences is known, implied consent is presumed and treatment should be given. This action is based on the ethical principle of beneficence. When a patient is initially intubated and subsequently it is demonstrated that the patient would have refused intubation, it is ethically supportable to withdraw life support. While withdrawing life support can be emotionally difficult, there is no ethical difference between withholding and withdrawing life support. Using the ethical principles of autonomy and beneficence, in most situations health care providers should be able to make proper decisions about intubation and airway management in the individual patient.

REFERENCES

1. *Textbook of Advanced Cardiac Life Support,* ed 2. Dallas, American Heart Association, 1987.
2. Smith JP, Bodai BI: Guidelines for discontinuing prehospital CPR in the emergency department—a review. *Ann Emerg Med* 1985; 14:1093.
3. Taffet GE, Teasdale TA, Luchi RJ: In-hospital cardiopulmonary resuscitation. *JAMA* 1988; 260:2069.
4. Schiedermayer DL: The decision to forgo CPR in the elderly patient. *JAMA* 1988; 260:2096.
5. American College of Physicians: American College of Physicians ethics manual. Part 2: The physician and society; research; life sustaining treatment, other issues. *Ann Intern Med* 1989; 111:327.
6. Siner DA: Advance directives in emergency medicine: Medical, legal and ethical implications. *Ann Emerg Med* 1989; 18:1364.
7. Rizzo RF: The living will: Does it protect the rights of the terminally ill? *N Y State J Med* 1989; 89:79.
8. Smedira NG, Evans BH, Grais LS, et al: Withholding and withdrawal of life support from the critically ill. *N Engl J Med* 1990; 322:309.
9. Jonsen AR, Siegler M, Winslade WJ: *Clinical Ethics— A Practical Approach to Ethical Decisions in Clinical Medicine,* ed 2. New York, Macmillan Publishing Co, 1986.
10. Lawrence VA, and Clark GM: Cancer resuscitation: Does the diagnosis affect the decision? *Arch Intern Med* 1987; 147:1637.
11. Appelbaum PS, Grisso T: Assessing patients' capacities to consent to treatment. *N Engl J Med* 1988; 319:1635.
12. Starr TJ, Pearlman RA, Uhlmann RF: Quality of life and resuscitation decisions in elderly patients. *J Gen Intern Med* 1986; 1:373.
13. Pearlman RA, Uhlmann RF: Quality of life in chronic diseases: Perceptions of elderly patients. *J Gerontol* 1988; 2:25.
14. Wachter RM, Luce JM, Hearst N, et al: Decisions about resuscitation: Inequities among patients with different diseases but similar prognoses. *Ann Intern Med* 1989; 111:525.
15. American College of Emergency Physicians: Guidelines for "do not resusciate" orders in the prehospital setting. *Ann Emerg Med* 1988; 17:1106.
16. Ayers RJ: Current controversies in prehospital resuscitation of the terminally ill patient. *Prehospital Disaster Med* 1990; 5:49.
17. Crimmins TJ: The need for a prehospital DNR sys-

tem. *Prehospital Disaster Med* 1990; 5:47.

18. Zimberg JM: AIDS: The duty to treat: A physician lawyer's perspective. *Mt Sinai J Med* 1989; 56:259.

19. Geraghty D: AIDS and the physician's duty to treat. *J Leg Med* 1989; 10:47.

20. Healy JM: Is there a duty to treat AIDS patients? *Conn Med* 1988; 52:187.

21. Healy JM: The duty to treat AIDS patients: Ethical and legal perspectives. *Conn Med* 1988; 52:249.

22. Patterson R: AIDS: The duty to treat: 1988 AMA position. *Mt Sinai J Med* 1989; 56:250.

23. Dunne RD: AIDS: The duty to treat: A patient advocate's perspective. *Mt Sinai J Med* 1989; 56:252.

24. Preus AP: AIDS: The duty to treat: A philosopher's perspective. *Mt Sinai J Med* 1989; 56:254.

25. Axelrod D: AIDS: The state of the New York State approach. *Mt Sinai J Med* 1989; 56:238.

26. American College of Emergency Physicians: AIDS—Statement of principles and interim recommendations for emergency department personnel and prehospital care providers. *Ann Emerg Med* 1988; 17:1249.

21

Terminal Shock and Cardiopulmonary Arrest

Barry Simon, M.D.

Charles V. Pollock, M.D.

The patient in terminal shock or cardiopulmonary arrest presents a significant challenge to the emergency physician. Establishment and maintenance of a definitive airway must be the initial goal in the resuscitation of these patients. Further efforts aimed at restoring adequate circulation and perfusion will be futile without efficacious airway management. There are many options and modalities available for the care of these seriously ill patients. The sequence in which they should be considered and employed is the primary emphasis of this chapter.

The clinical situations covered include patients that may present as alert and relatively stable but are hyperventilating with increased work of breathing. "Crashing" patients are those with altered mental status, inability to protect their airway, and yet continue to ventilate well. The most unstable, "crashed" scenario includes those who are hypoventilating in frank respiratory failure or those in overt cardiopulmonary arrest.

PATHOPHYSIOLOGY

Regardless of etiology or presentation, patients in shock eventually suffer an increased work of breathing. Hyperventilation is usually secondary to the lactic acidosis produced from the shock state. Factors leading to decreased pulmonary compliance or to reduced gas exchange add to the respiratory drive. The result is a significant respiratory alkalosis and metabolic acidosis. In addition, the exhausting mechanical task of breathing produces lactic acid from excessive diaphragmatic and accessory muscle

activity. This acidosis further complicates the complex acid-base abnormalities associated with hypoxia and ischemia from inadequate tissue perfusion.

Shock

Despite the existence of several primary causes of shock, the physiologic compensatory responses and the clinical manifestations are similar for most. The early response to shock is a neuroendocrine reflex mediated by the baroreceptors in the heart and great vessels. Epinephrine-induced venoconstriction will compensate for mild blood loss by augmenting venous return. Circulating epinephrine along with locally released norepinephrine will produce constriction of arteriolar smooth muscle to raise peripheral resistance and mean arterial pressure. Alteration of the forces which generally maintain fluid balance will develop as the systemic pressure falls. The decreasing hydrostatic pressure within the capillary occurs in early shock as a result of hypovolemia and precapillary arteriolar constriction. The effect is an influx of extracellular interstitial fluid into the capillaries and the systemic circulation. These mechanisms may compensate for the loss of as much as 25% of the circulating volume without clinical signs of deterioration. Undesirable cellular consequences of shock will not develop until these mechanisms have been overcome by overwhelming, persistent, or untreated blood loss.[1, 2]

Pulmonary tissues suffer from the same systemic and cellular consequences of shock as other organs and tissues of the body. Localized ischemia from inadequate perfusion leads to innumerable cellular consequences: (1) anaerobic metabolism is less efficient than aerobic metabolism resulting in lower levels of intracellular adenosine triphosphate (ATP) and the generation of metabolic acids; (2) failure of the sodium-potassium membrane pump causes sodium and water to enter the cell and potassium to escape; and (3) there is progressive impairment of intracellular organelles, especially the mitochondria and lysosomes. Damage or destruction of mitochondria impairs the cells' ability to utilize oxygen. Unless recovery from shock is rapid, the damaged mitochondria may be unable to function, resulting in cell death. Breakdown of the lysosomes causes the release of compounds such as histamine, serotonin, various kinins, and prostaglandins.[1, 2] Many of these substances will damage the capillary endothelium allowing for the escape of fluid and proteins into the interstitium and parenchyma of organs. Edema of pulmonary tissue and deteriorating compliance is a consequence of this sequence of events. Damage to the endothelium resulting in capillary leak may partially explain why resuscitation with colloids is particularly detrimental to pulmonary tissue. Further damage to the lung has been ascribed to complement activation and leukocyte aggregation, superoxide-induced injury from release of neutrophil byproducts of phagocytes, protease release with destruction of collagen, and platelet aggregation. Prostaglandins and thromboxane have been implicated in pulmonary damage in models of endotoxic shock. As the shock state progresses there is disruption of the pulmonary parenchyma, various degrees of microembolization, atelectasis, and hemorrhage. Shunting from the ventilation-perfusion mismatch becomes progressively more resistant to oxygen therapy. Positive end-expiratory pressure (PEEP) ventilation will be essential if the shock state persists. PEEP may help by increasing the functional residual capacity, reducing surfactant aggregation, and by allowing adequate oxygenation with lower inspired oxygen concentration.[3, 4]

Cellular function will continue to deteriorate as ischemia from inadequate perfusion persists, ATP production falls, the sodium-potassium pump fails, and systemic acidosis progresses. Ischemia of the liver and gastrointestinal tract may cause profound dysfunction of these organs. Damage to reticuloendothelial cell function can allow harmful substances to accumulate in the circulation. Bowel wall ischemia will cause sequestration of fluid in the lumen, complicating volume losses, and allow passage of bacteria and vasoactive amines. A myocardial depressant factor (MDF) may be released from ischemic pancreatic tissue, further complicat-

ing the direct myocardial depressant action of lactic acidosis.[5]

The severe shock state represents a cascade of events that will eventually become irreversible if not corrected in a timely fashion. Adequate perfusion and oxygenation must be maintained to protect cellular function and to prevent the sequence of events outlined above. Support of the cardiopulmonary system must take precedence in resuscitative efforts.

Airflow integrity is rarely a problem in the patient in shock regardless of the underlying process. The most notable exception is the patient with anaphylactic shock or with severe angioedema. Swelling of the tongue, uvula, and surrounding pharyngeal tissues may obstruct airflow. Any disease process resulting in obtundation of the mental status may allow the tongue to fall back and obstruct. Dentures can lose their support and fall to the back of the oropharynx and compromise airflow.

Exhaustion, hypoxia, and hypercarbia combine to produce a mental fatigue that eventually reaches obtundation. Without repositioning or mechanical airway adjuncts, the patient's tongue and secretions will compromise patency of the airway. Altered level of consciousness and loss of the protective gag reflex is common as the shock state progresses. Aspiration of stomach contents, oropharyngeal secretions, and the tongue are significant concerns.

Ventilation will eventually fail if the underlying problem is not corrected and poor tissue perfusion persists. Physiologically, patients in shock are driven to compensate for their hypoxia and acidosis by hyperventilating. Multiple feedback and regulatory mechanisms will enhance this response until there is improvement in oxygenation, or until hypoxia overcomes the respiratory center in the brainstem or there is loss of airway patency. Hypoventilation may occur during shock as a result of inadequate perfusion of the medullary respiratory center. Once respiratory drive is lost, hypoxia and acidosis worsen, and cardiopulmonary arrest ensues.

CLINICAL EVALUATION

The tools one uses to evaluate these patients will be the same regardless of the severity of the presentation. Yet the more critical the presentation, the less time and effort can be put into objective laboratory and radiographic tests. Clinical judgment is relatively easy in the stable and in the critically ill, but becomes the key in the "gray" patient. *Gestalt* is difficult to define and describe, yet it is the sense that physicians must call upon for critical decision making. Methods of airway control in shock patients will be determined by the overall wellness of the patient and not just by how well he or she may be moving air, etc. Skin signs, color and moisture, brightness of the eyes, affect, degree of apparent exhaustion, and vitality of the gag reflex are some of the more subtle clinical factors to consider. Baseline vital signs and their trends are essential and must be monitored continuously. A rise or fall in any of the parameters may be ominous and may herald respiratory failure. Etiology of the shock must also be figured in the decision-making equation. Anaphylaxis, for example, might be expected to respond readily to treatment and hemorrhagic shock will respond quickly to replacement therapy if the bleeding is controlled, but sepsis and cardiogenic shock are more likely to progress despite treatment.

Of the more objective bedside parameters available, pulse oximetry provides an excellent means of "at-a-glance" assessment of the patient. The results are accessible within seconds and provide continuous data on oxygenation. Arterial blood gas results, which are often available within minutes, may be helpful but should not be relied upon for final deci-

sion making. Laboratory results must never take the place of clinical judgment. The chest film can be helpful to rule out reversible causes of shock such as tension pneumothorax. Electrocardiography (ECG) exhibiting low voltage or electrical alternans, along with a suspicious chest film, may suggest cardiac tamponade. The ECG can also be helpful in diagnosing hyperkalemia as a cause of shock.

Routine laboratory studies such as complete blood count (CBC), chemistry panels, and urinalysis are performed as part of the overall patient evaluation. Rarely the results may uncover readily reversible causes of shock which may obviate the need for active airway management. Occult blood loss from a recent or ongoing gastrointestinal (GI) bleed may be discovered on the CBC. Hyperkalemia may have caused shock or cardiac arrest and profound hypocalcemia can cause severe hypoventilation. Marked increase of the anion gap might lead one to suspect the presence of substances other than lactate and stimulate a search for exogenous toxins. The natural history of shock leading to death is depicted in Figure 21–1. The management algorithm is Figure 21–2.

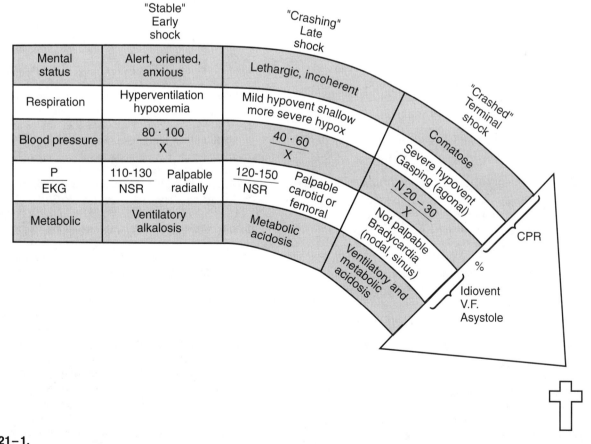

FIG 21–1.
Natural history of shock leading to death. (Adapted from Dailey RH: Approach to patient in emergency department, in Rosen P (ed): *Emergency Medicine,* ed 2. St Louis, Mosby–Year Book, Inc, 1987, p 37.)

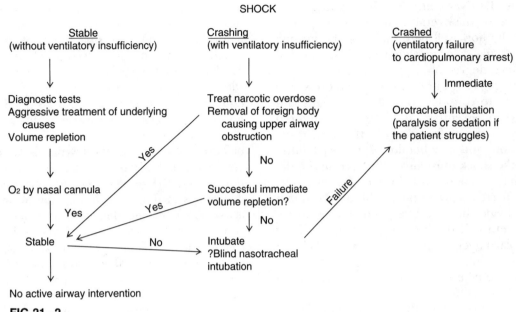

FIG 21–2.
Airway management algorithm for shock.

Scenario 1: The Stable Patient (Early Shock Without Ventilatory Insufficiency)

Patients in early shock may be alert and capable of protecting and maintaining their own airway. Yet they will be anxious and hyperventilating, demonstrating a ventilatory alkalosis and possibly a mild lactic acidosis. Their blood pressure will be 80 to 100 mm Hg systolic with a heart rate of 110 to 130 beats per minute. Their relative airway stability may be part of the initial presentation of rapidly progressive disease or it may be part of a less serious course. Clinical judgment becomes the crucial element in decision making. It is difficult for the most experienced physician to initiate aggressive invasive maneuvers in alert, talking patients. The ultimate question is: Should the patient be intubated in semielective fashion to prevent the sequelae of deterioration or can time be allowed for treatment modalities to be effective?

The airway of alert patients that appear stable may be treated with noninvasive modalities while diagnostic and therapeutic maneuvers (principally volume repletion) are underway. By definition, these patients are in shock with poor tissue perfusion. In other words, their skin, kidneys, and/or brain are not receiving adequate oxygenation. Yet the decision is being made that they are stable enough to leave the airway unprotected for a period of time. This judgmental decision is multifactorial and is constantly updated as conditions change and as information becomes available. Presumably, mental status is the major factor in the equation. Yet the other gestalt ingredients must also be factored. To be considered reasonably stable the vital signs must be steady or improving, the skin should be dry or drying, the patient should not have that look of fright or doom, and the patient must not appear or state that he or she is exhausted. Clinical judgment is confirmed by adequate pulse oximetry and arterial blood gas results.

The risk to airflow in these alert patients is generally not clinically significant. Aspiration remains a concern despite the level of consciousness because the vital signs demand that they remain supine. In their weakened state of health they may have difficulty handling secretions, especially if the stomach contents are regurgitated, while supine. Most patients with a critical illness or who are in shock will have an ileus with a significant likelihood of having a full stomach. Oxygenation and ventilation are generally adequate if one's judgment and the objective findings had determined the patient to be stable. Marginal levels of hypoxia may be present, especially if there is an underlying pulmonary pathologic condition. Excessive tachypnea or hypoxia might suggest early signs of shock lung. In this scenario, oxygenation is treatable with noninvasive techniques but with close monitoring for signs of deterioration.

Airflow, although patent, may be facilitated by using a nasopharyngeal airway ("trumpet"). Unlike oropharyngeal airways, trumpets are fairly well tolerated by awake patients, particularly if they are informed of the procedure and of its benefit. Aspiration is treated with anticipation and awareness. A large-bore, tonsil-tipped suction tube should be available at all times. Patients should be cautioned of the need to roll on their side and to ask for help if the urge to vomit is noted. Supplemental humidified oxygen is administered regardless of the pulse oximetry or arterial blood gas results. Supplemental oxygen administered by nasal cannula is generally sufficient for stable patients, but a nonrebreather mask may be used for those patients with significant hypoxia.

Many patients will respond quickly and effectively to these simple interventions. Yet the potentially severe nature of the underlying pathologic condition often progresses despite treatment. Deterioration of one or more of the elements noted above will place the patient in the scenario of the crashing patient.

Scenario 2: The Crashing Patient (Late Shock and Ventilatory Insufficiency)

The crashing patient in shock will be lethargic or incoherent with more shallow breathing. Systolic pressure is generally less than 60 mm Hg and the heart rate is 120 to 150. Shock in the patient with altered mental status and respiratory fatigue may be cause or effect. Yet airway concerns and management decisions are the same regardless of the underlying cause. All three airway pillars—integrity of airflow, protection from aspiration, and adequate ventilation and oxygenation—are threatened. The clinical judgment required to decide for whom and when active airway management is needed becomes much less of an issue. The difficult decision making in this scenario revolves around choosing the optimal method of intubation. (*Note:* All subsequent discussions assume that readily reversible airway problems such as narcotic overdose or upper airway foreign body have already been dealt with.)

Airflow integrity is threatened because the patient can no longer be counted on to support the tongue and pharyngeal tissues. As the gag reflex is lost and the level of consciousness falls, the chances of aspiration becomes greater. Some patients with a depressed level of consciousness will receive bag-valve-mask ventilation in the prehospital setting and in the emergency department (ED) which will increase the risk of gastric distention and aspiration of stomach contents. Oxygenation fails as the underlying pathologic condition is compounded by the development of alveolar shunting and faltering respiratory drive or exhaustion. Deteriorating pulmonary compliance is complicated by depressed cardiac activity and multiorgan failure. Respiratory failure is imminent unless the airway is aggressively managed. If shock is purely hypovolemic, vigorous immediate intravenous (IV) fluid repletion may improve circulation, mental status, and ventilation, and thus preclude the need for intubation. Otherwise, preparations are made to perform endotracheal intubation. A nasal or oropharyngeal airway can be placed to facilitate airflow. Suction should be readied and humidified

oxygen delivered with 100% nonrebreather mask. As the level of consciousness falls or as respirations begin to fail, ventilation should be assisted with bag-valve-mask. Care should be taken to "gently" bag the patient to avoid or minimize gastric distention.

Intubation options include the gamut of methods described elsewhere in this book. Discussion here is limited to the three most practical possibilities: (1) blind nasotracheal intubation (BNI), (2) conscious orotracheal intubation (COI), and (3) rapid-sequence intubation (RSI). Consideration must be for the method that will most quickly gain control of the airway with the least risk of decompensation during the process. BNI is an option because these patients are breathing, it avoids using paralyzing drugs, and it is ultimately more comfortable for the patient. The danger is that airway control is lost during the process of intubation, hypoxia worsens, the success rate is lower than with orotracheal intubation, and significant bleeding may complicate the overall situation. It is recommended that of this group needing active airway control, BNI should be attempted only in the most stable patients. Furthermore, only one attempt should be made before choosing another approach. It is perfectly acceptable to avoid this method altogether. COI is an option because it avoids the use of paralyzing drugs. Patients who are obtunded may or may not need additional sedation. Concerns of this approach include the added risk of vomiting when the oropharynx is stimulated in a conscious patient; less than optimal conditions for intubation in patients who continue to exert muscular control; and trismus, which prevents intubation and delays definitive management. RSI is an effective alternative should either of the above methods fail or be considered inappropriate. Hypoxia and hypercarbia will worsen during the intubation effort, and therefore no more than one or two attempts should be made before resorting to the more controlled methods. The rapid-sequence method provides maximum control and the most suitable intubating conditions. Caution must always be exercised when paralytic agents are being used. Ketamine may be considered the most suitable induction drug in these patients as it has minimal effect on the respiratory drive and it supports blood pressure.

In summary, conscious orotracheal intubation is recommended as the initial approach for definitive airway control. Induction and paralytic drugs should be readily available for RSI.

Scenario 3: The Crashed Patient (Terminal Shock: Ventilatory Failure to Cardiopulmonary Arrest)

The crashed patient is in terminal shock. Respiratory and cardiac arrest is imminent. Blood pressure is less than 40 mm Hg and the pulse is no longer palpable but the heart rate is generally slow, 60 or less. These patients are comatose with gasping or ag-onal respiratory efforts. Perfusion of the central respiratory center located in the medulla of the brainstem is maintained until the final stages of shock. Agonal respirations are the result of inadequate blood flow to this area of the brainstem. Ineffective ventilation will progress to cardiopulmonary arrest without immediate action. There is no doubt that immediate endotracheal intubation is indicated.

Risks to the airway are the same as in the prior scenario but with more urgency. These patients are completely unable to maintain the tone of their oropharynx, prevent aspiration, or to effectively ventilate and oxygenate. Patients with cardiopulmonary arrest have the same risks and concerns.

BNI should never be attempted in this setting even if some ventilatory effort is being made. Airway access has to be immediate, leaving no time for chance. If the patient is completely unconscious with relaxation of the facial muscles, then cricoid pressure can be applied, and orotracheal intubation attempted, without paralytic agents. Cricoid pressure should not be applied in conscious patients as it may increase the risk of vomiting, aspiration, and injury to the esophagus. RSI is preferred if the patient has trismus or continues to resist therapeutic interventions.

REFERENCES

1. Mannix FL: Hemorrhagic shock, in Rosen P (ed): *Emergency Medicine*, ed 2. St Louis, Mosby–Year Book, Inc, 1988, pp 179–202.
2. McCall D, O'Rourke RA: Hypotension and cardiogenic shock, in Stein JH (ed): *Internal Medicine*, ed 3. Boston, Little, Brown & Co, 1990, pp 97–103.
3. Billhardt RA, Rosenbush SW: Cardiogenic and hypovolemic shock. *Med Clin North Am* 1986; 70:853–877.
4. Moss GS, Saletta JD: Traumatic shock in man. *N Engl J Med* 1974; 290:724–726.
5. Passmore JM: Hemodynamic support of the critically ill patient, in Dantzker DR (ed): *Cardiopulmonary Critical Care*, ed 1. Orlando, Fla, Grune & Stratton, Inc, 1986, pp 387–395.

22

The Multiple Trauma Patient

Ron M. Walls, M.D., F.R.C.P.C.

There is little in emergency medicine that is as challenging as management of the patient who has been subjected to blunt multiple trauma or serious penetrating trauma. These patients often present as a paradigm of emergency medical care, requiring almost simultaneous assessment of airway, ventilation, circulation, integrity of body cavities and structures, status of the brain and spinal cord, and, frequently, behavioral disturbance. Many actions must be taken before complete information is available.[1-6]

Management of the multiply injured patient must first take into account the three pillars of the airway: (1) integrity of airflow; (2) protection from pulmonary aspiration; and (3) assurance of adequate ventilation and oxygenation. Consideration of these three pillars together constitutes the first fundamental principle of trauma airway management: control of the airway. There are two other fundamental principles of trauma airway management that will become implicitly or explicitly involved in all airway decisions in this group of patients. These are: control of the patient and facilitation of therapy. The complete concept of trauma airway management can be expressed as these three fundamental principles.

In the scenarios that follow, the patients have been divided on the basis of the mechanism and severity of their trauma, i.e., victims of blunt trauma are discussed separately from victims of penetrating trauma. Although the fundamental principles of airway management are identical in the two groups of patients, the application of these principles and the methods of airway control are significantly different. Dividing the patients in this manner, therefore, provides clarity to the management algorithms.

THE ROLE OF THE CERVICAL SPINE IN THE AIRWAY DECISION

There is great controversy concerning the possibility of injury to the cervical spinal cord during airway intubation. At the center of the controversy is the safety, or lack of safety, of oral endotracheal intubation in the patient with a potentially unstable cervical spine injury.[7-19] Correct management of the blunt trauma patient depends upon a consideration of:

- The potential for cervical spine injury.
- The role of cervical spine radiography.
- The available airway options.
- The safety of the airway maneuvers.
- The urgency of the situation.

The Potential for Cervical Spine Injury

The incidence of cervical spine fracture or injury in large populations of blunt trauma patients varies between 1% and 12%.[20-25] An attempt to predict cervical spine injury on the basis of clinical evidence was not successful.[26] A few studies have suggested that patients who are fully awake and alert, communicating well, not distracted by other significant injury, not intoxicated, and exhibiting no signs or symptoms of cervical spine or neurologic injury need not undergo cervical spine radiography, and can have cervical spine injury excluded solely on the grounds of these clinical findings.[20, 25, 27] However, these extremely low-risk patients will not require emergency airway management, so these recommendations are of no utility in the management of the multiple trauma patient. *It must be assumed that if a patient has sustained blunt injury of a magnitude sufficient to warrant airway management, that patient has a significant (up to 12%) risk of having a potentially unstable cervical spine injury.*

The Role of Cervical Spine Radiography

The standard initial radiographic assessment of the cervical spine in the multiply injured patient is the cross-table lateral cervical spine radiograph.[1, 22, 28–32] It is well established that 20% to 30% of cervical spine injuries are not detected by this view alone.[28, 29, 31, 33] In fact, even a three-view (lateral, anteroposterior, open mouth odontoid) or five-view (the same three views plus left and right oblique views) cervical spine series cannot definitively exclude cervical spine injury.[22, 31, 33] Only by using a combination of adequate radiographic study and thorough clinical assessment can one reliably exclude cervical spine injury.[22, 32] The thorough clinical assessment must include a neurologic examination and assessment of the degree of pain and the range of motion of the cervical spine. This detailed information will not be forthcoming in the circumstance of the blunt multiple trauma patient who requires active airway management. Therefore, only the incomplete information provided by the radiograph(s) will be available, identifying at most 80% of the injuries. In other words, if, say, 6% of all blunt trauma patients have cervical spine injuries, and lateral radiography identifies 80% of them, the remaining 20% or approximately 1.2% of all blunt trauma patients will have cervical spine injuries and normal lateral radiographs. *A significant probability of cervical spine injury persists, even after an adequate lateral radiograph has failed to demonstrate injury.*

The possibility of cervical spine injury with normal radiographs has led some authors to advocate that cervical spine radiography not be done in the trauma room, because it wastes time, exposes personnel to ionizing radiation, and is too unreliable to realistically influence subsequent management.[30, 34, 35] However, this approach negates the value of a *positive* study. The identification on initial lateral radiographs of a highly unstable injury, such as a fracture dislocation, may lead to a decision to undertake surgical airway management or to defer airway management until awake intubation or fiberoptic intubation can be achieved. The choice of a method for airway management in the blunt trauma patient is never simple. If more information has

been gathered, a wiser decision will be made. *The lateral cross-table cervical spine radiograph provides important, but not conclusive, information.*

The Available Airway Options

For the blunt trauma patient whose cervical spine status has not yet been established definitively, there is a long list of possible approaches to the airway:

1. Blind nasotracheal intubation with topical anesthesia.
2. Blind nasotracheal intubation with topical anesthesia, assisted by intravenous sedation.
3. Orotracheal intubation with local anaesthesia or no anesthesia.
4. Oral endotracheal intubation with local anesthesia and intravenous sedation.
5. Rapid-sequence induction (RSI) oral intubation.
6. Retrograde intubation.
7. Fiberoptic intubation.
8. Needle cricothyrotomy with percutaneous transtracheal ventilation (PTV).
9. Cricothyrotomy using a cricothyrotome.
10. Surgical cricothyrotomy.

Nasotracheal intubation with local anesthesia and topical vasoconstriction is widely practiced in the context of resuscitation of the victim of multiple trauma.[1, 36] This procedure is outlined in detail in Chapter 9. The addition of intravenous sedation to this technique will enhance the success rate and, provided the agent is appropriately chosen, should have no adverse effect on the patient.

Oral endotracheal intubation with local anesthesia alone (awake intubation) is not generally appropriate for the critically injured trauma patient. The presence of combative behavior contraindicates this approach. In fact, a high degree of patient cooperation is essential, especially in the context of the potentially injured cervical spine. A need for immediate intubation makes awake oral intubation a poor choice because both the administration of the topical anesthesia[37] and the intubation itself can be very time-consuming. Oral endotracheal intubation without neuromuscular blockade is of extremely limited use in the multiple trauma patient, whether or not topical anesthesia is used. In the context of the multiply injured patient, oral endotracheal intubation without full neuromuscular blockade is attempted in three settings: (1) awake intubation of the cooperative patient with anatomic disruption of the upper airway; (2) attempted orotracheal intubation using sedation as an alternative to neuromuscular blockade; and (3) cardiopulmonary arrest.

The patient with an anatomically disrupted airway should, in general, be intubated awake or undergo emergency tracheostomy, if possible.[38-40] This approach is outlined in Chapter 23. If there is impending airway compromise, however, and awake intubation or surgical airway management is not possible, immediate RSI with neuromuscular blockade should be undertaken. Although paralysis of the anatomically compromised airway is potentially perilous, further delay could result in complete airway obstruction and an inability to intubate by any means. Whenever paralysis is undertaken on a patient with the potential for anatomic disruption of the airway, equipment for surgical airway management should be readily available and close at hand. In the multiply injured patient, the need for immediate intubation and management of concomitant injuries, such as head injury, will most often militate against awake intubation. Oral endotracheal intubation using intravenous sedation as an alternative to paralysis is ill-advised.[41, 42] Induction of sedation to a degree sufficient to allow oral endotracheal intubation places the patient at risk for aspiration, hypoventilation, and hypoxemia, but does not create ideal circumstances for successful orotracheal intubation. Intubating conditions are vastly superior when neuromuscular blockade is used.[41, 42] In addition, controlled intubation in the context of the potentially injured cervical spine is virtually impossible without neuromuscular blockade. Therefore, the combination of inadequate conditions for intubation, and obtundation of protective airway reflexes and of ventilatory drive, make intravenous sedation for intubation of the multiple trauma patient a poor alternative to RSI with neuromuscular blockade.

Rapid-sequence induction intubation connotes a specific set of circumstances and a specific sequence of actions. The basic principles are preparation, preoxygenation, priming, and paralysis, the four "P's" of RSI intubation. This sequence can be compressed for use in the multiply injured patient, but the fundamental advantage remains the same. There is no other technique that provides the outstanding intubating conditions created by complete neuromuscular blockade.[41-47] Similarly, there is no other technique that affords the opportunity for optimal management of the overall patient and specific injuries, such as increased intracranial pressure (ICP), to the extent offered by RSI with neuromus-

cular blockade.[43, 48-51] Mastery of this technique is a prerequisite for the physician who manages critical trauma patients.

Retrograde intubation[52] requires some degree of patient cooperation or sedation, is not widely used, and has not been well studied in the context of resuscitation of the critically injured trauma patient. Its use in the general sense, therefore, should be restricted to those physicians with expertise and experience in the technique. Fiberoptic intubation[53] also requires some degree of patient cooperation, requires specialized equipment and expertise, and can be very time-consuming and difficult, even in experienced hands. Widespread use of this technique in the resuscitation of the multiple trauma patient, therefore, is not realistic. Again, this technique should be reserved for those centers and individuals who are experienced and proficient in its use.

Needle cricothyrotomy with PTV is frequently advocated as a "temporizing" measure in the resuscitation of critical patients.[54-57] Although many reports have described this technique, few have addressed the use of the technique in the critically injured patient. Because the use of PTV does not protect against aspiration and because these patients often have significant thoracic injuries, it is not easy to extrapolate the data to clinical resuscitation of the multiple trauma patient. Therefore, needle cricothyrotomy with PTV should be reserved for those few cases where no alternative method of airway control appears possible or where other techniques have been tried and have failed. Definitive airway management is still essential at the earliest possible opportunity (see also Chapter 15).

Surgical cricothyrotomy involves the insertion of a tube through a surgical incision in the cricothyroid membrane.[58] This is discussed in detail in Chapter 16. Some critically injured multiple trauma patients will require surgical airway management. Patients with extensive central facial destruction, complex mandibular fractures, or other anatomic disruptions of the upper airway may not be intubated successfully, orally or nasally. These patients will require surgical airway control.[1, 58-61] Also, patients with proven or strongly suspected unstable cervical spine injuries may be candidates for surgical cricothyrotomy. In addition, there is a population of patients for whom rapid establishment of a surgical airway would be vastly preferable to prolonged traumatic attempts at oral intubation in a difficult situation. Proficiency with surgical airway management, therefore, is an essential part of the armamentarium of the physician caring for critically injured trauma patients.

The list of potentially useful techniques is long and the amount of expertise required to master them is extensive. The "alternative" approaches are discussed in detail elsewhere in this book. Lack of familiarity with these techniques, complexity of performance, requirements for specialized equipment, and time delays in securing the airway relegate them to a minor role. There is a shorter list of "best choices" for airway management in the multiply injured patient. These choices are: (1) nasotracheal intubation with local anesthesia with or without intravenous sedation; (2) RSI intubation; and (3) cricothyrotomy.

The choice of approach is highly dependent on institutional practice and the preference of the bedside physician. With the exception of patients requiring immediate surgical airway management, most patients will be managed using nasotracheal intubation or RSI oral intubation. Each has benefits and disadvantages and these are discussed elsewhere in this book. There are certain circumstances, however, that argue very strongly in favor of one technique over another. Patients with significant head injury with suspicion of elevated ICP should be intubated using RSI intubation with careful attention to ICP[43] (see Chapter 24). Nasotracheal intubation stimulates a rise in ICP and is therefore potentially hazardous in this patient subgroup.[62–64] Nasotracheal intubation is difficult or impossible in the combative patient and the complication rate in this group is much higher. RSI oral intubation is preferable in these patients.[44] Patients who have been rendered hypoxemic because of respiratory injury are not ideal candidates for any of these approaches, and, prolonged attempts at nasal intubation may be distinctly harmful. Finally, the overall success and complication rates of nasotracheal intubation compare unfavorably with RSI oral intubation.[22] RSI intubation establishes a definitive airway much more rapidly than can be achieved with nasotracheal intubation, regardless of the adjuncts and aids used.[41, 42, 44] Therefore, in the vast majority of circumstances, consideration of the cervical spine, potential head injury, patient cooperation, and the urgency of the situation will favor RSI oral intubation over nasotracheal intubation. Nasotracheal intubation does not require paralysis of the patient or direct laryngoscopy, and in the hands of an inexperienced physician, this may be a benefit; however, physicians ought to be facile with the use of neuromuscular blockade and RSI intubation if they are to care for critically injured patients.

The Safety of Airway Maneuvers

The incidence of cervical spine injury in this patient population mandates that all patients be fully immobilized on a long spine board with an appropriate cervical collar, tape, and sandbags.[1, 7] The three approaches to airway management in these patients are discussed in the following paragraphs.

Blind Nasotracheal Intubation

Blind nasotracheal intubation is widely advocated as the optimal approach to airway management in the immobilized blunt trauma patient.[1] Because it does not require laryngoscopy, there is theoretically no leverage applied to the potentially injured cervical spine. This concept has not been studied adequately, although one study suggested that there was little shift of the cervical spine during nasotracheal intubation in an unstable cervical spine injury cadaver model.[7] The technique, contraindications, and complications of blind nasotracheal intubation are discussed in Chapter 9. In the multiple trauma patient, the essential elements of optimal management are timely establishment of the airway, avoidance of excessive agitation of the patient, and avoidance of stimulation of patients with known or suspected increased ICP. Nasotracheal intubation should be avoided in the combative patient unless adequate pharmacologic restraint (see patient scenarios below) can be accomplished. Similarly, the patient should not be subjected to prolonged or complicated attempts to secure the airway. Significant central facial trauma is a contraindication to the procedure.[36] Finally, nasotracheal intubation should probably be avoided in patients with elevated ICP.[43, 48, 62–64] If nasotracheal intubation must be used in such a patient, pharmacologic agents should be used to minimize exacerbation of the intracranial process[62–64] (see Chapter 24).

Oral Endotracheal Intubation with Cervical Spine Immobilization

This is the only one of the three principal airway approaches that requires insertion of a laryngoscope. The potential for application of distracting force to the site of the unstable cervical spine injury is the principal disadvantage of oral endotracheal intubation in the multiple trauma patient. In an elective intubation, the patient's head and neck are repositioned to facilitate visualization of the glottis. This repositioning is contraindicated in the blunt trauma patient.[11] There is no debate about the danger of repositioning the head and neck, flexing the neck, applying anterior traction on the neck, or other similar maneuvers in the context of the potentially injured cervical spine. The issue is whether oral endotracheal intubation is *ever safe* in the context of known or suspected cervical spine injury. Central to this argument is the role of manual cervical spine immobilization, with its frequently used misnomers: "cervical traction" and "axial traction." Bivens et al.[8] demonstrated that application of traction to the unstable cervical spine is capable of producing catastrophic subluxation or distraction. This limited study has led to well-meaning, but misguided, warnings about the dangers of manual cervical spine immobilization.[14, 18] Unfortunately, the distinction was not made between immobilization of the cervical spine and traction applied to the cervical spine. There would appear to be a consensus that *traction* should not be applied to the undiagnosed cervical spine, whether for intubation, or for any other purpose.[8, 10, 12, 14, 15, 18, 19]

The real issue is whether carefully applied manual *immobilization* of the head and neck, accompanied by skillful laryngoscopic technique, can achieve intubation without posing a threat to the unstable cervical spine. Holley and Jorden[13] reported on 29 patients with cervical spine injuries who sustained no neurologic deterioration when orotracheally intubated using manual cervical spine immobilization. These patients were intubated using awake technique, however, so extrapolation to the trauma room is not realistic. Rhee et al.[17] reported on 21 patients with cervical spine injuries who required airway management in the trauma room. None of the 15 patients that underwent orotracheal intubation with cervical immobilization and neuromuscular blockade demonstrated neurologic deterioration. Majernick et al.[65] studied cervical spine movement in normal patients during elective intubation for routine surgery. They reported significant reduction in the amount of cervical spine movement during laryngoscopy and intubation when cervical immobilization was applied. Crosby and Suderman[10] reported briefly on the oral intubation of 60 patients with incomplete cervical cord injury. They used cervical stabilization and neuromuscular blockade in the majority of these patients, with no increase in neurologic deficits. Other series that are cited in support of oral endotracheal intubation in this setting are difficult to evaluate because of the quality of the evidence presented.[11, 46] There does not appear to be a report in the literature, however, of a patient whose cervical cord was clearly and unequivocally injured during oral endotracheal intubation. Whether this represents a lack

of occurrence, or simply a lack of reporting, is not known.

The principal advantages of oral endotracheal intubation are the ability to use pharmacologic agents to protect the intracranial contents, the ability to completely control the patient and facilitate subsequent resuscitation and therapy, and familiarity with the technique.[43–47] In the majority of circumstances, when immediate intubation is required, oral intubation using RSI and neuromuscular blockade has the most favorable balance of advantages over disadvantages. The importance of establishing and maintaining strict cervical spine immobilization during intubation cannot be overemphasized. Failure to adhere to this standard carries devastating consequences for the patient and the physician. A few conclusions can be drawn about oral endotracheal intubation:

1. The cervical spine must be meticulously immobilized during oral endotracheal intubation. This immobilization must be maintained by a person other than the intubator. Laryngoscopy and intubation must be gentle and atraumatic, applying no traction or leverage to the cervical spine.

2. Unless awake intubation can be performed, RSI with neuromuscular blockade should be used for oral endotracheal intubation.

3. If careful oral intubation with immobilization is not successful, a surgical airway should be secured. Compromising the immobilization to achieve intubation is not acceptable, unless the operator is incapable of alternative airway techniques.

Cricothyrotomy

There have been no studies demonstrating that surgical cricothyrotomy can be performed without movement of an unstable cervical spine. However, descriptions of the technique[58] demonstrate convincingly that there is no significant leverage applied to the cervical spine. The only stress applied is a slight amount of traction to the airway itself—too little force to distract the elements of an injured, unstable cervical spine.[8, 15] However, the reports of the clinical use of cricothyrotomy in the emergency setting identify a significant complication rate ranging from 0% to 42%.[59–61, 66, 67] Analysis of these series suggests that the failure rate is less than 10%,[59–61, 66, 67] and that serious complications can be dramatically reduced or even eliminated with proper adherence to indications and technique.[59, 67] Nevertheless, there has not been widespread acceptance of this technique, and its use generally remains confined to major trauma centers and highly organized prehospital care systems.

A number of commercial kits or cricothyrotomes have been advocated as providing a more simple way of establishing a cricothyrotomy.[68-70] There are no conclusive data concerning the use of these sets (see Chapter 16). The following conclusions can be made about cricothyrotomy in the setting of the blunt trauma patient:

1. Widespread lack of familiarity with the technique and the lack of evidence that it is clearly safer make cricothyrotomy simply an alternative to blind nasotracheal intubation or oral endotracheal intubation with cervical spine immobilization in most settings. When either of the latter approaches is possible, and the physician performing the airway maneuver is significantly more competent with intubation than with surgical airway management, intubation should be considered the airway intervention of choice.

2. There are patients with massive facial or upper airway injury in whom oral or nasal intubation is not possible or should not be attempted. In these patients, cricothyrotomy is the procedure of choice.

3. There is inadequate information in the literature to recommend the use of a kit or cricothyrotome in lieu of surgical circothyrotomy.

The Urgency of the Situation

Despite the controversy surrounding airway management of the bluntly injured patient, there is one central theme that is neither controversial nor debated: *When a patient is in need of immediate airway management, the establishment of the airway itself is paramount, and takes precedence over all other considerations.* This is not to say that the cervical spine is not important, but the basic goal of immediately establishing an airway must never be obscured. It is necessary that the physician caring for critically injured patients be facile with airway maneuvers, and decisive when immediate action is called for.

Conclusion

Management of the airway in the immobilized, multiply injured patient presents one of the most difficult challenges in emergency medicine. The basic approach should maximize knowledge of the patient's injuries and integrate this knowledge with the urgency of the need for the airway and the expertise of the physician at the bedside. An algorithm for the role of cervical spine radiography and the individual physician's expertise is presented in Figure 22–1. The approach is as follows:

If airway management is indicated, the first decision is whether the airway must be managed immediately, or can be delayed for a few minutes to obtain a cross-table lateral cervical spine radiograph. If the lateral radiograph is adequate and demonstrates no abnormalities, the likelihood of cervical spine injury is reduced by about 80%. This allows the airway maneuver to be undertaken with a great deal more confidence, but full cervical spine protection is still required. More important, the demonstration of a highly unstable injury on the lateral radiograph may favor an alternative approach. In the absence of such injury, or if the lateral radiograph cannot be obtained, the patient's neurologic examination provides crucial information. If the screening neurologic examination is consistent with cervical cord injury, manipulation of the cervical spine must be avoided. If *immediate* airway management is indicated in such a patient, oral intubation should probably be avoided and blind nasotracheal intubation or cricothyrotomy should be performed. If blind nasal intubation is not possible and the physician is incapable of cricothyrotomy, oral intubation with meticulous manual cervical spine immobilization may be attempted. In a small minority of patients, this may be attempted with the patient awake, but usually RSI will be necessary. An alternative in selected cases is initiation of PTV as a temporizing measure, perhaps to allow for the arrival of a person with more airway expertise.

In the absence of suspected elevation of ICP, blind nasotracheal intubation is an appropriate initial choice of technique for trauma patients. The physician must also be capable of oral tracheal intubation using RSI technique and cervical spine immobilization. The presence of increased ICP, failure of nasotracheal intubation, a contraindication to nasal intubation, or personal preference will frequently make RSI with cervical spine immobilization the maneuver of first choice. When there is disruption of the face or mandible, or when oral intubation fails, cricothyrotomy is the preferred method of securing the airway.

Regardless of the airway maneuver under consideration, there is far more compelling evidence *in favor of* timely airway management than there is *against* any single airway maneuver. Detailed integration of this decision making into the overall management of the multiple trauma patient is presented in the patient scenarios below.

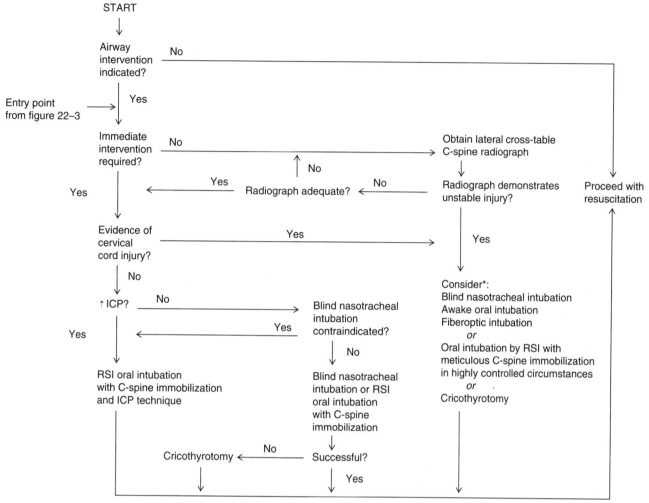

FIG 22–1.

Algorithm for interplay between airway management and cervical spine *(C-spine)* assessment. *ICP* = intracranial pressure; *RSI* = rapid-sequence induction.

THE BLUNT MULTIPLE TRAUMA PATIENT

Scenario 1: The Mildly Injured Patient

Many patients who have sustained significant blunt trauma do not have major injuries identified during prehospital assessment or early assessment in the emergency department (Fig 22–2). These patients are almost always immobilized on a long spine board, with a semirigid cervical collar, tape, and sandbags. During and following the initial assessment, the three fundamental principles of trauma airway management must be addressed. It is rarely necessary to take action based on control of the patient or facilitation of therapy. In fact, the very consideration of these issues would promote the patient to either the moderate or severely injured scenarios below. This leaves only the consideration of control of the airway itself, and hence the three pillars of airway management.

There are a number of possible threats to airflow. First, even a mildly injured patient may have injuries to the nose and mouth that prevent or interfere with normal passage of air. The nose may be contused, with extensive swelling, or fractured, with formation of intranasal hematomas or epistaxis. The alveolar ridge or teeth may be fractured, leading to significant intraoral hemorrhage. The tongue may be lacerated and may bleed briskly. Dentures or dental bridges may have been dislodged in the mouth. The cervical collar itself may prevent jaw opening, necessitating ventilation through the nares. Aspiration of blood from the oral or nasal pharynx may occur in patients who are immobilized in a supine position. Emesis may also occur with subsequent aspiration of

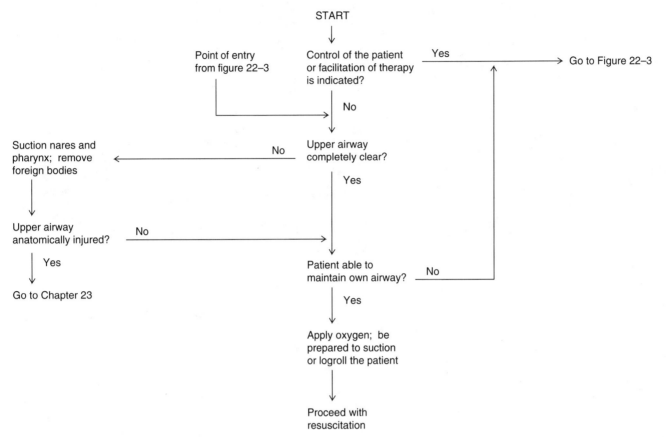

FIG 22–2.
The mildly injured patient algorithm.

the vomitus. In rare instances, portions of the dentition that have broken loose may be aspirated. Ventilation and oxygenation in these mildly injured patients is usually not an issue. Once the integrity of the upper airway is ensured and an airstream is established, ventilation and oxygenation will ensue.

Airway management in this setting consists of appropriate anticipation of problems, with specific interventions when indicated. Suctioning of the blood from the nares or oral pharynx can be accomplished using a suction catheter or Yankauer suction tip. Any obvious foreign bodies, including dentalwork, should be removed from the mouth if they are dislodged or interfere with airflow. Tongue lacerations can be controlled by suctioning or by direct pressure. If obstruction of the nares cannot easily be cleared, opening the front of the cervical collar will permit breathing through the mouth. It is appropriate to temporarily open or remove the anterior half of the cervical collar in any case to permit examination of the anterior neck (see Chapter 23).

Prevention of aspiration in the immobilized trauma patient is difficult and requires a combination of appropriate suctioning and, when necessary, logrolling the patient and placing the bed in a slightly head-down position. Even though these patients are alert and fully capable of protecting their airway, they are immobilized in the supine position and are therefore at risk for significant aspiration of emesis or blood. Whenever suctioning is not thought to have adequately removed this risk of aspiration, the patient should be logrolled in a controlled fashion. Early clinical and radiographic assessment to exclude injury to the cervical, thoracic, and lumbar spines will permit the patient to be repositioned such that self-protection of the airway can occur. Administration of low-flow nasal or mask oxygen is appropriate in all patients who have sustained significant trauma, but no additional support of ventilation or oxygenation is indicated. This approach is illustrated in the algorithm of Figure 22–2.

Scenario 2: The Moderately Injured Patient

This scenario (Fig 22–3) addresses the patient who has been subjected to a significant injury mechanism and arrives in the emergency department with evidence of significant, but not critical, injury. This includes all patients with head injury demonstrating agitation or obtundation (but without frank coma); moderate facial trauma; moderate chest trauma, including rib fractures, pneumothorax, or hemotho-

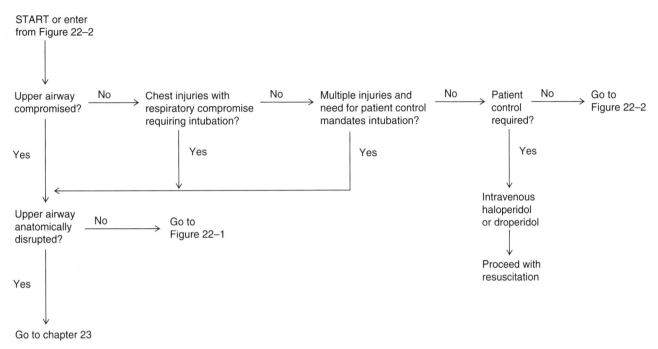

FIG 22–3.
The moderately injured patient algorithm.

rax; evidence of intraabdominal injury; pelvic or long bone fractures; or with some disturbance of vital signs, but not frank vascular collapse. In this scenario, management is much more complicated because all three of the fundamental principles of trauma airway management are operative.

Control of the Airway.—Control of the airway is best discussed using the concept of the three pillars of the airway. As in the preceding scenario, these patients are immobilized on a spine board with tape, sandbags, and a semirigid cervical collar. Evaluation of the upper airway for obstruction or interference with the airstream is virtually identical to that outlined above with the exception that patient cooperation may be limited. Although the patient may exhibit significantly altered mental status, self-protection of the airway is the rule rather than the exception. The immobilization in the supine position places the patient at risk for aspiration, and the patient must be observed closely. Ventilation and oxygenation may be significantly impaired. Isolated rib fractures can interfere with ventilation because of pain. This problem is compounded when multiple fractures are present. Pneumothorax of the simple or tension variety may interfere significantly with both ventilation and gas exchange. Mild hemothorax does not significantly alter thoracic dynamics or oxygenation, but massive hemothorax may cause lung compression and even lead to tension phenomena analogous to those seen in tension pneumothorax. Pulmonary contusion secondary to high-energy

blunt chest injury may lead to rapid formation of interstitial and alveolar fluid and dramatically reduce gas exchange. Pulmonary edema can also occur secondary to severe head injury, but that would promote the patient to the critical scenario. Ventilation and oxygenation may also be compromised by the ingestion or inhalation of toxic substances. These include illicit drugs, especially opiates or ethanol; and the products of combustion, such as carbon monoxide, chemical and particulate smoky matter, or cyanide, when both fire and blunt trauma are involved. Opiates depress ventilation and overdosage may cause pulmonary edema and thus inhibit gas exchange. Severe ethanol intoxication or ingestion of sedative-hypnotic drugs may significantly depress respiratory drive and decrease ventilation.

Restoration of airflow and relief of obstruction are undertaken in a manner similar to that described above. Again, the anterior neck should be inspected for evidence of blunt injury. Protection against aspiration will also follow the same approach as for the mildly injured patient. If the patient is combative or uncooperative, the principle of control of the patient will become operative (see below).

Assessment of ventilation and oxygenation encompasses all of the observations pertinent to the upper airway as well as the respiratory rate and careful inspection, palpation, and auscultation of the thoracic cavity. Arterial blood gases should be obtained. General observation of the patient's color and circulatory status is also important. Severe obtundation with depression of the respiratory rate to less than 10 breaths per minute will place the patient in the critical scenario as will evidence of profound respiratory dysfunction with elevation of the respiratory rate to greater than 40. For other patients, careful but prompt assessment of the integrity of the thoracic cage, the bellows function of the lung, and the integrity of the pulmonary parenchyma is central to management decisions. In the multiply injured patient with severe burns, circumferential thoracic eschar is an indication for immediate longitudinal escharotomy. Multiple rib fractures, even with a flail segment, is not an unequivocal indication for intubation. However, suspicion of accompanying pneumothorax or a significant pleural or pulmonary lesion is an indication for tube thoracostomy. Circumstantial evidence for hemothorax or pneumothorax is adequate. Therefore, presence of significant chest injury with hypotension, subcutaneous air, respiratory distress, tracheal shift, or increased or decreased resonance on percussion should be taken as evidence of a significant intrathoracic injury and a chest tube should be placed immediately. If chest injury is present bilaterally, and it is not clear which hemithorax is the problem, bilateral chest tubes should be placed. When the mechanical function of the thorax is restored, decisions regarding the need for intubation can be made more deliberately. If significant respiratory distress remains after exclusion of significant thoracic injury or insertion of bilateral chest tubes and administration of 100% oxygen by mask, intubation is indicated.

The technique chosen for intubation depends upon the presence of concomitant injury, the anatomic status of the upper airway, the expertise and preference of the bedside physician, and the perceived urgency of intervention. As previously described, for the purposes of simplicity in this highly complex situation, patients that require intubation on the basis of respiratory distress are promoted to the critical patient scenario outlined below.

Control of the Patient.—The second fundamental principle in trauma airway management is control of the patient. In this regard, we consider threats to the patient as a whole, rather than simply considering threats to the three pillars of the airway. The victim of blunt multiple trauma often exhibits substantial disturbances in behavior. These disturbances are usually multifactorial: brain injury, hypoxia, hypotension, intoxicants, pain, anxiety. Medically correctable causes, such as hypoglycemia, hypotension, and hypoxemia will generally be identified and corrected early in the course of trauma resuscitation. One is left with a need to control the patient in the remaining majority of circumstances when the cause of loss of control is not immediately reversible. In conjunction with physical restraint, there are three stages in the clinical response to the combative patient: (1) reassurance; (2) chemical restraint, and (3) paralysis.

In some cases, the patient's behavior can be controlled simply through good communication. If the patient is reassured that he or she is in a hospital and is safe, that the injuries are not serious, and that the caregivers are undertaking a number of helpful interventions, agitated or aberrant behavior may gradually subside and control of the patient will be regained. This approach should be taken early in the course of every multiple trauma resuscitation. If reassurance is unsuccessful, physical and pharmacologic restraint must be employed. Continued agitation and struggling impairs the resuscitative attempt and may be harmful to both patient and caregivers. Physical restraint usually involves the application of restraining devices to all four extremities. In addition, it is usually necessary to restrain the patient's head and neck against the spine board to maintain cervical spine immobilization. Tape and sandbags accompanied by limb restraint are, however, frequently inadequate to protect the violent patient from the possible consequences of disruption of an unstable spine injury. Therefore, in all but the most docile of patients, pharmacologic restraint is indicated.

This constitutes one of the most agonizing decision points in the course of management of the multiple trauma patient. Should the patient be sedated or should the patient be paralyzed and intubated? On the one hand, if sedation is used, sufficient control may be gained to permit rapid and thorough assessment of the patient's injuries and to obtain rapid radiographic studies and physical examination evidence to identify or exclude injury to the spine. Unnecessary intubation may thus be avoided. On the other hand, sedation can have significant drawbacks. Firstly, most sedative agents carry a risk of depression of respiration, blood pressure, and protective airway reflexes, thus threatening two of the three pillars of the airway. The sedating agent may be slow to act and may permit the patient to continue the dangerous behavior for a considerable period of time, often 15 minutes or longer. Fortunately, there are agents available that can be administered to gain timely control of the patient while allowing adequate protection of the airway and preserving ventilation and gas exchange. When control of combative behavior is desirable, but it is not felt to be necessary to paralyze and intubate the patient, intravenous sedation should be administered. The ideal sedative is one that is rapidly effective, does not depress respiration, has no adverse effects on the cardiovascular status of the hemodynamically compromised patient, or other adverse effects, has a relatively short duration of action, and is completely reversible by administration of a pharmacologic antagonist. Unfortunately, there is no agent that meets all of these criteria. The agent that most closely approximates the ideal is probably haloperidol. Haloperidol, given intravenously, acts within minutes, has virtually no respiratory depressant activity, is extremely safe in patients with cardiovascular compromise, and has no other adverse effects.[71-75] Haloperidol can be administered in incremental doses of 5 to 10 mg intravenously repeated every 3 to 5 minutes until adequate pharmacologic control is achieved. In general, the patient will be well controlled in less than 10 minutes with doses of 20 mg or less of intravenous haloperidol.[74, 76] Should larger doses be necessary, however, there are reports in the literature of patients receiving hundreds of milligrams of haloperidol over a 24-hour period without apparent adverse effect.[75] These patients received the drug while in coronary care units and exhibited no evidence of significant hypotension, respiratory compromise, or myocardial depression. There are numerous reports in the literature of the use of haloperidol as a sedating agent, and its ratio of effectiveness to adverse effects seems very high. An alternative agent is droperidol, which is approved for intravenous administration.

Paralysis of the patient, on the other hand, mandates definitive airway control. If it is apparent that the patient's injuries warrant intubation, early use of paralysis with intubation will optimize control of the patient and subsequent therapeutic efforts. *Paralysis with intubation is indicated when the patient's combative behavior requires pharmacologic control and it is believed that the nature of the patient's injuries are such that early intubation will be either necessary or beneficial.*

Paralysis and intubation solely for the purpose of controlling behavior is not justifiable.[77] If behavioral control is all that is needed, intravenous sedation is indicated. Paralysis and intubation for the combined purpose of controlling the patient's behavior and facilitating or optimizing management of the patient's multiple injuries, however, is one of the hallmarks of competent trauma management. Therefore, it is not the nature of the patient's combative behavior that will determine the need for intubation in this setting, rather it is the nature and severity of the accompanying injuries.

If the patient's combative behavior, when weighed in combination with concomitant injuries (e.g., significant head or chest injury; multiple orthopaedic injuries, including pelvic fracture; significant intraabdominal or retroperitoneal injury), mandates definitive airway control, it is appropriate to paralyze and intubate the patient rather than to temporize with sedation. Because of the risk of cervical spine injury, the intubation must be done in a highly controlled manner. The various considerations in the approach to the patient with cervical spine injury were outlined earlier in this chapter. In the context of the combative patient, however, paralysis and in-

tubation (RSI) is the method of choice. Alternative methods of intubation involving little or no sedation (blind nasotracheal intubation) or significant sedation, including topical airway anesthesia (awake orotracheal intubation), are not appropriate in this setting. After the patient is intubated, clinical assessment of the multiple injuries can continue in a controlled fashion and a decision can be made as to whether long-term paralysis is indicated.

Facilitation of Therapy.—The third fundamental principle of trauma airway management is facilitation of therapy. In this scenario, the facilitation of specific therapy is indicated only in two settings: serious head injury, and the combative patient with multiple injuries. If the patient has a serious or critical head injury, he or she is promoted to the critical patient scenario outlined below. If intubation is indicated on the basis of the combative patient with multiple injuries, proceed as discussed in the preceding paragraphs. Therefore, for the moderate injury scenario, this fundamental principle is easily dealt with. The approach to the moderately injured patient is illustrated in the algorithm of Figure 22–3.

Scenario 3: The Severe Multiple Trauma Patient (Critical Scenario)

This scenario (Fig 22–4) includes critically injured trauma patients with significant head injuries resulting in a Glasgow coma scale of 8 or less; multiply injured patients with shock or severe respiratory distress; combative patients with severe multiple injuries; and multiple trauma patients with direct anatomic threats to their upper airway or thoracic cage. Once again, discussion is facilitated by considering the three fundamental principles of trauma airway management.

The first principle is control of the airway. The threats to the three pillars of the airway—integrity of airflow, protection from aspiration, and assurance of ventilation-oxygenation—are virtually identical to those outlined in the scenario of the moderately injured patient. The principal difference between the moderately injured and the critically injured patient is that the latter forces the physician to act quickly. Indecisive management, temporizing, and hesitancy are potentially far more threatening to the critically injured patient than the possible complications of the procedures themselves. Immediate, definitive decisions are essential at the bedside of the critically injured patient. Within this group of critically injured patients is a subset of patients whose need for immediate airway management is readily apparent. These are the patients that present with upper airway obstruction or profound hypoventilation, including apnea. In all other cases, the decision to intubate is made partially on the basis of airway

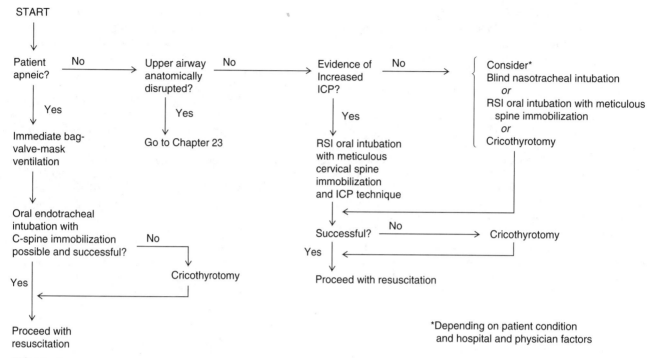

FIG 22–4.
The critical patient algorithm. For abbreviations, see legend, Figure 22–1.

considerations, but is heavily dependent on the overall status of the patient.

In many ways, management of the critically injured multiple trauma patient is simpler than management of the moderately injured patient. The extreme nature of the presentation makes the necessary airway decisions less elective and, therefore, more justified. Control of the patient and facilitation of therapy become linked in this setting. The critical patient requires a series of invasive resuscitative measures. Some of these measures, such as insertion of a chest tube, are both diagnostic and therapeutic. In the critical patient, therefore, the patient as a whole (i.e., control of the patient and facilitation of therapy) becomes the indicator for active airway management. The multiply injured patient with shock, significant head injury, severe agitation or obtundation, or severe respiratory distress unrelieved by bilateral tube thoracostomy is, therefore, a candidate for immediate active airway management (see Fig 22–4). The choice of airway maneuver is dependent on the nature of the patient's injuries, his or her mental status, the availability of resources within the institution, and the skills and preference of the physician. These issues have been addressed earlier in this chapter.

The approach to the severely multiply injured patient, therefore, involves, firstly, assessment of the upper airway with attention to the three pillars of the airway. Consideration of control of the patient and facilitation of therapy will almost always man-

date early or immediate intubation. In fact, it is perhaps the need for early or immediate intubation that most distinctly identifies the group of patients that belong in the critical scenario. Although the list of potential airway management choices is long and the variety of patients great, a basic algorithm for this group is presented in Figure 22–4. This algorithm reflects the philosophy that it is the control of the patient and facilitation of therapy, such as hyperventilation of head injury, that provides the impetus for active airway management in the majority of these patients. By definition, cervical spine radiography will usually not be possible.

THE PENETRATING TRAUMA PATIENT

Scenario 4: Penetrating Trauma

Patients who have sustained penetrating trauma (Fig 22–5), but arrive with an isolated injury and essentially normal vital signs, require only supportive airway management such as administration of supplemental oxygen. The management of the airway in the context of specific injuries, such as thoracic injury, head injury, or injury to the upper airway, is dealt with elsewhere in this book. Other than when there is a direct threat to the anatomic integrity of the airway, the principal role of active airway management in the penetrating trauma patient parallels that in the moderate or critically injured blunt

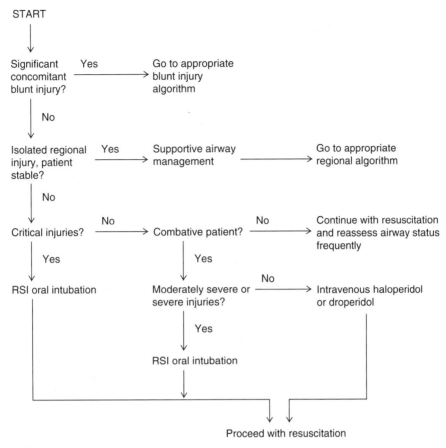

FIG 22–5.
The penetrating trauma patient algorithm. *RSI* = rapid-sequence induction.

trauma patient. That is, definitive airway control will be based on consideration of a combination of the patient's injuries, the need to control the patient's behavior, and the need for specific therapeutic interventions such as thoracostomy, thoracotomy, etc. Most victims of penetrating trauma that present with signs and symptoms of a regional injury and evidence of hemodynamic instability or compromise respond well to restoration of circulating blood volume and appropriate treatment of the injury. Active airway management in these patients is not necessary.

When the penetrating trauma patient's behavior interferes with assessment or therapy, pharmacologic control is essential. Once again, the choice is between intravenous sedation and paralysis. If the patient's injuries warrant early intubation in any case, immediate paralysis and orotracheal intubation is indicated. Injuries of this sort include most gunshot injuries to the head, neck, chest, or abdomen; stab wounds to the chest with significant hypotension, shock, or respiratory distress that persists after tube thoracostomy; stab wounds to the abdomen with persistent or refractory shock; or multiple penetrating injuries to various regions of the body. If one of these circumstances is present and the pa-

tient's combative or uncooperative behavior is inhibiting orderly assessment and resuscitation, immediate intubation should be undertaken. In the vast majority of patients, the optimal method will be RSI oral intubation with neuromuscular blockade. In the absence of these injuries, intravenous sedation with haloperidol or droperidol (see above) may be preferable. In these patients, sedation may permit orderly resuscitation and assessment, and intubation ultimately may not be required.

The other major difference between the victim of penetrating trauma and the victim of blunt trauma is that the cervical spine usually is not an issue in the penetrating trauma patient. If the penetrating trauma patient is believed to have sustained significant concomitant blunt injury, then the appropriate blunt injury algorithm should be followed. If the patient has not sustained blunt trauma in addition to the penetrating trauma, the principles of the appropriate blunt trauma scenario can be followed, but the cervical spine considerations outlined above may be disregarded. This increases the options for methods of intubation, but the same arguments in favor of RSI oral intubation in the blunt trauma patient can apply to this setting as well. Therefore, the majority of patients will undergo blind nasotracheal intubation or RSI oral intubation with neuromuscular blockade. The approach to the penetrating trauma patient is presented in the algorithm of Figure 22–5.

CONCLUSION

The enormous variety of possible injuries renders the discussion of airway management in the multiple trauma patient exceedingly complex. An attempt has been made to break the patient presentations down into discrete scenarios and an algorithm is presented for the management for each type of patient. The central role of appropriate intravenous sedation in milder cases and RSI oral intubation in more severe cases cannot be overemphasized. Induction agents may need to be modified to account for increased ICP or hypotension, and a thorough understanding of the basic principles and techniques involved in RSI oral intubation is essential for management of critically injured trauma patients.

REFERENCES

1. American College of Surgeons: *Advanced Trauma Life Support Instructors Manual.* Chicago, American College of Surgeons, 1988.
2. Cales RH, Trunkey DD: Preventable trauma deaths: A review of trauma care systems development. *JAMA* 1985; 254:1059–1063.
3. Collicott PE: Initial assessment of the trauma patient, in Mattox KL, Moore EE, Feliciano DV (eds): *Trauma.* East Norwalk, Conn, Appleton & Lange, 1988, pp 107–124.
4. Jorden RC, Barkin R: Multiple trauma, in Rosen P, Baker FJ II, Barkin R, et al (eds): *Emergency Medicine Concepts and Clinical Practice.* St Louis, Mosby–Year Book, Inc, 1988, pp 157–179.
5. Lowe DK, Gately HL, Goss JR, et al: Patterns of death, complication, and error in the management of motor vehicle accident victims: Implications for a regional system of trauma care. *J Trauma* 1983; 23:503–509.
6. Moylan JA, Detmer DE, Rose J, et al: Evaluation of the quality of hospital care for major trauma. *J Trauma* 1976; 16:517–523.
7. Aprahamian C, Thompson BM, Finger WA, et al: Experimental cervical spine injury model: Evaluation of airway management and splinting techniques. *Ann Emerg Med* 1984; 13:584–587.
8. Bivens HG, Ford S, Bezmalinovic Z, et al: The effect of axial traction during orotracheal intubation of the trauma victim with an unstable cervical spine. *Ann Emerg Med* 1988; 17:53–57.

9. Campbell WH: Editor's note. *J Emerg Med* 1989; 7:391.
10. Crosby E, Suderman V: Oral endotracheal intubation in cervical spine injured patients (letter). *J Emerg Med* 1989; 8:650–651.
11. Doolan LA, O'Brien JF: Safe intubation in cervical spine injury. *Anaesth Intensive Care* 1985; 13:319–324.
12. Fried LC: Cervical spinal cord injury during skeletal traction. *JAMA* 1974; 229:181–183.
13. Holley J, Jorden RC: Airway management in patients with unstable cervical spine fractures. *Ann Emerg Med* 1989; 18:151–153.
14. Joyce SM: Cervical immobilization during orotracheal intubation in trauma victims. *Ann Emerg Med* 1988; 17:145.
15. Kaufman HH, Harris JH, Spencer JA, et al: Danger of traction during radiography for cervical spine trauma. *JAMA* 1982; 247:2369.
16. Knopp RK: The safety of orotracheal intubation in patients with suspected cervical-spine injury. *Ann Emerg Med* 1990; 19:603–604.
17. Rhee KJ, Green W, Holcroft JW, et al: Oral intubation in the multiply injured patient: The risk of exacerbating spinal cord damage. *Ann Emerg Med* 1990; 19:511–514.
18. Turner LM: Cervical spine immobilization with axial traction: A practice to be discouraged. *J Emerg Med* 1989; 7:385–386.
19. Walls RM: Airway management in the blunt trauma patient: How important is the cervical spine? *Can J Surg,* in press.
20. Cadoux CG, White JD, Hedberg MC: High-yield roentgenographic criteria for cervical spine injury. *Ann Emerg Med* 1987; 16:738–742.
21. Gbaanador, GBM, Fruin AH, Taylon C: Role of routine emergency cervical radiography in head trauma. *Am J Surg* 1986; 152:643–648.
22. MacDonald RL, Schwartz ML, Mirich D, et al: Diagnosis of cervical spine injury in motor vehicle crash victims: How many x-rays are enough? *J Trauma* 1990; 30:392–397.
23. McNamara RM, O'Brien MC, Davidheiser S: Post-traumatic neck pain: A prospective and follow-up study. *Ann Emerg Med* 1988; 17:906–911.
24. Niefeld GL, Keene JG, Hevesy G, et al: Cervical injury in head trauma. *J Emerg Med* 1988; 6:203–207.
25. Roberge RJ, Wears RC, Kelly M, et al: Selective application of cervical spine radiography in alert victims of blunt trauma: A prospective study. *J Trauma* 1988; 28:784–788.
26. Jacobs LM, Schwartz R: Prospective analysis of acute cervical spine injury: A new methodology to predict injury. *Ann Emerg Med* 1986; 15:44–49.
27. Ringenberg BJ, Fisher AK, Urdaneta LF, et al: Rational ordering of cervical spine radiographs following trauma. *Ann Emerg Med* 1988; 17:792–796.
28. Blahd WH, Iserson KV, Bjelland JC: Efficacy of the posttraumatic cross-table lateral view of the cervical spine. *J Emerg Med* 1985; 2:243–249.

29. Shaffer MA, Doris PE: Limitation of the cross table lateral view in detecting cervical spine injuries: A retrospective analysis. *Ann Emerg Med* 1981; 10:508–513.

30. Spain DA, Trooskin SZ, Flancbaum L, et al: The adequacy and cost effectiveness of routine resuscitation-area cervical-spine radiographs. *Ann Emerg Med* 1990; 19:276–278.

31. Streitwieser DR, Knopp R, Wales LR, et al: Accuracy of standard radiographic views in detecting cervical spine fractures. *Ann Emerg Med* 1983; 12:538–542.

32. Walls RM, Connell DG: Multiple trauma, in Rosen P, Doris P, Barkin R, et al (eds): *Diagnostic Radiology in Emergency Medicine.* St Louis, Mosby–Year Book, Inc, 1991.

33. Freemyer B, Knopp R, Piche J, et al: Comparison of five-view and three-view cervical spine series in the evaluation of patients with cervical traumas. *Ann Emerg Med* 1989; 18:818–821.

34. Singer CM, Baraff LJ, Benedict SH, et al: Exposure of emergency medicine personnel to ionizing radiation during cervical spine radiography. *Ann Emerg Med* 1989; 18:822–825.

35. Weiss EL, Singer CM, Benedict SH, et al: Physician exposure to ionizing radiation during trauma resuscitation: A prospective clinical study. *Ann Emerg Med* 1990; 19:134–138.

36. Danzl DF, Thomas DM: Nasotracheal intubations in the emergency department. *Crit Care Med* 1980; 8:677–681.

37. Bourke DL, Katz J, Tonneson A: Nebulized anaesthesia for awake endotracheal intubation. *Anaesthesia* 1985; 63:690–692.

38. Fuhrman GM, Stieg FH, Buerk CA: Blunt laryngeal trauma: Classification and management protocol. *J Trauma* 1990; 30:87–92.

39. Gussack GS, Jurkovich GJ: Treatment dilemmas in laryngotracheal trauma. *J Trauma* 1988; 28:1439–1444.

40. Reece GP, Shatney CH: Blunt injuries of the cervical trachea: Review of 51 patients. *South Med J* 1988; 81:1542–1548.

41. Baumgarten RK, Carter CE, Reynolds WJ, et al: Priming with nondepolarizing relaxants for rapid tracheal intubation: A double-blind evaluation. *Can J Anaesth* 1988; 35:5–11.

42. Cicala R, Westbrook L: An alternative method of paralysis for rapid-sequence induction. *Anaesthesia* 1988; 69:983–986.

43. Ampel L, Hott KA, Sielaff GW, et al: An approach to airway management in the acutely head-injured patient. *J Emerg Med* 1988; 6:1–7.

44. Dronen SC, Merigian KS, Hedges JR, et al: A comparison of blind nasotracheal and succinylcholine-assisted intubation in the poisoned patient. *Ann Emerg Med* 1987; 16:650–652.

45. Hedges JR, Dronen SC, Feero S, et al: Succinylcholine-assisted intubations in prehospital care. *Ann Emerg Med* 1988; 17:469–472.

46. Talucci RC, Shaikh KA, Schwab CW: Rapid sequence induction with oral endotracheal intubation in the multiply injured patient. *Am Surg* 1988; 54:185–187.

47. Thompson JD, Fish S, Ruiz E: Succinylcholine for endotracheal intubation. *Ann Emerg Med* 1982; 11:526–529.

48. Hamill JF, Bedford RF, Weaver DC, et al: Lidocaine before endotracheal intubation: Intravenous or laryngotracheal? *Anaesthesia* 1981; 55:578–581.

49. McGillicuddy JE: Cerebral protection: Pathophysiology and treatment of increased intracranial pressure. *Chest* 1985; 87:85–93.

50. Minton MD, Grosslight K, Stirt JA, et al: Increases in intracranial pressure from succinylcholine: Prevention by prior nondepolarizing blockade. *Anaesthesiology* 1986; 65:165–169.

51. Stirt JA, Grosslight KR, Bedford RF, et al: "Defasciculation" with metocurine prevents succinylcholine-induced increases in intracranial pressure. *Anaesthesia* 1987; 67:50–53.

52. McNamara RM: Retrograde intubation of the trachea. *Ann Emerg Med* 1987; 16:680–682.

53. Delaney KA, Hessler R: Emergency flexible fiberoptic nasotracheal intubation: A report of 60 cases. *Ann Emerg Med* 1988; 17:919–926.

54. Campbell CT, Harris RC, Cook MH, et al: A new device for emergency percutaneous transtracheal ventilation in partial and complete airway obstruction. *Ann Emerg Med* 1988; 17:927–931.

55. Neff CC, Pfister RC, Van Sonnenberg E: Percutaneous transtracheal ventilation: Experimental and practical aspects. *J Trauma* 1983; 23:84–90.

56. Weymuller EA, Pavlin EG, Paugh D, et al: Management of difficult airway problems with percutaneous transtracheal ventilation. *Ann Otol Rhinol Laryngol* 1987; 96:34–37.

57. Yealy DM, Stewart RD, Kaplan RM: Myths and pitfalls in emergency translaryngeal ventilation: Correcting misimpressions. *Ann Emerg Med* 1988; 17:690–692.

58. Walls RM: Cricothyroidotomy. *Emerg Med Clin North Am* 1988; 6:725–735.

59. Erlandson MJ, Clinton JE, Ruiz E, et al: Cricothyrotomy in the emergency department revisited. *J Emerg Med* 1989; 7:115–118.

60. Miklus RM, Elliott C, Snow N: Surgical cricothyrotomy in the field: Experience of a helicopter transport team. *J Trauma* 1989; 29:506–508.

61. Spaite DW, Joseph M: Prehospital cricothyroidotomy: An investigation of indications, technique, complication, and patient outcome. *Ann Emerg Med* 1990; 19:279–285.

62. Fisher DM, Frewen T, Swedlow DB: Increase in intracranial pressure during suctioning—Stimulation vs. rise in $Paco_2$. *Anaesthesia* 1982; 57:416–417.

63. White PF, Schlobohm RM, Pitts LH, et al: A randomized study of drugs for preventing increases in intracranial pressure during endotracheal suctioning. *Anaesthesia* 1982; 57:242–244.

64. Yano M, Nishiyama H, Yokota H, et al: Effect of lidocaine on ICP response to endotracheal suctioning. *Anaesthesia* 1986; 64:651–653.
65. Majernick TG, Bieniek R, Houston JB, et al: Cervical spine movement during orotracheal intubation. *Ann Emerg Med* 1986; 15:417–420.
66. Boyd AD, Romita MC, Conlan AA, et al: A clinical evaluation of cricothyroidotomy. *Surg Gynecol Obstet* 1979; 149:365–368.
67. McGill J, Clinton JE, Ruiz E: Cricothyroidotomy in the emergency department. *Ann Emerg Med* 1982; 11:361–364.
68. Ravlo O, Bach V, Lybecker H, et al: A comparison between two emergency cricothyroidotomy instruments. *Acta Anaesthesiol Scand* 1987; 31:317–319.
69. Toye FJ, Weinstein JD: Clinical experience with percutaneous tracheostomy and cricothyroidotomy in 100 patients. 1986; 26:1034–1040.
70. Weiss S: A new emergency cricothyroidotomy instrument. *J Trauma* 1983; 23:155–157.
71. Adams F: Emergency intravenous sedation of the delirious, medically ill patient. *J Clin Psychiatry* 1988; 49(suppl):22–26.
72. Ayd FJ: Haloperidol: Twenty years clinical experience. *J Clin Psychiatry* 1978; 39:807–814.
73. Clinton JE, Sterner S, Steimachers A, et al: Haloperidol for sedation of disruptive emergency patients. *Ann Emerg Med* 1987; 16:319–322.
74. Silverstein S, Frommer DA, Marx JA, et al: Parenteral haloperidol in combative patients: A prospective study (abstract). Annual meeting of the University Association for Emergency Medicine, Portland, Ore, May 1–16, 1986.
75. Tesar GE, Murray GB, Cassem NH: Use of high-dose intravenous haloperidol in the treatment of agitated cardiac patients. *J Clin Psychopharmacol* 1985; 5:344–347.
76. Dudley DL, Rowlett DB, Loebel PJ: Emergency use of intravenous haloperidol. *Gen Hosp Psychiatry* 1979; 1:240–246.
77. Walls RM: The combative trauma patient: A paradigm of trauma leadership. *J Emerg Med* 1991; 9:67–68.

23

Massive Facial Trauma and Direct Neck Trauma

Stephen V. Cantrill, M.D.

Few situations evoke as much anxiety for an emergency physician as having to manage the airway of a patient with massive facial trauma or an actual or suspected neck injury. For those who have struggled through these situations, the memory remains vivid. These predicaments truly represent an opportunity for the emergency physician to make a significant impact upon the patient's potential outcome, but require the ultimate effort in rapid data acquisition and decision making.

Massive facial trauma is most often encountered as a result of motor vehicle accidents.[1] Auto-pedestrian and bicycle accidents also make up a significant percentage, especially in younger age groups.[2] The majority of patients suffering massive facial trauma will be male and in their 20s or 30s. These patients are often intoxicated, complicating their evaluation and treatment. Life-threatening concomitant injuries may accompany massive facial injuries, requiring rapid priority setting, evaluation, and treatment.

The major risks to the airway in patients with massive facial trauma are due to anatomic alteration of airway patency through bony disruption (e.g., nasal, maxillary, or mandibular fractures) or soft tissue swelling, and the increased potential for aspiration of body fluids or disrupted tissue (blood from epistaxis or intraoral trauma, saliva, teeth, etc.). The patient with massive facial trauma often presents a gruesome sight. The emergency physician must not, however, be distracted by the patient's presentation from the most immediate problem: the evaluation and care of the airway.

The neck is a marvel of construction. Encompassing the area from below the sternal notch to above the angle of the mandible, it is rife with vital structures, yet lacks a protective surrounding skeleton. This relative absence of protection places many structures at risk for injury. Vascular structures are particularly vulnerable owing to their number and location. Arterial structures at risk include the aortic arch, the common carotid, internal carotid, external carotid, subclavian, vertebral, and innominate arteries. Venous structures often injured include the internal jugular, the external jugular, the innominate, and the subclavian veins. Neurologic structures that may be injured include the spinal cord, the brachial plexus, and the vagus, phrenic, hypoglossal, spinal accessory, and recurrent laryngeal nerves. Other structures that may be injured include the pharynx, esophagus, larynx, trachea, lung, thyroid gland, hyoid bone, cervical vertebra, and the parotid and submandibular glands. Given their exposed positions, it is surprising that more injuries to these structures are not seen.

Of those tissues mentioned, injuries to the vascular structures along with the phrenic and recurrent laryngeal nerves, the pharynx, larynx, and the trachea will directly and immediately impact efforts made to secure a viable airway in the traumatized patient. Any of these structures may be injured by either a blunt or penetrating mechanism.

In this chapter, four specific classes of injuries are addressed: (1) massive facial trauma, (2) blunt neck trauma, (3) hanging and strangulation trauma, and (4) penetrating neck trauma. For each mechanism, three scenarios are presented: the "stable" patient, the deteriorating ("crashing") patient, and the moribund ("crashed") patient.

ANATOMY

Anatomy of the Face

It is mainly the areas of the mid- and lower face that are important when considering the airway. Anteriorly this area is composed of the nasal bones, the maxillary bones, and the mandible (Fig 23–1). Significant fractures involving these structures may compromise the airway, either directly through obstruction or indirectly through hemorrhage or soft tissue swelling. Maxillary fractures which can lead to airway compromise include the Le Fort II fracture, which involves the maxilla, nasal bones, and the medial aspects of the orbits, and the Le Fort III fracture in which the lower face is separated from the calvarium at the level of the orbits (Fig 23–2). Bilateral mandibular fractures may result in loss of support for the tongue, causing it to fall toward the back of the oropharynx, occluding the airway.

Anatomy of the Neck

The neck contains a vast array of crucial anatomic structures with the greatest concentration of vulnerable structures lying in the anterior portion. The most superficial and anterior muscle layer in this area is the platysma, beneath which runs the external jugular vein. Deep to this layer run the other muscle groups, including the sternocleidomastoid, sternohyoid, and sternothyroid. These muscles afford some protection to the deeper structures at the

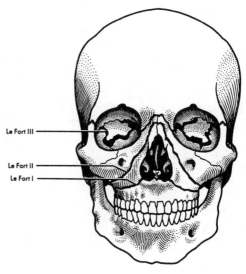

FIG 23–2.
Le Fort classification of facial fractures. Le Fort I: palate facial dysfunction. Le Fort II: pyramidal dysfunction. Le Fort III: craniofacial dysfunction. (From Rosen P, Baker FJ II, Barkin RM, et al (eds): *Emergency Medicine: Concepts and Clinical Practice,* ed 2. St Louis, Mosby–Year Book, Inc, 1988, p 408. Used by permission.)

base of the neck, but afford little protection in the more cephalad portion.

Anteriorly, progressing from cephalad to caudad along the midline of the neck, can be found the hyoid bone (opposite to C3), the thyroid cartilage (anterior to C4), the cricoid cartilage (anterior to C6), and the trachea, all encasing the airway (Fig 23–3). Any trauma to these structures can result in direct compromise of the airway. Continuing caudad, the isthmus of the thyroid gland is encountered, lying anterior to the second, third, and fourth tracheal rings. These rings, which maintain tracheal patency, are U-shaped, permitting compression (and therefore compromise) by force exerted posteriorly from external masses, such as hematoma or soft tissue swelling.

Posterior to the trachea lies the esophagus. The recurrent laryngeal nerves run immediately lateral to the esophagus, near the trachea. Lateral to the esophagus on either side is the carotid sheath, a fascial layer which surrounds the carotid artery (common and internal), the internal jugular vein, and the vagus nerve. Injury to these vessels may cause airway compromise through airway compression by a resulting hematoma. Interruption of the vagus or the superior laryngeal or recurrent laryngeal nerve branches of the vagus may compromise the airway by creating difficulty in swallowing (and therefore clearing secretions) or moving the vocal cords. In the area above the angle of the mandible, the glossopharyngeal (cranial nerve IX) and spinal accessory (XI)

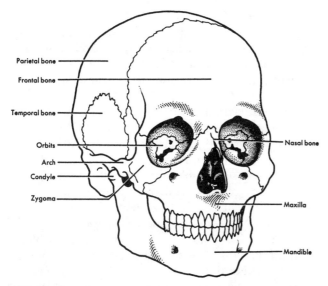

FIG 23–1.
Bones making up facial skeleton. (From Rosen P, Baker FJ II, Barkin RM, et al (eds): *Emergency Medicine: Concepts and Clinical Practice,* ed 2. St Louis, Mosby–Year Book, Inc, 1988, p 406. Used by permission.)

Parietal bone
Frontal bone
Temporal bone
Orbits
Arch
Condyle
Zygoma
Nasal bone
Maxilla
Mandible

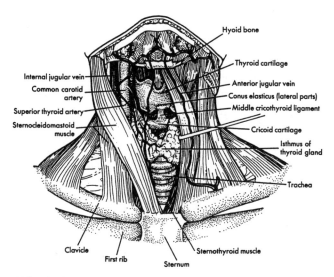

FIG 23–3.
Anterior aspect of neck with relative anatomic structures. (From Rosen P, Baker FJ II, Barkin RM, et al (eds): *Emergency Medicine: Concepts and Clinical Practice,* ed 2. St Louis, Mosby–Year Book, Inc, 1988. Used by permission.)

nerves run in close proximity to the vagus. Interruption of either of these may also compromise the airway by interfering with the swallowing mechanism. The hypoglossal nerve (XII) also runs in this area and innervates the intrinsic and extrinsic movements of the tongue. Disruption of this nerve may result in difficulty maintaining a patent airway owing to occlusion of the posterior oropharynx by the tongue.

Posterior to the carotid sheath lie the vertebral artery and vein. Lateral to these structures, in the lower part of the neck, lies the brachial plexus. Trauma to the upper section of the brachial plexus (area of C5) may injure the accessory phrenic nerve which gives variable motor innervation to the diaphragm. Superior to the brachial plexus lies the cervical plexus, composed of the anterior rami of the first four cervical nerves. The phrenic nerve, the major motor innervation of the diaphragm, arises from this plexus, running in proximity to the internal jugular vein. Injury to this nerve will cause obvious compromise in airflow via paralysis or paresis of the ipsilateral hemidiaphragm.

In the lower neck, the major vessels of the right innominate and subclavian arteries and veins, the left subclavian artery and vein, and the left innominate vein are present and vulnerable. Injury to any of these vessels may result in exsanguinating hemorrhage or hematoma formation which may cause airway obstruction by extension into the neck and compression of the trachea.

The bony support of the neck, the cervical spine,

protects the spinal cord, the disruption of which may have grave consequences for airflow. Injury to the spinal cord in the area of the lower neck may compromise air exchange via interruption of intercostal muscle activity, resulting in diaphragmatic ("abdominal") breathing. *Interruption of the cervical spinal cord at the level of C4 or above will result in cessation of all spontaneous breathing efforts, causing a respiratory death unless immediate intervention and support are initiated.*

MASSIVE FACIAL TRAUMA

The patient presenting with presumably isolated massive facial trauma can be an airway disaster waiting to happen. These patients may have several threats to their normal airflow. A nasal fracture and accompanying epistaxis may deprive them of their normal nasal air path. The accumulation of saliva or blood from epistaxis or other oropharyngeal lacerations may increase the level of airflow obstruction. Dislodged teeth may be present in the oropharynx and cause obstruction. Because it is standard practice to immobilize the cervical spine of these patients in a supine position until a cervical spine fracture has been excluded, active effort is required on the part of the patient to avoid having the tongue interfere with airflow. This may be difficult for the patient to accomplish in the presence of a mandibular fracture, which can rob the tongue of its support, leaving it free to fall posteriorly, occluding the posterior oropharynx.

Aspiration is always a risk in patients with massive facial trauma, especially early in their evaluation while the cervical spine is immobilized. In the supine position, the patient may not be able to adequately deal with the rate of fluid collection in the oropharynx, resulting in aspiration. Teeth or denture material that were dislodged as a result of the trauma also represent a high risk for aspiration. Aspiration of vomitus is always a potential problem. Trauma patients may vomit at any time owing to previous (excessive) ethanol ingestion or gastric irritation induced by swallowing large amounts of blood.

In cases of isolated massive facial trauma, impairment of ventilation and oxygenation is due to disruption of airflow and aspiration. If ventilatory or oxygenation problems are present without evidence of obstruction, other associated injuries must be sought in an expeditious fashion. In this case, the patient does *not* have *isolated* facial trauma, but rather is actually a multiple trauma patient requiring complete evaluation.

Stability

As with all trauma patients the stability of the airway will be dependent on the type and urgency of intervention required. Although many patients with massive facial trauma may present as stable—alert, moving air easily, with a stable mandible and tongue, an airway free of debris, secretions, and hematoma or edema—the physician must never completely relax as deterioration may occur without warning. Defining the crashing patient is more straightforward as it becomes evident that the patient is having difficulty or is unable to protect his or her airway. Most often a combination of factors will produce these unstable conditions: decreasing level of consciousness, massive pooling of blood, loss of tongue support, etc. The patient that has crashed has upper airway obstruction and has suffered from a respiratory arrest or arrest is imminent. Obstruction may be from any one of the causes enumerated earlier in this paragraph. An algorithm for management of massive facial trauma is presented in Figure 23–4.

Scenario 1: The Stable Patient: Massive Facial Trauma Without Airway Compromise

Airway treatment in the stable patient with isolated massive facial trauma is straightforward. Pa-

tients who are conscious and alert with massive facial trauma will attempt, if possible, to assume the position which gives them an unobstructed airway. This is most often a sitting position leaning forward. Unfortunately, if there is concern about the integrity of the cervical spine, the patient is prohibited from assuming this position. If radiographic clearance of the cervical spine is indicated, then the process must be expedited and the patient carefully monitored until this has been accomplished. Once the cervical spine has been cleared, the patient should be allowed to assume the position of maximum comfort.

In the patient with massive facial trauma, part of the early evaluation should be to assess the presence of any material, either native (teeth) or foreign (denture material), which may be obstructing the posterior oropharynx. If missing teeth or denture material cannot be accounted for, they must be assumed to have been aspirated or lodged in the posterior hypopharynx until this is radiographically disproved. In the cooperative patient, potential obstruction of the airway by body fluids may be ameliorated by providing the patient with a Yankauer (tonsil) suction catheter and instructing him or her on its use in suctioning the oropharynx. In cases of massive, unresolving epistaxis, immediate attention to achieving hemostasis is warranted through the placement of a nasal pack.

In the stable patient with facial trauma, ventilation and oxygenation are usually normal. However,

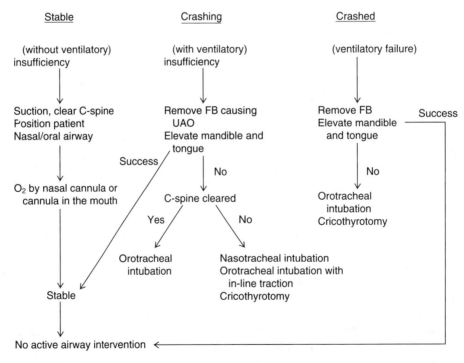

FIG 23–4.
Algorithm for airway management of massive facial trauma. *C-spine* = cervical spine; *FB* = fiberoptic bronchoscope; *UAO* = upper airway obstruction.

supplemental oxygen via nasal cannula is still warranted, as airway compromise may develop during the patient's evaluation and treatment in the emergency department. In those cases where nasal airflow is compromised, the cannula should be placed in the mouth to augment the patient's fractional concentration of oxygen in inspired gas (FiO_2).

As with all patients who are stable, but who represent a potential airway management problem, part of the initial intervention should be planning what to do if the patient should deteriorate. In the patient with massive facial trauma, a careful physical examination will assist in that process. Presence of a nasal fracture or any evidence of a possible basilar skull fracture (cerebrospinal fluid rhinorrhea, raccoon eyes, midface mobility when grasping the upper incisors) argues against the use of nasotracheal intubation. Attempting to pass an endotracheal tube through a nose with distorted anatomy could increase the injury. Nasal intubation in the face of a basilar skull fracture creates the risk, although small, of intracranial penetration by the endotracheal tube.[3] Mandibular fractures are not a contraindication to oral intubation. In fact, the presence of a mandibular fracture may make oral intubation technically easier, although it can be impossible to obtain the necessary seal for bag-mask ventilation of a patient with such an injury.

After assessing the patient and planning the approach for possible active airway management, the necessary implements should be acquired and made ready, if this has not already been done.

Scenario 2: The Crashing Patient: Massive Facial Trauma With Respiratory Distress

The patient with massive facial trauma in respiratory distress represents an imminent airway disaster. The challenge to the emergency physician is to expeditiously evaluate the cause of the airway distress and deal with the problem. As noted above, obstruction to airflow may be present due to the accumulation of body fluids in the posterior hypopharynx. Airflow may also be occluded by teeth, foreign material, or by the tongue simply falling to the back of the oropharynx. Aspiration may have already occurred, resulting either directly or indirectly (via laryngospasm) in compromise of ventilation and oxygenation.

The intervention in patients with massive facial trauma with respiratory distress is straightforward: actively manage the patient's airway as quickly as possible. The first step is to evaluate the patient for airway obstruction, correcting the problem if possible: open the mouth and elevate the mandible by grasping the symphysis and lifting. In the case of a severe mandible fracture, this may alleviate the obstruction. Sweep the mouth of any foreign material

and use a Yankauer suction catheter to remove any liquid material from the posterior oropharynx. (Two or more catheters may be needed in cases of extremely brisk bleeding.) Concurrent with these actions, the patient should be placed on a cardiac monitor and, if possible, a pulse oximeter. If excessive, unchecked epistaxis is present, the situation may be somewhat improved by quickly occluding the posterior nasopharynx with an intranasal balloon device or a Foley catheter inflated with saline. This may not stop the epistaxis, but should decrease the amount of blood in the hypopharynx.

At this time, an oral airway should be inserted and the patient's mouth and ventilations assisted with a bag-valve-mask on 100% oxygen. Getting the mask to seal well around the mouth may be a problem, especially if the patient has sustained a midface or mandibular fracture. This problem can often be solved by having one person hold the mask with two hands around the patient's face and jaw while a second person does the actual bagging.

The decision must then be made as to how endotracheal intubation should be attempted. Nasotracheal intubation (either "blind" or over a fiberoptic intubating bronchoscope or a lighted stylet) is an option if it is not excluded by the presence of a nasal, midface, or basilar skull fracture or excessive bleeding into the oropharynx. If this approach is attempted prior to excluding cervical spine injury, the patient's neck should remain immobilized and the position of the head must not be altered during the procedure. If the integrity of the cervical spine has been established, orotracheal intubation may be attempted. If integrity has not been established, current thinking is that oral intubation may be accomplished with some degree of safety if in-line stabilization of the head, neck, and shoulders is carefully maintained throughout the procedure (see Chapter 22, for a discussion of this subject). Cricothyrotomy is also an option in this situation, and has the advantage of permitting bag-valve ventilatory assistance during performance of the procedure. Oral fiberoptic intubation, retrograde wire-guided intubation, and lighted stylet intubation are possible options. Percutaneous transtracheal ventilation (PTV) is also a possibility, but this should only be considered as a temporizing measure.

If oral intubation is elected, an additional complication is present if the trauma makes it impossible for the patient to receive bag-valve-mask ventilation (e.g., midface instability or mandibular fracture). In this situation, paralysis via rapid-sequence induction is relatively contraindicated. Should the intubation attempt fail, the emergency physician will have no way to ventilate the patient. Mild sedation with a short-acting benzodiazepine or barbiturate (see Chapter 14) may allow an awake oral intubation to be performed. In the rare instance where rapid-sequence induction is to be used under these circumstances, the neck should be prepared and a team should be present (with the necessary implements in hand) to perform an immediate cricothyrotomy if any difficulties are encountered with the intubation.

Scenario 3: The Crashed Patient: Massive Facial Trauma in Respiratory Arrest

The crashed patient with massive facial trauma presenting in respiratory arrest represents an airway disaster that has occurred. Only the most rapid and aggressive approach to airway management can wrest this situation from its most common outcome: death. This patient may still succumb to associated injuries, but this scenario often represents a potentially avoidable airway demise.

The threats to the patient's airway, in terms of obstruction of airflow, aspiration, and problems with ventilation and oxygenation, were discussed in the previous section and will not be enumerated here. The intervention must be quick and decisive. The approach is initially the same as in the crashing patient with massive facial trauma in terms of clearing the airway and attempting to establish ventilation with a bag-valve-mask. However, in this circumstance there is no time for any possible radiographic evaluation of the cervical spine. If the cervical spine is not felt to be at risk in this situation (which is rarely the case), orotracheal intubation should be attempted. If the cervical spine has not been cleared, oral intubation with in-line stabilization of the head, neck, and shoulders may be attempted or an immediate cricothyrotomy should be performed.

BLUNT NECK TRAUMA AND HANGING AND STRANGULATION INJURIES

Blunt Trauma

Blunt trauma to the neck may result in minor contusion or abrasion with no impact on the airway or it can produce life-threatening destruction of the larynx and surrounding tissues. Laryngotracheal trauma is one of the most common injuries associated with blunt neck trauma, and poses multiple immediate potential airflow problems. An injury to this area may result in a hematoma which can compress and distort the anatomy of the trachea or larynx. Supraglottic, glottic, and subglottic injuries may occur which compromise airflow: avulsion of the epiglottis; avulsion of the false vocal cords; thyroid cartilage fracture; avulsion of the true vocal cords; vocal cord paralysis due to local disruption or recurrent laryngeal nerve injury; tracheal separation from the cricoid cartilage; mucosal tears; subglottic edema; sub-

glottic hematoma formation; and esophageal tears.[4] Thyroid cartilage fractures and esophageal tears may cause the development of expanding emphysema in the neck, further compromising airflow. Laryngotracheal injury may also result in hemoptysis which, on occasion, can be massive. Resultant accumulation of blood and edema in the laryngeal submucosa can cause stridor that can progress to complete airway obstruction. It is important to note that many of these life-threatening injuries may exist without any evidence of external neck trauma.[5]

Aspiration, while always a risk, is not as significant a problem with blunt neck trauma as it is with massive facial trauma. Aspiration of blood is a concern in those cases in which massive hemoptysis is present. Aspiration of saliva may be a problem owing to the patient's inability to handle normal secretions secondary to dysphagia, which is commonly seen with blunt neck trauma. As with all other trauma patients, aspiration of vomitus is a potential problem, again complicated by the necessity for prophylactic cervical spine immobilization.

Ventilation and oxygenation difficulties may be seen as a result of any of the problems mentioned above. When ventilation problems are encountered, however, a pneumothorax must be suspected. This may result from the dissection of air along the respiratory tree from a tear in the trachea or larynx. Hanging and strangulation patients may develop ventilatory difficulty from noncardiac pulmonary edema secondary to severe anoxic brain injury.

Hanging and Strangulation

Hangings and strangulations result in approximately 3,500 deaths each year in the United States.[6] These may be classified by mechanism and by the setting in which the patient is found.[7] The possible mechanisms include hanging (partial or complete suspension of the body from the neck—the most common), ligature strangulation, manual strangulation, and postural strangulation (the neck placed over an object with body weight causing pressure on the neck—seen usually in very young children). Classification is also possible based on the setting: suicidal, accidental, homicidal, or (in the past) judicial, with the majority being a suicide setting. Information concerning the setting is important since it is usually only the judicial hanging that results in significant cervical spine or spinal cord injury. In this type of hanging, the subject is forced to fall at least one body length before having downward progress suddenly halted. This creates a significant distraction force at the level of the noose, with resultant fracture of the spine or fracture of the base of the skull and subsequent spinal cord disruption. These injuries are very rare in other forms of hanging (less than 1% in one study[8]) because of the short fall and subsequent small deceleration impulse.

Death in hangings involving a fall greater than body height is due to disruption of the upper cervical spinal cord or brain stem. In these cases, the pharynx and carotid arteries are often also injured. Unconsciousness is immediate, but full cardiopulmonary arrest may not occur for up to 15 minutes. The sequence of events leading to death is less clear with other mechanisms. Simple asphyxiation is not the major cause (as once was believed) as evidenced by successful suicides by persons with tracheostomy sites below the ligature and the frequent finding of vomitus in the tracheobronchial tree of victims of suicidal hangings. Current evidence indicates that the sequence of events culminating in death in most nonjudicial hangings and strangulations begins with obstruction of venous return from the head. This results in stagnant hypoxia, leading to loss of consciousness. This in turn results in decreased muscle tone with subsequent arterial occlusion, airway obstruction, and death.[9]

In patients presenting after nonfatal hanging or strangulation, injuries to the thyroid cartilage or the hyoid bone may be seen, but are often not of clinical significance. A small percentage may also sustain minor injuries to the carotid arteries. Tardieu's spots, petechial hemorrhages of the skin and subconjunctival tissues, may be seen as a result of venous occlusion. Patients that are conscious after their injury may present with aphonia, dysphonia, or dysphagia. Superficial injuries of the neck are sometimes seen as a result of the direct trauma. Patients that survive the initial injury but subsequently succumb most often do so because of pulmonary edema or bronchopneumonia which develops during their hospital course.[9]

Stability

Patients with isolated blunt trauma to the neck will often present with a stable airway. Air will be moving easily without evidence of obstruction. Stability also implies that the anatomy of the neck is near normal. Minor ecchymosis or edema may be present but without evidence that it is progressing. Slight hoarseness and small amounts of subcutaneous air may be present without impacting the airway. Once again the unstable, crashing patient is easier to

define as threats to airflow become greater. Any factors which produce stridor (obstruction) or distort neck anatomy qualify as deteriorating or unstable conditions. Progression of swelling, hoarseness, or subcutaneous emphysema may exist alone or in concert to cause rapid deterioration. The crashed patient has obstructed the airway from massive damage to tissues in the neck. Blood, air, edema, and distorted anatomy combine to obstruct airflow. Crashed patients may be making respiratory efforts but arrest is imminent. An algorithm for management of neck trauma is presented in Figure 23–5.

Scenario 1: The Stable Patient: Blunt Neck Trauma With No Acute Airway Distress

Similar to the stable patient with massive facial trauma, the patient who has sustained blunt neck trauma and arrives without airway compromise may, during the stay in the emergency department, deteriorate into a true airway challenge. The patient who has survived the initial insult from hanging or strangulation can present anywhere on the spectrum from asymptomatic to unconscious. These patients all warrant careful evaluation and monitoring until it can be assured that the natural history of the injury will not mandate active airway management.

Airway management in the blunt neck trauma patient who shows no signs of respiratory compromise is supportive and expectant. Airflow should be carefully monitored for evidence of deterioration during the patient's stay in the emergency department. Patients with dysphagia may be more comfortable using a suction catheter to rid themselves of their normal accumulating secretions. As with all major trauma patients, ventilatory augmentation with oxygen administered by nasal cannula is appropriate. Rapid evaluation of the cervical spine is also indicated to ensure safety with orotracheal intubation should active airway management become necessary.

Most important, in stable patients with blunt neck trauma it is necessary to be aware of what signs and symptoms to watch for that would be indicators for active airway management. Absolute indications include stridor, severe subcutaneous emphysema, rapidly expanding neck hematoma, severe or progressive hoarseness, respiratory distress not resolved by correction of lower respiratory tract disorders (e.g., pneumothorax), and agitation due to hypoxia.[10] Relative indications for active airway intervention include slight hoarseness, a small amount of subcutaneous emphysema, and a small neck hematoma. In these cases, the patient must be monitored constantly and ongoing consideration given to eventual intubation. If any worsening in the patient's condition is noted (e.g., increase in hematoma size or degree of hoarseness), the emergency physician should

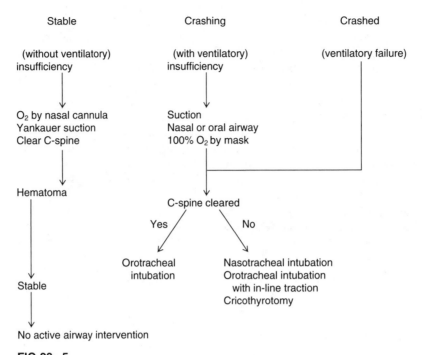

FIG 23–5.
Algorithm for airway mangement of neck trauma. *C-spine* = cervical spine.

proceed with active airway management. Any delay could result in having to manage a severely compromised airway, a problem which could have been avoided by more aggressive intervention earlier.

The unconscious, stable posthanging or poststrangulation patient is likely to be suffering from anoxic cerebral injury and therefore active airway management is mandated to avoid potential aspiration and to treat increased intracranial pressure and any developing pulmonary edema. High-flow oxygen should be supplied to the patient and cervical spine radiographs obtained, if indicated by the mechanism of injury. Intubation may then proceed. Orotracheal intubation is probably the best approach, allowing the operator to observe and avoid any potential disrupted anatomy from the hanging or strangulation. A comatose patient should have the airway managed quickly, as the patient can become more responsive and combative as time passes, complicating the procedure. If orotracheal intubation is not technically possible owing to anatomic disruption, a semielective surgical airway should be established. After intubation, these patients should be hyperventilated. Developing pulmonary edema can be treated with positive end-expiratory pressure (PEEP) (see Chapter 30).

Scenario 2: The Crashing Patient: Blunt Neck Trauma With Respiratory Distress

The crashing patient with blunt neck trauma represents a true airway emergency. Temporizing mea-

sures will buy little; definitive airway management must be carried out with dispatch.

The airway threats from blunt neck trauma have been enumerated above. In terms of intervention, the upper airway should be checked for obstruction due to blood or saliva, using suction as necessary. An oral or nasopharyngeal airway should be placed and 100% oxygen administered to the patient via bag-valve-mask (although this may worsen any subcutaneous emphysema, if present). Presence of a pneumothorax should be considered and treated if suspected. The patient's anterior neck should be prepared for the possibility of a surgical airway. Again, the decision must be made as to whether time permits clearing the cervical spine, providing added safety with orotracheal intubation. The options for active airway management should then be considered: orotracheal intubation is the initial procedure of choice if cervical spine injury has been excluded. Evaluation of the prehospital history should indicate to the emergency physician the degree of risk of a cervical spine injury being present if the patient was involved in a hanging. If the mechanism did not involve a drop of at least body height, the likelihood of a concomitant bony injury is low. If the cervical spine has not been evaluated and the risk of fracture is believed to be low, it is the opinion of many that orotracheal intubation can proceed after establishing careful in-line head, neck, and shoulder stabilization. Nasotracheal intubation may be attempted in the nonapneic patient who does not have extensive facial trauma. Yet concern for exacerbating injuries to structures in the neck with blind nasotracheal intubation requires the practitioner to proceed with caution. Cricothyrotomy may be utilized if the oral or nasal approaches are contraindicated or attempts to use them fail. This may be technically an extremely difficult procedure if there is alteration of the normal landmarks of the neck by swelling or hematoma. Some prefer to perform a tracheostomy in this setting,[11] although this can also be difficult and time-consuming. This procedure, however, may be the only option for active airway management if an injury is present below the cricoid cartilage. If orotracheal intubation is attempted, rapid-sequence induction is often required in the agitated patient.

Variations of the above approaches (oral or nasal fiberoptic intubation, retrograde wire-guided intubation, etc.) may also be considered if the equipment and expertise are readily available and the procedure can be rapidly performed. PTV should be considered as a temporizing measure if all other approaches have failed and the patient becomes apneic, has no injuries below the cricothyroid membrane, and has no complete upper airway obstruction.

After establishment of the airway, the patient should be hyperventilated on 100% oxygen. Tube placement should, of course, be evaluated radiographically. This must be followed by assessment of respiratory status via arterial blood gases. If hypooxygenation is detected, noncardiac pulmonary edema should be suspected. In this case, oxygenation may be improved by ventilating the patient with PEEP, although it is unclear if this has any long-term positive effect on outcome. If a spinal cord injury is present, administration of steroids may be indicated.[12]

Scenario 3: The Crashed Patient: Blunt Neck Trauma in Respiratory Arrest

Even more than the patient with massive facial trauma in respiratory arrest, the patient with blunt neck trauma in respiratory arrest has an extremely poor prognosis. The approach to this patient should be the same as that with the blunt neck trauma patient with respiratory distress in terms of clearing the airway and attempting to ventilate the patient. The patient should then be immediately orally intubated while simultaneous preparations are made for a potential cricothyrotomy. If the cervical spine has not been cleared prior to attempts at oral intubation, this procedure should be done with in-line stabilization of the head, neck, and shoulders.

PENETRATING NECK TRAUMA

Patients with penetrating trauma to the neck often appear deceivingly stable at the time of their arrival in the emergency department, especially if the prehospital time has been short, only to rapidly decompensate. In all but the most minor injuries, active airway intervention must be prepared for and implemented early in the patient's course.

The mechanism of injury should alert the emergency physician to be watchful. Gunshot wounds, especially from high-velocity weapons (AK-47, M-16) or with dum-dum or frangible bullets, have a higher likelihood of causing indirect injury owing to the kinetic energy imparted to the surrounding area.[13] This is also true of shotgun injuries at close range.[14, 15]

The most common cause of disruption of airflow in the patient sustaining penetrating neck trauma is by hematoma formation with subsequent compression of the trachea or hypopharynx. Anatomic disruption of the airway via direct laryngotracheal trauma may also cause disruption of airflow. Although not common, nerve injury can disrupt airflow via injury to either the phrenic or recurrent laryngeal nerves. Any wound which penetrates the esophagus, trachea, or hypopharyngeal areas may result in injection of air into the soft tissues of the neck which further compromises airflow. As noted for blunt neck trauma, the accumulation of blood and edema in the laryngeal submucosal area may produce stridor and subsequent complete airway obstruction.

Concerns of aspiration and vomiting are the same as in prior neck trauma scenarios. The risk in patients with penetrating trauma may be somewhat greater because of the extent of anatomic disruption. Threats to ventilation and oxygenation are also similar to those described earlier. Yet the likelihood of a pneumothorax, hemothorax, or both, resulting in problems with ventilation are greater. This is especially true with a penetrating injury in zone I of the neck, the area below the cricoid cartilage. In this instance, direct violation of the pleural cavity or of the subclavian vessels is of high potential. Dissection of air down the neck into the lower respiratory tree may also cause a pneumothorax.

Scenarios

Definitions of various stages of stability are similar to patients with blunt neck injuries. The major difference is that stability is more tenuous in this group and a more expectant aggressive posture is required.

The Stable Patient: Penetrating Neck Trauma With No Acute Airway Distress

More than with any other stable patient with facial or neck trauma, it is the stable patient with a penetrating neck injury who is the most worrisome and the most likely to deteriorate into the stage of respiratory distress. The management of the airway in the stable patient with penetrating neck trauma requires careful observation with willingness to actively manage the airway at the slightest provocation. Many emergency physicians seriously consider prophylactic active airway management in these patients, since the actual magnitude of the injury may be initially masked by the innocuous appearance of the wound, especially if the time since injury has been short. This does not mean that every patient with a scratch on the neck is intubated, but rather, that one's threshold for airway intervention should be the lowest of all stable patients.

Stable patients with penetrating neck trauma must have their airflow carefully monitored and their secretions attended to. Administration of oxygen by nasal cannula is advisable. The initial appearance of the wound and the patient as a whole must not lull the emergency physician into a false sense of security. Many cases presenting as innocent neck wounds have subsequently ended up as airway disasters. At the first indication of any respiratory distress following penetrating neck injury, active airway management must be implemented. This includes evidence of expanding neck hematoma, stridor, hoarseness, significant subcutaneous emphysema, or any obvious signs of hypoxia. The presence of any hematoma in the neck is cause for concern. Prophylactic active airway management should be considered if there is *any* increase in the size of the hematoma. Cervical spine immobilization must not interfere with treatment and evaluation of these patients. Penetrating injuries of the bony spine are rarely unstable and immobilization may make definitive management more difficult.[14–16]

An additional reason for the increased level of concern with these patients is the necessary course of their emergent evaluation: they often will require angiographic evaluation of the neck vessels, requiring an extended period of time outside of the emergency department in a relatively uncontrolled and unmonitored environment. A darkened angiographic suite is a difficult place to have to actively manage a deteriorating airway. Prophylactic intubation in a more controlled setting prior to leaving for angiography should be seriously considered.

The Crashing Patient: Penetrating Neck Trauma With Respiratory Distress

The patient with respiratory distress due to penetrating neck trauma represents one of the most anxiety-provoking situations encountered in the emergency department. This crashing patient is on a precipitous downhill course that requires immediate intervention for patient salvage. These patients often have isolated injuries and are therefore conscious but markedly agitated owing to their impending (or already present) hypoxic state. Speed and carefully orchestrated efforts of the trauma team are of the utmost importance.

The causes of potential airway distress have been covered above. Simultaneous actions include placement of the patient on 100% oxygen, attachment to a cardiac monitor (and pulse oximeter, if possible), and immediate assessment of the airway. The patient's neck should also be prepared at this time for a potential surgical airway.

Most often, the cause of this airway compromise will be immediately obvious: a large hematoma of the neck. If this is not the case, more subtle causes such as blood or vomitus in the pharynx or pneumothorax should be sought. The posterior oropharynx should be suctioned free of liquid. Massive hemorrhage may be discovered, mandating the use of multiple Yankauer suction catheters. Orotracheal intubation should then immediately be attempted.[14] Rapid-sequence induction is an option, but may complicate the situation by removing what little respiratory drive is present. During intubation, the patient's heart rate, and, if possible, his or her oxygen saturation, should be monitored. Frequently in these situations, the emergency physician will encounter markedly distorted anatomy upon passing the laryngoscope, adding further difficulty to the situation. In these cases, it should be appreciated that excessive attempts at oral intubation will not improve the likelihood of success and the decision to move quickly to a surgical airway should be made. Cricothyrotomy, although difficult in these cases, may represent the only possible approach for patient airway salvage. If the injury is below the cricoid cartilage, a more difficult (and time-consuming) tracheostomy may be necessary and lifesaving. Wire-guided retrograde intubation may be attempted with difficulty but fiberoptic intubation has little utility in this setting owing to the disruption of anatomic landmarks and the presence of copious amounts of blood. PTV is contraindicated if any possibility of upper airway obstruction exists. Nasotracheal intubation is an option, although there is a theoretical potential for exacerbating any already existent penetrating injury in the hypopharynx.

If, after active airway management, the patient with penetrating neck injury continues to have difficulty with ventilation or oxygenation, pneumothorax must be immediately considered. If this is a significant problem, immediate chest tube placement should be undertaken.

The Crashed Patient: Penetrating Neck Trauma in Respiratory Arrest

The patient with penetrating neck trauma in respiratory arrest can be salvaged only through the most heroic of measures. The approach to this patient is the same as that to the crashing patient, with a few caveats. First, bag-valve-mask ventilation may be impossible owing to injury-caused airway obstruction. If the patient cannot be bagged, move quickly on to intubation. Initial attempts at orotracheal intubation may reveal grossly distorted anatomy, precluding this approach to active airway management. During the emergency physician's attempts at oral intubation, others should be preparing the neck for a surgical airway. If oral intubation is not immediately successful, attempts should be made to establish an airway surgically.

In these cases, the emergency physician's efforts may be truly lifesaving. Many patients are alive today who arrived in the emergency department in respiratory arrest but who were saved by the timely airway intervention performed by an emergency physician. Patients with neck and facial injuries present the emergency physician with among the most difficult of airway challenges. Understanding the potential for airway problems and having a full grasp of the technical options available will assist the emergency physician in dealing successfully with these challenging patients.

REFERENCES

1. Davidoff G, Jakubowski M, Thomas D, et al: The spectrum of closed-head injuries in facial trauma victims: Incidence and impact. *Ann Emerg Med* 1988; 17:6–9.

2. Haymond C, Nicholson C, Kiyak A, et al: Age differences in responses to facial trauma. *Special Care Dent* 1988; 8:115–221.

3. Donnelly WH: Histopathology of endotracheal intubation. *Arch Pathol* 1969; 88:511.

4. Reece GP, Shatney CH: Blunt injuries of the cervical trachea: Review of 51 patients. *South Med J* 1988; 81:1542–1548.

5. Myers EM, Iko BO: The management of acute laryngeal trauma. *J Trauma* 1987; 27:448–452.

6. *Statistical Abstract of the United States,* ed 101. Washington, DC, US Bureau of the Census, 1980, pp 178, 187.

7. Iserson KV: Strangulation: A review of ligature, manual, and postural neck compression injuries. *Ann Emerg Med* 1984; 13:179–185.

8. Sen Gupta BK: Studies on 101 cases of death due to hanging. *J Indian Med Assoc* 1965; 45:135–140.

9. Fishman CM, Goldstein MS, Gardner LB: Suicidal hanging: An association with the adult respiratory distress' syndrome. *Chest* 1977; 71:225–227.

10. Flancbaum L, Wright J, Trooskin SZ, et al: Orotracheal intubation in suspected laryngeal injuries. *Am J Emerg Med* 1986; 4:167–169.

11. Schaefer SD, Close LG: Acute management of laryngeal trauma: Update. *Ann Otol Rhinol Laryngol* 1989; 98:98–104.

12. Bracken MB, Shepard MJ, Collins WF, et al: A randomized, controlled trial of methylprednisolone or naloxone in the treatment of acute spinal-cord injury. Results of the Second National Acute Spinal Cord Injury Study. *N Engl J Med* 1990; 322:1405–1411.

13. Sykes LN Jr, Champion HR, Fouty WJ: Dum-dums, hollow-points, and devastators: Techniques designed to increase wounding potential of bullets. *J Trauma* 1988; 28:618–623.

14. Wilson J: Shotgun ballistics and shotgun injuries. *West J Med* 1978; 129:149.

15. Kupcha PC, An HS, Cotler JM: Gunshot wounds to the cervical spine. *Spine* 1990; 15:1058–1063.

16. Arishita GI, Vayer JS, Bellamy RF: Cervical spine immobilization of penetrating neck wounds in a hostile environment. *J Trauma* 1989; 29:332–337.

24

Increased Intracranial Pressure

Michael F. Murphy, M.D., F.R.C.P.C.

When and how to manage the airway is of paramount importance in the patient with an intracranial pathologic condition. On the one hand, the issues of airway patency, airway protection, and ventilation and oxygenation must be addressed. On the other hand, the clinician may believe that active intervention is required as a therapeutic maneuver to reduce arterial carbon dioxide partial pressure ($PaCO_2$) and intracranial pressure (ICP). Most often the distinctions are blurred and the intervention is indicated for *all* of these reasons.

It has long been recognized that laryngoscopy and endotracheal intubation produce a sympathetic response characterized by tachycardia, hypertension, and elevations in ICP.[1] This response has been shown to produce neurologic deterioration and jeopardize outcome.[2] Pharmacologic intervention, coupled with aggressive management of hypoxia, hypercarbia, hypotension, and acidosis are indicated to optimize the neurologic outcome.

The relationship between airway management and neurologic compromise is complex. The neurologic compromise may be due to any number of medical or surgical conditions such as meningitis, brain tumors, or trauma. Although the clinical scenarios are many and varied, the emergency physician must not only recognize when to intervene, but how to intervene. The "when" is an amalgamation of clinical acumen, experience, and an adequate database. When do you intubate and hyperventilate the head-injured patient with a decreased level of consciousness, but intact airway protective reflexes?

Other questions arise: Is the cervical spine intact? What is the pace of deterioration? What is my skill level in securing an airway? Will I do more damage than good by intervening now? Do I need to transfer the patient to another facility? Or to the computed tomography (CT) scanner? Is paralysis necessary to facilitate investigations, management, or ICP control? Finally, if I do need to intervene in the airway, how do I minimize the adverse effects on the central nervous system (CNS)?

The goal of this chapter is to establish, expand, or reinforce a database that allows rational clinical decision making in the setting of the patient with an elevated ICP requiring endotracheal intubation. Much of the discussion utilizes head trauma as a model owing to its frequency of presentation. However, the principles of airway management and neurologic preservation apply equally to medical and traumatic conditions.

It is estimated that more than 1 million Americans sustain major closed head injuries each year.[3] In most published series on trauma, head injuries account for half the fatalities, over 5 million days of hospitalization, and over 30 million days of lost work annually in the United States.[4] The frequency of the problem coupled with the potential for appropriate early care to optimize neurologic outcome presents an enormous challenge to emergency physicians. In fact, it has been demonstrated that appropriate emergency care can reduce the mortality of acute severe head injury by as much as 52%.[5] Effective management of the head-injured patient is predicated upon the early identification of surgically correctable mass lesions and the mitigation of further neuronal injury by hypoxia, hypercarbia, hypotension, and elevations in ICP. The deleterious influence of hypoxia, hypercarbia, and endotracheal intubation on ICP are well-known, and an appropriate focus for this chapter.

Optimum outcome of the patient with CNS compromise is dependent upon the emergency physician having a firm grasp of the physiology, pathophysiology, and principles of management of elevated ICP, particularly as it relates to active airway intervention.

PHYSIOLOGY

Neurons are the primary functional units of the brain and spinal cord, and are the focus of efforts to maintain CNS integrity. Their function is dependent upon a continuous supply of glucose and oxygen and the removal of metabolic by-products. Ischemia results when blood flow is inadequate to meet the metabolic demands of brain tissue, leading to potentially irreversible neuronal damage. Brain stores of oxygen and glucose are minimal, highlighting the critical nature of adequate cerebral blood flow (CBF) and continuous substrate supply. The CBF below which cerebral ischemia occurs is termed the *critical cerebral blood flow*.[6]

CBF and ICP are intimately related.

Ohm's law:

$$I = V/R$$

where I = amperage (flow)
V = voltage (pressure)
R = resistance (ohms)

Hemodynamic application

$$Q = \delta P/R$$

where Q = flow
δP = pressure gradient
R = resistance

Cerebral blood flow (CBF)

$$CBF = CPP/CVR$$

where CPP = cerebral perfusion pressure
CVR = cerebrovascular resistance
CPP = MAP − ICP
MAP = mean arterial pressure
= diastolic pressure
+ ⅓ pulse pressure (PP)

CBF is directly proportional to the driving pressure across the cerebrovascular bed (cerebral perfusion pressure, CPP), and inversely proportional to the cerebrovascular resistance (CVR). CPP, in turn, is determined by the mean arterial pressure (MAP) less the ICP.[7, 8]

ICP is a distinct parameter produced by a complex interplay between arterial pressure and intracranial volume. An elevation in ICP, for whatever reason, may lead to a reduction in cerebral perfusion. Should flow fall below critical CBF, ischemia

results. In extreme circumstances ICP may exceed MAP, virtually eliminating CBF. Permanent and lethal neurologic injury may result. Now let us analyze in more detail CBF, intracranial volume, and ICP.

A number of mechanisms serve to regulate CBF in normal brain.[9] By and large, these control mechanisms predominantly affect CVR and rely on the organism to supply an adequate head of pressure to allow perfusion. It is important to appreciate that these mechanisms may fail, to varying degrees, in ill or injured brain, both regionally and globally. The four main methods of CBF control include: autoregulation, blood gas changes, metabolic regulation, and neurogenic control.[7, 9]

Autoregulation refers to the ability of the normal brain to maintain a constant CBF despite considerable variations in CPP. It is generally thought that the range of CPPs over which autoregulation operates normally is 50 to 130 mm Hg.[10, 11] Above and below these limits CBF varies passively in normal brain. The mechanism is unclear. It is important to understand that the integrity of this mechanism may not be intact in ill or injured areas of brain, and that CBF may be "pressure passive" in these areas. The implications for intracranial volume and ICP with therapeutic maneuvers such as endotracheal intubation are obvious. The attendant hypertension and cerebral alerting lead to increases in cerebral blood volume and ICP.

Alterations in the arterial tensions of carbon dioxide ($PaCO_2$) and oxygen (PaO_2) have profound effects on CBF. Hypercapnia produces cerebrovasodilation and increased CBF, whereas hypocapnia produces the opposite effect. Within the physiologic range ($PaCO_2$ 20–80 mm Hg) the relationship between $PaCO_2$ and CBF is linear, CBF altering by about 4% per millimeter of mercury change in $PaCO_2$. This effect is mediated by alterations in hydrogen ion concentration at the cerebral arteriolar level. The cerebral vasculature is less sensitive to changes in PaO_2 although significant vasodilation and increases in CBF occur at PaO_2 values of less than 50 mm Hg. Lactic acid production by ischemic brain likely mediates the effect. High concentrations of oxygen lead to cerebral vasoconstriction by unknown mechanisms. CBF falls by about 10% at a fractional concentration of oxygen in inspired gas (FiO_2) of 1.0, and by 20% at 2 atm.[9]

Induced hypocarbia not only reduces cerebral blood volume and ICP but confers a degree of protection against surges in arterial pressure such as that seen with intubation. Bag-mask hyperventilation routinely precedes active airway intervention in patients when compromised intracranial compliance is suspected.

The metabolic rate of the brain and CBF remains relatively high and constant over time, whether awake or asleep. However, localized areas of brain may be more active than others, demanding increased blood flow and substrate delivery. Global increases occur with pain, anxiety, or grand mal seizures. The upper airway and larynx are heavily populated with sensory receptors. The surge in cerebral metabolic activity that accompanies stimulation of these receptors by endotracheal intubation can be appreciated. The accompanying increase in CBF may lead to excessive increases in ICP, particularly in areas of brain with impaired autoregulation secondary to injury or disease. CNS stimulants such as amphetamines, cocaine, and ketamine increase the metabolic rate and CBF. It is of interest that most inhalation anesthetics (e.g., halothane, enflurane) uncouple this relationship, depressing metabolism and increasing CBF. Induced hypocarbia mitigates this effect.[9]

Neurogenic control by autonomic pathways exerts a small (<10%) but measurable effect on CBF.[10] Sympathetic activity causes cerebral vasoconstriction and a fall in CBF, whereas parasympathetic activity leads to cerebral vasodilation and an increase in CBF.[11] It is probable that the cerebral vasoconstriction of increased sympathetic tone mitigates to some extent the surge in CBF due to the rise in systemic blood pressure. This balancing act to provide "appropriate" flow is heavily dependent on intact autoregulation, which in turn relies on a normal brain and normal PaO_2 and $PaCO_2$. Sympathomimetic drugs such as ketamine, pancuronium, cocaine, and α-agonists may be hazardous in the setting of compromised intracranial compliance because the net effect may be increased CBF, cerebral blood volume, and ICP. Some therapeutic maneuvers are aimed at obtunding this sympathetic response. Medications such as lidocaine, opioids, barbiturates, and β-blockers are used. It is exceedingly difficult to determine whether the beneficial effects of these agents are related to their ability to reduce cerebral metabolic rate or obtund the sympathetic response. The likelihood is that they have effects to varying degrees on both control mechanisms. The sum leads to improved ICP control during endotracheal intubation. Other therapeutic maneuvers are directed toward improving the brain's ability to protect itself from an increase in sympathetic activity and blood pressure.

Induced hypocarbia, maintenance of oxygenation, and optimizing jugular venous flow (head elevation) are examples.

Three components constitute the intracranial contents: brain, blood, and cerebrospinal fluid (CSF). Each is essentially liquid, incompressible, and occupies a particular volume. Blood is forced into the cranium under arterial pressure, generating a distinct ICP. CSF and blood are, ordinarily, displaceable from the intracranial space, serving as important compensatory mechanisms to an increase in the volume of one of the other components. There is, however, a limit to the extent that the extrusion of blood and CSF can accommodate an increase in some other volume. When this compensatory mechanism becomes exhausted, ICP can rise rapidly to high levels, perhaps exceeding MAP. Massive elevations in ICP may lead to brain-stem compression or ischemia resulting in the classic cushing response of bradycardia, arterial hypertension, and respiratory irregularity.[12] The relationship of intracranial volume to ICP is known as *intracranial compliance*.[9] The "break point" of the curve where unit changes in volume produce larger and larger changes in ICP occurs at an ICP of around 15 mm Hg.[12, 13]

To summarize, CBF and the delivery of essential nutrients for neural activity and integrity is especially dependent upon CPP. Either falls in MAP or elevations in ICP may cause CPP to fall below the critical CBF and result in cerebral ischemia. In addition, the brain's ability to regulate the amount of blood in the cranial vault may be compromised by a disturbance of autoregulation or a disorder of arterial blood gases (ABGs) leading to intracranial hypervolemia, and increases in ICP.

Whether cause or effect, airflow integrity, adequate ventilation and oxygenation, and airway protection are crucial to an optimum neurologic outcome.

PATHOPHYSIOLOGY

The potential consequence of an increased ICP is ischemia, and ultimately neural demise. Initially, the cerebral vessels dilate in response to an increase in ICP as an autoregulatory mechanism to maintain CBF. However, as ICP continues to rise, CPP begins to suffer, and once ICP exceeds 30 to 40 mm Hg, CBF falls progressively, leading to a cycle of ischemia, increased ICP, and decreased CBF.[6, 14]

Episodes of prolonged ICP elevation may occur

when intracranial compression is advanced and control of CBF has become unstable.[9, 15, 16] CPP may be greatly reduced at such times. Various types of stimuli, such as endotracheal intubation or painful procedures, may provoke devastating rises in ICP. The patient with moderate to severe head trauma, a decreased level of consciousness, or known intracranial lesions that present with acute deterioration must be considered at the limits of intracranial compensation and prone to exaggerated ICP responses to stimulation.

Elevations in ICP may be related to an increase in the volume of blood, brain, or CSF in the cranial vault. Only one disorder leads to an increase in the absolute volume of CSF: obstructive hydrocephalus of whatever etiology. It is unusual for these patients to present to the emergency department with sufficient CNS depression to compromise ventilation, or to require intubation and hyperventilation as a therapeutic maneuver.

An increase in intracranial blood volume may be intravascular or extravascular (e.g., intracranial hematoma). The former may be related to an extracranial (e.g., hypertension) or an intracranial etiology. All of the common intracranial, intravascular causes relate to a failure of autoregulation, either globally (postanoxic encephalopathy) or regionally (tumor, abscess, trauma). The compounding effects of primary or secondary ventilatory failure potentiate the intracranial hypervolemia, as may maneuvers such as endotracheal intubation with its attendant sympathetic stimulation and hypertension.

An increase in brain tissue volume may be due to mass lesions, brain edema, or a combination of the two. Brain (cerebral) edema implies an increase in the water content of the brain and is of three varieties: interstitial, cytotoxic, and vasogenic.[17] Interstitial edema results from obstructive hydrocephalus leading to increased water and electrolytes in the periventricular white matter. Cytotoxic edema is an intracellular form of edema that occurs in hypo-osmolar and postanoxic situations. Vasogenic edema is the most common type and is associated with brain tumors, abscesses, infarctions, trauma, and other disorders. Increased capillary permeability permits the leakage of plasma filtrate into extracellular brain, primarily white matter.

The relationships among cerebral perfusion, intracranial volume, intracranial pressure, and neuronal integrity have been presented. Now let us utilize acute *severe* head injury as a model for understanding the priorities of patient management, and the impact of airway and ventilatory management on ICP and neurologic outcome.

The commonest cause of elevated ICP presenting to emergency departments is head injury. The emergency physician must recognize the entity, understand its pathophysiology, estimate its severity, and design a management scheme to optimize outcome. Airway management is crucial not only because of the threat posed to the airway and ventilation but also because of the potential adverse effects that airway maintenance maneuvers may have on ICP and neuronal survival. Additionally, ventilatory management is an essential therapeutic aspect of ICP control in these patients.

The pathophysiology of acute severe head injury is divided temporally into three phases: immediate, intermediate, and late.[18] The immediate phase occurs within minutes and is characterized by an acute rise in systemic and intracranial pressure, apnea, and an isoelectric electroencephalogram (EEG).[19] All of these disturbances abate after about 1 minute.

The intermediate phase occurs over minutes to hours and is associated with two pathologic entities. The first is diffuse axonal injury due to shear or stretch forces. Similar injuries to vessels produce intracranial hematomas. The second is discrete lesions produced by direct CNS trauma such as cerebral lacerations and contusions. These are termed *primary brain injury*. The emergency physician can have no impact on primary brain injury, save from the preventive aspect. However, superimposed on the primary injury are those factors leading to *secondary brain injury* that occur during this phase. These include hypotension, hypoxemia, and intracranial hypertension.

Hypotension (systolic blood pressure <90 mm Hg) coupled with severe head injury quadruples mortality. A cardiac output that maintains cerebral perfusion is crucial.[20] Hypoxemia (PaO$_2$ <60) is associated with a doubling of mortality for a variety of reasons[21] including intracranial hypertension, vital organ ischemia, and clotting disorders. Intracranial hypertension (ICP >20 mm Hg) is associated with a doubling of mortality that can be mitigated by aggressive management.[22] It is typically related to intracranial hematomas, congestive brain swelling, and traumatic subarachnoid hemorrhage. The prevention and management of those factors that lead to secondary brain injury are intimately related to rational airway management.

The late phase of acute severe head injury occurs within hours to days. Cytotoxic edema occurs in areas of brain damage.[23] Vasogenic edema escalates over the first 24 to 36 hours and then settles.[23] Post-traumatic epilepsy,[24] arterial hypertension, and dysfunctional cerebral circulatory control also occur.[25]

The patient with an acute severe head injury is critically ill and active airway intervention is mandatory. It is essential that the issue of hemodynamic stability be assessed as this will determine the time frame one has to work with as well as the techniques, classes, and doses of medications to be used in attenuating the adverse responses to intubation.

CEREBRAL PROTECTION

There are three prime goals of airway management: (1) the maintenance of airway integrity; (2) the maintenance of oxygenation and ventilation; and (3) airway protection. In the patient with a neurologic disorder one must attempt to attenuate the circulatory and ICP responses to intubation as well. A variety of nonpharmacologic and pharmacologic strategies should be considered.

The nonpharmacologic strategies include: (1) bag-mask ventilation to optimize PaO_2, maximize functional residual capacity (FRC) oxygenation, and reduce $PaCO_2$ (30 ± 2 mm Hg); (2) management of hypotension; (3) optimizing venous drainage from the cranium by elevating the head of the stretcher 15 degrees, if possible, and avoiding constricting devices around the neck, e.g., cervical collars and ties that secure tubes.

Several medications and techniques have been reported to attenuate the sympathetic and ICP responses to intubation: (1) local anaesthetic agents, administered topically or by nerve block, to produce laryngeal anesthesia; lidocaine has been used intravenously (IV) to attenuate rises in blood pressure and ICP; (2) barbiturates, particularly thiopental sodium; (3) opioids (fentanyl and alfentanil); (4) nitrates (sodium nitroprusside); (5) benzodiazepines (midazolam and diazepam); (6) muscle relaxants (succinylcholine, pancuronium, atracurium); (7) β-blockers (metoprolol, esmolol).

PHARMACOLOGIC AIDS

Local Anesthetic Agents

A variety of local anesthetic agents may be used to block afferent sensory traffic from the oral cavity, larynx, and trachea. This may be accomplished by a combination of topical applications (gargle, spray, aerosolized or transtracheal injection) and blockade of the superior laryngeal nerve (topically or by injection). These techniques have been shown to attenuate increases in heart rate and blood pressure associated with laryngoscopy and endotracheal intubation.[26]

Intravenous lidocaine has been shown to attenuate the rise in ICP associated with endotracheal intubation. The precise mechanism, optimal dose, and interval from administration to intubation are all unclear. Intravenous lidocaine has been reported to block the cough reflex[27-30] and in so doing attenuate rises in ICP. The data here, however, are conflicting. Lidocaine also depresses cortical electrical activity, decreasing cerebral metabolism,[6] and increasing CVR.[31, 32] It may also attenuate the rise in ICP associated with endotracheal suctioning,[33] although the intratracheal route appears to be more effective than the IV one. The literature is confusing as to how effective IV lidocaine is in obtunding the sympathetic response to intubation.[34-37] A general consensus is that it *is* effective. How much this effect contributes to an attenuation in ICP response has not been investigated. The dose of lidocaine to produce an effective blood level of 3 to 6 μg/mL is 1.5 to 2.0 mg/kg.[28, 35] The time from administration of the bolus dose of lidocaine to endotracheal intubation is generally 90 seconds to 3 minutes, with one study finding optimal attenuation at 3 minutes.[37]

In summary, IV lidocaine is indicated to attenuate a rise in ICP associated with endotracheal intubation in the patient with a neurologic disorder. The dose is 1.5 mg/kg and it should be given 3 minutes prior to intubation. Potential complications associated with the administration of lidocaine include hypotension, a lowered seizure threshold, and sedation. The administering physician must balance risks and benefits and prepare to manage these complications.

Barbiturates

The epileptogenic potential of methohexital has left thiopental sodium as the preeminent anesthesia induction agent for the patient with a neurologic disorder.[38] Several features of this drug are desirable. It causes sedation and a dose-related decrease in cerebral metabolic rate and blood flow.[39, 40] It also attenuates the hemodynamic responses to intubation owing to direct myocardial depression.[41, 42] Its anticonvulsant properties are also desirable.

In the intubation sequence thiopental sodium

should be administered immediately before intubation as a bolus. It is effective in one arm-heart-brain circulation time and the effect abates rapidly. The dose should be matched with the hemodynamic status of the patient but should not exceed 3 mg/kg as a bolus. Repeated small doses (50–100 mg) to control postintubation hypertension are useful. The grossly unstable, hypotensive, "crashed" patient should not be administered thiopental sodium. The stable patient is given 3 mg/kg. The crashing patient receives 0 to 3 mg/kg, depending on the degree of instability, the pace of deterioration, and the judgment of the physician.

Complications associated with thiopental sodium include apnea and hypotension. Damage to cutaneous structures may occur if the alkaline (pH $\simeq$ 10) solution extravasates from the vein on injection. The usual preparation of the drug is a 2.5% solution, giving 25 mg of thiopental per milliliter of solution.

Opioids

The effects of opioids on cerebral metabolism and blood flow are not well defined.[6] Metabolic rate and CBF are not altered by small doses, provided $PaCO_2$ does not rise. However, in large doses (fentanyl 25–400 µg/kg) a dose-related decrease in rate and flow does occur.[43]

Fentanyl and alfentanil are synthetic opioids that possess several desirable features related to airway management of the patient with a neurologic disorder: they have remarkable cardiovascular stability, effectively obtund the sympathetic response to noxious stimuli, have a rapid onset of action, and abate quickly. The dose of fentanyl is 5 to 8 µg/kg[35, 44] given 3 minutes before intubation. Although the higher dose is more effective at blunting the sympathetic response, it is also more often associated with muscular rigidity, particularly if injected rapidly. Alfentanil 30 µg/kg as a bolus 2 minutes before intubation is also reliable and effective, and probably preferable to fentanyl.

Whether or not one administers an opioid in the intubation sequence will be a function of the time frame available and the analysis of the risk-benefit ratio. Respiratory depression, a rising $PaCO_2$, and muscular rigidity are potential hazards.

Nitrates

Sodium nitroprusside has been used in doses of 1 to 2 µg/kg IV before laryngoscopy to attenuate the rise in systolic blood pressure.[45] The difficulty with this technique in the patient with a neurologic disorder is that is causes cerebral vasodilation, and a remarkable increase in ICP.[46] For this reason it is relatively contraindicated in this clinical scenario.

Benzodiazepines

Benzodiazepines decrease both cerebral metabolic rate and blood flow; midazolam does so in a dose-related fashion.[47] Although this suggests that midazolam may be a useful adjunct in patients with compromised intracranial compliance, at a dose of 0.15 mg/kg it does not protect against increases in ICP with intubation.[48, 49] It is unknown whether higher doses would confer protection. Although midazolam may block the sympathetic responses to intubation, the 2-minute delay from administration to peak effect make its clinical use awkward in the rapid-sequence intubation (RSI) setting.

Muscle Relaxants

Coughing, straining, and combative behavior during the intubation sequence, or subsequently on the ventilator, all produce significant ICP elevations. The ideal relaxant should produce profound paralysis rapidly with no significant cardiovascular side effects. The depolarizing agent succinylcholine and the nondepolarizers vecuronium, atracurium, and pancuronium may all be useful.

In the past it was believed that reported increases in ICP after succinylcholine were a relative contraindication to its use in the neurologic patient.[9] Fasciculations were the supposed culprit, leading to increased CVP and thus ICP. However, recent reports of the use of succinylcholine in patients with elevated ICP, and in animal experiments,[9, 50–52] suggest that succinylcholine can be used provided the patient is sufficiently sedated, has his or her blood pressure and $PaCO_2$ controlled,[9, 52] and has had a pretreatment (defasciculating) dose of a nondepolarizer.[53, 54] The dose of succinylcholine is 1.5 mg/kg. Both atracurium, (0.5 mg/kg) and vecuronium (0.1 mg/kg) appear to have clinically insignificant cardiovascular effects compared to the sympathomimetic effects of pancuronium (0.1 mg/kg).[6] However, all have a significantly greater time to total paralysis compared with succinylcholine.

β-Blockers

Cardioselective (metoprolol)[55] and ultra-short-acting (esmolol)[56–59] β-blockers have been used to attenuate the hypertensive response to intubation. The relatively slow onset and long duration of action of metoprolol have allowed esmolol to emerge as the leading candidate. Esmolol is a water-soluble, cardioselective β-adrenergic blocker with a rapid onset and ultrashort duration of action with a half-life of 9 minutes.[60] The effective dose is 1.5 to 3.0 mg/kg administered over 15 seconds, 90 to 120 seconds prior to intubation.[57–59] The drug effectively attenuates the surge in blood pressure without adverse effects in *otherwise healthy patients.*

Caution must be exercised in volume-depleted patients, patients with bradyarrhythmias and reactive airway disease. The use of this agent in the setting of multiple trauma warrants careful consideration by the administering physician.

AIRWAY MANAGEMENT

Airway management in the patient with CNS illness or injury must be analyzed from two perspectives: the patient with an isolated CNS disorder, and the patient with a CNS disorder coupled with varying degrees of hemodynamic stability. In either case the emergency physician must be mindful of CBF and CPP, and how they are affected by airway interventions and the use of adjuvant medications. The challenge is categorizing the patient with a CNS disorder as "stable," "crashing," or "crashed" from the neurologic perspective, attempting to define the thresholds that motivate active airway intervention, and managing the hemodynamics appropriately. The literature is unable to guide us definitively in these decision-making processes.

The indications for active airway intervention are relatively clear-cut and include inability to maintain a patent airway, protect the airway, or maintain reasonable ABG values. The presence of any of these indications demands airway intervention independent of neurologic status and is consistent with the accepted priorities of resuscitation. That the patient with a combined airway-ventilation and CNS problem demands even more meticulous attention to the details of airway management is axiomatic.

The real question to be answered is: When does the CNS status independently demand active airway intervention (i.e., intubation and hyperventilation) as a therapeutic maneuver? In other words, is there some way to "clinically" determine when the limits of intracranial compliance have been exceeded and manual hyperventilation is required? The precise measurement of ICP and CPP is neither practical

nor reasonable in the emergency department (ED). There are no definitive parameters to precisely define the crashed patient in the ED. However a consensus does allow some reasonable suggestions. The Glasgow coma scale is widely used to grade severity, identify changes in clinical status, and prognosticate in the patient with a CNS disorder. The patient with a coma score of 8 or less is generally considered to be severely ill and likely at the limits of, or exceeding, intracranial accommodation. Patients with coma scores of less than 8 or who exhibit a pace of neurologic deterioration anticipated to lead to such a score will require active airway intervention and hyperventilation. Patients with mild (coma score 13–15) and moderate (coma score 9–12) neurologic dysfunction do not ordinarily require intubation and hyperventilation as a therapeutic maneuver, and airway management is dictated by threats to airway maintenance, airway protection, and the maintenance of oxygenation and ventilation.

Scenario 1: The Stable Patient

The patient with a "mild" neurologic disorder is stable neurologically and has a coma score of 13 to 15. This is not to say that this patient could not have a serious intracranial pathologic condition and does not bear close observation and perhaps investigation. Rather, such patients do not require specific therapeutic interventions to control ICP. A typical patient has sustained a closed head injury with a brief loss of consciousness, and on presentation is drowsy but rousable, cooperative, generally orientated, but with a definite defect in short-term memory. In other words, this patient has a reversible, nonstructural neurologic injury that is also known as a concussion. Intracranial pressure and its control mechanisms are intact. Should active airway intervention be required, the obtundation of adverse cardiovascular reflexes should be attended to as with any other intubation.

Scenario 2: The Crashing Patient

The patient with a coma score between 9 and 12 is in a precarious neurologic situation, is certainly neurologically unstable, and should deterioration be evident, crashing. The typical patient in this category has had significant blunt head trauma and presents as combative, confused, and very difficult to evaluate and manage. The CNS examination is usually nonfocal. Alcohol, other injuries, and vomiting confound the picture. This patient should be considered to be at the limits of intracranial compensation. The indications for active airway intervention should be meticulously monitored by clinical observation, pulse oximetry, and ABG sampling. Endotracheal intubation and hyperventilation are indicated if airway maintenance or protection is compromised, or if ABG values are not absolutely normal. The procedure must meticulously attend to the principles of RSI: maintenance of adequate oxygenation, airway protection, and the obtundation of adverse cardiovascular and ICP responses. In addition, bag-mask hyperventilation to produce hypocarbia should precede intubation. This modification of the RSI algorithm is performed with cricoid pressure in place and without generating upper airway pressures sufficient to inflate the stomach. Evaluation of the ABGs will determine the need for active airway intervention unless the coma score falls to 8 or below. Optimal patient management often requires that sedative medications be administered. The most appropriate medications are those with minimal respiratory and cardiovascular depression such as haloperidol. Should the administration of sedative medications produce an indication for intubation, it should be performed according to the principles of RSI.

Scenario 3: The Crashed Patient

The patient who presents with a coma score of 8 or less is in dire condition and is neurologically crashed. The cause may be any medical or surgical condition and is of no consequence from the perspective of airway management. Endotracheal intubation by RSI (see Fig 24–1) with hyperventilation to a $PaCO_2$ of 30 mm Hg is indicated. Initial ventilator settings of 10 mL/kg of tidal volume at a rate of 12 to 14 breaths per minute should approximate this $PaCO_2$ in patients with normal lungs. Following intubation, additional principles of ICP management such as head-up tilt, pharmacologic paralysis, and the use of osmotic agents and steroids are administered as indicated.

Modification of Rapid-Sequence Intubation by Hemodynamic Instability

Perhaps the most daunting task facing the emergency physician about to intubate the patient with a neurologic disorder is integrating the hemodynamic status of the patient with the RSI algorithm, particularly if the patient is incipiently or actually unstable. Whether the patient has a mild, moderate, or severe neurologic disorder, as long as hemodynamic stability is present, the full RSI algorithm is utilized.

How then is the intubation algorithm modified for the patient with a neurologic disorder who is *hemodynamically* crashing or crashed? The algorithm for RSI in the stable, crashed, and crashing patient is presented in Figure 24–1.

The Hemodynamically Stable Patient

The equipment needed is prepared and checked, and suction is made available. The patient is preoxygenated with 100% O_2 with assisted ventilation synchronized with his or her own respirations for 3 to 5 minutes. The goal is to replace as much FRC with O_2 as possible and attain a $PaCO_2$ of 30 mm Hg. The patient is pretreated with 0.01 mg/kg of pancuronium, 1.5 mg/kg of lidocaine, and if appropriate, 30 μg/kg of alfentanil. Two to three minutes later 3 mg/kg of thiopental sodium as a bolus is followed by 1.5 mg/kg of succinylcholine. When the gag reflex is lost, cricoid pressure is applied. Ventilation should be avoided to prevent inflation of the stomach unless a lower $PaCO_2$ is required in the patient with a moderate or severe neurologic status. Laryngoscopy is performed, intubation of the trachea accomplished, and the tube position verified. Cricoid pressure is then released. The patient is ventilated to achieve a $PaCO_2$ of 30 ±2 mm Hg.

Surges in blood pressure after intubation may be attenuated with 50- to 100-mg bolus doses of thiopental sodium,[61] or 50- to 100-mg bolus doses of esmolol. The pretreatment doses of lidocaine and alfentanil may be replaced with 1.5 to 3.0 mg/kg of esmolol 90 to 120 seconds prior to intubation. Succinylcholine, if contraindicated, may be replaced by vecuronium 0.1 mg/kg or atracuronium 0.5 mg/kg. The sympathomimetic effects and long duration of action of pancuronium 0.1 mg/kg make it less desirable in this situation.

The Hemodynamically Crashing Patient

The equipment needed is prepared and checked, and suction is made available. The pace of deterioration and adequacy of perfusion determine the time frames between drug administration and intubation. Preoxygenation and assisted ventilation, as feasible, is performed. The patient is pretreated with a nondepolarizer and lidocaine. Three minutes later 1 to 2 mg/kg of thiopental sodium is given, followed by 1.5 mg/kg of succinylcholine. The patient is intubated, once paralyzed, and cricoid pressure is applied. Tube position is verified and the cricoid pressure is released. Surges in blood pressure can be managed with 50- to 100-mg bolus doses of thiopental sodium.

The Hemodynamically Crashed Patient

The equipment is readied and suction prepared while bag-mask ventilation is undertaken. Should time permit, and if orotracheal intubation is anticipated, the cross-table lateral cervical spine film is ob-

Stable patient	Crashing patient	Crashed patient

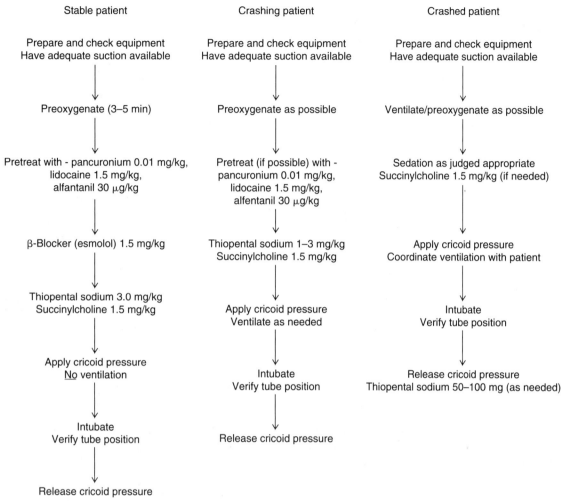

FIG 24–1.
Algorithm for rapid-sequence intubation modified by hemodynamic instability.

tained. If not, or if the film is abnormal, the appropriate algorithm is followed (see Fig 24–1). In the hemodynamically unstable patient, when time is of the essence, many features of the standard algorithm will be abbreviated or aborted. However, manual hyperventilation is continued and cricoid pressure is initiated. Pretreatment with a nondepolarizer, opiates, lidocaine, or a β-blocker will likely be impractical. Small doses (50–100 mg of thiopental sodium) may be required to obtund consciousness or treat surges in blood pressure but is generally contraindicated. Succinylcholine 1.5 mg/kg is indicated for the struggling patient with intact laryngeal or cough reflexes. Ongoing bag-mask hyperventilation may be useful in minimizing any rise in ICP due to the succinylcholine. Cricoid pressure is maintained until the correct tube position is verified.

In all cases, particularly where increased ICP is suspected, caution must be exercised that the method of securing the endotracheal tube in place does not obstruct jugular venous flow.

REFERENCES

1. Fox EJ, Sklar GS, Hill CH, et al: Complications related to the pressor response to endotracheal intubation. *Anesthesiology* 1977; 47:524–525.
2. Shapiro HM: Intracranial hypertension: Therapeutic and anesthetic considerations. *Anesthesiology* 1975; 43:445–471.
3. Caveness WF: Incidence of craniocerebral trauma in the United States from 1970–1975, in Thompson RA, Green JR (eds): *Advances in Neurology*, vol 22. New York, Raven Press, 1979, pp 1–3.
4. Pitts LH, Martin N: Head injuries. *Surg Clin North Am* 1982; 62:47–60.
5. Klauber MR, Marshall LF, Toole BM, et al: Cause of decline in head injury mortality rate in San Diego

County, California. *J Neurosurg* 1985; 62:528–531.

6. Messick JM, Newberg LA, Nugent M, et al: Principles of neuroanesthesia for the non-neurosurgical patient with CNS pathophysiology. *Anesth Analg* 1985; 64:143–174.

7. Lassen NA, Christensen MS: Physiology of cerebral blood flow. *Br J Anaesth* 1976; 48:719–734.

8. Michenfelder JD: The cerebral circulation, in Prys-Roberts C (ed): *The Circulation in Anesthesia: Applied Physiology and Pharmacology.* Oxford, Blackwell Scientific Publishing, 1980, pp 209–225.

9. Campkin TV, Turner JM: *Neurosurgical Anesthesia and Intensive Care,* ed 1. London, Butterworths & Co Ltd, 1980, pp 5–11.

10. Meyer MW, Klassen AC: Regional brain blood flow during sympathetic stimulation (abstract). *Stroke* 1973; 4:370.

11. McDowall DG: Neurosurgical anesthesia and intensive care, in Hewer CL, Atkinson RS (eds): *Recent Advances in Anesthesia and Analgesia.* Edinburgh, Churchill Livingstone Ltd, 1976, p 16.

12. Cushing H: Some experimental and clinical observations concerning states of increased intracranial tension. *Am J Med Sci* 1902; 124:375.

13. Miller JD: Intracranial pressure monitoring. *Br J Hosp Med* 1978; 19:497.

14. Shapiro HM: Intracranial hypertension: Therapeutic and anesthetic considerations. *Anesthesiology* 1975; 43:445–471.

15. Lundberg N: Continuous recording and control of ventricular fluid pressure in neurosurgical practice. *Acta Psychiatr Neurol Scand Suppl* 1960; 36:149.

16. Turner JM, McDowall DG: The measurement of intracranial pressure. *Br J Anaesth* 1976; 48:735.

17. Fishman RA: Brain edema. *N Engl J Med* 1975; 293:706–711.

18. Miller JD: Head injury and brain ischemia implications for therapy. *Br J Anaesth* 1985; 57:120–129.

19. Sullivan HG, Martinez J, Becker DP, et al: Fluid percussion model of mechanical brain injury in the cat. *J Neurosurg* 1976; 45:520–534.

20. Davis DH, Sundt TM: Relationship of cerebral blood flow to cardiac output, mean arterial pressure, blood volume, and alpha and beta blockade in cats. *J Neurosurg* 1980; 52:745–754.

21. Miller SD, Butterworth JF: Gudeman SK, et al: Further experience in the management of severe head injury. *J Neurosurg* 1981; 54:289–299.

22. Saul TG, Ducker TB: Effect of intracranial pressure monitoring and aggressive treatment on mortality in secure head injury. *J Neurosurg* 1982; 56:498–503.

23. Overgaard J, Tweed WA: Cerebral circulation after head injury. *J Neurosurg* 1976; 45:292–300.

24. Jennett B: Epilepsy after non-missile head injuries. *Scott Med J* 1973; 18:8–13.

25. Obrist WD, Langfitt TW, Jagge JL, et al: Cerebral blood flow and metabolism in comatose patients with acute head injury: Relationship to intracranial hypertension. *J Neurosurg* 1984; 61:241–256.

26. Denlinger JK, Ellison N, Ominsky AJ: Effects of intratracheal lidocaine on circulatory responses to tracheal intubation. *Anesthesiology* 1974; 41:409–412.

27. Bedford RF, Winn HR, Tuson G, et al: Lidocaine prevents increased ICP after endotracheal intubation, in Shulman K, Mamarou A, Miller JD, et al (eds): *Intracranial Pressure,* vol 4. Berlin, Springer-Verlag, 1980; pp 595–598.

28. Hamill JF, Bedford RF, Weaver DC, et al: Lidocaine before intubation: Intravenous or laryngotracheal. *Anesthesiology* 1981; 55:578–581.

29. Poulton TJ, James FM: Cough suppression by lidocaine. *Anesthesiology* 1979; 50:470–472.

30. Steinhaus JE, Gaskin L: A study of lidocaine as a suppressant of cough reflex. *Anesthesiology* 1963; 24:285–290.

31. White PF, Schlobohm RM, Pitts LH, et al: A randomized study of drugs for preventing increases in intracranial pressure during suctioning. *Anesthesiology* 1982; 57:242–244.

32. Sakabe T, Maekawa T, Ishikawa T, et al: The effects of lidocaine on cerebral metabolism and circulation related to the electroencephalogram. *Anesthesiology* 1974; 40:433–441.

33. Yano M, Nishiyama H, Yokota H, et al: Effect of lidocaine on ICP response to endotracheal suctioning. *Anesthesiology* 1986; 64:651–653.

34. Abou-Madi MN, Keszler H, Yacoub JM: Cardiovascular reactions to laryngoscopy and tracheal intubation following small and large intravenous doses of lidocaine. *Can Anaesth Soc J* 1977; 24:12–19.

35. Payne KA, Murray UB, Oosthuizen JHC: Obtunding the sympathetic response to intubation. *S Afr Med J* 1988; 73:584–586.

36. Splinter WM: Intravenous lidocaine does not attenuate the hemodynamic response of children to laryngoscopy and tracheal intubation. *Can J Anaesth* 1990; 37:440–443.

37. Tam S, Chung F, Campbell JM: Attenuation of circulatory responses to endotracheal intubation using intravenous lidocaine: A determination of the optimal time of injection (abstract). *Can Anaesth Soc J* 1985; 32(suppl):565.

38. Dundee JW: Abnormal responses to barbiturates. *Br J Anaesth* 1957; 29:440.

39. Siesjo BK: *Brain Energy Metabolism.* New York, John Wiley & Sons, Inc, 1978.

40. Steen PA, Neuberg L, Milde JH, et al: Hypothermia and barbiturates: Individual and combined effects on canine cerebral oxygen consumption. *Anesthesiology* 1983; 58:527–532.

41. Sonntag H, Hellborg K, Schenk HD, et al: Effects of thiopental on coronary blood flow and myocardial metabolism in man. *Acta Anaesthesiol Scand* 1975; 19:69.

42. Conway CM, Ellis DB: The hemodynamic effects of short acting barbiturates. *Br J Anaesth* 1969; 41:534.

43. Carlsson C, Smith DS, Keykhah MM, et al: The effects of high dose fentanyl in cerebral circulation and

metabolism in rats. *Anesthesiology* 1982; 57:375–380.

44. Martin DE, Rosengerg H, Aukburg SJ, et al: Low dose fentanyl blunts circulatory responses to tracheal intubation. *Anesth Analg* 1982; 61:680.

45. Stoelting RK: Attenuation of blood pressure response to laryngoscopy and tracheal intubation with sodium nitorprusside. *Anesth Analg* 1979; 58:116.

46. Turner JM, Powell D, Gibson RM, et al: Intracranial pressure changes in neurosurgical patients during hypotension induced with sodium nitroprusside or trimethaphan. *Br J Anaesth* 1977; 49:419.

47. Reves JG, Fragen RJ, Vinik HR, et al: Midazolam: Pharmacology and uses. *Anesthesiology* 1985; 62:310–324.

48. Belopavlovic M, Buchthal A: Modification of ketamine-induced intracranial hypertension in neurosurgical patients by pre-treatment with midazolam. *Acta Anaesthesiol Scand* 1982; 26:458–462.

49. Cottrell JE, Giffin JP, Lim K, et al: Intracranial pressure, mean arterial pressure and heart rate following midazolam or thiopental in humans with intracranial masses (abstract). *Anesthesiology* 1982; 57:A323.

50. Bormann BE, Smith RB, Bunegin L, et al: Does succinlycholine raise intracranial pressure? (abstract). *Anesthesiology* 1980; 53(suppl):5262.

51. Paul WL, Bishko JR, Woodham B: Succinylcholine *d*-tubocurarine, dimethyl-tubocurarine and intracranial pressure in dogs. *Anesth Analg* 1981; 60:269.

52. Lam AM, Nicholas JF, Mannien PH: Influence of succinlycholine on lumbar cerebral spinal pressure in man (abstract). International Anesthesia Research Society 1984, p 102.

53. Minton MD, Crosslight KR, Stirt JA, et al: Increases in intracranial pressure from succinlycholine: Prevention by prior nondepolarizing blockade. *Anesthesiology* 1986; 65:165–169.

54. Stirt JA, Crosslight KR, Bedford RF, et al: Defasciculation with metocurine prevents succinlycholine-induced increases in intracranial pressure. *Anesthesiology* 1987; 67:50–53.

55. Magnusson J, Thulin T, Werner O, et al: Hemodynamic effects of pre-treatment with metoprolol in hypertensive patients undergoing surgery. *Br J Anaesth* 1986; 58:251–60.

56. Cucchiara RF, Benefiel DJ, Matteo RS, et al: Evaluation of esmolol in controlling increases in heart rate and blood pressure during endotracheal intubation in patients undergoing carotid endarterectomy. *Anesthesiology* 1986; 65:528–531.

57. Miller DR, Martineau RJ: Esmolol for control of hemodynamic responses during anesthetic induction (abstract). *Can J Anaesth* 1989; 36:5164–5165.

58. Knox JWD, Oxorn DC: Esmolol is efficient in controlling post intubation tachycardia and hypertension (abstract). *Can J Anaesth* 1989; 36:5165–5166.

59. Withington DE, Ramsay JG, Ralley FE, et al: Attenuation of the heart rate response to intubation by bolus doses of esmolol (abstract). *Can J Anaesth* 1989; 36:5166–5167.

60. Sum CY, Yacobi A, Kartzinec R: Kinetics of esmolol, an ultra-short-acting beta blocker, and of its major metabolite. *Clin Pharmacol Ther* 1983; 34:427–434.

61. Unni VKN, Johnston RA, Young HSA, et al: Prevention of intracranial hypertension during laryngoscopy and endotracheal intubation: Use of a second dose of thiopentone. *Br J Anaesth* 1984; 56:1219–1223.

25

Chest Injuries

Sarah K. Scott, M.D.

All significant chest trauma impacts the airway by altering the ventilatory system. The chest wall and its contents are major components of the ventilatory system. Normal airflow occurs only if all components of the airway, from the oral pharynx to the alveoli, are clear. The chest wall and the diaphragm, both functionally and structurally, must be sound for normal ventilation to occur. The pleural surfaces of the lung, as well as the lung parenchyma, must be intact for normal lung function and gas exchange.

Specific chest injuries which variably alter the ventilatory system and form the clinical scenarios to be discussed are: pneumothorax, hemothorax, pulmonary contusion, flail chest, and tracheobronchial disruption. Each of these injuries alone, by virtue of its impact on the cardiopulmonary system, may lead to a fatal outcome if rapid, accurate evaluation and treatment are not carried out. The evaluation begins with removal of all clothing, noting the level of patient alertness, and assessing the adequacy of air exchange by listening at the nose and mouth. Next, the relationship of the trachea to the midline is examined and the chest wall is observed for paradoxical movement. The chest is palpated and auscultated bilaterally for the presence of subcutaneous emphysema, rib fractures, and the quality of breath and heart sounds. The circulatory status is noted grossly by assessing vital signs, neck vein fullness, and peripheral pulses.

This initial approach to the patient with chest trauma and potential cardiorespiratory compromise will detect life-threatening conditions. The choice of additional management strategies depends upon the type and severity of the chest wound, as well as the presence and significance of associated injuries. Reassessment of the patient's condition at intervals af-

ter beginning initial therapy allows management adjustment as needed.

PNEUMOTHORAX AND HEMOTHORAX

Pneumothorax and hemothorax are the accumulation of air or blood, respectively, in the pleural space. The pleural space is conceptualized as a potential space that exists between the visceral and parietal lung pleura. Pneumothorax occurs in approximately 30% of major chest injuries and is classified as closed, open, or tension, depending upon the ability of atmospheric air to enter and to exit the pleural space.[1] A simple closed pneumothorax commonly occurs after a deceleration injury such as a fall or motor vehicle accident, but also may result from a self-sealing penetrating injury as from a small-caliber bullet or knife wound.[2, 3] There is no free communication of air between the pleural space and the environment via the chest wall; thus the terms *closed* or *noncommunicating*. True, open, sucking chest wounds are rare in the civilian emergency department (ED).[4] With the exception of shotgun wounds or other large, penetrating, open defects, they are primarily seen in military combat. Tension pneumothorax may result from any type of penetrating or blunt chest injury that allows continuous air entry into the pleural space without exit. Accumulation of air without exit leads to increased positive pressure or "tension" in association with the pneumothorax. Hemothorax occurs in about 20% to 30% of both major blunt and penetrating chest injuries. Inclusion of hemopneumothorax increases the overall incidence to 40% to 50%.[3, 5, 6]

Trauma significant enough to create a pneumothorax or hemothorax causes pain. Pain blunts cough effectiveness causing secretions to pool in both large and small airways. Abnormal ventilation results in dyspnea, tachypnea, and hypoventilation. Functional dead space, carbon dioxide retention, and work of breathing increase. Further ventilation and oxygenation defects occur as a result of alveolar rupture or tracheobronchial injury associated specifically with pneumothorax. With air entrance into the pleural space, intrapleural and alveolar pressures become more positive. This, in concert with retained secretions, causes lung collapse with small to moderate airway and alveolar closure. Decreased vital capacity and increased intrapulmonary shunt result.[3, 7] The magnitude of this effect depends upon the size of the pneumothorax and the degree of tension in the thoracic cavity.

With tension pneumothorax, accumulation of air under pressure leads to compression of the ipsilateral lung, mediastinal shift, and contralateral lung compression. It is generally believed that cardiopulmonary collapse occurs as a result of decreased venous return, secondary to the positive pressure effects of the tension pneumothorax.[3, 8] However, the true mechanism(s) is debated.[9, 10] With open pneumothorax, rapid equilibration of intrapleural and atmospheric pressure occurs, allowing air entry into the pleural space during inspiration. The ipsilateral lung will collapse with some shift of the mediastinum, but to a lesser degree than with a tension pneumothorax.

The pleural space can accommodate 2 to 3 L of fluid.[3] Blood in the pleural space compromises airflow, ventilation, and oxygenation similar to tension pneumothorax by compressing the ipsilateral lung and causing mediastinal shift. These airway threats may be compounded by shock and decreased venous return secondary to massive hemothorax. Bronchial or pulmonary laceration may allow aspiration of blood.[3, 5, 6, 8] In all but 5% to 10% of cases, the source of pleural blood is the intercostal or internal mammary vessels. Bleeding from the pulmonary vasculature is uncommon and blood loss from the aorta, heart, or hilar vessels is often rapidly fatal.[3, 5, 6]

Diagnosis of a simple, noncommunicating pneumothorax is based on clinical signs and symptoms, including shortness of breath and chest pain, physical examination, and chest radiography. Yet, clinical findings do not necessarily correlate with the presence, size, or degree of increased intrathoracic pressure associated with a pneumothorax. Physical examination findings may include increased respiratory rate, normal to decreased breath sounds with possible hyperresonance, and subcutaneous emphysema. Simple closed pneumothoraces are graded by size approximations based on posteroanterior (PA) chest radiographs. Air in less than 20% of the lung field on the PA chest film is considered to be small; 20% to 50%, moderate; and greater than 50%, large.

A small pneumothorax may be missed both clinically and radiographically, particularly if pleural air is sought only in the apical lateral areas of the film. In upright chest films, the apical lateral area is most likely to demonstrate free pleural air. However, in the supine position, free air may only be visible in the inferior aspect of the film.[11] Lordotic or upright expiratory chest films may be useful diagnostic options in stable patients with small pneumothoraces.

Computed tomography (CT) is more sensitive and specific than plain radiographs in the evaluation of subcutaneous or pleural air or fluid and lung parenchymal abnormalities.[11] Yet, in the emergency department evaluation of the acutely injured trauma patient, there is little role for CT during the initial patient evaluation. Currently, CT studies are reserved for more stable patients with specific diagnostic dilemmas.

Tension pneumothorax may be diagnosed by auscultation of decreased or absent breath sounds and hyperresonance to percussion over the affected lung field. Tracheal deviation may occur, but is a late finding. Neck vein distention and subcutaneous emphysema may be noted. Shock, with hypotension and tachycardia or bradycardia, may be dramatic clinical evidence of tension pneumothorax. In intubated and ventilated patients, difficult bag-valve-mask ventilation or increasing airway pressures may indicate tension pneumothorax. Intubation of the right mainstem bronchus and reactive airway disease may produce similar findings. However, it is a management error to obtain a chest film solely to diagnose tension pneumothorax, as it is a clinical diagnosis. Determination of open pneumothorax is also clinical. Respiratory distress with an apparent open chest wall defect and the presence of bubbling or sucking air sounds make the diagnosis obvious.

Diagnosis of a hemothorax based upon signs, symptoms, and physical examination may reveal a stable patient without obvious complaint. Evidence of chest injury by history or visual inspection and decreased breath sounds with dullness to percussion over the affected area suggest the diagnosis. Yet, patients may also present in hypovolemic shock with rapidly deteriorating cardiorespiratory status requiring immediate therapy. In initially stable patients, chest radiography is the diagnostic tool of choice.

Patients without tachycardia or hypotension may be placed in the upright position for an anteroposterior (AP) chest film. In this position, 250 to 400 mL of blood are required to demonstrate blunting of the costophrenic angle. In the supine position, fluid in the chest layers over a greater area and up to a liter may be missed.[3, 5, 6] In either instance, lateral decubitus films or ultrasonography may confirm the presence and location of free blood.[12] In the "crashing" patient with suspected hemothorax, a chest tube should be placed without preliminary chest films.

Although there is debate, the mainstay of therapy for pneumothorax and hemothorax is tube thoracostomy. It is generally agreed that pneumothoraces of at least moderate size, i.e., 20% to 25% of the lung field, should be evacuated by chest tube.[3, 13] However, in the setting of trauma, thoracostomy drainage of even small (<20%) pneumothoraces is common practice. This is particularly the case in the setting of major trauma, patients with multiple injuries, or in patients requiring positive pressure ventilation. The latter may convert a simple pneumothorax to a tension pneumothorax.

For adequate drainage in the adult trauma patient with pneumo- or hemothorax, a 36 to 40F chest tube is selected. In patients with spontaneous simple pneumothorax, smaller tubes, 24 to 28F, may be used. Tube thoracostomy is performed at approximately the fourth intercostal space, from the mid- to the anterior axillary line, observing sterile technique. If adhesions are encountered that are not easily removed during digital exploration prior to placement of the chest tube, a new site may be established one to two spaces away. Another quickly recognizable landmark for chest tube placement is the position of the nipple extended to the axillary line.[2, 3, 12] In trauma patients, during insertion, chest tubes should be directed apically and posteriorly to most effectively evacuate air and blood. For lung reexpansion, secured chest tubes should be attached via water seal to a suction source of −10 to −15 cm H_2O. On follow-up chest film, if reexpansion fails to occur, changing to higher suction of −20 to −25 cm H_2O or placement of a second chest tube may be considered. If these therapies fail, a tracheobronchial injury should be considered (see Fig 25–5).[3] Suction is contraindicated in patients in whom a large pneumothorax has been present for more than 24 hours. Significant pulmonary edema may develop following rapid lung reexpansion. This group should undergo slow lung reexpansion using water seal alone.[14]

Selected patients with small spontaneous pneumothoraces may be treated with needle aspiration or simple observation. These patients should be admitted and followed with repeat chest films. Small-caliber, 9 to 12F thoracostomy tubes with a flutter valve attachment have also been utilized for evacuation of pneumothorax but in some instances have been unable to maintain lung reexpansion. Chest tubes utilizing a trocar for insertion are not recommended, as they are blindly inserted and may be placed inadvertently into lung or abdominal organs.[2, 15] Treatment of hemothorax is less controversial as most factors favor the routine use of large-bore chest tube drainage for complete evacuation of the blood.[5, 6, 16–18] Needle aspiration results in ineffective drainage and is not an acceptable treatment choice.[3, 13] Observation of patients with blood in the pleural space leads to several unacceptable complications: fibrothorax with decreased vital capacity, empyema ultimately necessitating decortication, and increased hospital stay.

Complications of chest tube placement include persistent pneumothorax, hemothorax as a result of injury to intracostal vessels, empyema if a hemothorax occurs and is then incompletely evacuated, and infection. The use of prophylactic antibiotics in conjunction with chest tube placement to theoretically prevent subsequent infection is an area of unresolved controversy. Studies considering antibiotic treatment after chest tube placement in trauma and nontrauma patients with isolated and multiple injuries have had mixed outcomes.[19–21] There is no firm consensus as to the efficacy of prophylactic antibiotics in patients undergoing tube thoracostomy. At present, they are not recommended.

Scenario 1: The Stable Patient

The stable patient with a pneumo- or hemothorax has isolated chest trauma, normal vital signs, and no respiratory distress (Figs 25–1 and 25–2). The hematocrit is stable and the total chest tube output is less than 300 mL (see Fig 25–2). Therapeutic decisions are based on multiple factors: size, type, and cause of the injury (traumatic, spontaneous, iatrogenic) and the presence of underlying pulmonary disease.[12] In the emergency department, all patients with known pneumothorax or hemothorax should be placed on oxygen, preferably 100% by nonrebreather mask, a monitor, and have one to two 14-gauge intravenous (IV) lines of lactated Ringer's or normal saline established. Patients with underlying lung disease may require more individually tailored oxygen therapy. For patients with hemo- or hemopneumothorax, a hematocrit should be spun, and a type and hold sent to the blood bank. Initial IV volume deficits should be replaced by crystalloid and, when necessary, blood. The chest film should con-

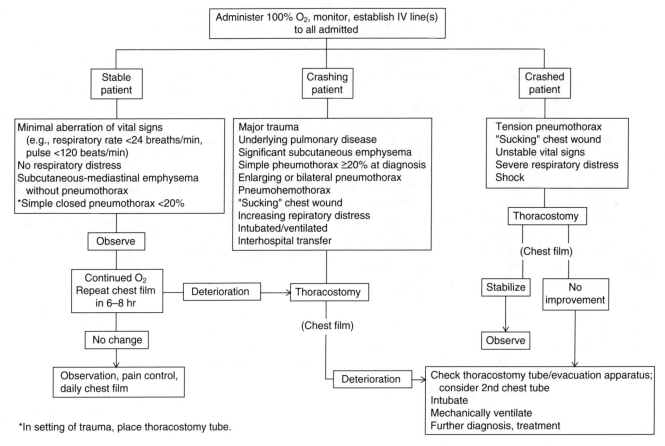

FIG 25–1.
Algorithm for management of pneumothorax.

firm the diagnosis before methods of intervention are considered.

Stable patients with isolated penetrating chest injuries above the nipple who have normal inspiratory and expiratory chest films should be observed for 4 to 6 hours. If repeat films after this period of observation are normal, the patient may be discharged.[4] Uncomplicated patients with minor chest trauma that present with minimal subcutaneous or mediastinal emphysema and no demonstrable pneumothorax may be observed in the hospital without tube thoracostomy.[14] These patients should continue to receive supportive care and repeat chest films every 6 to 8 hours. Subsequent daily chest films are sufficient to monitor resolution of the extrapleural air. Evidence of expansion of the subcutaneous air or the development of a pneumothorax will demand placement of a chest tube.

As noted above, selected patients with small uncomplicated spontaneous or iatrogenic pneumothoraces may be treated with alternative methods. Patients who are being transported to other hospitals are not candidates for observation alone because of the risk of decompensation en route. This is espe-

cially true if air transport systems are utilized. However all traumatic hemo- and pneumothoraces, regardless of the stability of the patient, must be evacuated with a chest tube. This approach will prevent the development of a life-threatening tension pneumothorax.[8] In addition, most bleeding from lung parenchyma will subside with lung reexpansion.[3, 19, 20] Post tube placement, all patients should receive a follow-up chest film to evaluate tube position, lung reexpansion, and evacuation of blood.

Scenario 2: The Crashing Patient

On initial inspection it is often difficult to determine exactly why a patient suffering from multiple trauma is crashing. (Chapter 22 gives a broader discussion of the subject.) Regardless of whether there is isolated chest trauma or generalized trauma with chest injuries, these patients should be treated as if their hypotension and agitation is all or in part secondary to a chest pathologic condition (tension pneumothorax, open pneumothorax, or a moderate to large hemothorax). Crashing patients with major chest trauma will exhibit increasing respiratory dis-

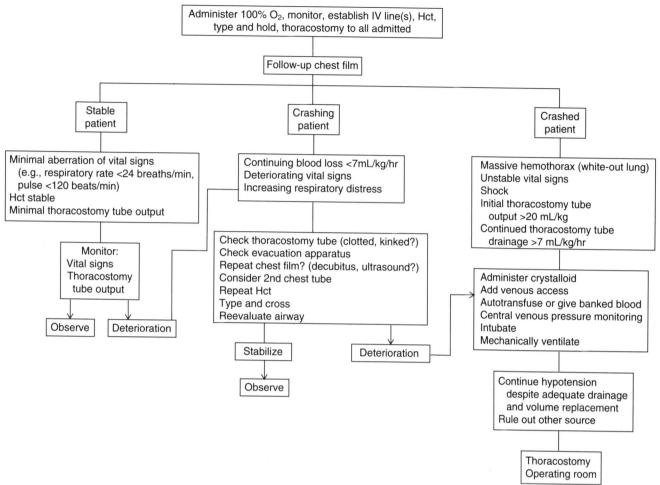

FIG 25–2.
Algorithm for management of hemothorax.

tress including an increased respiratory rate, dia-phoresis hypoxemia, a rapid heart rate, and hyper-carbia, singly or in combination. The blood pressure may be high, normal, or low, depending on the type and extent of injury. With isolated chest injury the blood pressure may eventually fall from blood loss, decreased venous return, or hypoxia. Underlying pulmonary disease may predispose patients with simple, closed pneumothorax to precipitous respiratory embarrassment. All of these patients should have expeditious chest tube placement. Chest radiography is not necessary prior to tube placement and must never delay treatment in deteriorating patients. In some instances, if time and stability allow, the chest film may be taken for documentation purposes, but with the tube placed prior to development of the film. In addition to routine laboratory studies, an early blood gas determination should be obtained. As with stable patients, 100% oxygen is administered by nonrebreather mask and cardiac and pulse oximetry monitors are attached.

Thoracostomy tube placement may fail to correct the problem or may malfunction at a later time. Reevaluation includes physical examination of the chest, repeat chest film, and inspection of the tube and the evacuation system. Expanding subcutaneous emphysema suggests that the proximal hole of the chest tube may be outside the pleural space. Cessation of drainage of blood or air in the crashing patient may indicate that the tube is kinked, that there is a blood clot in the tube, or that a connection hose has become loose or disconnected. Increasing size of the hemothorax or loculation of a collection of blood may require a second chest tube. Patients who are unresponsive to tube therapy may have an occult or missed hemothorax on the opposite side. Once again, the unstable or deteriorating patient should have a second tube placed on the opposite side regardless of a chest film having documented the abnormality. Ongoing collection of blood for autotransfusion should be routine for all victims of isolated chest trauma.[2] If ventilation and oxygenation defects are unresolved by proper chest tube placement, then intubation and active airway management are required.

In patients with bleeding in the thoracic cavity, controversy has surrounded the amount of blood loss which mandates thoracotomy. An initial output of 20 mL/kg with continued blood drainage of more than 7 mL/kg/hr are guidelines commonly referred to.[3, 5, 6, 16] At the very least, these patients are monitored closely with placement of a central venous pressure catheter. Their response to crystalloid, and to autotransfused or banked blood should be assessed along with various hemodynamic and clinical parameters. The decision for thoracotomy is best made using a combination of all factors rather than just the volume of blood drainage from the chest tube.

Treatment of open, sucking chest injuries requires immediate occlusion of the open wound with any available dressing to convert the injury to a closed pneumothorax. The dressing should be left open on one side or a chest tube placed to prevent formation of a tension pneumothorax. Another option in more unstable patients is to intubate and ventilate the patient leaving the chest wall defect open and uncovered until operative repair.[3, 8, 14]

Scenario 3: The Crashed Patient

The "crashed" patient is similar to the crashing patient. Yet, in this scenario, the patient has ventilatory failure and is either arrested or arrest is imminent. Just prior to loss of vital signs these patients are often severely agitated, hypotensive, bradycardiac, and cold and clammy. Unless the patient has deteriorated in the ED after arriving in stable condition, radiography will never be a part of the pretreatment evaluation. The only crucial decisions that must be made are whether to intubate first and on which side the chest tube is to be placed. The decision will be based on the availability of ancillary personnel, such as a respiratory therapist; on how definite the diagnosis of major chest injury is; on the presence of associated injuries; and on the state of the patient.

The arrested patient must be ventilated and oxygenated first. If the respiratory therapist is present and able to effectively administer bag-mask ventilation, then the physician is free to place the chest tube before actively managing the airway. If the physician must control the upper airway alone, then a nurse might be instructed to attempt decompression of a tension pneumothorax by placing a 14-gauge angiocatheter in the second intercostal space on the affected side.[3, 8] Severely agitated patients will have to be paralyzed and intubated prior to tube placement simply because of the logistical problem of placing the tube in a thrashing patient. If the pa-

tient is not thrashing about, yet is ventilating, the chest tube may be placed immediately. If the deterioration was secondary to isolated tension pneumothorax, there will be a rapid return of vital signs and overall stability after the air is evacuated. Once again, failure to respond to chest tube placement demands that a second tube be placed on the opposite side. In the patient without vital signs, time should not be spent meticulously preparing the patient or in using delicate surgical technique. Povidone-iodine (Betadine) may be splashed over the skin just as an aggressive 5- or 6-cm incision is made. It is also not necessary to tunnel two interspaces up from the initial incision to prevent a pneumothorax from redeveloping when the tube is removed.

PULMONARY CONTUSION AND FLAIL CHEST

Contusion of the lung is a frequent complication of motor vehicle accidents, falls, and blast injuries. It results from compression-decompression, shearing, or deceleration forces that accompany severe blunt chest trauma.[8, 22, 23] *Flail chest* is defined as paradoxical chest wall motion during respiration caused by sequential, double fractures of three or more ribs, or the sternum and ribs, resulting in a free-floating section of chest wall.[24, 25] It continues to be an important injury, occurring in 1 in 13 patients with rib fractures, with a mortality ranging from 5% to 50%, depending on the series. It has long-term morbidity consisting of chest pain, compromised pulmonary function, as measured by spirometric testing, and lost employment.[26-28] Because of the continued high morbidity and mortality, current investigations concerning the success of therapies have tried to elucidate the influence of all the major factors that determine the outcome of therapy.[26]

Pulmonary contusion and flail chest compromise ventilation and oxygenation. At the cellular level, contusion produces interstitial and intraalveolar hemorrhage and edema. This causes small airway collapse, decreased pulmonary vascular flow, decreased alveolar gas perfusion, increased pulmonary vascular resistance, and reduced lung compliance. With extensive pulmonary contusion, secretions and blood may also cause small airway atelectasis and obstruct airflow. Intrapulmonary shunt and systemic hypoxemia result.[14, 22, 23, 29] Flail chest, in particular, causes pain and altered chest wall mechanics secondary to paradoxical movement of the flail segment. There is increased splinting and decreased cough effectiveness. Secretions accumulate, increasing the work of respiration. Fatigue and possible pulmonary contusion underlying the flail segment can exacerbate ventilation and oxygenation mismatch leading to further respiratory decompensation. Aspiration is not an initial concern in awake, alert patients. However, in patients with severe associated injuries, in particular head injury, protective airway reflexes may be lost and aspiration of oral and gastric contents can occur.

Diagnostic evidence of pulmonary contusion may be lacking at the time of admission to the emergency department. Its onset may be insidious and optimal therapy relies on early diagnosis. It is important for the clinician to suspect pulmonary contusion when reviewing chest films, as a contusion may be masked by overlying subcutaneous emphysema, pneumohemothorax, rib fractures, or other distracting pathologic conditions. The mechanism of injury and other historical details may excite clinical suspicion.

Clinical signs and symptoms may range from none to external evidence of chest wall trauma, pain, dyspnea, tachypnea, hypotension, and in 50% of patients, mild hemoptysis.[23] Chest auscultation may reveal rales or decreased breath sounds over the area of injury. Initially, chest films may or may not show evidence of pulmonary contusion. However, radiographic changes are usually apparent by 6 hours postinjury and, in simple cases, begin to resolve within 24 to 48 hours. Complete resolution of uncomplicated cases takes several days.[23] The magnitude of contusion seen on serial chest radiographs has not been predictive of the impact of the injury upon ventilation or oxygenation or the need for subsequent intubation.

Arterial blood gas (ABG) determinations may be helpful in making the diagnosis of pulmonary contusion in suspect patients. ABGs should be drawn, if possible, on room air and early in the patient's course to aid expeditious institution of therapy. Hypoxemia alone may be evidence of contusion. The alveolar-arterial oxygen gradient [$P(A-a)O_2$] has been used as a more sensitive indicator of respiratory distress.[7] A similar, frequently used measure of the presence of pulmonary injury is the ratio of arterial oxygen pressure to the fractional concentration of inspired oxygen (PaO_2/FiO_2). This is an indirect measurement of intrapulmonary shunt. Though values vary, a PaO_2/FiO_2 ratio of less than 300 has been associated significantly with the need for intubation and increased mortality.[29] While PaO_2 measurements may easily be obtained from ABGs for estimating the PaO_2/FiO_2 ratio, it is difficult to get an

accurate measure of FiO_2 when oxygen masks and cannulas instead of endotracheal tubes are used for oxygen delivery. Falsely high estimates of the FiO_2 may lead to false-positive identification of serious intrapulmonary shunt.[29]

Recently, there has been increased interest in assessing the utility of CT in the diagnosis and evaluation of pulmonary contusion. Several interesting observations have been made. CT is the most sensitive method for assessing the presence and extent of pulmonary contusion. It has called into question the long-standing definition of pulmonary contusion as damage to lung tissue that results in hemorrhage and edema *without laceration*. In one study assessing pulmonary contusion with plain radiographs and chest CT, the infiltrates seen on plain chest radiographs which were classically consistent with pulmonary contusion were found on CT to be pulmonary lacerations surrounded by intraalveolar hemorrhage.[30] Emergent chest CT is being examined as a tool in the management of blunt trauma. In one small study, CT identified ten pulmonary contusions, while chest films detected only four and falsely identified an additional three contusions not seen on CT. However, no significant therapeutic changes were made based on these findings.[31] Despite the increased diagnostic sensitivity and early diagnostic potential of CT, its utility in the evaluation of pulmonary contusion may be limited by its high cost, lack of specific criteria for its use, and its questionable influence on management. Further investigation is necessary.

Emergency department diagnosis of flail chest is made by direct observation of a flail segment during active breathing or by chest radiograph. Posterior flail segments may not be obvious on physical examination because of support by an underlying gurney or backboard. Lateral flail segments are most common.[32] Palpation and auscultation of the chest may reveal evidence of subcutaneous emphysema, rib fractures, and pneumo- or hemothorax. Complete primary and secondary surveys with attention to the adequacy of ventilation should be performed. ABG samples should be obtained early on all patients to evaluate respiratory function, particularly to rule out hypoxemia and hypercapnia.

Management of pulmonary contusion and flail chest is controversial. Both continue to have a high morbidity and mortality, ranging from 13% to 50%, despite major advances in pulmonary care.[3, 7, 26, 29] The main areas of controversy include respiratory and fluid management, the use of steroids, and prophylactic antibiotics.

Treatment of flail chest has evolved from the uniform practice of surgical chest wall stabilization or mechanical ventilation (pneumatic splinting) to a more selective approach.[26, 28, 33–35] Changes in therapy are based on the belief that underlying pulmonary contusion (75%–90%)[26] is responsible for the respiratory failure in patients with flail chest.[7, 26, 36] Pulmonary contusion in patients without respiratory decompensation can be managed effectively without intubation. Increased morbidity is associated with ventilator therapy, particularly when prolonged, as it is complicated by a high incidence of pulmonary infection and other complications.[14, 26, 37] At present, respiratory and fluid management of patients with pulmonary contusion with or without a flail segment is essentially the same. Paradoxical chest wall movement alone, without respiratory failure (see Fig 25–4) is not an indication for intubation and mechanical ventilation.[35] As demonstrated by the anecdotal report of the recovery of a Roman soldier's skeleton from the fourth century B.C., which had 16 healed, bilateral rib fractures, even without modern respiratory intervention severe flail chest injuries may not lead to death.[35] In patients requiring intubation, investigators have shown that intermittent mandatory ventilation (IMV) is preferred over controlled mechanical ventilation (CMV) for the treatment of pulmonary contusion. IMV improves oxygen transport to a greater extent than does CMV.[38] Initially, an IMV rate of 6 to 12 breaths per minute with a tidal volume of 10 to 15 mL/kg should be tried in the emergency department. Ventilator settings should be adjusted to maintain a pH of approximately 7.35 or greater while trying to keep spontaneous respirations to less than 30 breaths per minute.[39]

If oxygenation continues to be inadequate positive end-expiratory pressure (PEEP) may be added. An alternative is continuous positive airway pressure (CPAP) via endotracheal tube. It may be tried initially in place of PEEP to maintain a PaO_2 greater than 60 to 65 mm Hg with an FiO_2 less than 50%.[14, 39] If PEEP is selected, the exact level necessary to improve pulmonary gas exchange is controversial. PEEP is usually added in the emergency department in small increments to prevent hypoxemia.[32] Eventually, central monitoring will be necessary to balance the negative cardiac effects of PEEP against its pulmonary benefits.

High-frequency positive pressure ventilation (HFPPV), has been advocated in place of conventional PEEP. HFPPV interferes less with cardiac function and provides adequate oxygenation at lower peak airway pressures, lessening pulmonary barotrauma.[40] In patients with severe unilateral pulmonary contusion not responsive to the above methods, synchronized independent lung ventilation (SILV) applied through a double lumen endotracheal tube has proved useful. By allowing independent ventilation of each lung, SILV prevents hyperexpansion of the normal lung. This occurs when high airway pressures are needed to expand the injured lung, but are delivered by a single lumen endotracheal tube indiscriminately to both injured and noninjured lungs. Hyperexpansion increases capillary resistance and enhances blood flow to the damaged lung promoting increased pulmonary shunt and ventilation-perfusion mismatch.[41] At present, SILV is not routinely used in the emergency department. It is more likely to be instituted in the intensive care unit.

Fluid therapy in the management of isolated pulmonary contusion or in association with flail chest has been debated. Investigators theorized that judicious fluid restriction and the use of colloids and diuretics to dry out areas of edema would prevent respiratory insufficiency and avoid the need for mechanical ventilation.[8, 22, 36] Experimental evidence has not uniformly supported this approach. Current recommendations are to resuscitate hypovolemic shock with crystalloid solutions and blood products.[14, 29, 42, 43] Packed red blood cells should be administered to maintain a hematocrit above 21% to 23% to ensure adequate oxygen-carrying capacity. Large infusions of crystalloids have not been correlated with worsening of pulmonary contusion, increased likelihood of intubation, or with mortality when used to resuscitate patients from hypovolemic shock.[22] Colloids may aggravate pulmonary edema, as increasing hydrostatic pressure causes leaking of colloid and fluid through damaged capillaries.[43] Diuretics are not routinely recommended, as hypovolemia may decrease perfusion and exacerbate hypoxemia.[44]

Steroid therapy is another area of controversy.[45] At present steroids are not advocated. In the setting of pulmonary contusion they have been associated with increased risk of infection and with aggravating shock-related pulmonary failure.[29] Prophylactic antibiotics are not recommended. They do not alter the incidence of pneumonia and they may select for resistant organisms.[11]

Scenario 1: The Stable Patient

The stable patient with flail chest or pulmonary contusion, or both, will have near-normal vital signs

(Figs 25–3 and 25–4). Some tachypnea and tachycardia will be present from anxiety and pain but not from respiratory distress. The skin will be dry and pink. The pulse oximeter should read greater than 95%. ABG samples will document a PaO_2 greater than 60 mm Hg on room air and the arterial carbon dioxide tension ($PaCO_2$) will be less than 40 mm Hg.[3, 7, 14] Pulmonary function testing will generally document a tidal volume of greater than 5 mL/kg and a vital capacity of greater than 10 mL/kg.[14] In the absence of head trauma and intoxicants, these patients are generally awake and alert with little risk of aspiration.

The greatest concern in these patients is to watch for early signs of deterioration. Pulmonary contusion can progress rapidly over the first few hours post trauma, especially as fluid is administered during resuscitation. Routine trauma laboratory tests, monitoring, IV access, chest films, and oxygen administration are part of the standard early evaluation and treatment. Pain control and chest physiotherapy are important to prevent splinting, atelectasis, and retained secretions which can cause obstruction to airflow and increase the risk of infection. Parenteral pain medication may be supplemented by intercostal blocks or epidural anesthesia.[7, 42] Respiratory mechanics and function are optimized when pain medication is administered to the point of abolishing paradoxical chest wall motion. The best respiratory management of pulmonary contusion is supportive without intubation. Active airway control should be reserved for patients who develop respiratory insufficiency.[3, 29, 37, 42]

Following the initial evaluation and resuscitation, fluid management should be optimized to prevent volume overload. Central venous pressure or Swan-Ganz catheter monitoring should supplement clinical indicators such as vital signs and urine output.[7, 42] These patients must be admitted to an intensive care bed to optimize pulmonary toilet and monitoring of fluids. ABGs and the chest film are used to assess daily progress.

Scenario 2: The Crashing Patient

The crashing patient with pulmonary contusion or flail chest will present with respiratory distress or will clearly deteriorate while in the resuscitation room. Respiratory rate and heart rate are generally increased greater than would be expected from pain alone. These patients are in great pain; they may be diaphoretic and working very hard to breath. The PaO_2 is less than 60 mm Hg on room air or has fallen substantially from initial values obtained in the ED. The $PaCO_2$ may be rising and is greater than 40 mm Hg. Other factors which have been associated

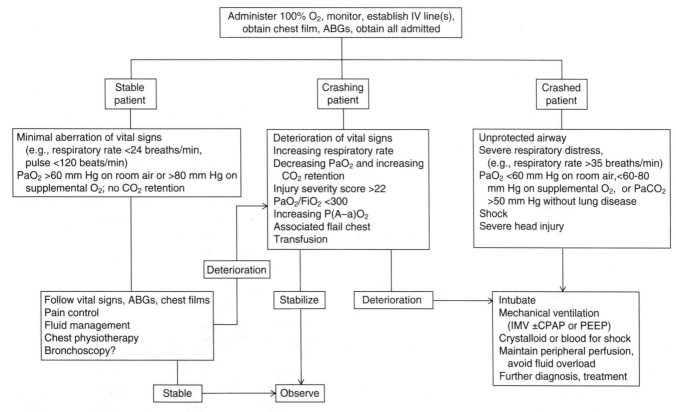

FIG 25–3.
Algorithm for management of pulmonary contusion.

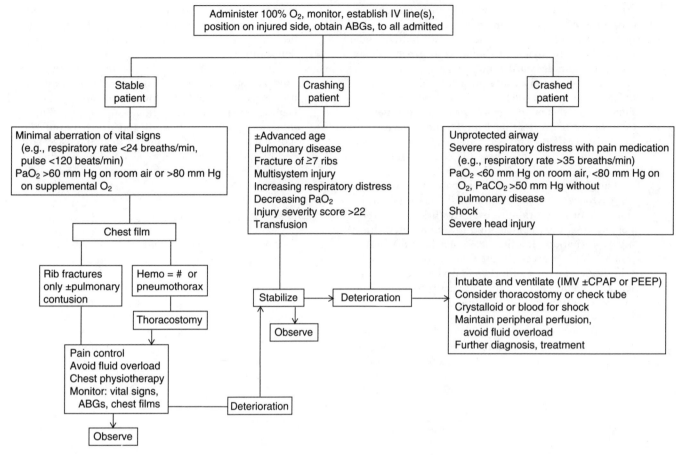

FIG 25–4.
Algorithm for management of flail chest.

with the eventual need for intubation and with increased morbidity and mortality include: an injury severity score (ISS) greater than 22; a PaO_2/FiO_2 ratio of less than 300; an increasing $P(A-a)O_2$; blood transfusions for shock; flail chest; extrathoracic fractures; underlying pulmonary disease; and injuries requiring thoracotomy or laparotomy.[3, 7, 26, 27, 29, 37]

Most patients described here will require intubation. However an attempt may be made to resuscitate and oxygenate prior to active airway management. CPAP by face mask may be tried prior to intubation and mechanical ventilation. CPAP will increase thoracic compliance and decrease respiratory work to improve oxygenation.[11, 39] If the patient's condition continues to worsen despite supportive efforts, then the airway should be secured with an endotracheal tube.

Scenario 3: The Crashed Patient

Crashed patients are in severe respiratory distress or have significant head injuries and are close to cardiopulmonary arrest. These patients are severely agitated, hypotensive, tachycardic, or bradycardic and

tachypneic. Rapid-sequence intubation is critical and there is little room for error. These patients will have no oxygen reserve when they are paralyzed, they will be impossible to hyperoxygenate, and it may be very difficult to administer bag-mask ventilation. Preparation for a surgical airway should be made when a difficult intubation is anticipated.

The goal of mechanical ventilation and oxygenation is to maintain a PaO_2 of greater than 60 mm Hg. The lowest FiO_2 necessary to obtain this level of oxygenation should be used. As discussed above, the patient should be placed on IMV. Other modalities available to aid oxygenation include PEEP, HFPPV, and SILV.

TRACHEOBRONCHIAL INJURY AND AIR EMBOLISM

Injury to the intrathoracic tracheobronchial tree may result from either blunt or penetrating trauma to the chest. Tracheobronchial tears are more common than complete ruptures. Intrathoracic injuries outnumber cervical tracheal injuries. Eighty percent to 90% of all tracheal injuries occur within 2.5 cm of the carina.[14, 46, 47] Overall mortality ranges from 10% to 30%.[3, 48] Traumatic air emboli resulting from injuries which allow air to escape into the pulmonary vascular system are rare, but catastrophic. Without immediate therapy, disability or death is probable. In one series of 61 patients with air embolus, overall mortality was 56%.[47] Because signs, symptoms, and diagnostic findings are nonspecific, physicians must initially suspect these injuries in all patients with significant blunt or penetrating chest trauma.

A tracheobronchial injury causing a partial tear or complete rupture threatens the airway by allowing escape of air into the mediastinum or pleural space, disrupting airflow. Massive subcutaneous emphysema resulting from these injuries, particularly if under pressure, may obstruct airflow. Pneumothorax may develop from intrapleural airway rupture. Curtailed airflow, lung collapse, and loss of normal intrathoracic pressure gradients secondary to pneumothorax may severely compromise gas exchange. Injury to the lung vasculature may result in hemoptysis.[49] Aspiration of blood can further compromise

airflow, ventilation, and perfusion. Unrecognized tracheobronchial injuries, frequently extrapleural ruptures, may be diagnosed when previously discharged patients return to the ED with atelectasis or pulmonary infection. Airway complications develop secondary to granulation tissue formation and airway narrowing at the healing wound site.[14] Airflow and gas exchange are impaired at the affected site.

On presentation, patients (Fig 25–5) may be relatively asymptomatic and thus difficult to diagnose. Those with extrapleural or mediastinal airway ruptures fall into this group. Physical examination in suspect patients should include palpation and auscultation of the soft tissues of the neck and chest, looking for subcutaneous emphysema and Hamman's crunch.[3, 49–52] Subcutaneous emphysema is the most common physical and radiographic finding, occurring in approximately 75% to 85% of patients.[49, 51] Chest films may reveal pneumomediastinum, subcutaneous emphysema, pneumothorax, deep cervical emphysema, parabronchial air, or sudden loss of continuity of an air-filled bronchus.[14, 50, 52] With complete tracheal transection, and injury to tissues that support airway structures, the pulmonary hilum may seem to drop toward the dia-

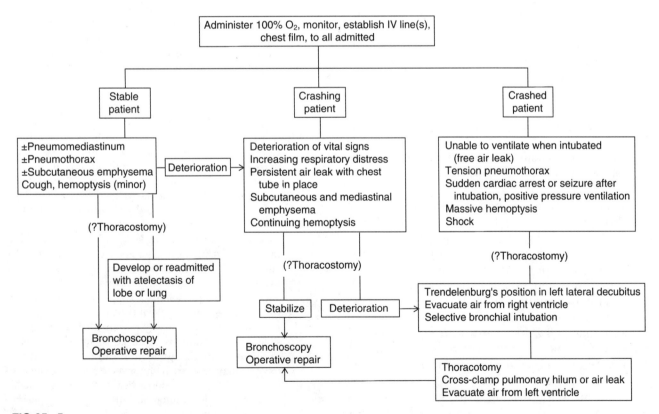

FIG 25–5.
Algorithm for management of tracheobronchial injury and air embolism.

phragm.[50] Unrecognized tracheobronchial injuries often present 1 to 4 weeks after the initial event, with postobstructive atelectasis of a lobe or lung on chest film.[3, 14]

Pneumothorax is common and is caused by intrapleural airway rupture. A pneumothorax that fails to reexpand, or which has a continued air leak after chest tube placement, strongly suggests a tracheobronchial injury.[3, 52] A follow-up chest radiograph after thoracotomy tube placement will assure proper position and tube configuration, and lung reexpansion. Assessment of function of chest tube drainage equipment and suction apparatus assures that inability to reexpand the affected lung is not the result of equipment malfunction. If doubt remains, a second chest tube may be placed (see under Pneumothorax and Hemothorax above).

Patients may present with other signs and symptoms in addition to the above, including cough, respiratory distress, and hemoptysis.[3, 49–51] Injury to bronchial vessels was the most common vascular injury found in one review of pediatric tracheobronchial injuries.[49] Massive hemoptysis is rare.[3] Tension pneumothorax is unusual in adults but may be more common in children.[49]

Tracheobronchial injuries in unstable patients (see Fig 25–5) are often missed. Instability is often attributed to associated injuries of the chest or elsewhere. A high degree of suspicion by caretakers, based on the mechanism of injury, the prehospital course, the presence of blunt or penetrating chest injury, or recognition of symptom complexes, is imperative. Unstable patients may present with rapidly deteriorating vital signs, significant respiratory distress, or hemodynamic shock. These patients may be impossible to ventilate adequately because of massive air leakage worsened by positive pressure ventilation.

Patients with air embolism resulting from tracheobronchial injury (see Fig 25–5) are critically unstable. In the setting of chest injury, sudden dramatic cardiac arrest, loss of consciousness, seizure, or confusion, particularly after intubation and positive pressure ventilation, or shock that is unresponsive to resuscitation, should immediately suggest air embolism.[3, 14] A series of 61 patients with air embolism showed that 100% had cardiac arrest or shock.[53] Other cardiac aberrations may result from the effects of air embolism on the heart and brain. Patients may present with tachycardia, bradycardia, new murmurs, or distant heart sounds.[54] Rarely, free air in the arterial and venous systems of the heart may be seen on the chest radiograph.[54] Occa-

sionally, the diagnosis in unstable patients is made by visualizing air bubbles in the coronary arteries during emergency thoracotomy.[3, 54]

Scenario 1: The Stable Patient

The stable patient has near-normal vital signs and is in no acute distress (see Fig 25–5). Symptoms may include cough, pleuritic chest pain, and mild hemoptysis. Physical examination may be normal or may reveal subcutaneous air about the chest or neck and/or air in the mediastinum (Hamman's crunch). Routine laboratory work, monitoring, and initial resuscitation should be initiated. Chest radiography is the only ED study that will be helpful in making the diagnosis. Once the diagnosis is suspected, the patient should be placed on 100% oxygen. Studies suggest that the outcome is better with air embolism if the embolized gas is oxygen rather than air.[55]

Provided that the patient remains stable and has no associated trauma, no other studies or treatment is necessary in the ED. Rigid or flexible fiberoptic bronchoscopy is the diagnostic tool of choice.[3, 12, 51, 56] It is preferable to perform the procedure in the operating room where complications can be dealt with expeditiously. The bronchoscope can be used to identify and evaluate the injury.[56, 57] In addition, intubation can be performed over the bronchoscope. Single and double lumen endotracheal tube placement, selective right or mainstem intubation, and ventilation may be performed with the aid of the bronchoscope. Arteriography should also be performed to identify or rule out significant vascular injuries.[49]

Scenario 2: The Crashing Patient

Crashing patients are those with significant respiratory distress, ongoing hemodynamic deterioration, massive emphysema, and pneumothorax unrelieved by thoracostomy tubes. As with other respiratory emergencies these patients are generally agitated, diaphoretic, tachypneic, and tachycardic. Oxygen is administered and a second chest tube is placed if there is a persistent air leak. All forms of airway management in these patients are dangerous, difficult, and wrought with complicating factors. Positive pressure ventilation may aggravate air leaks and subcutaneous emphysema. Passage of endotracheal tubes can convert a partial tracheal tear into a complete tear. Surgical airway placement may be impossible if the anatomy is obscured by massive amounts of air in the neck. Ventilation can be ineffective, as oxygen may not reach the affected lung because of injury distal to the endotracheal tube, uncontrollable air leak, or tension pneumothorax caused by positive pressure ventilation.[15]

Alternative methods of airway management may

be attempted in the most difficult cases. High-frequency transtracheal jet ventilation (HFJV) may be lifesaving in patients with air leaks.[47, 57] This approach may provide adequate oxygenation and ventilation until operative evaluation and repair. Concerns with HFJV include carbon dioxide retention and exacerbating preexisting barotrauma, particularly subcutaneous emphysema.[57] Independent lung ventilation is another option. In the ED, selective bronchial intubation may be the most practical lifesaving tool in crashing patients. Emergency physicians trained to use a fiberoptic intubating bronchoscope may find tracheobronchial injuries ideal settings for their method. The bronchoscope may be used to guide the endotracheal tube past damaged tissues and ultimately into either bronchus if desired.

Scenario 3: The Crashed Patient

Patients who have crashed are those with suspected air embolism or respiratory failure from substantial air leak or massive subcutaneous emphysema. In addition to maneuvers used in the crashing scenario, the patient should be placed in Trendelenburg's position in left lateral decubitus. This positioning is an attempt to keep air emboli in the right side of the heart and away from the brain and the systemic circulation. One hundred percent oxygen should be administered. These tactics should be followed by needle aspiration of the right ventricle and then thoracotomy to allow cross-clamping of the involved pulmonary hilum. Needle evacuation of air from the left ventricle should then follow along with expeditious operative repair.[14, 53]

Securing the airway is once again the number one priority. All of the options and concerns discussed in the crashing scenario apply to the crashed patient. Patients with isolated tracheobronchial injuries most commonly arrest from pure respiratory embarrassment. Successful control of the airway in a timely fashion, although difficult, is often lifesaving.

PREHOSPITAL CARE OF CHEST INJURIES

Many emergency therapies and stabilization procedures may readily be performed in the prehospital setting. Prehospital personnel can secure airway access, institute oxygen therapy, and administer ventilation and initial fluid resuscitation. Patients with lateral flail chest, by selective positioning on the affected side, can have their flail segment stabilized during transport. Prior to chest tube placement, tension pneumothorax can be evacuated with a 14-gauge angiocatheter. Prehospital caretakers can alert the ED team of possible air embolism by relating the occurrence of sudden cardiac arrest or seizure. With suspicion of air embolism, further emboli may be prevented by positioning the patient in Trendelenburg's position, in left lateral decubitus, during transport to the hospital.

REFERENCES

1. Vukich DJ: Pneumothorax, hemothorax, and other abnormalities of the pleural space. *Emerg Med Clin North Am* 1983; 1:431.
2. Mattox KL, Allen MK: Systematic approach to pneumothorax, hemothorax, pneumomediastinum and subcutaneous emphysema. *Injury* 1986; 17:309.
3. Carrero R, Wayne M: Chest trauma. *Emerg Med Clin North Am* 1989; 7:389.
4. Karanfilian R, Machiedo GW, Bolanowski PJ: Management of nonpenetrating stab and gunshot wounds of the chest. *Surg Gynecol Obstet* 1981; 153:395.
5. Richardson JD: Indications for thoracotomy in thoracic trauma. *Curr Surg* 1985; 42:361.
6. Burrington JD: Chest injuries in children. *Can J Surg* 1984; 27:466.
7. Pate JW: Chest wall injuries. *Surg Clin North Am* 1989; 69:59.
8. Jones KW: Thoracic trauma. *Surg Clin North Am* 1980; 60:957.
9. Bitto T, Mannion JD, Stephenson LW, et al: Pneumothorax during positive pressure mechanical ventilation. *J Thorac Cardiovasc Surg* 1985; 89:585.
10. Hurewitz AN, Sidhu U, Bergofsky EH, et al: Cardiovascular and respiratory consequences of tension pneumothorax. *Bull Eur Physiopathol Respir* 1986; 22:545.
11. Clemmer TP, Fairfax WR: Critical care management of chest injury. *Crit Care Clin* 1986; 2:759.
12. Glinz W: Priorities in diagnosis and treatment of blunt chest injuries. *Injury* 1986; 17:318.
13. Vukich DJ: Disease of the pleural space. *Emerg Med Clin North Am* 1989; 7:309.
14. Mattox KL, Moore EE, Feliciano DV: *Trauma*, ed 1. San Mateo, Calif, Appleton & Lange, 1988.
15. Mattox KL, Allen MK: Penetrating wounds of the thorax. *Injury* 1986; 17:313.
16. Weil PH, Margolis IB: Systematic approach to traumatic hemothorax. *Am J Surg* 1981; 142:692.
17. Moorehead RJ, Spence RJ, McAdam WD, et al: Hemothorax—the importance of adequate drainage. *Injury* 1985; 16:387.
18. Coselli JS, Mattox KL, Beall AC: Reevaluation of early evacuation of clotted hemothorax. *Am J Surg* 1984; 148:786.
19. Grover FL, Richardson JD, Fewel JG, et al: Prophylactic antibiotics in the treatment of penetrating chest wounds. *J Thorac Cardiovasc Surg* 1977; 74:528.

20. LeBlanc KA, Tucker WY: Prophylactic antibiotics and closed tube thoracostomy. *Surg Gynecol Obstet* 1985; 160:259.

21. LoCurto JJ, Tischler CD, Swan KG, et al: Tube thoracostomy and trauma—antibiotics or not? *J Trauma* 1986; 26:1067.

22. Mulder DS: Chest trauma: Current concepts. *Can J Surg* 1980; 23:340.

23. Hill JW, Deluca SA: Pulmonary contusion. *Am Fam Physician* 1988; 38:219.

24. Beal SL, Oreskovich MR: Long-term disability associated with flail chest injury. *Am J Surg* 1985; 150:324.

25. Schmit-Neuerburg KP, Weiss H, Labitzke R: Indication for thoracotomy and chest wall stabilization. *Injury* 1982; 14:26.

26. Freedland M, Wilson RF, Bender JS, et al: The management of flail chest injury: Factors affecting outcome. *J Trauma* 1990; 30:1460.

27. Schulpen MJ, Doesburg WH, Lemmens WJ, et al: Epidemiology and prognostic signs of chest injury patients, *Injury* 1986; 17:305.

28. Landercasper J, Cogbill TH, Lindesmith LA: Long-term disability after flail chest injury. *J Trauma* 1984; 24:410.

29. Johnson JA, Cogbill TH, Winga ER: Determination of outcome after pulmonary contusion. *J Trauma* 1986; 26:695.

30. Wagner RB, Jamieson PM: Pulmonary contusion evaluation and classification by computed tomography. *Surg Clin North Am* 1989; 69:31.

31. McGonigal MD, Schwab CW, Kauder DR, et al: Supplemental emergent chest computed tomography in the management of blunt torso trauma. *J Trauma* 1990; 30:1431.

32. Carroll GC, Tuman KJ, Braverman B, et al: Minimal positive end-expiratory pressure (PEEP) may be "best PEEP." *Chest* 1988; 93:1020.

33. Carpintero JL, Rodriguez Diez A, Ruiz Elvira MJ, et al: Methods of management of flail chest. *Intensive Care Med* 1980; 6:217.

34. Christensson P, Gisselsson L, Lecerof H, et al: Early and late results of controlled ventilation in flail chest. *Chest* 1979; 75:456.

35. Glinz W: Problems caused by the unstable thoracic wall and by cardiac injury due to blunt injury. *Injury* 1986; 17:322.

36. Trinkle JK, Richardson JD, Franz JL, et al: Management of flail chest without mechanical ventilation. *Ann Thorac Surg* 1975; 19:355.

37. Richardson JD, Adams L, Flint LM: Selective management of flail chest and pulmonary contusion. *Ann Surg* 1982; 196:481.

38. Pinilla JC: Acute respiratory failure in severe blunt chest trauma. *J Trauma* 1982; 22:221.

39. Shackford SR, Virgilio RW, Peters RM: Selective use of ventilator therapy in flail chest injury. *J Thorac Cardiovasc Surg* 1981; 81:194.

40. Barzilay E, Lev A, Ibrahim M, et al: Traumatic respiratory insufficiency: Comparison of conventional mechanical ventilation to high frequency positive pressure with low-rate ventilation. *Crit Care Med* 1987; 15:118.

41. Frame SB, Marshall WJ, Clifford TG: Synchronized independent lung ventilation in the management of pediatric unilateral pulmonary contusion: Case report. *J Trauma* 1989; 29:395.

42. Clark GC, Schecter WP, Trunkey DD: Variables affecting outcome in blunt chest trauma: Flail chest vs. pulmonary contusion. *J Trauma* 1988; 28:298.

43. Wisner DH, Sturm JA: Controversies in the fluid management of post-traumatic lung disease. *Injury* 1986; 17:295.

44. Trinkle JK: Management of major thoracic wall trauma. *Curr Surg* 1985; 42:181.

45. Svennevig JL, Pillgram-Larsen J, Fjeld NB, et al: Early use of corticosteroids in severe closed chest injuries: A 10-year experience. *Injury* 1987; 18:309.

46. Ecker RR, Libertini RV, Rea WJ, et al: Injuries of the trachea and bronchi. *Ann Thorac Surg* 1971; 11:289.

47. Maull KI, Cleveland HC, Strauch GO, et al: *Advances in Trauma*, vol 1. St Louis, Mosby–Year Book, Inc, 1986.

48. Burke JF: Early diagnosis of traumatic rupture of the bronchus. *JAMA* 1962; 181:682.

49. Nakayama DK, Rowe MI: Intrathoracic thracheo-bronchial injuries in childhood. *Int Anesthesiol Clin* 1988; 26:42.

50. Lazar HL, Thomashow B, King TC: Complete transection of the intrathoracic trachea due to blunt trauma. *Ann Thorac Surg* 1984; 37:505.

51. Jones WS, Mavroudis C, Richardson JD, et al: Management of tracheobronchial disruption resulting from blunt trauma. *Surgery* 1983; 95:319.

52. Grover FL, Ellestad C, Arom KV, et al: Diagnosis and management of major tracheobronchial injuries. *Ann Thorac Surg* 1979; 28:384.

53. Yee ES, Verrier ED, Thomas AN: Management of air embolism in blunt and penetrating thoracic trauma. *J Thorac Cardiovasc Surg* 1983; 85:661.

54. Lee SK, Transwell AK: Pulmonary vascular air embolism in the newborn. *Arch Dis Child* 1989; 64:507.

55. Fries CC, Levoweitz B, Adler S, et al: Experimental cerebral gas embolism. *Ann Surg* 1957; 145:461.

56. Hara KS, Prakash US: Fiberoptic bronchoscopy in the evaluation of acute chest and upper airway trauma. *Chest* 1989; 96:627.

57. Shimazu T, Sugimoto H, Nishide K, et al: Tracheobronchial rupture caused by blunt chest trauma: Acute respiratory management. *Am J Emerg Med* 1988; 6:427.

26

Airway Burns and Toxic Gas Inhalation

David Gough, D.O.

Gary Young, M.D.

Airway burns and inhalation exposure present a spectrum of threats to the three pillars of the airway which can be immediate or delayed.[1-18] Inhalation injury develops in three clinical stages (Table 26–1).[1, 3, 9, 12, 16, 19, 20] The first stage involves potential airway compromise primarily from upper airway edema and bronchospasm. Symptoms may be absent or marked by overt dyspnea occurring at the time of exposure or delayed for up to 24 hours. The second stage of respiratory injury occurs at 24 to 48 hours and results from pulmonary edema. The final stage is due to the complications of pneumonia and develops 2 to 3 days following exposure.

Heat injury is usually confined to the upper airway; the low specific heat capacity of air and the efficient heat-exchanging capacity of the upper airway sufficiently cools inhaled smoke before it reaches the lower airways.[21] Also, the vocal cords close reflexively when exposed to heat which further provides lower airway protection.[8] Superheated steam, which has a much higher specific heat capacity than air, often causes thermal injury to the lower airways.[13, 17, 21] Additionally, inhaled particulates cause airway irritation (potentially inducing bronchospasm), and can carry toxic chemicals to the lower respiratory tract resulting in irritation and pulmonary edema.[8]

Airflow obstruction secondary to airway burns and toxic inhalations results from airway edema, mucous plugging, atelectasis, tracheobronchitis, laryngospasm, and bronchospasm.[4, 5, 9, 12, 17-20] Aspiration results from emesis coupled with altered mental status. Excessive tracheobronchial secretions and carbonaceous particulates are poorly cleared secondary to ciliary dysfunction. Embarrassment of ventilation and oxygenation attends all significant thermal,

smoke, or chemical inhalation. Noncardiogenic pulmonary edema or pneumonitis from pulmonary vascular and parenchymal injury results in ventilation-perfusion ($\dot{V}/\dot{Q}$) mismatching, increased work of breathing, and mental obtundation.[2, 7, 19, 20] Hypoxia from asphyxiants that displace oxygen (e.g., carbon dioxide, carbon monoxide) or systemic asphyxiants that cause cellular poisoning (e.g., cyanide) lead to anaerobic metabolism and metabolic acidosis (Table 26–2).[20, 22, 23,] Asphyxiant gases are likely to play a major role in the burn patient who arrives comatose or in respiratory arrest.

There are a number of chemicals or gases that are involved in the smoke inhalation victim. Chemical injury occurs from irritant gases coming in contact with the airway mucosa.[1, 2, 4, 8, 24] Gases of high solubility (i.e., chlorine, ammonia, acrolein, tear gas) are rapidly absorbed on the moist surfaces of the eyes, nose, mouth, and upper airway. An intense inflammatory response occurs that may lead to upper airway obstruction from edema. Gases of low solubility (e.g., phosgene, nitrogen and sulfur oxides) dissolve more slowly allowing passage beyond protective upper airway mucosa to the lower respiratory tract. Bronchitis and alveolitis may develop (see Table 26–2).

The main gases found in smoke, in addition to CO and CN, are oxygen and CO_2.[8] The process of combustion in a fire rapidly consumes O_2, exposing the victim to decreasing levels of fractional concentration of oxygen in inspired gas (FiO_2).[25] Hypoxia is the leading cause of death at the fire scene.[24] Inhalation of CO_2 causes two problems. First, it stimulates respiration which leads to further smoke inhalation. Second, elevated carbon dioxide partial

TABLE 26–1.

Clinical Stages of Inhalation Injury

Stage 1 (0–24 hr)	Stage 2 (24–48 hr)	Stage 3 (48–72 hr)
Airway compromise	Pulmonary edema	Pneumonia
Upper airway edema	Symptomatic ±	Progressive pulmonary
Bronchospasm	respiratory distress	compromise
Alveolitis	Alveolar-capillary	Fever, sepsis
	membrane injury	

pressure (PCO_2), as a direct result of inhalation or from retention stemming from altered consciousness, will compound the metabolic acidosis caused by cellular toxins in smoke.[8] Carbon monoxide is another common by-product of fire. It is produced by incomplete combustion of carbon-containing materials. The high affinity of CO for hemoglobin displaces O_2.[26] The shift of the oxygen-hemoglobin dissociation curve to the left further prevents release of O_2 to the tissues.[27] Carbon monoxide also causes direct cellular poisoning by disabling the cytochrome oxidase system.[28, 29] Multiple organ systems are involved, particularly the central nervous system (CNS). In order of increasing severity, CNS symptoms are headache, nausea, vomiting, lethargy, visual disturbances, ataxia, confusion, seizures, and deep coma. The degree of clinical manifestations and mortality correlate poorly with the blood carboxyhemoglobin (COHb) level.[30, 31] A severe lactic acidosis may be confused with that produced by sei-

zure activity. Unfortunately, too often it is the coroner that makes the diagnosis of CO poisoning.[32]

The combustion of natural and synthetic nitrogen-containing polymers found in household furnishings produces CN.[2, 23] Cyanide is a direct cellular poison which interferes with the cytochrome oxidase system, leading to cellular hypoxia and worsening metabolic acidosis. Symptom onset is very rapid, and significant CN exposure usually results in rapid loss of consciousness. With exposure to high concentrations, collapse and death can occur almost immediately! Patients who actually arrive awake at the emergency treatment facility have probably sustained sublethal exposure. Manifestations of CN poisoning overlap with those of CO intoxication, especially the finding of a severe lactic acidosis. Although CN levels have been shown not to correlate with COHb levels in inhalation patients,[33] a low COHb level obtained shortly following the exposure implies a low probability of significant CN poisoning.[8] Cyanide poisoning does not occur without concomitant CO poisoning in house fire victims.[23]

TABLE 26–2.

Agents of Airway Burns and Inhalation

Irritant Gases
  High solubility
    Ammonia
    Chlorine
    Sulfur oxides/dioxides
  Low solubility
    Phosgene
    Nitrogen oxides/dioxides

Asphyxiant Gases
  Oxygen displacement
    Carbon dioxide
    Nitrogen
  Cellular poisoning
    Carbon monoxide
    Hydrogen cyanide
    Hydrogen sulfide
    Oxidizing agents
      Nitrates
      Aniline dyes
      Nitrobenzenes
      Nitrous gases

SCENARIOS

The clinical scenarios of patients presenting with airway burns and inhalation injuries are:

Scenario 1. The asymptomatic patient with a potential airway burn

Scenario 2. The mildly symptomatic patient without overt respiratory distress

Scenario 3. The very symptomatic patient with impending or actual acute respiratory failure

Scenario 4. The patient with severe hypoventilation or coma

Scenario 1: The Asymptomatic Patient

Most patients with a history of inhalation exposure will be either asymptomatic, or will have only symptoms of local upper airway irritation. Prolonged exposure, closed space, toxic combustibles, or major underlying illness constitute potentially significant airway exposures.

Although there may be no immediate threat to airflow in the asymptomatic patient, delayed obstructive symptoms can occur from thermal or chemical inhalation exposure.[9] Oral, nasopharyngeal, and upper airway edema as a consequence of thermal or chemical injury usually occurs rapidly but may be delayed for 12 to 24 hours.[1, 3, 6, 9] Lower airway inhalation injury does not correlate well with upper airway findings (facial burns, soot in the mouth or nose, singed nasal vibrissae, and conjunctival or mucosal erythema).[26, 30, 34, 35]

Aspiration is not found in the asymptomatic patient. The risk for aspiration of particulates and excessive secretions is small. Vomiting is not seen in the patient with normal mental status and no other trauma unless there is an underlying reason for emesis (e.g., toxic inhalation, CO or CN poisoning, alcohol or drug intoxication).

Impairment of ventilation and oxygenation may not be clinically apparent in asymptomatic patients, yet may occur.[1, 3, 9, 12, 16, 20, 36] Dyspnea, tachypnea, or tachycardia usually do not occur until the oxygen partial pressure (PO_2) and O_2 saturation levels fall below 80 mm Hg and 95%, respectively.[20, 37] Exposure to CO or CN, or to both, is unlikely to be clinically significant in the asymptomatic patient.[8, 36]

Management

In asymptomatic patients, management involves primarily clinical monitoring and supportive care. Physical examination will typically reveal normal vital signs and no evidence of airflow obstruction. Nevertheless, baseline testing is suggested, including digital oximetry, arterial blood gas (ABG) determinations, the COHb level, chest radiograph (CXR), and possibly bedside spirometry (Table 26–3).[10, 25, 38, 39] Humidified O_2 may be given. However, because delayed airway obstruction does occur, prolonged observation is necessary, including monitoring with serial oximetry and repeated ABG sampling.[25, 38] Should clinical deterioration occur, the patient must be admitted for bronchoscopy. This is performed both to assess the airway for injuries and to administer treatment, such as suctioning and removal of debris (and endotracheal intubation if airway damage is marked).[9, 14, 34, 40, 41]

There are, unfortunately, no universally agreed-upon criteria for admission of asymptomatic patients. Previously well patients without prolonged or closed-spaced exposure who present without clinical or laboratory evidence of significant exposure may be discharged with close follow-up and instructions

TABLE 26–3.

Recommended Baseline Tests for Patients With Airway Burns and Inhalation Injuries

Laboratory	Bedside
Complete blood count	Oximetry
Electrolytes	Spirometry
Arterial blood gases	Chest radiograph
Carboxyhemoglobin	?Bronchoscopy

to return or telephone at the first sign of any respiratory symptoms. Patients who are asymptomatic with normal laboratory values but who, by history, have sustained a significant exposure or are at increased risk of complications (e.g., patients with chronic cardiopulmonary disease) should be admitted for observation.

Scenario 2: The Mildly Symptomatic Patient Without Respiratory Distress (Stable, But Symptomatic)

This clinical scenario is common. In these "intermediate" patients, the clinical course may improve or worsen, often unpredictably. The individual patient may manifest only transient symptoms, including increased secretions, sore throat, hoarseness, and cough. This same patient, however, may go on to develop significant upper airway edema, manifested by dysphagia, drooling, croupy cough, and stridor followed by hypoxia and hypercarbia.[4, 8, 19, 40] This patient may progress rapidly to full-blown ventilatory failure and upper airway obstruction.[40]

Again, burns to the face, nose, lips, tongue, palate, and uvula should be sought.[5] If present, significant upper airway damage and subsequent airflow obstruction should be anticipated. When respiratory symptoms progress, then more frequent monitoring of the patient's symptoms, airway patency, and vital signs must be performed.

Lower airway burns are manifested by central chest discomfort or tightness, dyspnea, cough, and wheezing. Rhonchi, rales, and especially wheezing may be noted.

Aspiration of gastric contents must be suspected if the patient had temporary loss of consciousness (with or without overt emesis) and presents with cough.

Oxygenation and ventilation impairment should be suspected if any of the aforementioned symptoms occur or if the respiratory rate is increased (>20–24 breaths/min).

Management

Provided the patient rapidly and spontaneously improves, the measures followed in the first scenario (the asymptomatic, stable patient) should be adequate. To enhance airflow, expectoration should be facilitated (i.e., by humidified O_2, deep breathing, coughing). If upper airway edema is suspected, aerosolized racemic epinephrine may be given (see under Bronchodilators below).[6] Consultation for bronchoscopy is indicated when these clinical findings are present, especially if facial burns are also evident.[14, 40] Aspiration would not be probable in this patient while under observation in the emergency department (ED). Ventilation-oxygen impairment warrants therapy. If wheezing persists after the inhalation of racemic epinephrine, an aerosoized β-adrenergic bronchodilator should be administered.[4, 5, 8, 9] The use of steroids is controversial (see below).[16, 42-47] Some clinicians recommend steroid use for inhalation injury, particularly with persistent bronchospasm unrelieved by bronchodilators.[4] Unnecessary intravenous (IV) fluids should be avoided so as not to aggravate pulmonary edema, which may respond to judicious use of diuretics (see below). Antibiotics should not be administered "prophylactically" but rather should be reserved for objective evidence of infection (i.e., fever, purulent sputum, pleuritic chest pain corroborated by a positive CXR).[4, 5, 8, 9, 12, 18] Pneumonia, of course, would be a late complication, not seen upon initial presentation to the ED.

Scenario 3: The Very Symptomatic Patient With Impending or Actual Respiratory Failure (Crashing)

In this scenario, the burn or chemical inhalation victim clearly has complications which threaten the three pillars of the airway.[5, 19, 24, 36] Burns to the upper airway pose a threat to airflow. The patient may have stridor, develop a croupy cough, and may drool. The presence of facial and oropharyngeal burns together with these manifestations heralds serious upper airway obstruction. The patient will often produce thick, carbonaceous sputum. The mental status of the patient may be impaired, which threatens the ability of the patient to protect the airway from aspiration. Ventilation and oxygenation are significantly impaired. Impending respiratory failure is manifested by frank dyspnea, poor color or cyanosis, diaphoresis, and mental obtundation. There is respiratory distress, tachypnea, tachycardia, wheezes, rhonchi, or rales. Truncal burns may contribute to inadequate respiratory excursions.

ABG assessment is mandatory. It is important to recognize, however, that ABGs cannot directly reflect CO poisoning! The arterial oxygen partial pressure (PaO_2) may be near-normal despite significant

O_2 displacement from hemoglobin by CO, and the O_2 saturation reported by blood gas analyzers is calculated from the PaO_2, not directly measured.[5, 11] (Continuous oximetry is more useful as a direct measurement of tissue oxygen saturation.[20, 48]) Likewise, the PaCO_2 may not be a true indicator of the degree of ventilatory insufficiency. Elevated PaCO_2 levels may be due to inhalation of CO_2 itself rather than from CO_2 retention.[8] The pH and base deficit are very useful in detecting lactic acidosis which occurs in significant CO and CN poisoning.

Carboxyhemoglobin levels, or CO oximetry, if available, should be obtained to establish a definite diagnosis of CO poisoning.[11] However, although COHb levels provide important information on the extent and severity of the smoke inhalation exposure, COHb levels elevated on ED arrival will be lower than at rescue, giving the impression of a less significant exposure. This is particularly true if the patient receives supplemental high-flow O_2 administration en route. A nomogram has been developed that allows extrapolation of the COHb level back to the prerescue level (Figure 26–1).[23] This value is useful in predicting outcome and planning hyperbaric O_2 therapy (see below).

Cyanide levels are technically difficult to obtain and require hours for reporting, so they are not

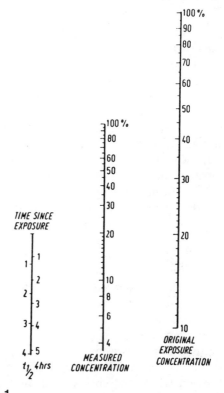

FIG 26–1.
Nomogram for calculating carboxyhemoglobin concentration at time of exposure. (From Clark CJ, Campbell D, Reid WH: *Lancet* 1981; 1:1332. Used with permission.)

helpful in the acute setting. As previously discussed, CN toxicity presents with a similar clinical picture and ABG findings as does CO toxicity. Cyanide poisoning should be suspected in any smoke inhalation victim because it is produced in many structural fires and requires specific therapy (see below).

The majority of patients will have normal chest films, but early changes of pulmonary edema or pneumonitis may be detected.[49, 50] Other associated injuries for which fire victims are at risk (e.g., fractured ribs, pneumothorax) may be discovered with a CXR. Caution should be exercised in sending a patient to the radiology suite. Delayed symptoms can rapidly appear and a patient may "crash out of sight" and away from an area of appropriate resuscitation! Thus, the treating physician may have to settle for a portable CXR.

Management

Treatment of impending respiratory failure must be prompt and aggressive.[2, 4, 8, 9] The patient should be given high-concentration O_2 via a nonrebreather mask. Preparations must be made for possible endotracheal intubation, and cricothyrotomy equipment should be at the bedside. If the patient clinically appears to have a lower airway obstructive respiratory pattern (wheezes, prolonged expiration), then a trial of aerosolized bronchodilators is warranted (see below); however, their effectiveness may be decreased in damaged airways where absorption may be limited.[39] Intravenous bronchodilators (aminophylline in adults and, occasionally, isoproterenol therapy, especially in children) may be tried.[1, 3, 5, 9] Diuretics are usually ineffective in treating pulmonary edema associated with adult respiratory distress syndrome (ARDS).[8, 51]

Early intubation is mandatory in the patient who has respiratory failure or who has not responded to initial therapy or who has impending upper airway obstruction (see Fig 26–2).[15, 52] Those patients who develop a pattern of acute respiratory distress will also require intubation and mechanical ventilation with positive end-expiratory pressure (PEEP).[12, 19, 53, 54] How should the patient be intubated? Blind nasotracheal intubation may be appropriate in awake victims,[9, 58, 59] but there is always a risk of epistaxis that may further threaten the airway. However, if nasopharyngeal burns are not present and edema is minimal, then nasotracheal intubation may be ideal since

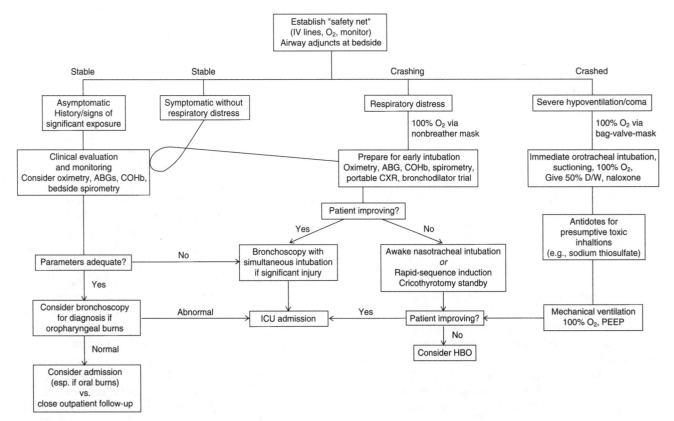

FIG 26–2.
Algorithm for management of the patient with airway burns and inhalation exposure. *ABGs* = arterial blood gases; *COHb* = carboxyhemoglobin; *CXR* = chest x-ray film; *HBO* = hyperbaric oxygen; *PEEP* = positive end-expiratory pressure.

the lower airway can be both assessed and well suctioned. For the patient with severe upper or lower airway compromise, intubation should be performed without delay.[2, 4, 5, 16, 55] Intubation of awake patients with nasopharyngeal edema or those with CNS depression or increased motor activity can be accomplished with rapid-sequence intubation (see Chapter 6).[57] Of course, the use of muscle relaxants requires personnel knowledgeable in their use and skilled in alternative procedures should intubation fail. Succinylcholine has been shown to cause precipitous elevations in serum potassium in patients with major trauma and cutaneous burns. Pseudocholinesterase, which rapidly degrades succinylcholine, is depleted as a consequence of liver dysfunction in burn patients. The result is an intense and sustained effect of this muscle relaxant. Both of these phenomena occur after the initial ED stay and with subsequent administrations of the drug.[58, 59] Therefore, succinylcholine is not contraindicated in the ED for "fresh" burn victims. The short-acting barbiturates sodium pentobarbital and methohexital theoretically may cause laryngospasm and bronchospasm,[60] potentially worsening the patient's underlying inhalation injury and burn-induced airway bronchospasm. A safer alternative would be a rapid-acting benzodiazepine (e.g., midazolam).

Once the patient is intubated, a nasogastric tube is placed, both to prevent regurgitation and aspiration and to titrate the gastric pH to protect against the development of stress ulcers.[61, 62] If truncal burns are present and eschars are preventing adequate respiratory excursions, then escharotomy may be necessary immediately after admission. The possible role of steroids, antibiotics, and diuretics in these acutely ill inhalation victims are discussed under Controversies below.

Poisoning from one or more of the common toxic gases previously mentioned must be presumed in the unconscious smoke inhalation victim. If significantly elevated COHb levels are found (>30%–40%), regardless of clinical symptoms, then hyperbaric O_2 therapy, although controversial, should be considered if readily available.[31, 63–66] The presence of severe neurologic symptoms, including coma, seizures, or neuropsychiatric deficits; cardiovascular compromise manifested by angina, electrocardiographic (ECG) abnormalities, or shock; and severe metabolic acidosis unresponsive to supplemental O_2 (implying mixed CO and CN poisoning) should prompt strong consideration for immediate transfer to a hyperbaric oxygen (HBO) facility.[31, 64] Since CN levels are not easily obtained, the antidotal treatment of smoke inhalation victims must be based on clinical

grounds and a high index of suspicion for CN poisoning, as previously discussed.[23, 67] The traditional cyanide antidote kit (containing nitrite and thiosulfate) has been questioned as the standard antidotal measure owing to its possibility of inducing severe methemoglobinemia.[11, 38, 68–70] Remembering that patients rescued alive from fires tend to survive with only O_2 and good supportive care,[11, 26] it is probably safer to administer only sodium thiosulfate (see below), in addition to 100% O_2, via nonrebreather mask or endotracheal intubation and consider transfer to an HBO facility for concomitant CO poisoning.[64, 66] Consultation with a regional poison control center should be considered.

Scenario 4: The Patient With Severe Hypoventilation or Coma (Crashed)

Patients presenting with severe hypoventilation or coma following thermal or toxic inhalation require aggressive airway management. The same factors that threatened airflow in the last (crashing) scenario are present to major degrees in the comatose patient. Aspiration may have already happened in these patients, depending upon whether emesis (which frequently accompanies CO and CN poisoning) occurred.[2, 5] Ventilatory failure with attendant hypoxia and acidosis (both respiratory and metabolic) must be assumed.[1, 2, 5, 6, 29]

Management

The cornerstone of resuscitation in the apneic or comatose victim is immediate endotracheal intubation (see the previous scenario). If initial intubation is unsuccessful because of associated trauma or upper airway burn or edema, then alternative techniques must be used. Many patients can be supported for extended periods with a nasopharyngeal or oropharyngeal airway with a tight-fitting mask connected to 100% O_2.[57] This technique should be rigidly maintained until more advanced airway adjuncts are ready. Difficult intubations secondary to distorted landmarks can be aided by fiberoptic laryngoscopy (see Chapter 12). Other techniques that can be considered include digital intubation (see Chapter 10), use of a lighted stylet (Chapter 11), and retrograde intubation (Chapter 13). Should these measures fail, then a surgical approach (percutaneous transtracheal ventilation, cricothyrotomy, cricotomes) must be undertaken (see Chapters 15, 16, and 17). Once intubation is completed and 100% O_2 delivered, the patient should be suctioned. Since emesis frequently occurs, especially with toxic inhalations, a good seal of the endotracheal tube cuff should be assured and a nasogastric tube inserted—

both procedures performed to avoid aspiration.[61] Bronchoscopy through the endotracheal tube may be required not only to assess the extent of airway injury but to facilitate suctioning for debridement.[4, 15, 40]

The patient is then placed on a ventilator (see Appendix). Continuous positive airway pressure (CPAP) or PEEP may also be required if the patient is in pulmonary edema from ARDS or if oxygenation is not improved even with high FiO_2 settings (i.e., >50%–60%).[4, 5, 12, 19, 53, 54] The standard drugs to treat any coma victim (dextrose, thiamine, and naloxone) should not be forgotten. The use of HBO and antidotal therapies for chemical inhalations are described in the preceding scenario.

CONTROVERSIES IN MANAGEMENT OF AIRWAY BURNS AND SMOKE OR CHEMICAL INHALATION

Antibiotics

Intervention with antibiotics is not indicated in the acute management of airway burns and smoke inhalation. Prophylactic administration of antibiotics has not been shown to beneficially alter the burn victim's course and, in fact, may result in colonization or pneumonia with resistant strains.[34, 71] Only when such a patient develops clinical evidence of pneumonia should narrow-spectrum antibiotic therapy be ordered, based upon results of sputum Gram's stain obtained by suctioning or bronchoscopy.[2, 4, 5, 8, 9, 18, 44, 72]

Corticosteroids

The only controlled studies that have shown a beneficial use of steroids in inhalation injury have been confined to animal models with isolated smoke inhalation (without concomitant cutaneous burns).[42, 46] However, a well-designed prospective human study showed a fourfold increase in mortality as a result of sepsis in patients treated with steroids.[73] A more recent study found no beneficial effect upon pulmonary-related mortality in isolated smoke inhalation injury.[44] The Falkland Islands conflict is frequently cited in suggesting the potential benefits of corticosteroids.[74] Sixty-nine victims of the *Sir Gallahad* fire received steroids for smoke inhalation injuries. The degree of respiratory involvement was not quantified and various amounts of steroids were administered. There were no reported deaths and none of the patients went on to develop sepsis or ARDS. However, these results must be viewed

cautiously as all the victims were in excellent physical condition and the observations made were uncontrolled. The obvious concern is that corticosteroids suppress the immune response to infection and may reduce pulmonary bacterial clearance.[45] The anti-inflammatory property of steroids may have a role in treating persistent bronchospasm unresponsive to inhaled or parenteral bronchodilators. However, the use of steroids in patients with parenchymal lung injury and coexistent burns is not warranted based on current literature data. If administered, steroids should probably be given only very early and as a single large IV dose (1–2 g of methylprednisolone).[4, 75]

Diuretics

The judicious use of diuretics (e.g., furosemide 40 mg IV) may be indicated in the presence of mild pulmonary edema in smoke inhalation victims.[3, 5, 12, 34] In addition, osmotic diuresis (e.g., mannitol 0.25–1.0 g/kg IV) may be necessary to maintain adequate urinary output in patients with associated tissue burns at risk for renal failure secondary to rhabdomyolysis.[76] In patients with significant burns where fluid therapy is critical, then pulmonary artery pressure monitoring should be considered.

Bronchodilators

Airflow obstruction may be due to inflammatory edema rather than true bronchospasm. Therefore, bronchodilators may have a variable effect on wheezing. If inflammatory edema is suspected, then aerosolized racemic epinephrine (2.25%, 0.5 mL in 3 mL normal saline) may be tried.[3, 6]

If bronchospasm is suspected, then aerosolized β-adrenergies (e.g., albuterol, metaproterenol, terbutaline) are indicated.[4, 5, 8, 9, 52, 77] When airway damage is significant, or excessive, thick secretions are present, decreased absorption of these inhaled medications may limit their efficacy. Intravenous bronchodilators such as aminophylline (theophylline) may then be warranted. Subcutaneous administration of epinephrine or terbutaline is another option. In the severely ill child, IV isoproterenol may be tried if a satisfactory response is not obtained with other bronchodilators.

Nonsteroidal Anti-inflammatory Drugs (NSAIDs)

Ibuprofen, a cyclooxygenase inhibitor, has been studied in the setting of smoke inhalation injury.[78, 79] In inhalation injury, pulmonary changes and increased lung lymph flow appear to be associated with elevations of the metabolites of arachidonic acid, such as thromboxane and prostaglandins. Ibuprofen has been shown to diminish pulmonary lung lymph flow and microvascular permeability in animal models of inhalation injury.[78] However, human studies are lacking, and even if NSAIDs are found to be clinically important, their relevance in the emergency setting is doubtful. Finally, burn victims are at significant risk for stress gastric ulcer formation.[61, 62]

Dimethyl Sulfoxide (DMSO)

Similar results as those described above for NSAIDs have been reported in studies using the oxygen free radical scavenger DMSO in sheep exposed to inhalation injury.[80] There was less extravascular lung fluid formation (less microvascular permeability) in those animals receiving DMSO, implying that oxygen free radicals are responsible for the pulmonary edema seen with inhalation injury. Again, human studies have not yet been reported and its applicability to emergency care is not apparent.

Hyperbaric Oxygen Therapy

Hyperbaric oxygen therapy should be considered early in patients suspected of having significant CO poisoning with or without CN toxicity. Clinical effects and laboratory measurements do not correlate well with acute manifestations or long-term sequelae.[23, 81] Improved outcomes have been reported even when transfer to an HBO facility was delayed.[31, 63, 64] The half-life of COHb can be shortened from 4 hours at room air ($FiO_2 = 21\%$) to 40 to 60 minutes (applying 100% O_2 at 1 atm) to 20 to 30 minutes (HBO at 2–3 atm).[31] Even so, no human clinical controlled trials have documented the efficacy of HBO therapy compared with 100% normobaric O_2 in preventing late neuropyschiatric sequelae in CO- or CN-intoxicated patients. However, there is systemic and cardiovascular compromise, persistent metabolic acidosis, and combined CO and CN poisoning.[7, 63, 64, 65] Hyperbaric oxygen therapy should therefore be considered for any severely poisoned patient or even in the less severely intoxicated patient who has not responded to standard 100% O_2 administration within 2 to 4 hours. Accessibility of an HBO facility, associated injuries, and the transfer of a potentially unstable patient must be considered when making this therapeutic decision.

Antidotal Therapy for Cyanide Toxicity

In patients who present from a closed-space fire with elevated COHb levels, decreased arterial O_2 saturation, metabolic acidosis, and significant CNS symptoms, presumptive therapy for coexistent CN poisoning should also be given. Judicious use of the CN antidote kit (i.e., administration of IV thiosulfate with or without the inhalation of amyl nitrite pearls) is usually preferable (and avoids altogether the administration of IV sodium nitrite). The recommended dose of IV thiosulfate in adults is 12.5 g or 50 mL of the 25% solution; in children, 1.65 mL/kg of the 25% solution is given.[52] Thiosulfate is nontoxic; the amyl nitrite pearl produces a tolerable 5% methemoglobinemia. However, substituting an iatrogenic and potentially lethal level of methemoglobinemia with the administration of IV sodium nitrite for the presumptive diagnosis of an environmental cyanide toxicity is probably not reasonable management in the great majority of these patients.[64, 69] Initial transport or secondary transfer to an HBO facility is reasonable, if the patient can tolerate the transfer and such a facility is readily available and able to handle an unstable patient.

PREHOSPITAL PERSPECTIVES

Because there is frequently a delay in onset of respiratory symptoms from inhalation injuries, all patients with a history of significant exposure must be transported for evaluation at an emergency facility, even if they are asymptomatic at the time of rescue.[1-16] Paramedical personnel should take careful note of the fire scene (including open or closed spaces and types of structure or materials burned) and relate these observations to the emergency physician. Once the victim is removed from the fire, the primary diagnostic survey with concurrent resuscitative maneuvers for airway, breathing, and circulation should be rapidly accomplished. The patient must be evaluated for associated trauma while the cervical spine is protected, especially if a fall or blast was involved. The airway must be maintained which may simply involve proper positioning of the patient, placement of a nasopharyngeal or oropharyngeal airway, or immediate orotracheal or nasotracheal intubation with a firm "tonsil" suction tip available. Alternatives for difficult intubations were discussed earlier in this chapter. Once the airway is established, then vigorous correction of hypoxemia and presumed acidosis must begin with the application of high-concentration O_2 (nonrebreather mask). To ventilate effectively, suctioning with a flexible catheter may be required to remove excessive secretions, mucus, and other debris from the respiratory tract. Oximetry, if available, may provide useful information about the patient's condition, but results should not supplant the need for high-flow O_2 administration. The safety net is completed by establishing at least one IV access of crystalloid at a "to keep open" rate in order to avoid pulmonary or cerebral fluid overload (unless hypovolemia is present). The patient should be placed on a cardiac monitor. If there is evidence of closed-space exposure with loss of consciousness in a fire involving synthetic materials (plastic, upholstery, etc.) and the patient is in extremis, the receiving physician must be forewarned that the patient may have either CO or CN poisoning, in which case transport to a facility with an HBO chamber may be indicated.[52] Despite the often dramatic setting in which fire victims are found, other unrelated conditions (alcohol intoxication, injuries, etc.) must not be overlooked. Also, altered mental status should prompt routine administration of thiamine, naloxone, and glucose.

PEDIATRIC PERSPECTIVES

The same three pillars of successful airway management that support adult burn and inhalation victims are also operative in children. The assessment of children uses the same approaches as those for adults. Oximetry, ABG assessment, COHb levels, and CXR should be accomplished early in the patient's evaluation. Small children will not be able to perform bedside spirometry. Therefore, close and repeated clinical monitoring for development of airway obstruction (falling O_2 saturation, increased use of accessory muscles, tachypnea, tachycardia) must be diligently performed.

Management principles are also similar.[2, 24] Children with respiratory injury tend to mouth-breathe, bypassing the normal humidifying capabilities of the nose and nasopharynx. Tachypnea further aggravates airway water loss. High-flow, humidified O_2 should be applied in the prehospital setting and continued in the ED. The threat of obstruction to airflow must be removed with proper positioning, appropriately sized airway adjuncts, and tracheal intubations if respiratory failure is imminent. Uncuffed endotracheal tubes are used in children under 8 years of age; the cricoid cartilage is the narrowest portion of the pediatric upper airway and

effectively serves as the "cuff" for an endotracheal tube. Protection against aspiration is accomplished with frequent suctioning, placement of a nasogastric tube, and possibly endotracheal intubation following the same clinical criteria as those for adults. Ventilatory support with CPAP or application of PEEP on a volume-limited ventilator may be required.[2] Children are just as susceptible to poisoning from toxic inhalation as adults. In children toxicologic guidelines similar to those recommended for adults should govern the use of supportive care, laboratory tests, antidotal treatment of CN exposure, and consideration of transport to an HBO facility for CO toxicity. The emergency physician must ensure that the emotional and informational needs of the parents or guardians are satisfied by all emergency care personnel.

REFERENCES

1. Cahalane M, Demling RH: Early respiratory abnormalities from smoke inhalation. *JAMA* 1984; 251:771.
2. Carnock EL, Meehan JJ: Postburn respiratory injuries in children. *Pediatr Clin North Am* 1980; 17:661.
3. Chu C: New concepts of pulmonary burn injury. *J Trauma* 1981; 21:958.
4. Clark RJ, Beeley MJ: Smoke inhalation. *Br J Hosp Med* 1989; 41:252.
5. Crapo RO: Smoke inhalation injuries. *JAMA* 1981; 246:1694.
6. Demling RH: Smoke inhalation injury. *Postgrad Med* 1987; 82:63.
7. Herndon DN, Barrow RE, Lanares HA, et al: Inhalation injury in burned patients: Effects and treatment. *Burns* 1988; 14:349.
8. Kinsella J: Smoke inhalation. *Burns* 1988; 14:269.
9. Moylan JA: Smoke inhalation and burn injury. *Surg Clin North Am* 1980; 60:1533.
10. Petroff PA, Hander EW, Clayton WH, et al: Pulmonary function after smoke inhalation. *Am J Surg* 1976; 132:346.
11. Prien T: Toxic smoke compounds and inhalation injury—a review. *Burns* 1988; 14:451.
12. Stone HH, Martin JD: Pulmonary injury associated with thermal burns. *Surg Gynecol Obstet* 1969; 129:1242.
13. Wang CZ, Li A, Zhu PF, et al: Dynamic changes of lung lymph flow and the release of lysosomal enzyme from the lungs after severe steam inhalation injury in goats. *Burns* 1986; 12:415.
14. Hunt JL, Agee RN, Pruitt BA, et al: Fiberoptic bronchoscopy in acute inhalation injury. *J Trauma* 1975; 15:641.
15. Moylan JA, Chan CK: Inhalation injury: An increasing problem. *Ann Surg* 1978; 188:34.

16. O'Hickey SP, Pickering CA, Jones PE, et al: Manchester air disaster. *Br Med J* 1987; 294:1663.
17. Stone HH, Rhame DW, Corbitt JD: Respiratory burns: A correlation of clinical and laboratory results. *Ann Surg* 1967; 165:157.
18. Clark WR: Smoke inhalation. *Burns* 1988; 14:473.
19. Demling RH, Wong C, Liu LG: Early lung dysfunction after major burns: Role of edema and vasoactive mediators. *J Trauma* 1985; 25:949.
20. Stevenson SF, Esrig BC, Polk HC: The pathophysiology of smoke inhalation injury. *Ann Surg* 1975; 182:652.
21. Moritz AR, Henriques FC, McLean R: The effect of inhaled heat on the air passages and lungs. *Am J Pathol* 1945; 21:311.
22. Buehler JH, Burns AS, Webster JR : Lactic acidosis from carboxyhemoglobin after smoke inhalation. *Ann Intern Med* 1975; 82:803.
23. Clark CJ, Campbell D, Reid WH: Blood carboxyhaemoglobin and cyanide levels in fire survivors. *Lancet* 1981; 1:1332.
24. Mellins RB, Parks S: Respiratory complications of smoke inhalation in victims of fires. *J Pediatr* 1975; 87:1–7.
25. Dressler DP: Laboratory background on smoke inhalation. *J Trauma* 1979; 19:913.
26. Larkin JM, Brahos GJ, Moylan JA: Treatment of carbon monoxide poisoning: prognostic factors. *J Trauma* 1976; 16:111.
27. Jackson DL, Menges HM: Accidental carbon monoxide poisoning. *JAMA* 1980; 243:772.
28. Piantades CA: Carbon monoxide, oxygen transport, and oxygen metabolism. *J Hyperbaric Med* 1987; 2:27.
29. Goldbaum LR, Ramirez RG, Absalon KB: What is the mechanism of carbon monoxide toxicity? *Aviat Space Environ Med* 1975; 46:1289.
30. Clark WR, Bonaventura M, Myers W: Smoke inhalation and airway management at a regional burn unit: 1974–1983, part I. *J Burn Care Rehabil* 1989; 10:52.
31. Myers RAM, Snyder S, Lindberg S: Value of hyperbaric oxygen in suspected carbon monoxide poisoning. *JAMA* 1981; 246:2478.
32. Zikria BA, Weston GC, Chodoff M: Smoke and carbon monoxide poisoning in fire victims. *J Trauma* 1972; 12:641.
33. Barillo DI, Good R, Rush BF, et al: Lack of correlation between carboxyhemaglobin and cyanide in smoke inhalation injury. *Curr Surg* 1986.
34. Moylan JA, Alexander LG: Diagnosis and treatment of inhalation injury. *World J Surg* 1978; 2:185.
35. Moylan JA: Inhalation injury. *J Trauma* 1981; 21:720.
36. Peters WJ: Inhalation injury caused by the products of combustion. *Can Med Assoc J* 1981; 125:249.
37. Urokinase pulmonary embolism trial: A national cooperative study. *Circulation* 1973; 47(suppl 2):II–81.
38. Garnier R, Bismuth C, Riboulet-Delmas G: Poisoning from fumes from polystyrene fire. *Br Med J* 1981; 283:1610.
39. Haponik EF, Crapo RO, Herndon DN, et al: Smoke inhalations. *Am Rev Respir Dis* 1988; 138:1060.
40. Clark CJ, Reid WH, Telfer ABM, et al: Respiratory injury in the burned patient—the role of flexible bronchoscopy. *Anaesthesia* 1983; 38:35.
41. Harvey JS, Watkins GM, Sherman RT: Emergency burn care. *South Med J* 1984; 77:204.
42. Beeley JM, Crow J, Jones JG, et al: Mortality and lung histopathology after inhalation lung injury: The effect of corticosteroids. *Am Rev Respir Dis* 1986; 133:191.
43. Levene BA, Petroff PA, Slade CL, et al: Prospective trails of dexamethasone and aerosolized gentamicin in the treatment of inhalation injury in burned patients. *J Trauma* 1978; 18:188.
44. Robinson NB: Steroid therapy following isolated smoke inhalation injury. *J Trauma* 1982; 22:876.
45. Skornik WA, Dressler DP: The effects of short term steroid therapy on lung bacterial clearance and survival in rats. *Ann Surg* 1974; 179:415.
46. Dressler DP, Skornik WA, Kupersmith S: Corticosteroid treatment of experimental smoke inhalation. *Ann Surg* 1976; 183:46.
47. Welch GW, Loull RJ, Petroff PA: The use of steroids in inhalation injury. *Surg Gynecol Obstet* 1977; 145:539.
48. Barker SI, Tremper KK, Hufstedler S: The effects of carbon monoxide on noninvasive oxygen monitoring. *Anesth Analg* 1986; 65(suppl):S12.
49. Putnam CE, Loke J, Mathay RA, et al: Radiographic manifestations of acute smoke inhalation. *AJR* 1977; 129:865.
50. Trexidor HS, Rubin E, Novick GS, et al: Smoke inhalation: Radiologic manifestations. *Radiology* 1983; 149:383.
51. Sataloff DM, Sataloff RT: Tracheotomy and inhalation injury. *Head Neck Surg* 1984; 6:1024.
52. Dinerman N, Huber JA: Inhalation injuries, In Rosen P, et al (eds): *Emergency Medicine: Concepts and Clinical practice*, ed 2. St Louis, Mosby–Year Book, Inc, 1988, pp 585–607.
53. Davies LK, Poulton TJ, Modell JH: Continuous positive airway pressure is beneficial in the treatment of smoke inhalation. *Crit Care Med* 1983; 11:726.
54. Mathru M, Venus B, Rao TLK, et al: Noncardiac pulmonary edema precipitated by tracheal intubation in patients with inhalation injury. *Crit Care Med* 1983; 11:804.
55. Bartlett RH, Niccole M, Travis MJ, et al: Acute management of the upper airway in facial burns and smoke inhalation. *Arch Surg* 1976; 111:744.
56. Cuono CB: Early management of severe thermal injury. *Surg Clin North Am* 1980; 60:1021.
57. Morris IR: Pharmacologic aids to intubation and the rapid sequence induction. *Emerg Med Clin North Am* 1988; 6:753.

58. Bush GH, Graham HAP, Littlewood AHM, et al: Danger of suxamethonium and endotracheal intubation in anesthesia for burns. *Br Med J* 1962; 2:1081–1085.

59. Dripps RD, Eckenhoff JE, Vandam LD: *Introduction to Anesthesia: The Principles of Safe Practice*, ed 5. Philadelphia, WB Saunders Co, 1977, pp 195–215.

60. Harvey SC: Hypnotics and sedatives, in Goodman LS, Gilman A (eds): *The Pharmacological Basis of Therapeutics*, ed 5. New York, Macmillan Publishing Co, 1975, pp 102–123.

61. Weimer SL, Barrett J: Burn injury and management, in Weimer SL, Barrett J (eds): *Trauma Management for Civilian and Military Physicians*. Philadelphia, WB Saunders Co, 1986, pp 53–76.

62. Pruitt BA, Foley FD, Moncrief JA: Curling's ulcer: A clinical pathology study of 323 cases. *Ann Surg* 1970; 172:523.

63. Harris M, Young D: Hyperbaric medicine. *Indiana Med* 1987; 258.

64. Hart GB, Strauss MB, Lennon PA, et al: Treatment of smoke inhalation by hyperbaric oxygen. *J Emerg Med* 1985; 3:211.

65. Kindwall EP: Carbon monoxide poisoning, in Davis JC, Hunt TK (eds): *Hyperbaric Oxygen Therapy*. Rockville, Md, Undersea Medical Society, Inc, 1977, pp 177–190.

66. Myers RAM, Schnitzer B: Hyperbaric oxygen use: Update 1984. *Postgrad Med* 1984; 76:83.

67. Jones J, et al: Toxic smoke inhalation: Cyanide poisoning in fire victims. *Am J Emerg Med* 1987; 5:317.

68. Cohen MA, Guzzardi LJ: Toxic smoke inhalation and cyanide poisoning, editorial. *Am J Emerg Med* 1988; 6:203.

69. Hall AH, Kulig KW, Rumack BH: Toxic smoke inhalation (editorial). *Am J Emerg Med* 1989; 7:121.

70. Ivankovich AD, Braverman B, Kanuru RP: Cyanide antidotes and methods of their administration in dogs. *Anesthesiology* 1980; 52:210.

71. Lund T, Goodwin CW, McManus WF, et al: Upper airway sequelae in burn patients requiring endotracheal intubation or tracheostomy. *Ann Surg* 1985; 201:374.

72. Moylan JA, Alexander G Jr: Diagnosis and treatment of inhalation injury. *World J Surg* 1978; 2:185.

73. Moylan JA: Smoke inhalation: Diagnostic techniques and steroids. *J Trauma* 1979; 19(suppl):917.

74. Williams JG, Ridley TRD, Moody RA: Resuscitation experience in the Falkland Islands campaign. *Br Med J* 1983; 286:775.

75. Stone HH: Commentary on: Diagnosis and treatment of inhalation injury. *World J Surg* 1978; 2:190.

76. Pruitt BA Jr, Goodwin CW Jr: Current treatment of the extensively burned patient. *Surg Ann* 1983; 15:331.

77. Pruitt BA: The burn patient. I. Initial care. *Probl Surg* 1979; 16:42.

78. Kimura R, Traber LD, Herndon DN, et al: Ibuprofen reduces the lung lymph flow changes associated with inhalation injury. *Circ Shock* 1988; 24:183.

79. Shinozawa Y, Hales C, Jung W, et al: Ibuprofen prevents synthetic smoke induced pulmonary edema. *Am Rev Respir Dis* 1986; 134:1145.

80. Kimura R, Traber LD, Herndon DN, et al: Treatment of smoke induced pulmonary injury with nebulized dimethylsulfoxide. *Circ Shock* 1988; 25:333.

81. Broome JR, Skrine H, Pearson RR: Carbon monoxide poisoning—forgotten not gone! *Br J Hosp Med* 1988; 39:298.

27

Atraumatic Upper Airway Obstruction

Robert H. Dailey, M.D.

Steven Pace, M.D.

Acute upper airway obstruction (UAO) is one of the most critical clinical situations that a physician can face in the practice of medicine. The major pillar of the airway, airflow, is directly imperiled. Uncorrected, UAO leads to asphyxia. *Asphyxia* is defined as cardiopulmonary arrest secondary to deprivation of oxygen and accumulation of carbon dioxide, which in turn produce severe tissue hypoxia and ventilatory and metabolic acidoses. In the dog model,[1] asphyxia occurs in about 10 minutes following complete UAO. If interventions are delayed or resuscitation attempts only partially successful, a vegetative state may be the dreaded outcome, arguably "a fate worse than death."

UAO is one of the few conditions that (1) is an immediate threat to life which, undiagnosed, leads inevitably and rapidly to death; (2) is usually totally curable or reversible; and (3) often occurs in otherwise healthy young people. In these respects it travels in the exclusive company of such lethal conditions as pericardial tamponade, tension pneumothorax, meningococcal meningitis, and acute hyperkalemia.

UAO can occur anywhere from the mouth to the trachea. However, the most critical area is the glottic opening at the larynx. It is narrowest there in the adult, is most susceptible to lodgment of foreign material, and the structures are rigid—allowing no possibility of increasing the lumen size.

Three physiologic principles obtain in UAO. First, as with all organs, there is built into the airway a large functional reserve; thus, airflow can be impaired to a large degree without affecting ventilation. However, there is a critical point at which the natural functional reserve is exceeded. Second,

Pouseille's law states that flow through a lumen is directly proportional to the fourth power of the radius of the lumen. This means not only that flow increases geometrically with increases in the lumen size, which is pertinent to intravenous (IV) flow rates, but that also, and more germane here, *flow is geometrically decreased as the lumen is narrowed.* These two concepts, then, explain why a patient will be functionally quite stable over time despite a progressive lesion, but then "crash" suddenly when the critical decrease in lumen size is reached. A third concept illustrates how this process can become a negative feedback loop. Once extrathoracic (upper) airway obstruction occurs, inspiration produces an increase in transmural pressure on the upper airway, thus further diminishing its lumen upon inspiration[2] (Fig 27–1). *These three factors serve to illustrate the inherent instability of even "stable" patients with slowly progressive lesions!*

We approach UAO in this chapter as we would approach it at the bedside, i.e., (a) identifying the defining clinical manifestations, (b) determining both the degree of UAO and its tempo of progression, (c) formulating a differential diagnosis, (d) choosing tests to clarify both the pathophysiology and diagnosis as appropriate to the individual clinical circumstance, and finally (e), devising appropriate therapeutic stratagems.

CLINICAL MANIFESTATIONS AND EVALUATION

Clinical manifestations will be discussed in the order of progressive severity. In this manner they

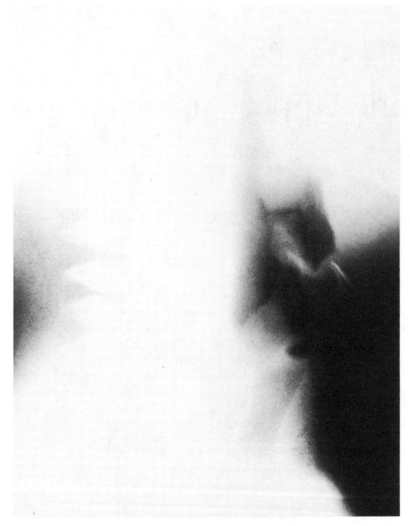

FIG 27–1.
Normal epiglottis.

define, roughly and respectively, the degree of airway obstruction in the stable, crashing, and crashed patient.

The earliest manifestations of UAO often escape detection. Some sort of coarse *noisy breathing* short of stridor occurs; at first it is intermittent, later constant. These sounds are relatively low-pitched and can sound like rhonchi, wheezes, uncleared secretions, or are simply very difficult to describe. The patient is concerned about a respiratory abnormality, but more often than not, is unable to ascribe it to the upper airway. Since these sounds can be heard upon auscultation of the chest, the lungs inappropriately become the suspected culprit. However, careful observation will invariably reveal the noisy breathing to be present *primarily upon inspiration.* As the degree

of obstruction increases, so too will the pitch of the abnormal sound, becoming harsh, rasping, or grating. Dysphonia of any degree indicates a lesion involving the vocal cords; the voice may be hoarse, husky, muffled, or absent. If an acute inflamatory process is present, pain may be the overriding feature, usually occurring well before any of the above-mentioned symptoms. With this minimal degree of obstruction, the airway is not immediately threatened, and the patient can be said to be *relatively* stable.

More marked and obvious symptoms of UAO should prompt great concern; they are characteristic of the crashing patient. True stridor is readily identifiable as a high-pitched sound emanating from the larynx in both inspiration and expiration; it has been characterized as "crowing," and it can be produced voluntarily by breathing against a partially closed glottis. The patient is concerned and often anxious, sensing impairment of respiration. Mild tachypnea and tachycardia may, but may not (!), be present. The breathing is only mildly labored—accessory muscles are not in use, and there are no retractions.

The crashed patient is clearly having a major ventilatory emergency: asphyxia is imminent. There will be some disturbance in consciousness due to hypercarbia and hypoxia; marked anxiety, disorientation, uncooperativeness, or even combativeness is common. Stridor is obvious and loud. Breathing is labored, with retractions, use of accessory muscles, and often diaphoresis. There will be tachypnea and tachycardia. If oxygen is not being administered the patient may be cyanotic, and O_2 desaturation will be apparent upon oximetry.

In the terminal phase of asphyxia, there is loss of consciousness altogether, the pulse and respirations slow, and severe hypoxia and acidosis culminate in full respiratory and then cardiac arrest (see Prehospital Perspective below).

This classification is arbitrary. The careful reader will note that, by comparison with other clinical situations in this book, lesser degrees of apparent clinical acuity have been accorded more serious classifications. (That is, clinical manifestations here accorded "crashing" status have been referred to as "stable" in other disease processes.) We have done this "upgrade" because, even though UAO patients may not appear acutely ill, their airways have exceeded the airflow reserve discussed above. Thus, *they are closer to catastrophe than they appear* and are inherently highly unstable!

If observation suggests a diagnosis of UAO, and time permits, a history should be taken with two very specific objectives in mind: (1) How fast have the UAO symptoms been progressing? and (2), What are the most likely causes? The answer to the first question (in concert with the current observed degree of UAO) informs us how much time we have before the patient is likely to crash. The answer to the second question dictates our best diagnostic and therapeutic options.

Further evaluation is rather straightforward. Pulse oximetry should ordinarily be applied at the outset, before initiating O_2 therapy. It best documents change on the steep slope of the O_2 saturation curve, and so is insensitive to early stages of UAO! And the routine administration of O_2 will also blunt its sensitivity to clinical change. A portable chest film

and soft tissue lateral film of the neck should be routine. If a subglottic process is suspected, the tracheal shadow should be carefully examined on the frontal chest film. *Under no circumstances should the patient with UAO of any degree ever be sent to the radiology suite,* even if it is located in the department! An arterial blood gas determination (ABG) should be performed to define the adequacy of alveolar ventilation. If, however, this is likely to worsen anxiety and promote hyperventilation (as with young children), the test should be waived. The same holds for obtaining a complete blood count (CBC).

Diagnosis usually awaits direct or indirect visualization of the oropharynx and larynx. Time availability dictates the method. The stable patient can often await fiberoptic examination. Both the stable and the crashing patient will usually tolerate indirect laryngoscopy. The crashed patient will require direct laryngoscopy. (see The Crashed Patient under Clinical Scenarios). *The more advanced and rapidly advancing the UAO, the more aggressive must be attempts at diagnosis and airway establishment,* and the less do contraindications pertain!

CAUSES OF UPPER AIRWAY OBSTRUCTION

The causes of UAO will also be discussed in the order of progressive severity, from stable to crashed (Table 27–1). *Chronic UAO* may be thought of as evolving over a period of greater than days (more often many weeks or months). Thus the underlying pathologic processes would be tumors, congenital malformations, indolent infections or inflammations, or cicatrization following injury or surgery. Unless some acute process were superimposed, such conditions would be only very slowly progressive (if at all) and so would not ordinarily present as airway emergencies. They are diagnosed in nonacute environments. Little more need be said about them in the context of this chapter.

Subacute UAO may be said to evolve over a period of hours to a few days. Acute infection or abscesses with swelling of structures adjoining the airway constitute the majority of cases, e.g., Ludwig's angina, retropharyngeal or peritonsillar abscess, acute upon chronic tonsillitis, diphtheria, etc.[3, 4] These entities are usually easily diagnosed and present well before significant UAO occurs. Croup and acute tracheitis constitute the infectious causes of subglottic UAO (see Chapter 34); although tra-

TABLE 27–1.

Causes of Upper Airway Obstruction Classified by Rapidity of Evolution

Stable
  Chronic (>days)
    Tumors
    Congenital malformations/dysfunctions
    Posttracheostomy subglottic stenosis
    Chronic inflammatory diseases (sarcoid, Wegener's
      granulomatosis, erythema nodosum, Sjögren's syndrome,
      etc.)
    Sleep apnea syndrome
  Subacute (hours to a few days)
    Infections of oropharynx
    High esophageal foreign bodies
    Stevens-Johnson syndrome
    Croup, tracheitis
Crashing
  Acute (minutes to a few hours)
    Burns (thermal, chemical)
    Hematomas secondary to warfarin
    Epigottitis supraglottitis
    Allergic/hereditary angioneurotic edema
    Psychogenic
Crashed
  Hyperacute (seconds to a few minutes)
    Laryngospasm
    Foreign body

cheitis is generally limited to children, it has been reported in adults.[5] The Stevens-Johnson syndrome, a variant of erythema multiforme, may produce massive swelling and desquamation intraorally.[6] All emergency physicians should be familiar with this entity because it is often misdiagnosed as an infectious disease; the distinction is important since proper treatment is IV corticosteroids. Foreign bodies impacted in the upper esophagus can compress the posterior wall of the trachea, producing UAO[7] (remember that the first few tracheal rings are not cartilaginous posteriorly). Large fruit pits are particularly likely to lodge there,[7, 8] and may not be appreciated at the time of ingestion owing to old age, alcohol ingestion, central nervous system (CNS) disease, etc; thus, at presentation, the initiating event may not be recognized. A kinked esophageal obturator tube has been reported to produce UAO by the same mechanism.[9] Tracheal obstruction secondary to esophageal foreign bodies can also make tracheal intubation impossible!

Acute UAO evolves over a period of minutes to a few hours. Severe chemical or thermal burns of the upper airway do not present a diagnostic challenge (see Chapter 26), but it is often not clear at the outset whether there has been a burn significant enough to cause acute swelling of upper airway

structures. Therefore, it is imperative that the oropharynx be carefully inspected initially, and that the patient be monitored for several hours thereafter for signs of UAO!

Bleeding into upper airway structures is usually secondary to trauma, but Warfarin (Coumadin) has been implicated in spontaneous bleeding into the tongue or parapharyngeal structures.[10]

One of the most dreaded causes of acute UAO is adult epiglottitis, and the incidence of this infection appears to be increasing.[11, 12] *Haemophilus influenzae* is the most common causative organism, but *Staphylococcus aureus, Streptococcus pneumoniae,* and other streptococci have also been implicated.[13] Inflammation usually involves all of the supraglottic structures, though some part of the epiglottis may be spared; also, abscesses can form. There is intense laryngeal pain, dysphagia and drooling, and usually significant fever; the voice may be muffled, but not hoarse (since the vocal cords are generally spared). The diagnosis can be made by a soft tissue lateral film of the neck, which demonstrates the swollen epiglottis as a thumblike projection[14] (Figs 27–1 and 27–2). However, gentle indirect or direct laryngoscopy is more accurate. The likelihood of laryngoscopy worsening the UAO in adults is much less than in children since the adult glottis is larger.[15, 16] Too often the diagnosis is missed on the first visit, and the victim returns to the emergency department (ED) dead on arrival (DOA) or in extremis. *Epiglottitis must be ruled out in all febrile patients who complain of throat pain or dysphagia, but have normal pharyngeal examinations!*

Acute allergic angioedema is quite commonly seen in acute care facilities. It usually affects the lips or other external organs and is then of little significance. However, in the rare instance of glottic swelling, it becomes life-threatening. When in conjunction with anaphylaxis, one is faced with a threat to the integrity of both airway and circulation. If the glottis is the only structure affected, there is no clue to the underlying cause of UAO.

One of the most confusing and interesting causes of acute UAO is functional or psychogenic stridor, called variously Munchausen's stridor,[17] pseudoasthma,[18] factitious asthma,[19] nonorganic UAO,[20] or simply functional UAO.[21] Such fanciful terminology refers to the simple act of involuntary partial glottic closure. This syndrome is usually seen in young women, and is often accompanied by hyperventilation, tears, and considerable emotion, in response to some acutely disturbing life event. However, it may be an isolated event without these

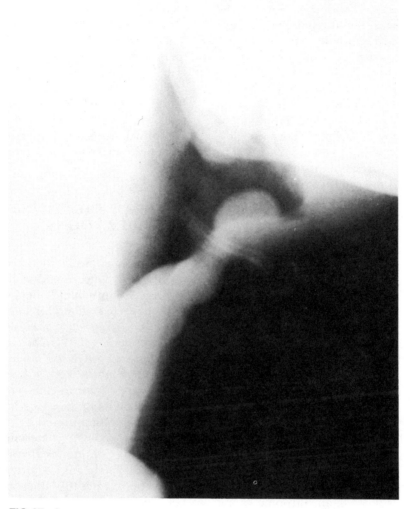

FIG 27–2.
Swollen epiglottis.

clearly defining associated features. One must be careful not to overreact: precipitant, dangerous, and wholly unnecessary tracheostomies have been performed![22]

Hyperacute UAO occurs over time lines of seconds to a few minutes. Although foreign bodies and laryngospasm are the only two causes listed in Table 27–1, *any of the less acute etiologies can present in this hyperacute state if they have evolved to the point of near-obstruction.* Thus the differential diagnosis would be limited to these two entities *only* if the total elapsed time of symptom evolution spanned seconds to a few minutes.

Laryngospasm rarely occurs except with direct physical stimulation of the glottic structures. Thus, for all practical purposes, it is usually due to traumatic attempts at endotracheal intubation. The un-relenting complete or partial apposition of the vocal cords is recognized either by severe stridor and other symptoms of high-grade UAO, or by direct laryngoscopic observation.

Foreign body obstruction of the upper airway has nightmare possibilities for the unwary or unprepared physician. It may be conveniently divided into the extremes of age. Part of the development of toddlers is assessing interesting objects by placing them in their mouths. Because they are mobile and active, this is frequently done without parental observation or permission. Thus, many objects of no interest to an adult are mouthed by the toddler. Also, the toddler is sometimes inappropriately given food that cannot be properly masticated (especially hot dogs, candy, grapes, or nuts).[23] Should the foreign object fall into the glottic opening, partial or complete

UAO will result. This event will induce a spasmodic coughing or choking episode with some sort of respiratory distress. Usually the foreign body is expelled successfully, and the whole event may pass virtually unnoticed. However, in a small minority of instances, the foreign body causes obvious manifestations of hyperacute UAO, and the emergency medical services (EMS) system is called. A still more unusual eventuality is the incomplete expulsion of the foreign body, leaving it "lurking" above the glottis, often in one of the piriform sinuses, ready to obstruct again. Upon ED evaluation, if there has been a suspicious event, and the child is in no respiratory distress, the first action would be to gently visualize the oropharynx. This examination would most often be unrewarding. Since it would be difficult to obtain the cooperation necessary to perform indirect laryngoscopy, the next step would be a soft tissue lateral film of the neck. Although the majority of foreign bodies are radiopaque, a few are not! Therefore, if the suspicion of foreign body is high enough (a tough judgment call sometimes), emergency consultation with the appropriate endoscopist must be sought before the child is released! *Any episode of coughing or choking in a toddler which produces symptoms alarming enough to precipitate an ED visit is reason for the physician to suspect an unexpelled foreign body, and mandates an exhaustive search for it!*

Foreign bodies also plague the elderly. The predisposing factors are well known[7, 24, 25]: (1) CNS diseases impairing the swallowing mechanism (bulbar palsies, especially secondary to old basilar artery cerebrovascular accidents (CVAs), amyotrophic lateral sclerosis, multiple sclerosis, Parkinson's disease, tardive dyskinesia, etc.; (2) impaired level of consciousness that is primary (organic brain disease) or secondary (alcohol, anticholinergic, or sedating psychotropic drugs); (3) dentures or dehydration (preventing adequate mastication); (4) foodstuffs that are hard to chew or swallow (at one extreme would be steak or hard rolls; at the other, sticky, viscous foods such as peanut butter); and (5) an inciting incident, such as laughing, which produces gasping and other upper airway motions which "compete" with the coordinated act of swallowing. The last four mechanisms are particularly germane to the so-called cafe coronary, wherein the elderly restaurant diner suddenly becomes speechless, grasps his throat (universal choking sign), turns blue, and quickly collapses—comatose, apneic, and then pulseless.[24]

A three-phase negative feedback loop model for foreign body obstruction or aspiration proposed by Harris et al.[23] seems logical: (1) The foreign body or material occludes or stimulates the glottis, producing (2) a cough to attempt expulsion, followed by (3) a quick gasping inspiration which may promote further aspiration or obstruction from uncleared material. Particularly with thin sticky foods, pulmonary aspiration may complicate UAO. In this instance, however, the aspirate is not the low-pH gastric contents which causes severe pulmonary edema; rather, the principal insult is short-term UAO and long-term pulmonary inflammation and atelectasis.

GENERAL TREATMENT CONSIDERATIONS

Upper airway obstruction of any degree is a matter of grave concern and as has been emphasized is intrinsically unstable: "unexpected" deterioration is to be expected! Therefore: (1) *These patients must be placed in a resuscitation room with materials for surgical airway at the bedside.* (2) *There must be a nurse or physician always present during this time monitoring the patient until a stable airway is established!* (3) An IV line should be routine, except in children that have high-grade UAO which might be exacerbated by the procedure. (4) Oxygen administered by nasal cannula, after an initial pulse oximetry determination, is generally indicated. (5) Continuous rhythm monitoring will detect immediately any important increase or slowing of the pulse rate. (6) Other ancillary measures may be important in particular situations, *but are always secondary* to airway management.

Since most causes of UAO presenting to an ED will be inflamatory or infectious, or both, antibiotic therapy must be begun as soon as an infection is identified. Abscesses should be drained at the earliest possible moment.

Steroid therapy is always an issue in most acute inflamatory conditions. It is usually difficult to demonstrate any benefit from steroid administration. However, we propose that even a small possible benefit must not be withheld in critical situations such as acute UAO. And since any benefit from steroids will be delayed several hours, they should be administered immediately. Also, the adverse effects of steroids are only from longer-term therapy, to which one is not committed by giving a single initial IV dose. It is important to realize, though, that *whatever the effect of steroids, they will never be the primary or definitive mode of therapy in any condition causing UAO!*

Scenario 1: The Stable Patient

The clinical manifestations of early UAO have been described above. In summary, there are only the most meager signs and symptoms; the situation may well not even be diagnosed. However, the situation is only stable if the manifestations have evolved subacutely or chronically, i.e., over hours to days. If, using these criteria, the patient is stable, no immediate definitive therapy is necessary, and the evaluation may proceed in a deliberate fashion. The broad categories of subacute and chronic causes listed in Table 27–1 should be considered. Except for hidden tumors, various congenital abnormalities, and rare chronic inflammatory diseases, even a cursory evaluation should quickly establish a diagnosis.

These patients are alert with intact oropharyngeal reflexes, have only mild and slowly progressive UAO, are at virtually no risk of aspiration, and disturbances of ventilation and oxygenation are not an issue. Active airway management is not required. However, while attempts to determine the cause are being pursued, the patients must be kept in a room equipped for full resuscitation. And patients must be observed frequently for manifestations of increased UAO. They are only to be labeled stable as long as their symptoms and signs are stable! The studies discussed under Clinical Manifestations and Evaluation should be pursued. Among these studies fiberoptic laryngoscopy deserves special mention since it has, as well, a therapeutic use: intubation over the fiberoptic endoscope (see Chapter 12).

Certainly, pulse oximetry and O_2 by nasal cannula are appropriate, though not mandatory.

Scenario 2: The Crashing Patient

Upper airway obstruction in the crashing patient is acute, and is evolving over a period of minutes to a few hours. The clinical manifestations have been described above. In summary, this patient has obvious but mild UAO and is alert and cooperative; the obstruction is not yet severe enough to produce impressive respiratory distress or any ventilatory compromise. One must plan less than an hour for definitive evaluation and therapy and assume the worst case: that the patient will deteriorate suddenly and without warning.

Airway management must be aggressive without being precipitous. Most of the conditions categorized as *acute* (or upgraded from *subacute* or *chronic*) in Table 27–1 will not be able to be controlled within safe time spans with drug treatment alone. This means, specifically, that active intervention to establish both a diagnosis and a definitive airway is to be anticipated.

A general approach that covers most situations is as follows: Gentle visualization of the oropharynx with a tongue blade is a simple first step with virtually no contraindications. In cases of oropharyngeal burns, hematomas, and infections, a reasonable assessment can be made of the severity of the process and the chances of successful orotracheal intubation. If direct oropharyngeal visualization fails to define the cause of the UAO, indirect laryngoscopy (mirror) is a next logical step. The procedure should be carefully explained to the patient, and the posterior oropharynx anesthetized with a topical anesthetic. If luck prevails, a foreign body is found that can be plucked out with a curved Kelly or Magill forceps. If one can see the glottis well, the diagnosis and the way to proceed is usually apparent. Normal supraglottic structures, but with partial apposition of the vocal cords occurring in inspiration, indicates a functional (psychological) basis.[26] Bland edema of the supraglottis indicates allergic angioedema. Intense inflammation clinches a diagnosis of acute epiglottitis or supraglottitis.

One must now proceed with preparations for airway establishment. In unusual circumstances temporizing measures may avert the necessity for intubation. An example might be the patient with nonexplosive allergic glottic edema. There is a reasonable chance that IV epinephrine, antihistamines, and cimetidine might reverse the UAO in minutes (steroids will not). However, one must always weigh against such temporization the awful possibility of clinical deterioration to a crashed status, with its perilous intubating conditions! No simple guidelines can be advanced for making a decision; each such situation is a wrenching judgment call.

The intubation technique of choice will usually be orotracheal. *Blind* nasotracheal intubation has no place here; it cannot establish a diagnosis, must be attempted in the face of an impaired airstream, is almost sure to fail because of the obstruction, and has a high likelihood of exacerbating the cause of the obstruction. However, nasotracheal intubation with simultaneous laryngoscopic cord visualization, using Magill forceps to guide the tube, is a possible alternative. But regardless of the choice, *direct visualization of the glottis is all-important!*

Fiberoptic endoscopic intubation is an option only if the emergency physician is accomplished in the technique, or a qualified endoscopist is *immediately* available. Otherwise, one should proceed with orotracheal intubation.

Since the patient is not in severe respiratory distress or ventilatory failure, sedation with an ultrashort-acting sedative can be administered carefully IV. The choice of tube size will vary with the pathologic condition, but adequacy of airflow must be balanced against successful tube passage.

If, for whatever reason, orotracheal intubation

fails, *and obstructive symptoms do not worsen,* secondary techniques can be considered. One such is retrograde transtracheal intubation. This ingenious and simple, but rarely attempted, technique can theoretically be performed in a matter of a few minutes. And the stiff end of the tube-guiding Seldinger wire, gently advanced, should traverse most incomplete obstructions unimpeded, given the steeple configuration of the subglottic anatomy. However, we know of no partial UAO cases in which it has been used, and such techniques in inexperienced hands are invariably fraught with unexpected difficulties.

If intubation is still unsuccessful, and the patient continues to deteriorate, one must consider the crashed patient options.

Scenario 3: The Crashed Patient

Upper airway obstruction in the crashed patient is hyperacute and evolves over a period of seconds to few minutes. Only two conditions that arise so explosively de novo come to mind: laryngospasm and foreign body lodgment. The former occurs virtually only as a complication of intubation, and so it rarely provides a problem in diagnosis (see Chapter 6 for its management). This leaves foreign body obstruction as the working diagnosis in any patient exhibiting hyperacute UAO *without any prodromal symptoms.* But one must remember that any of the causes of subacute or acute UAO may be upgraded to hyperacute. To review: the crashed patient is in extremis. UAO is high-grade, but not complete, with marked stridor in both inspiration and expiration; there is labored breathing and ventilatory insufficiency; patient cooperation is unlikely—disorientation and combative behavior may be present.

One must immediately diagnose and treat the cause of the UAO. Yet a real dilemma exists: the next logical step is direct laryngoscopy to both visualize the glottis and attempt intubation, but the patient cannot cooperate and any such manipulation of the upper airway may precipitate worsening of the obstruction! This is the worst possible circumstance in medicine: an "uncontrolled" situation combined with an immediate threat to life. All authorities would agree that the correct way to proceed in this desperate situation is to "do the right thing immediately"; beyond that, we doubt there is any measure of consensus. The following recommendations are submitted only on the basis of experience mixed with some measure of logic, but without a shred of substantiation from the literature.

Nothing can be done until the patient is controlled! An IV line must be secured; possibly physical restraint will be necessary. Then definitive chemical control is achieved by paralysis with IV succinylcholine or ultrarapid-acting sedation, or

both. But one has now traded control of the patient for control of the airway—the patient has been rendered iatrogenically apneic! But initially one did *not* have control of the airway, and further, *could not achieve it.* The upper airway is now visualized laryngoscopically. (One may preventilate with bag and mask and 100% O_2 only if it is likely that significant oxygenation can be achieved.) In the best case, a removable supraglottic foreign body will be found. In all other cases, depending upon what is seen, a decision must be made whether to perform an airway from below or whether to attempt intubation. In the preponderance of cases *one or two* attempts at intubation would be warranted: the attempts should take only seconds; the equipment is immediately at hand and the operator has far more experience with oral intubation than with any other technique. But the attempts should take no more than 10 to 15 seconds! That failing, one must perform the most rapid and simple airway-from-below procedure possible. In the hands of most operators, this would be the wire-guided percutaneous transtracheal catheter (Cook Inc., Bloomington, Ind.). This technique involves exactly the same steps as IV placement of wire-guided catheters; it provides a lumen large enough for adequate ventilation as well as oxygenation and its complication rate would be far less than that with cricotomes, cricothyrotomy, or tracheostomy. It will not, however, provide protection against aspiration since it is cuffless. But once the crisis has passed, the percutaneous catheter site in the trachea or cricothyroid membrane can easily be converted to a cuffed tracheostomy tube semielectively, if desired.

A discussion of UAO is not complete without dealing with the patient with essentially complete UAO who is comatose but still has a pulse. This patient will not resist treatment and needs no preparation for the definitive procedure: immediate laryngoscopic examination of the airway. Thereafter, he is managed as discussed above.

An algorithm for ER management of UAO is given in Figure 27–3.

PREHOSPITAL PERSPECTIVE

Prehospital training for UAO in most areas of the United States is either (or sometimes both) basic life support (BLS) or advanced cardiac life support (ACLS), i.e., emergency medical technician (EMT) I or EMT III (paramedical), respectively. Most paramedical personnel are trained, as well, to perform percutaneous transtracheal ventilation (PTV). The prehospital treatment of partial and complete UAO has engendered an enormous amount of interest,

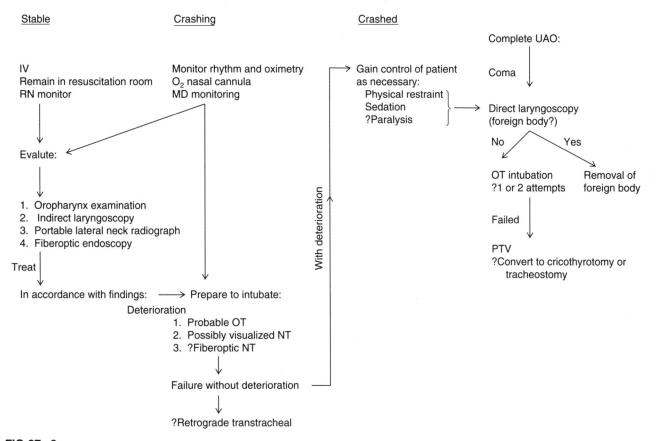

Stable   Crashing   Crashed

FIG 27–3.
Algorithm for emergency department management of upper airway obstruction *(UAO)*. OT = orotracheal; *NT* = nasotracheal; *PTV* = percutaneous transtracheal ventilation.

speculation, and controversy in the literature.[27–31] The interest in the subject has been fueled by a number of factors: the ascendancy of modern-day prehospital care; the "discovery" of the "cafe coronary" as a clinical entity; and the introduction of the so-called Heimlich manuever.

In fact, the hyperacute nature of foreign body obstruction makes it appropriately a prehospital care problem: the patient will often truly live or die depending on the skill of lay or prehospital personnel. It is, therefore, worth examining in detail the evolution of hyperacute UAO, with especial emphasis on the presumed foreign body scenario (Table 27–2). From both a diagnostic and therapeutic point of view, it is useful to divide UAO secondary to presumed foreign bodies into incomplete and complete obstruction.

The signs of incomplete UAO have been described in detail above; they may, of course, be of any degree of severity. As long as the patient is conscious (i.e., achieving sufficient oxygenation to support life), the management is very simple: (1) En-

courage cough; it provides the best combination of both force and airstream volume to expel the foreign body. (2) Try to calm the patient: struggling respirations cause collapse of upper airway structures (see above) and may impact the foreign body further. (3) Encourage the "sniffing" position of the patient's head and neck; it aligns the three axes of the airway to optimize airway patency. (4) Do not attempt any active airway interventions; they are unnecessary and possibly harmful. (5) Initiate code III transport to the nearest appropriate ED.

Complete UAO from foreign bodies has three phases: First, in sudden complete UAO the patient will often exhibit the "universal choking sign" (raise a hand to the throat), become aphonic, demonstrate struggling paradoxical respirations (severe inspiratory retractions), and will be tachypneic and tachycardic. In the second phase, the patient has become sufficiently hypoxic to lose consciousness and have depressed respirations, pulse, and blood pressure. In the third stage, the patient becomes comatose, apneic, loses circulation, and develops dilated pupils.

TABLE 27–2.

Summary of Prehospital Assessment and Management of Acute Upper Airway Obstruction*

Problem	Signs and Symptoms	Field Management†
Incomplete	Conscious; inspiratory and expiratory stridor; respiratory distress; cyanosis	Encourage cough and "sniffing" position of head and neck; no active intervention!; to emergency department immediately
Complete		
First phase	Conscious; universal choking sign; struggling paradoxic respirations without air movement or voice; increased blood pressure and pulse	Activate EMS (2nd person); back blows; abdominal/chest thrusts
Second phase	Loss of consciousness; decreased respiration, blood pressure, and pulse	*EMT I:* in succession, as necessary: airway opening "rescue" breathing; back blows (head down) and abdominal/chest thrusts; examination and finger sweep of oropharynx
Third phase	Coma; absent vital signs; pupils dilated	*EMT III:* laryngoscopy, PTV, ?cricothyrotomy

*Adapted from Dailey RH: *Emerg Med Clin North Am* 1983; 1:261–277.
†EMS = emergency medical services; EMT = emergency medical technician; PTV = percutaneous transtracheal ventilation.

The management of all phases of complete UAO is the same since the underlying pathologic condition is the same. The American Academy of Pediatrics[32] and current BLS recommendations[30] are based on a number of factors: (1) the Heimlich manuevers (either chest or abdominal thrusts) produce a high-pressure but low-volume stream of air to eject an impacted foreign body. (2) Back blows produce higher pressures but lower volumes than the Heimlich manuevers. (3) Heimlich manuevers have complications that can be severe, and in infants abdominal thrusts are not recommended.[31] (4) Back blows in the upright position and blind oral finger sweeps both run the risk of further impacting obstructing foreign bodies.

Collating this and other information, recommendations for out-of-hospital actions are as follows[30]; first, four back blows with the patient in a "torso-down" position; second, that failing, chest or abdominal thrusts; third, those failing, an oropharyngeal sweep with the index finger. If these BLS measures fail, optional bag-mask ventilation with 100% O_2 can be initiated, given the possibility that some oxygenation may occur. However, gastric distention will invariably occur with this manuever so that a nasogastric tube must be inserted in the ED as soon as practicable to prevent aspiration!

Paramedical personnel have further options available to them. In turn, as appropriate, they are: direct laryngoscopy (this should be the procedure of FIRST choice in the comatose patient!); that failing, PTV; that failing, some form of cricothyrotomy, depending upon training and local EMS-approved protocols. Prehospital surgical airways must, of course, be a last-ditch recourse, given the anticipated low success rates and high incidence of lethal complications under field conditions.

PEDIATRIC PERSPECTIVE

Upper airway obstruction is more explosive and dangerous in children than in adults. First, the airway is smaller; thus a tiny decrement in airway diameter, which in an adult would be well tolerated, could be catastrophic in a child. Second, the airway structures are more pliable; thus high inspiratory pressures associated with obstruction cause more collapse of the airway, exacerbatinging obstruction. Third, the infant's proportionally larger head exaggerates flexion of the head on the neck, malaligning that airway axis, and so causing obstruction. Fourth, the child's tongue is large in relation to the mandible. Fifth, relative adenoidal hypertrophy produces nasal obstruction. Sixth, the child's airway is narrowest in the subglottic area at the level of the cricoid ring, at a point inaccessible to therapeutic manuevers from above. Sixth, certain features of the young child's airway anatomy make intubation more difficult: the larynx is more anterior, and the epiglottis is longer. Seventh, aspiration is more likely, oropharyngeal secretions are more profuse, and protective airway reflexes are immature. Eighth, UAO in the young child is more likely to produce reflex bronchospasm, impairing ventilation and drawing attention away from the upper airway. Ninth, O_2 consumption per kilogram of body weight is higher in children; thus they are more susceptible to hypoxia. Last, respiratory reserve, or the ratio of functional residual capacity to alveolar gas volume, is lower in children.

Although the differential diagnosis of acute UAO in children is similar to that in the adult, there is a different emphasis (Table 27–3). Foreign bodies, croup and epiglottitis, and other oropharyngeal infections would make up the clear majority of cases.

TABLE 27–3.

Serious Acute Upper Airway Obstruction in the Infant and Child*

Infections
    Acute laryngotracheobronchitis
    Supraglottitis (epiglottitis)
    Diphtheria
    Bacterial tracheitis (pseudomembranous croup)
    Pharyngeal abscesses (e.g., retropharyngeal)
    Tonsillitis, tonsillar hypertrophy
Accidents/trauma
    Glottic, subglottic, or esophageal foreign body
    External trauma to neck
    Burns to upper airway
    Iatrogenic
        Postintubation
        Postinstrumentation
Others
    Angioedema
    Spasmodic croup
    Tumors (e.g., lymphoma in anterior mediastinum)

*From Kilham H, Gillis J, Benjamin B: *Pediatr Clin North Am* 1987; 34:2. Used by permission.

They have been adequately addressed above and in Chapter 34 and need no more attention here.

REFERENCES

1. Kristoffersen MB, Rattenborg CC, Holaday PA: Asphyxial death: The roles of acute anoxia, hypercarbia, and acidosis. *Anesthesiology* 1967; 28:488.
2. Brookes GB, Fairfax AJ: Upper airway obstruction. *J R Soc Med* 1982; 75:425.
3. Whiting JL, Chow AW: Life-threatening infections of the mouth and throat. *J Crit Illness* 1987; 87:36–56.
4. Boster SR, Martinez SA: Acute UAO in the adult. *Postgrad Med* 1982; 72:50–57.
5. Campbell TP, Paris PM, Stewart RS: Tracheitis: The other cause of UAO. *Ann Emerg Med* 1988; 17:66–68.
6. Koch W, McDonald GA: Steven-Johnson syndrome with supraglottic laryngeal obstruction. *Arch Otolaryngol* 1989; 115:1381–1383.
7. Handler SD, Beaugard ME, Canalis RF, et al: Unsuspected esophageal foreign bodies in adults with UAO. *Chest* 1981; 80:234–236.
8. Schofferman J, Oill PA: UAO. *J Am Coll Emerg Physicians* 1976; 5:706–709.
9. Low RB: Marked anterior displacement of the trachea and larynx from an esophageal obturator airway. *Ann Emerg Med* 1982; 11:670.
10. Cohen AF, Warman SP: UAO secondary to warfarin-induced hematoma. *Arch Otolaryngol* 1989; 115:718–720.
11. Stair TO, Hirsch BE: Adult supraglottitis. *Am J Emerg Med* 1985; 3:512–518.
12. Fontanarosa PB, Polsky SS, Goldman GE: Adult epiglottitis. *J Emerg Med* 1989; 7:223–231.
13. Warner JA, Finaly WE: Fulminating epiglottitis in adults. *Anaesthesia* 1985; 40:348–352.
14. Assael LA, McCravy LL: Use of soft tissue radiographs for assessing impending UAO in head and neck infections. *J Oral Maxillofac Surg* 1986; 44:398–401.
15. Ossoff RN, Wolff AP: Acute epiglottitis in adults. *JAMA* 1980; 244:2639–2640.
16. Cohen E: Epiglottitis in adults. *Ann Emerg Med* 1984; 13:620–623.
17. Patterson R, Schatz M, Horton M: Munchausen's stridor: Non-organic laryngeal obstruction. *Clin Allergy* 1974; 4:307–310.
18. Dailey RH, Pseudoasthma: A new clinical entity? *J Am Coll Emerg Physicians* 1976; 5:192–193.
19. Downing ET, Braman SS, Fox MJ, et al: Factitious asthma. *JAMA* 1982; 248:2878–2881.
20. Cormier YF, Camus P, Desmeules MJ: Non-organic UAO. *Am Rev Respir Dis* 1980; 121:147–150.
21. Heiser J, Kahn M, Schmidt T: Functional airway obstruction presenting as stridor: A case report and literature review. *J Emerg Med* 1990; 285–289.
22. Appelblatt NH, Baker SR: Functional UAO—A new syndrome. *Arch Otolaryngol* 1981; 107:305–306.
23. Harris CS, Baker SP, Smith GA, et al: Childhood asphyxiation by food. A national analysis and overview. *JAMA* 1984; 251:2231–2235.
24. Mittelman R, Wetli C: Fatal cafe coronary. Foreign body airway obstruction. *JAMA* 1982; 247:1285–1288.
25. Craig TJ, Richardson MA: Cafe coronaries in psychiatric patients (letter) *JAMA* 1982; 248:2114.
26. Christopher KL, Wood RP, Eckert RC, et al: Vocal cord dysfunction presenting as asthma. *N Engl J Med* 1983; 308:1566–1570.
27. Abman S, Fan L, Cotton E: Emergency treatment of foreign body obstruction of the upper airway in children. *J Emerg Med* 1984; 2:7–12.
28. Heimlich H: First aid for choking children: Back blows and chest thrusts cause complications and death. *Pediatrics* 1982; 70:120–125.
29. Heimlich H, Patrick E: The Heimlich maneuver. *Postgrad Med* 1990; 87:38–53.
30. American Heart Association: Standards and guidelines for cardiopulmonary resuscitation and emergency cardiac care. *JAMA* 1986; 255:2843–2989.
31. Greensher J, Mofenson HC: Emergency treatment of the choking child. *Pediatrics* 1982; 70:110–112.
32. Committee on Accident and Poison Prevention, American Academy of Pediatrics: First aid for the choking child. *Pediatrics* 1981; 67:744.

28

Airway Management of Asthma

Robert H. Dailey, M.D.

Frederick B. Carlton, Jr., M.D.

Asthma affects approximately 5% of the population of industrialized countries[1] and is the most common airway problem seen in the emergency department (ED). Although mortality from this disease can approach 2%,[2] nearly 90% of exacerbations respond to simple therapeutic measures, permitting safe discharge home[3] from the ED for most patients. Asthma scenarios to be considered in this chapter are: (1) the stable (but severe) asthmatic patient; (2) the "crashing" (severe and unstable) asthmatic patient, and (3) the "crashed" (premorbid) asthmatic patient.

PATHOPHYSIOLOGY

A number of pathophysiologic changes occur during an asthma exacerbation (Table 28–1). The major change is obstruction to airflow, especially during expiration. Although there is variability among subjects, acute asthma exacerbations appear to have increased resistance in both the large and peripheral airways with the former being more rapidly reversible. Bronchoconstriction, mucous plugging, and bronchial inflammation are the principle causes of the increased resistance. The relative contributions of these factors are variable, explaining the differences observed in clinical courses and treatment.

Early airway closure on expiration and a compensatory increase in inspiratory muscle tone results in increased lung volumes. These increased volumes open the peripheral airways and increase the diffusion capacity. However, these higher volumes also shorten the diaphragm and decrease the force that it can generate. There is also a decrease in the elastic recoil of the lungs during asthma exacerbations and this contributes to the hyperinflation.

As the obstruction to airflow worsens, ventilation-perfusion inequality becomes more severe and produces hypoxemia. When respiratory muscles are unable to compensate for airway narrowing, hypercapnia results. With increased metabolic demands and hypoxemia, the respiratory muscles fatigue and unless the cycle is interrupted ventilatory failure worsens.

The greatest threat then in asthma exacerbations is airway obstruction leading to inadequate ventilation and oxygenation. Aspiration usually does not become a significant problem until the patient is moribund.

ASSESSMENT

Assessment of the severity of asthma exacerbation begins immediately upon presentation.

History

Particularly useful historical points to be sought include precipitating and exacerbating factors (e.g., infection, aspirin, inhalants, etc.); severity and duration of symptoms of the current exacerbation; steroid treatment, especially recent discontinuance; frequency and duration of hospitalizations, particularly intensive care unit (ICU) stays; adequacy of current medication regimen, compliance, and therapeutic response; and, especially, prior episodes requiring endotracheal intubation.

TABLE 28–1.
Pathophysiology of Asthma

Increased airway resistance
  Bronchoconstriction
  Mucous plugging
  Bronchial inflammation
Hyperinflation
Ventilation-perfusion inequality
Hypoxemia
Respiratory muscle fatigue
Hypercarbia
Respiratory and metabolic acidosis
Pulmonary hypertension

Physical Examination

A host of physical signs have been touted to be useful to assess severity at the bedside. However, no single one (or combination, for that matter) has been found to be consistently predictive of either severity or as an admission criterion.[3, 4]

1. Pulse rate: There is a rough correlation between severity and pulse rates above 120 to 130 beats per minute[5] but terminal hypoxemia will be associated with pulse rate "normalization" and finally bradycardia.[6]
2. Respiratory rate: Like the pulse rate there is only a general direct relationship to exacerbation severity.[7] Similarly, there is terminal slowing of respirations.
3. Wheezing: Generally there is a continuum of mild to severe wheezing, as follows: expiratory, low-pitched; expiratory and inspiratory, high-pitched; distant; near-absent. However, studies have been unable to document consistency in these findings.[8]
4. Use of accessory muscles: Although it is a hallmark indicator of severity, in unusual cases use of accessory muscles may be absent.
5. Pulsus paradoxicus is limited by many observers to inability to perform this maneuver, but, more important, it is quite inconstant, even in very severe episodes.[5]
6. Number of words spoken: This sign has quietly gained great usage, despite virtually no mention of it in the asthma literature. Experienced clinicians consciously or unconsciously appreciate the progression in severity from full sentences, to phrases, to single words.
7. Diaphoresis (indicative of both marked sympathetic outflow and work of breathing) is generally an indicator of severity.[9]
8. Mental status: Lethargy, combativeness, and disorientation bespeak end-stage ventilatory failure

and impending cardiopulmonary arrest, and constitute one of the principal indications for immediate intubation (see below).

Objective Studies

1. Direct measurements of outflow obstruction (spirometry) have been extensively studied and used in many institutions.[10–12] The two most common modalities are peak expiratory flow (PEF) and forced expiratory volume in 1 second (FEV_1). Twenty percent to 30% of predicted normal values (PEF <200 L/min, FEV_1 <1 L) correlates roughly with hypercapnia and significant hypoxemia (arterial oxygen partial pressure [PaO_2] <60 mm Hg).[13, 14] Improvement to 60% of predicted values has been correlated with successful discharge from the ED.[12] These measurements have the advantage of being objective, although the sickest patients may not be able to cooperate with the testing. As one would expect, the most success with, and confidence in these tests is in institutions with considerable experience with them.
2. Pulse oximetry (percent oxygen saturation) has stormed emergency medicine in the last year or two as a means to monitor pulmonary and cardiac conditions. It has, however, been little studied in this setting. An initial reading did not successfully predict ultimate hospital admission.[15] Certainly, it is clearly useful in detecting subtle improvement or deterioration in ventilatory status.
3. Arterial blood gas (ABG) determinations have the advantage of exactly determining oxygenation and ventilation (carbon dioxide tension [$PaCO_2$]). However, the time required to draw and perform this test limits its utility in minute-to-minute patient evaluation.
4. Chest films are useful only if a specific pathologic condition is suspected, e.g., pneumonia, pneumothorax, or if the patient does not clear sufficiently to permit discharge.

PHARMACOLOGIC THERAPY

All patients with significant acute asthma must be placed in an appropriate acute care room with airway equipment, oxygen, intubation tray and drugs, and electrocardiogram (ECG) and pulse oximetry monitoring. An intravenous line should be established. Depending on the degree of severity, such patients should be continuously observed by either an experienced nurse or an emergency physician.

For the sake of discussion it is convenient to divide pharmacologic therapy into two groups: standard (established, first-line, primary) and adjunctive (second-line, secondary) (Table 28–2). This division is somewhat artificial and certainly fluid; today's standard drugs may become obsolete, and other drugs that are now adjunctive may become first-line. And even authorities on asthma cannot agree on which drugs should today be primary and which secondary. But the division is useful since one tends to use them "grouped." That is, the first-line drugs are usually used upon the patient's initial presentation, and the second-line drugs used only if the patient has not then responded clinically (see Fig 28–1).

Standard Drugs

Oxygen

Severe asthmatic patients should have a baseline room air pulse oximetry performed upon entry. Supplemental O_2 should then be administered by nasal cannula. If ventilatory failure is suspected, it is probably wise to administer O_2 at flows to produce only an acceptable O_2 saturation by oximetry (>90%–95%), since occasionally unrestricted O_2 may worsen the ventilatory failure. But all severe asthmatic patients have significant hypoxemia and must receive O_2!

Aerosolized β-Adrenergics

There are many effective drugs in this category, and despite the theoretical advantages of the newer agents, none has a clear superiority over the others in all patients.[16] It is often useful to ask the patient which drug provides optimal relief. A rough order of choice of the three in most common usage in the

TABLE 28–2.

Pharmacologic Therapy of Asthma

Standard (first-line, primary) drugs
  Oxygen
  Aerosolized β-adrenergics
  Glucocorticoids
  Subcutaneous adrenergics
  Parasympatholytics (anticholinergics)
  Aminophylline
Adjunctive (second-line, secondary) drugs
  Magnesium sulfate
  Sodium bicarbonate
  ?IV isoproterenol
  ?Ketamine
  ?Nonsedating antihistamines

United States today is as follows: albuterol (Ventolin, Proventil), metaproterenol (Alupent, Metaprel), and isoetherine (Bronkosol). They are packaged conveniently in unit doses for use by power-driven nebulization. Although multidose inhalers (MDIs) with spacers can be quite effective, nebulizers are better tolerated by the severe asthmatic patient. Near-continuous therapy can be given as long as toric side effects do not supervene (tachycardia, tremulousness, dysrhythmias, undue anxiety, etc.); no limiting number of unit doses or optimal time period between doses has been established.

Subcutaneous Adrenergics

Patients who have very intense bronchospasm may not be able to get enough inhaled β-adrenergic medication to their alveolar-capillary interface to be effective. If this situation is believed to obtain, subcutaneous adrenergics should be administered. Terbutaline (0.2 mg) or epinephrine (0.3 or 0.4 mL of 1:1,000 solution) are both effective. Massaging the injection site may hasten absorption.

Glucocorticoids

This group of drugs is routinely administered in virtually all severe exacerbations of asthma. Their many unique actions take hours to be clinically significant, so they should be given immediately.[17] Even if the patient subsequently clears rapidly and completely so that it is deemed unnecessary to continue them, no harm has been done. Although both oral and intramuscular[18] administration have been shown to be effective, an intravenous (IV) bolus injection of 125 mg of methylprednisolone (Solu-Medrol) is in current general use.

Parasympatholytics (Anticholinergics)

This class of drug has achieved greater prominence in the past few years in the treatment of acute asthma.[19, 20] The most effective is ipratropium bromide (Atrovent), but it is currently available in the United States only in MDI form; therefore, in the ED a spacer should be used. Alternatively, and in more common usage, 2 mg atropine sulfate can be given by nebulization. One or two such treatments can be interpolated between β-adrenergic nebulizations. Onset of action typically is not seen for 60 to 90 minutes, and duration is up to 6 hours. Atropine can cause anticholinergic side effects (mydriasis, urinary retention, dry mouth, and tachycardia) since it is systemically absorbed to some degree; however, these undesirable effects are seldom seen. More recently success with glycopyrrolate (Robinul), a quaternary ammonium anticholinergic compound, has been reported.[21] Although usually administered by aerosolization (2.0-mg dose), success with its use IV (0.2 mg) has been cited.[22]

Aminophylline

The use of aminophylline is currently undergoing painstaking reevaluation. Its place as *the* principal drug in acute asthma has long since rightfully been usurped by the inhaled β-adrenergics. Indeed, it has been difficult to demonstrate any benefit additive to the β-adrenergics. Additionally, undesirable side effects have been emphasized. However, a recent blinded and controlled study has demonstrated a decrease in the rate of admissions in acute asthmatics receiving aminophylline.[23] For the time being, it is probably prudent to maintain low therapeutic levels (about 10–15 mg/L). This should confer any possible benefit without the risk of significant toxicity.

Adjunctive Drugs

Magnesium Sulfate

In the last few years a number of studies, all with small numbers of patients, have appeared examining the use of this compound in acute asthma.[24–27] Most have demonstrated benefit given alone or in addition to inhaled β-adrenergics[24–26]; others have not.[27] About 1 to 3 g in 50 to 100 mL of diluent is infused over about 15 minutes.

Sodium Bicarbonate

The use of this compound is shrouded in the mists of time and has received little notice in the literature. However, anecdotal accounts are often glowing about its use in the asthmatic patient who is in severe ventilatory failure and refractory to adrenergic drugs.[28–30] The theoretical basis of its action is restoration of the reactivity of β-adrenergic sites that have been inactivated by acidosis.[31] The recommended dosing is quite aggressive: 100 mEq over 5 to 10 minutes, repeated every 15 to 20 minutes as necessary to achieve either near-normalization of pH or improved ventilation.[29] Controlled studies are much needed to clarify the use of this compound in asthma.

Intravenous Isoproterenol

Isoproterenol has largely been reserved for refractory asthma in infants.[32] It has been only rarely used in adult asthma because of the likelihood of dysrhythmias and myocardial ischemia.[33] (Thus, it should not be used in any adult with the possible presence of coronary artery disease!) However, there are anecdotal accounts of its success, and its use can be considered in extreme circumstances in the younger adult.[34] Isoproterenol 1 mg is diluted in 500 mL 5% D/W and infused at 1 to 3 μg/min. It should be used for as short a period as possible.

Ketamine

Ketamine is discussed below under Intubation of the Unstable Asthmatic.

Nonsedating Antihistamines

No place has been found for *sedating* antihistamines in severe asthma. The danger of sedation worsening respiratory failure is well recognized. Recent work with newer, *non*sedating antihistamines (cetirizine, terfenadine, azelastine), however, has demonstrated bronchodilation approximating that of β-adrenergics.[35–37] These drugs are not yet commercially available in the United States, and they have not been studied in the ED setting.

Scenario 1: The Stable (but Severe) Asthmatic Patient

This patient presents in marked distress: quite tachypneic and tachycardic; alert, oriented, and very anxious; sweating; with labored but strong respirations with use of accessory muscles; able to speak only in phrases; and with audible moderately high-pitched inspiratory and expiratory wheezes. The room air pulse oximetry reading is in the range of 85% to 90% saturation, a $PaCO_2$ (if measured) would be 40 to 60 mm Hg, and spirometry would show less than 20% to 25% of predicted values.

Although very sick, this patient is not terminal and is strong enough to breathe without intubation. But aggressive standard pharmacologic therapy must be immediately instituted. This therapy (see Table 28–2) includes O_2 by nasal cannula, nebulization of β-adrenergic and parasympatholytic drugs, ıV corticosteroids, and optimization of theophylline levels. If there is any doubt that nebulized medications are reaching the alveolar-capillary interface, subcutaneous epinephrine or terbutaline should be administered. During this treatment the patient must be observed carefully and continuously (by an experienced emergency nurse) until definitely improving. Lack of improvement (or, indeed, deterioration!) over the first half to 1 hour defines the patient as crashing, and requires additional therapeutic measures (see Fig 28–1 and below).

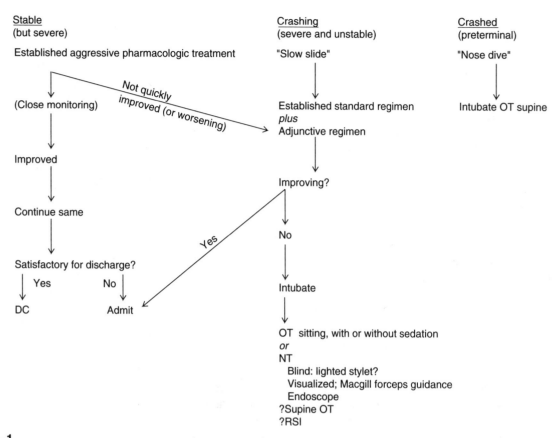

FIG 28–1.
Algorithm for airway management of asthma. *DC* = discharge; *OT* = orotracheal; *NT* = nasotracheal; *RSI* = rapid-sequence intubation.

Scenario 2: The Crashing (Severe and Unstable) Asthmatic Patient

This patient is in extremis and, without immediate relief, is at risk of dying in the ED! He may be alert and extremely anxious, but may also be showing signs of "CO_2 narcosis," i.e., lethargy or disorientation, or both. Tachypnea and tachycardia are marked; respirations are labored and *tiring;* all accessory muscles are in maximal use; sweating is likely to be generalized instead of just facial; speech is limited to a word or two; there is little air movement, and wheezing is very high-pitched and distant; the room air pulse oximetry reading is probably less than 85% saturation; $PaCO_2$ would exceed 65 mm Hg; and the patient is unlikely to be able to cooperate with spirometry.

Unless improvement can be achieved within minutes, this patient will need to be intubated and mechanically ventilated. Both primary and secondary forms of pharmacologic therapy should be instituted *at the outset* (see Table 28–2). Practically, this means addition of IV magnesium sulfate and sodium bicarbonate to the first-line drugs. *The emergency physician must not leave the bedside of this patient until unequivocal and substantial improvement is demonstrated!!* This is one of the most discomfiting situations in emergency medicine: the patient at risk of dying of a reversible disease. Intubating conditions are the worst possible: a sitting patient who is likely to be uncooperative or combative, a nonexistent margin of error (just a brief and small decrease in ventilation may precipitate cardiopulmonary arrest), and a technically difficult intubation. Worse, intubation will not necessary solve the ventilatory problems: it will not, in and of itself, provide any bronchodilation; and the unavoidable high ventilation pressures will (1) produce barotrauma, (2) decrease right heart blood return, producing hypotension, and (3) worst, risk producing a fatal pneumothorax. Therefore, the decision to intubate should not be made lightly. On the other hand, if intubation is unduly delayed, the patient is likely to arrest, *and then be nonresuscitable!* Risks and difficulties aside, the unimproved or deteriorating unstable asthmatic patient, as described above, must be intubated and ventilated.

Intubation of the Unstable Asthmatic Patient

Once the decision to intubate has been made, the procedure should be completed without delay, within approximately 5 minutes. Equipment for all intubating options should be available and readied, and one should have a clear idea of not only the procedure of first choice but also the alternatives in the event of initial failure to intubate.

The procedure of first choice will not be the same for all operators, and should depend on the specific skills and prior experience of the physician, the equipment and time available, and the ability of the patient to cooperate. If the patient is confused and combative, some method of control is necessary. Restraints on the patient's hands are helpful, but no method of restraint will keep the patient from turning and twisting his head and fighting the laryngoscope with the muscles of deglutition. Therefore, some other method of control is often necessary. The use of ketamine (Ketalar) is often considered in this circumstance, but it has seldom been used because emergency physicians have virtually no familiarity with it. Its use is usually restricted to the operating room. However, there is a scattering of reports of single case successes.[38–40] It is a powerful bronchodilator, and renders the patient immediately unconscious and immobile yet *without depressing respiration!* The adult dose is 2 mg/kg (about 150–200 mg), given as an IV bolus; its duration of action is about 45 to 60 minutes. Hallucinatory emergence phenomena are frequent in adults (it is a phencyclidine congener!), but this undesirable side effect can be mitigated by coadministration of a benzodiazepine.[41]

Otherwise, to maintain patient control and improve intubating conditions, sedation must be used. And, unfortunately, the better the sedation the greater the risk of exacerbating ventilatory failure. One is left walking a fine line here. We advise slowly injecting an ultra-rapid-acting sedative (midazolam [Versed], methohexital [Brevital], etc.) into the Y port of a rapidly running IV line. Thus a diluted bolus is delivered quickly, and its effects on consciousness and breathing can be titrated carefully. The least amount that will prevent struggling is the correct amount. But remember that *some* hypoventilation is the price one must unavoidably pay for sedation!

Blind Nasotracheal Intubation.—This procedure would probably be the first chosen by most emergency physicians today. Most are familiar and comfortable with the procedure; it needs no special equipment; it can be done with the patient in the sitting position; and it is quickly performed. However, it is blind, and the *realistic* success rate probably does not exceed 75% to 80%. If unsuccessful on the first pass or two, further passes are usually futile and often result in epistaxis, laryngospasm, and damage to upper airway structures. Use of a lighted stylet may increase slightly the success rate for those familiar with its use, but the procedure is still blind.

Visualized Nasotracheal Intubation.—If blind nasotracheal (NT) intubation fails, one can use a laryngoscope and Macgill forceps to enhance NT intubation. The operator stands on a stool, leaning over the right side of the patient's head. Leaving the NT tube in the nose with its tip just above the cords, the laryngoscope is inserted into the mouth in the usual manner, and then the Macgill forceps (in the right hand) is used to grasp the distal tube (take care not to rupture the cuff!) and guide it through the cords. A helper is necessary to advance the tube upon command as the operator guides it. This simple adjunct to NT intubation is often overlooked. More's the pity, since all intubators have the requisite skills. It quickly turns a blind technique into a sighted one.

Endoscopic Nasotracheal Intubation.—Use of the fiberoptic laryngoscope or bronchoscope is an elegant technique with a very high success rate in skilled hands. Unfortunately, it requires training and experience that few emergency physicians have, and it takes more time to perform than most asthmatic patients in desperate circumstances can tolerate. Certainly, this is a technique that emergency physicians should acquaint themselves with, for it has great promise in many emergency airway situations.

Sitting Orotracheal Intubation.—This technique should be considered as an alternative to blind NT intubation. It is only because most physicians have not considered it that it is not used more frequently. It is performed in the same manner as described above under Visualized Nasotracheal Intubation. Stated simply, the technique is virtually the same as standard supine orotracheal (OT) intubation, except that the patient is sitting and the physician is standing above and behind the patient.

Rapid-Sequence Intubation (RSI).—All else failing one may be tempted to paralyze the unstable asthmatic. It is a temptation to be resisted! Sedation can be pushed to improve intubating conditions without rendering the patient apneic. If paralysis is produced one must be assured that the patient can be adequately ventilated, and that he or she can be successfully intubated. Unfortunately, interim bag-mask ventilation in the patient with very high airway resistance is unlikely to be adequate and, using the requisite high ventilation pressures, one risks gastric insufflation and thus aspiration (even with careful and correctly applied cricoid pressure). We are avowed enthusiasts of RSI, but find it difficult to recommend in any asthmatic patient.

The Crashed (Premorbid) Asthmatic Patient

This patient is preterminal; moribund. He or she is bradypneic, bradycardic, has gasping ineffective respirations, is comatose or nearly so, and will die within a few minutes if heroic measures are not immediately undertaken. Decision making is as easy in this case as it is difficult in the crashing patient.

The patient must be immediately intubated orotracheally, generally without prior preventilation or pharmacologic therapy. This patient usually resists very little, but sedation may be necessary if the patient fights the procedure.

POSTINTUBATION VENTILATION AND CARE

Most airway emergencies are brought under control by endotracheal intubation. Not so with the asthmatic patient! The principal problem—bronchoconstriction—remains, and may indeed even be exacerbated by the high airway pressures needed to maintain adequate ventilation. On-line, nebulized β-adrenergic therapy must be immediately instituted.[42] And one must begin all other first- and second-line drugs.

The patient should be ventilated with a volume-cycled ventilator that is capable of generating high peak inspiratory pressures. A relatively slow respiratory rate of 8 to 12 breaths per minute and tidal volume of 10 to 15 mL/kg should be used. Because these patients tend to be hyperinflated and have prolonged expiratory phases, the ratio of inspiration to expiration should be approximately 1:3. Initial fractional concentration of oxygen in inspired air (FiO_2) should be 100%, with reduction based on subsequent blood gas determinations. Positive end-expiratory pressure (PEEP) and continuous positive airway pressure (CPAP) have been suggested as useful adjuncts in ventilator management of asthma patients, but their exact role is yet to be defined.[43, 44]

REFERENCES

1. Barnes PJ: The changing face of asthma. *Q J Med* 1987; 63:359–365.
2. Santiago SM Jr, Klaustermeyer WB: Mortality in status asthmaticus: A nine-year experience in a respiratory intensive care unit. *J Asthma Res* 1980; 17:75–79.
3. Rose CC, Murphy JG, Schwartz JS: Performance of an index predicting the response of patients with acute bronchial asthma to intensive emergency department treatment. *N Engl J Med* 1984; 310:573.
4. Centor RM, Yarbrough B, Wood JP: Inability to predict relapse in acute asthma. *N Engl J Med* 1984; 310:577.
5. Carden DL, Nowak RM, Sarkar D, et al: Vital signs including pulsus paradoxus in the assessment of acute bronchial asthma. *Ann Emerg Med* 1983; 12:80.
6. Rebuck AS, Read J: Assessment and management of severe asthma. *Am J Med* 1971; 51:788.
7. Rees HA, Millar JS, Donald KW: A study of the clinical course and arterial blood gas tensions of patients in status asthmaticus. *Q J Med* 1967; 148:541.
8. Shim CS, Williams MH: Relationships of wheezing to the severity of obstruction in asthma. *Arch Intern Med* 1983; 143:890.
9. Brenner BE, Abraham E, Simon RR: Position and diaphoresis in acute asthma. *Am J Med* 1983; 74:1005.
10. Avery WG: Maximizing spirometry in reversible airways disease. *Ann Allergy* 1981; 47:410.
11. Boggs PB, Bhat KD, Vekovius WA, et al: The clinical significance of volume-adjusted maximal mid-expiratory flow (isovolume FEF 25%–75%) in assessing airway responsiveness to inhaled bronchodilator in asthmatics. *Ann Allergy* 1981; 47:307.
12. Nowak RM, Pensler MI, Sarkar DD, et al: Comparison of peak expiratory flow and FEV_1 admission criteria for acute bronchial asthma. *Ann Emerg Med* 1982; 11:64.
13. Nowak RM, Tomlanovich MC, Sarkar DD, et al: Arterial blood gases and pulmonary function testing in acute bronchial asthma. *JAMA* 1983; 249:2043.
14. Martin TG, Elenbaas RM, Pingleton SH: Use of peak expiratory flow rates to eliminate unnecessary arterial blood gases in acute asthma. *Ann Emerg Med* 1982; 11:70.
15. Hedges JR, Amsterdam JT, Cionni DJ, et al: Oxygen saturation as a marker for admission or relapse with acute bronchospasm. *Am J Emerg Med* 1987; 5:196–200.
16. Emerman CL, Cydulka RK, Effron D, et al: A randomized, controlled comparison of isoetharine and albuterol in the treatment of acute asthma. *Ann Emerg Med* 1991; 20:1090–1093.
17. Arnaud A, Charpin J: Interaction between corticosteroids and beta-agonists in acute asthma. *Eur J Respir Dis* 1982; 122(suppl):126.
18. Ogirala RG, Aldrich TK, Prezant DJ, et al: High-dose intramuscular triamcinolone in severe, chronic life-threatening asthma. *N Engl J Med* 1991; 324:585–589.
19. Gross NJ, Skorodin MS: Anticholinergic, antimuscarinic bronchodilation. *Am Rev Respir Dis* 1984; 129:856–870.

20. Gross NJ: Ipratropium bromide. *N Engl J Med* 1988; 319:486–494.

21. Gilman MJ, Meyer L, Carter J, et al: Comparison of aerosolized glycopyrrolate and metaproterenol in acute asthma. *Chest* 1990; 98:1095–1098.

22. Slovis CM, Daniels GM, Wharton DR: Intravenous use of glycopyrrolate in acute respiratory distress due to bronchospastic pulmonary disease. *Ann Emerg Med* 1987; 16:898–900.

23. Wrenn K, Slovis CM, Murphy F, et al: Aminophylline therapy for acute bronchospastic disease in the emergency department. *Ann Intern Med* 1991; 115:241–247.

24. Noppen M, Vanmaele L: Bronchodilating effect of intravenous magnesium sulfate in acute severe asthma. *Chest* 1990; 97:373–376.

25. McNamara RM, Spivey WH, Skobeloff E, et al: Intravenous magnesium sulfate in the management of acute respiratory failure complicating asthma. *Ann Emerg Med* 1989; 18:197–199.

26. Okayama H, Aikawa T, Okayama M, et al: Bronchodilating effect of intravenous magnesium sulfate in bronchial asthma. *JAMA* 1987; 257:1076–1078.

27. Green SM, Rothrock SG: IV magnesium for acute asthma: Failure to decrease emergency treatment duration or need for hospitalization (abstract). *Ann Emerg Med* 1991; 20:952.

28. Mithoefer JC, Runser RH, Karetzky MS. The use of sodium bicarbonate in the treatment of acute bronchial asthma. *N Engl J Med* 1965; 272:1200–1203.

29. Mithoefer JC, Porter WF, Karetzky MS: Indications for the use of sodium bicarbonate in the treatment of intractable asthma. *Respiration* 1968; 25:2201–2215.

30. Menitove SM, Goldring RM: Combined ventilator and bicarbonate strategy in the management of status asthmaticus. *Am J Med* 1983; 74:898–901.

31. Barton M, Lake CR, Rainey TG, et al: Is catecholamine release pH-mediated? *Crit Care Med* 1982; 10:751.

32. Parry W, Martorano F, Cotton E: Management of life-threatening asthma with intravenous isoproterenol infusions. *Am J Dis Child* 1976; 130:39–42.

33. Van Metre T Jr: Adverse effects of inhalation of excessive amounts of nebulized isoproterenol in status asthmaticus. *J Allergy* 1969; 43:101–103.

34. Schwartz SH: Treatment of status asthmaticus (letter). *N Engl J Med* 1985; 253:343.

35. Patel KR: Effect of terfenadine on methacholine-induced bronchoconstriction in asthma. *J Allergy Clin Immunol* 1987; 79:355–358.

36. Kemp JP, Metzer EO, Orgel HA, et al: A dose response study of the bronchodilator action of azelastine in asthma. *J Allergy Clin Immunol* 1979; 79:893–899.

37. Taskin DP, Brik A, Gong H: Cetirizine inhibition of histamine induced bronchospasm. *Ann Allergy* 1987; 59:49–52.

38. Rock MJ, Reyes DeLa Rocha S, L'Hommedieu CS, et al: Use of ketamine in asthmatic children to treat respiratory failure refractory to conventional therapy. *Crit Care Med* 1986; 14:514–516.

39. L'Hommedieu CS, Arens JJ: The use of ketamine for the emergency intubation of patients with status asthmaticus. *Ann Emerg Med* 1987; 16:568–571.

40. Fisher MM: Ketamine hydrochloride in severe bronchospasm. *Anaesthesia* 1977; 32:771–772.

41. Kothary SP, Zsigmond EK: A double-blind study of the effective antihallucinatory doses of diazepam prior to ketamine anesthesia. *Clin Pharmacol Ther* 1977; 21:108–109.

42. MacIntyre NR, Silver RM, Miller CW, et al: Aerosol delivery in intubated, mechanically ventilated patients. *Crit Care Med* 1985; 13:81–84.

43. Quist J: High level PEEP in severe asthma (letter). *N Engl J Med* 1981; 305:1398; 1982; 307:1347.

44. Martin JG, Shore S, Engel LA: Effect of continuous positive airway pressure on respiratory mechanics and pattern of breathing in induced asthma. *Am Rev Respir Dis* 1982; 126:812.

29

Chronic Obstructive Pulmonary Disease

Glenn F. Tokarski, M.D.

Robert H. Dailey, M.D.

Airway management of patients with chronic obstructive pulmonary disease (COPD) can be challenging and complex. Appropriate and successful management of the airway requires a thorough understanding of the associated pathophysiologic principles. COPD in this chapter will deal with pulmonary emphysema and chronic bronchitis. (Bronchospasm due to asthma is dealt with in Chapter 28). Both entities are responsible for a wide spectrum of disease, ranging from mild to life-threatening episodes. Our scenarios for discussion include (1) the "stable" COPD patient with mild to moderate exacerbation of respiratory symptoms but who does not have an immediate threat to life, (2) the "crashing" COPD patient with a severe exacerbation of respiratory symptoms who requires immediate therapy to maintain adequate independent airway control and who may require endotracheal intubation and mechanical ventilation, and (3) the "crashed" patient who demands immediate airway control and management lest death be a rapid consequence.

PATHOLOGY AND PATHOPHYSIOLOGY

In emphysema, abnormal permanent enlargement of the air spaces distal to the terminal bronchioles is accompanied by destruction of alveolar walls.[1] The alveolar septa are responsible for support of bronchial walls and their destruction leads to bronchial collapse which clinically results in expiratory airflow obstruction. Chronic bronchitis affects both large- and small-caliber airways and is characterized by inflamed and edematous airways filled with secretions from hypertrophied goblet cells and submucosal glands. These copious respiratory secretions contribute to expiratory obstruction.

Pathophysiologically, patients with COPD walk a constant pulmonary tightrope. They maintain adequate ventilation by balancing the mechanical load on the lung with adequate respiratory muscle strength.[2] Mechanical overload or diminished muscle strength can tip this precarious balance and result in acute ventilatory failure.

Alterations in mechanical load may be due to changes in resistance in the airways or elasticity of the lung or chest wall. Increases in airway resistance (e.g., bronchospasm, tracheal stenosis from previous intubations resulting in upper airway obstruction[3]) result in further expiratory obstruction superimposed on the chronic obstruction of the primary pulmonary disease process. This increased resistance makes expiration an active and energy-requiring process (normally only inspiration is active). Increased airway obstruction can also increase the elastic load on the lung. Dynamic airway obstruction increases the time required for full expiration to occur. If tachypnea is present, less time is spent in expiration. The combination of airway obstruction and tachypnea results in dynamic air trapping such that alveolar pressure remains positive at the end of expiration (known as intrinsic positive end-expiratory pressure, or intrinsic PEEP). The air trapping results in an increase in lung volume as well as an increased elastic load on the lungs and puts the respiratory musculature at a mechanical disadvantage. More energy is required by the respiratory muscles to overcome the positive end-expiratory pressure as well as to generate the normal negative intrathoracic pressure required for inspiration. Both obstruction and intrinsic PEEP increase the work and therefore the energy requirements of the respiratory muscles.

Alterations in respiratory muscle strength in a patient with COPD can also result in acute ventilatory failure. Depressed central nervous system (CNS) output (e.g., stroke or drug overdose) and faulty neuromuscular transmission (e.g., aminoglycoside toxicity or spinal cord lesions) may diminish respiratory muscle strength. Primary respiratory muscle dysfunction also can occur with malnutrition or electrolyte disturbances such as hypokalemia or hypocalcemia.

The three pillars of successful airway management are important when applied to patients with COPD. The above-mentioned derangements in inspiratory and expiratory airflow will ultimately result in rapid deterioration progressing to death if appropriate recognition and intervention are not provided.

Aspiration is not a major threat to the airway in patients with stable or mild respiratory exacerbations unless other disease entities (e.g., stroke, depressed level of consciousness) impair the gag reflex. In the crashing or crashed patient, secretions and stomach contents may physically obstruct the upper airway and, if aspirated, contribute to impaired gas exchange.

Changes in ventilation and oxygenation are intricately related in patients with COPD and their interrelationships have major implications for airway maintenance and therapy. Chronic hypoxemia in COPD patients results from impaired ventilation-perfusion ($\dot{V}/\dot{Q}$) relationships. Superimposed acute insults such as bronchospasm, mucous plugging, or alveolar disease impair the $\dot{V}/\dot{Q}$ relationship further, leading to greater decreases in gas exchange and worsening hypoxemia. Impaired $\dot{V}/\dot{Q}$ relationships also effect carbon dioxide exchange. COPD patients who maintain normal arterial carbon dioxide partial pressure ($PaCO_2$) levels achieve this by increasing minute ventilation to compensate for the CO_2 retention. The inability to maintain an increased minute ventilation results in hypercapnia.[4] As a patient with COPD progresses from a stable to a crashing to a crashed status, $\dot{V}/\dot{Q}$ relationships likewise progressively deteriorate and ultimately result in severe hypoxemia and hypercapnia. Chronic hypoxemia and hypercapnia produce increased pulmonary artery pressures, which in turn over time cause right heart strain and hypertrophy (i.e., cor pulmonale). In turn, with left heart failure $\dot{V}/\dot{Q}$ abnormalities are further worsened. The whole process constitutes a negative feedback loop.

ASSESSMENT

The acuity of the COPD patient must be determined before a treatment plan can be formulated. Is the patient stable, crashing, or crashed? A preliminary history precedes a more careful physical assessment. Does the dyspneic patient have pulmonary disease, cardiac, or other? Is the diagnosis of COPD secure? Are there other associated pulmonary symptoms, and if so, of what severity and rapidity of progression? Most critically, how much time do we have to evaluate the patient before we need to act?

A careful physical examination follows, keeping in mind the pathophysiologic features of COPD. Although we have sophisticated means to quantify ventilatory function, the most important part of the immediate clinical assessment consists of observation of the patient's general appearance and mental status, vital signs, breathing pattern, and the chest examination.

COPD patients tend to be more comfortable upright and leaning forward than recumbent, since the abdominal organs aid diaphragmatic motion and the work of accessory muscles is lessened.[5] The lips are sometimes pursed, especially in patients with predominant emphysema, to increase intrabronchial pressure upon expiration and thus prevent collapse of unsupported terminal bronchioles. Since speech occurs in expiration, marked airway obstruction causes multiple pauses in speech (words or phrases instead of fluid sentences) or even gasping monosyllabic speech. Sweating is a good indicator of increased work of breathing.

The mental status is of paramount importance in assessing the acuity of the COPD patient. Hypoxemia and hypercapnia alter higher cognitive function; the most common signs are inappropriate responses to history taking, anxiety, confusion, and a peculiar irritable lethargy. Obtundation or coma (if purely on the basis of COPD) indicates progressively more severe degrees of ventilatory failure.

Vital signs must be checked carefully! Blood pressure and the pulse and respiratory rates generally rise in proportion to the severity of COPD. The degree of elevation of the respiratory rate is proportional to the severity of the underlying disease[6] and an elevated respiratory rate is often the earliest sign of an imminent respiratory disaster.[7] However, the moribund patient has contrary findings: decreased respirations, blood pressure, and pulse terminating in shock and apnea.

One should always carefully observe the breathing pattern of the COPD patient with bared chest.

The deteriorating patient, in whom pure diaphragmatic effort is insufficient, recruits accessory muscle groups (i.e., sternocleidomastoids, intercostals, and scalenes) to aid ventilation. Thoracoabdominal paradoxical breathing (inward movement of the abdomen with inspiration) has been noted to herald respiratory collapse[8] in some but not all COPD patients. Respiratory alternans denotes alternating periods of diaphragmatic and accessory respiratory muscle activity. This pattern may allow the respective muscle groups short periods of rest, allowing intermittent periods of recovery, and thus prolong endurance,[9] although other investigations suggest this pattern represents increased respiratory load[10] or muscle fatigue.

The physical examination should focus on the chest. The combination of an increased anteroposterior diameter and low diaphragm (so-called barrel chest) suggests the hyperinflation of emphysema. Wheezing occurs in all COPD patients regardless of pathophysiologic cause (bronchospasm, emphysema, or bronchial secretions). Increased degrees of airway obstruction are indicated as one progresses from "loose" low-pitched, solely inspiratory wheezes to "tight" high-pitched inspiratory and expiratory wheezes to inaudible or nearly inaudible wheezing.

Findings of cor pulmonale should be sought: right ventricular gallops or heave (found retrosternally or subxiphoid), distended neck veins, tender and enlarged liver, and peripheral edema. One must be sure that the right ventricular failure is secondary to pulmonary disease, and not (as more commonly occurs) on the basis of left ventricular failure (a differentiation that is always difficult and often impossible to make at the bedside of the acutely ill patient).

Time and patient acuity permitting, after the above cursory evaluation, a more thorough history must be undertaken. It should document the natural history of the patient's COPD and the nature of the current acute episode. Special attention must be given to the myriad of factors that can complicate or exacerbate COPD (Table 29–1). Any clues must then be followed by appropriate specific physical examination and laboratory and radiologic studies.

Next, appropriate pulmonary function testing should be considered. Although measurements of forced expiratory volume in 1 second (FEV_1) and peak expiratory flow rate (PEFR) have been shown to correlate with hypoxemia in asthmatics,[11] these pulmonary function studies are of limited utility in patients with COPD exacerbations as it is difficult to obtain accurate measurements in the acutely ill and

TABLE 29–1.

Precipitating Causes of Worsening COPD

I. Pulmonary
  A. Obstruction
    1. Anatomic (e.g., foreign body, mucus plug)
    2. Dynamic (e.g., bronchoconstriction)
  B. Infection
  C. Aspiration
II. Cardiac
  A. Ischemic heart disease
  B. Left ventricular failure
  C. Valvular insufficiency
  D. Dysrhythmias
  E. Hypertension
III. Vascular
  A. Pulmonary embolus
  B. Anemia
IV. Metabolic
  A. Hypokalemia
  B. Hypocalcemia
  C. Hypophosphatemia
  D. Hypomagnesemia
V. Drugs
  A. Beta blockers
  B. Cholinergic agents
  C. Prostaglandin inhibitors
  D. CNS depressants
VI. Anatomic
  A. Pneumothorax
  B. Rib fracture
  C. Pleural effusion
  D. Ascites
VII. Miscellaneous
  A. Recent surgery
  B. Noncompliance
  C. Total parenteral nutrition

often uncooperative COPD patient. In addition, even small and seemingly insignificant improvements in pulmonary function may be associated with a marked subjective improvement in dyspnea if a patient has poor baseline parameters.

Digital pulse oximeters are being used increasingly in the emergency department (ED) to monitor arterial oxygen saturation. They are easy to set up, calibrate, and read. Although these devices are accurate under steady-state conditions, little has been done to determine their accuracy in detecting dynamic changes in oxygen saturation.[12] In addition, multiple factors (carboxyhemoglobin, motion, low perfusion states) may affect the accuracy of these devices. Currently there is little to suggest that these devices alter mortality and morbidity in COPD patients and their exact role in the monitoring of COPD patients remains to be defined.

Arterial blood gas (ABG) measurements are the gold standard in defining and quantifying oxygenation and ventilation in COPD patients. If patients have no complicating metabolic abnormalities, ABGs are interpreted with relative ease. For the purposes of this chapter, the emergency physician needs to understand the ABG patterns of hypoxemia, oxygen desaturation, acute ventilatory failure, chronic ventilatory failure, and *acute on chronic* ventilatory failure. The reader must be conversant with ABG interpretation. However, even ABG determinations have their limitations: they are painful to the patient and sometimes difficult to obtain (multiple sequential determinations require an indwelling arterial catheter); the clinical status of the patient may change faster than the laboratory turnaround time; and ABGs must be considered in the context of the entire clinical situation. *ABG values alone cannot be used as a criterion for endotracheal intubation!* Indeed, some clinicians suggest the decision to intubate patients with COPD should be made on clinical criteria alone.[2, 13]

All patients with severe exacerbation of COPD and the possibility of hospital admission should have a complete blood count, electrolyte profile, and (where appropriate) a theophylline level determined, as hematologic and metabolic derangements may precipitate or contribute to deteriorations in pulmonary function. A chest radiograph should likewise be obtained to determine if pneumonitis, pneumothorax, or alveolar edema is present. Electrocardiography may indicate acute ischemia precipitating or associated with a COPD exacerbation.

GENERAL TREATMENT: GOALS AND METHODS

The treatment goals in patients with COPD in exacerbation are improved oxygenation, decreased expiratory obstruction, and detection and correction of factors responsible for acute declines from baseline pulmonary function. Although abnormalities in airflow, the possibility of aspiration, and changes in ventilation and oxygenation each require specific attention, their relative importance may differ in individual patients. There are, however, several treatment modalities which must be addressed in all patients with COPD exacerbations.

Oxygen should be administered to all hypoxemic COPD patients. As well as increasing tissue oxygenation, other salutary effects are realized. Raising the partial pressure of oxygen (PO_2) in severely hypoxemic patients to 50 to 60 mm Hg reduces pulmonary artery vasoconstriction and pulmonary hyperten-

sion[14]; this relieves the right heart strain of cor pulmonale and increases flow through the pulmonary vascular bed. Left ventricular and respiratory muscle function are also improved by increasing tissue oxygenation.

Despite the beneficial effect of O_2 administration to the hypercapnic and hypoxemic COPD patient in exacerbation, physicians are frequently reluctant to administer O_2 for fear that O_2 may suppress respiratory drive, increasing the partial pressure of carbon dioxide (PCO_2), thus worsening ventilatory acidosis and possibly resulting in a need for mechanical ventilation. The common explanation for this phenomenon is that the medullary chemoreceptors of patients with chronic CO_2 retention are insensitive to further increases in PCO_2 owing to increased bicarbonate levels surrounding these receptors.[4] These patients have been thought to depend upon their hypoxemic drive for ventilation and that suppression of this drive will occur if excess O_2 is administered. It appears, however, that the phenomenon of O_2-induced hypercapnia is not as great and yet more complex than previously thought. Aubier et al.[15] found that administration of 100% O_2 to patients with COPD in acute respiratory failure resulted in an average increase of the PCO_2 of 23 mm Hg. Yet, despite this major increase, minute ventilation fell by only 7% (not enough to account for the total increase in PCO_2). Other investigations have yielded similar results.[16, 17] Further studies have shown that other mechanisms accounting for the increase in PCO_2 include a mild depression of minute ventilation, a change of the binding of CO_2 to hemoglobin (Haldane effect), and most important, changing $\dot{V}/\dot{Q}$ relationships which effectively increase dead space ventilation.[15–17]

The goal of O_2 therapy is to produce adequate tissue oxygenation by providing an arterial O_2 saturation of 90%; adjusting the inspired O_2 concentration just high enough to achieve a PO_2 of 50 to 60 mm Hg will yield this result. Nothing is gained by raising the inspired O_2 concentration to higher levels since O_2 content is little changed and there is a risk of significant hypercapnia.

Bronchodilators are the mainstay of treatment for bronchospasm. Currently recommended agents include β_2-specific agonists, aminophylline, and anticholinergics. β_2-Agonists are preferred over nonselective β-agonists since they have less cardiovascular side effects. Nebulization further minimizes these side effects as it allows delivery directly to the target organ. Oxygen-powered nebulizing devices are commonplace as these devices require no hand-breathing coordination (as contrasted to metered dose inhalers). Terbutaline is a β_2-agonist which may be administered subcutaneously if there is poor delivery of nebulized agents due to extreme bronchospasm or lack of appropriate equipment. Although the mechanism of action of theophylline is currently debated, it remains useful in bronchodilator therapy. Full therapeutic levels should be achieved intravenously once the baseline blood level has been ascertained. Anticholinergics have been shown to be beneficial in COPD patients. The most potent, ipratropium bromide, is currently only available in metered dose inhaler form. Alternatively, atropine (2–3 mg) may be administered by nebulization.

Corticosteroid use in COPD is beneficial.[18] Intravenous administration is indicated for most patients with exacerbations of COPD.

Finally, a search for, and appropriate treatment of, factors responsible for aggravating or precipitating exacerbations complete the general approach for these patients (see Table 29–1). Most important are those factors which can be reversed in the ED (e.g., bronchospasm, hypokalemia, left ventricular failure) or which must not be missed (e.g., pneumothorax, pulmonary embolus).

An algorithm for airway management of the patient with COPD in exacerbation is presented in Figure 29–1.

Scenario 1: The Stable Patient With COPD in Exacerbation (Respiratory Insufficiency)

This patient complains of worsening of chronic respiratory complaints, but is not in any immediate danger. The patient is alert and orientated and is generally able to speak in short sentences or long phrases. Most important though, is that his *ventilatory status is stable* and acute ventilatory failure is not present. Chronic ventilatory failure may be present, but it is generally of only mild degree (pH normal, PCO_2 usually not greater than 50–55 mm Hg). Hypoxemia, however, is usually more pronounced than baseline status.

Although ventilatory status is essentially stable and near baseline, the patient is clearly not baseline clinically; he or she has, after all, sought care for an acute exacerbation of some respiratory complaint. In this particular patient, time permits (and demands) a thorough evaluation. Especially useful are the following general screening questions: What percent of your baseline are you at now? In what way are you worse than usual? (Short of breath? Increased sputum? Increased wheezing? Fever?,

etc.). Further clinical evaluation should be directed specifically toward ruling in or out specific aggravating or precipitating factors (see Table 29–1). Also, specific information should be sought from the old chart or regular physician about ABG values during acute episodes of decompensation and during stability as well as the need for previous mechanical ventilation.

If the patient has only mild COPD, never has been intubated, rarely has been hospitalized, is without cor pulmonale, and without evidence of either chronic or acute ventilatory failure, he or she may not require intensive therapy or hospital admission. If, however, some of these factors do pertain, the patient must be thoroughly evaluated (as outlined under Assessment) and treated.

Treatment

Emergency physicians are often frustrated by their inability to effect dramatic improvement in the stable COPD patient. Indeed, it is true that only the acute portions of the patient's deterioration can be reversed in the ED. For practical purposes, these portions are most commonly hypoxemia and bronchospasm.

Mild hypoxemia that is baseline for the patient and which approaches normal arterial O_2 saturation may not require specific treatment. Otherwise, O_2 should be given as a matter of routine. It is preferable to draw a baseline ABG sample prior to O_2 administration so that the baseline level of hypoxemia can be ascertained. The stable patient needs only a modest increase in inspired O_2 concentration to approximate full arterial O_2 concentration. Oxygen delivery at 2 to 3 L/min via nasal cannula usually suffices. Although a Venturi mask delivers more predictable percentages of inspired concentration, the stable patient does not need such precision. In addition, the Venturi mask uses considerable amounts of O_2, is not well accepted by patients, is expensive, and is ill suited for chronic use. The physician should avoid high-flow oxygen (>3 L/min) until it is clear that respiratory drive is unlikely to be suppressed. It is easy to overlook the fact that O_2-powered (as opposed to motor-powered) nebulization has this potential hazard.

Bronchospasm is the only cause of lower airway obstruction that can be improved over short ED time frames. Full dosing with inhaled β-agonists and anticholinergics should be instituted as needed. Inhaled β-agonist therapy may be required as frequently as every 1 to 2 hours depending on patient response. Therapeutic blood levels of theophylline should be

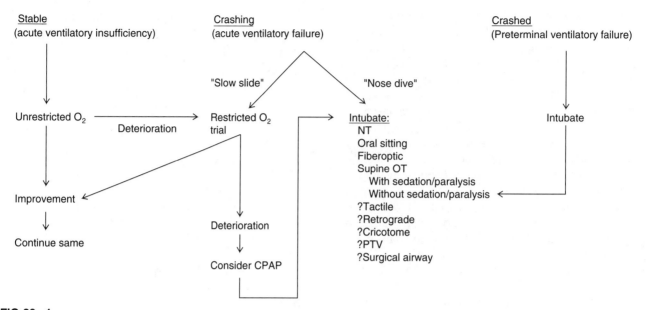

FIG 29–1.
Algorithm for airway management in the patient with COPD in exacerbation. *CPAP* = continuous positive airway pressure; *NT* = nasotracheal; *OR* = orotracheal; *PTV* = percutaneous transtracheal ventilation.

attained intravenously. Corticosteroids may also be indicated.

Scenario 2: The Crashing Patient With COPD in Exacerbation (Acute Ventilatory Failure)

This patient is clearly in major respiratory distress. He or she may be alert and orientated but may also be lethargic, irritable, or have other subtle mental status changes such as irrationality, uncooperativeness, or mild confusion. The patient may be anxious and diaphoretic and usually speaks in short phrases or monosyllables. Profound dyspnea, tachypnea, and tachycardia are noted. Labored breathing is clearly evidenced by accessory muscle use and there may be evidence of respiratory fatigue as well. Instability is revealed by ABGs which demonstrate acute ventilatory failure (i.e., elevated PCO_2 with a corresponding lowered pH). Usually (but not universally), chronic ventilatory failure preexists as shown by an elevated bicarbonate level. Severe hypoxemia is present ($PO_2 < 50-55$ mm Hg) resulting in marked arterial O_2 desaturation.

Airflow obstruction is usually associated with some degree of bronchospasm and often with poorly cleared bronchial secretions. Increased levels of patient-generated intrinsic PEEP also impair inspiratory flow. Respiratory effort cannot match ventilatory demands, heralding possible respiratory collapse.

Treatment

Adequate ventilation and oxygenation are the principal therapeutic objectives. Most crashing pa-

tients will tolerate a "trial of oxygen." After baseline ABG samples have been drawn, low O_2 (1–2 L/min by nasal cannula or 24% Venturi mask) is administered and the clinical status (respiratory effort, mental status, and ABG values) is closely followed. Aggressive bronchodilator therapy is concurrently administered. If hypoxemia is satisfactorily improved (to a level of approximately 50 mm Hg) and adequate respiratory effort is noted, the patient "passes the test": he does not need artificial ventilatory support. If, however, there is respiratory deterioration, two alternatives may be considered.

If deterioration is minimal and the patient maintains his or her ability to cooperate and can tolerate a tightly fitting mask, noninvasive positive pressure ventilation techniques may be attempted. These techniques utilize a tight-fitting face mask attached to a ventilator or a positive pressure assistance device[19, 20] to provide positive airway pressure during inspiration only (note this is not continuous positive airway pressure [CPAP]). This method of noninvasive ventilation reduces the work of the inspiratory muscles by mechanically providing the pressure required to overcome intrinsic PEEP. Although only a small number of patients have been studied, increases in PO_2 and pH and decreases in PCO_2 have been observed and the need for tracheal intubation obviated. It remains to be seen whether noninvasive face mask ventilation will become a practical alternative to intubation in the crashing COPD patient.

If clinical deterioration occurs during low-flow O_2 therapy or noninvasive face mask ventilation, endotracheal intubation and mechanical ventilation become mandatory. One must not equivocate or tarry at this critical juncture! Intubating a critically ill, often uncooperative COPD patient leaves little room for error. It is daunting to even the most experienced clinician, but failure to do so places the patient's life in immediate jeopardy. There is a perception that endotracheal intubation should be a last-ditch measure in the COPD patient because of the difficulty in weaning these patients from mechanical ventilation. However, a recent report revealed that over three fourths of such patients could be successfully weaned even after 2 weeks of mechanical ventilation.[21]

Intubation of the Crashing COPD Patient

Intubation of the crashing COPD patient requires the ultimate sophistication in clinical judgment and skills. There are two general approaches taken, depending upon the rapidity and degree of the patient's deterioration. The patient who has deteriorated over hours or fails to improve in the ED after intensive medical therapy is in a "slow slide." Very careful continuous ED bedside clinical and ABG monitoring are necessary before a decision to intubate is made. A different approach is needed for the patient who arrives clearly needing intubation or who deteriorated acutely over a period of minutes; he is in a "nose dive." This patient requires immediate successful intubation.

The slow-slide patient should be intubated before needing crash intubation, so that the procedure can be carried out in a planned, structured, and orderly fashion. The procedure may be performed in several ways, but an upright body position is preferred because ventilatory function is optimal, the risk of aspiration is diminished, and because the patient will actively fight recumbency. Three alternatives may be considered. The most commonly used method is blind nasotracheal intubation. A no. 8 tube should be used to allow adequate suctioning and minimize airflow resistance. This procedure is familiar to most emergency physicians, can be done quickly, and is well tolerated by the patient if careful instructions and good topical analgesia are provided. Also, sedation (which will further diminish ventilation) is not necessary. Once placed, the tube is stable, well tolerated, and allows the patient oral alimentation. Unfortunately, long-term use results in a high incidence of sinusitis.

A second method of upright intubation is sitting oral intubation (see Chapter 6). This procedure has only recently been described in the emergency medicine literature[22] and few physicians are familiar with it. However, it differs little from traditional recumbent orotracheal intubation, so that theoretically most acute care physicians should gain proficiency quickly. It has the advantages of blind nasotracheal intubation without its disadvantages. The cords are directly visualized, topical nasal analgesia is unnecessary, and sinusitis does not occur. Certainly, this procedure should be tried more often, and there is every reason to believe that it will find an important place in the management of patients requiring sitting intubation.

A third technique to be considered in the slow-slide patient is fiberoptic assisted intubation (see Chapter 12). This elegant technique is often appropriate, but usually time-consuming. Also, it takes considerable experience to gain proficiency, and few physicians are fluent in its use.

The nose-dive patient, who requires near-crash intubation, is still more difficult to handle. He is gasping, and—most important—uncooperative. This patient is the true test! If time permits and the patient is sufficiently fatigued and unable to fight the procedure, blind nasotracheal or sitting orotracheal intubation may be quickly tried. However, if he can and does fight intubation, sedation or paralysis, or both, will be necessary. There is an intrinsic conflict in this situation: sedation or paralysis makes intubation possible but also renders the patient's respirations ineffective. The answer is found in accepting the undesirable hypoventilation for only the brief moments necessary for rapid successful intubation. Often, intravenous sedation alone (without paralysis) is sufficient.

A number of sedative-hypnotic agents have been used with success. Rapid-acting barbiturates (e.g., methohexital) provide excellent sedation but little muscle relaxation. Benzodiazepines (e.g., midazolam, lorazepam) provide both sedation and muscle relaxation of variable duration. Morphine may result in histamine release and increased bronchospasm but has been used with success for many years. Droperidol and ketamine have bronchodilator as well as sedative properties. Any of these agents are effective sedatives and the emergency physician should be familiar with one or two of them for use in daily clinical practice.

If it is felt that successful intubation may not be achievable with sedation alone, paralysis should be induced in concert with sedation. Succinylcholine is a rapid-acting and effective short-term paralyzing agent (see the discussion of rapid-sequence intubation in Chapter 14). Vecuronium, an analogue of pancuronium but lacking cardiovascular side effects, is another option.

Once adequate paralysis or sedation has been achieved, artificial ventilation must be provided. Temporary use of bag-mask ventilation may not be effective in this situation as tight fit of the mask may be impaired by secretions, and adequate ventilation may be thwarted by airflow obstruction and decreased pulmonary compliance. Thus, definitive endotracheal intubation is mandatory as soon as possible. One must be prepared for a difficult intubation in the crashing COPD patient. The "bull neck" so often found includes a short and muscular neck, stiff osteoarthritic cervical spine, small mouth, and large tongue.

If the sedated or paralyzed nose-dive patient cannot be intubated successfully, the options narrow. Lighted or tactile intubation can be quickly attempted. The retrograde transtracheal technique can actually be performed surprisingly quickly by the experienced operator. Percutaneous transtracheal ventilation might be considered, but without a tracheal cuff aspiration cannot be avoided and adequate ventilation would be difficult to achieve. The Pertrach cricotome could be considered because of its speed of use, but only if the operator had previous experience with it. Finally, the much-discussed but seldom performed surgical airways from below (cricothyrotomy and tracheostomy) have to be entertained. Unfortunately, once other means have failed in this iatrogenically apneic patient, only a rapid successful airway from below can save the patient. However, the success rate under these circumstances is exceedingly small (especially in the bull-neck patient) and the complications fearsome (pneumothorax, massive hemorrhage, subcutaneous emphysema, etc.). It is obvious that patient care will be most benefited if the physician is totally expert in orotracheal intubation techniques rather than partially competent in seldom utilized surgical airway techniques.

Scenario 3: The Crashed Patient With COPD in Exacerbation (Terminal Acute Ventilatory Failure Superimposed on Chronic Ventilatory Failure)

At a glance it is clear that this patient is moribund and that without immediate intubation will die within a period of minutes. Respirations are ineffective: at best they are paradoxical (thoracoabdominal) or alternans in character; at worst they are gasping or agonal. The patient is stuporous, unaware of his surroundings, and unable to respond intelligibly. He is cyanotic and diaphoretic. If bradycardia and hypotension are observed, cardiopulmonary arrest is imminent. ABG measurements show severe hypoxemia and hypercapnia (values will depend on whether O_2 is being administered and in what concentration); resultant ventilatory acidosis will be severe. A metabolic acidosis is also likely due to anaerobic metabolism and cardiovascular collapse.

All three pillars of the airway are in jeopardy, and for the first time, aspiration is a real threat; if emesis occurs, this patient's airway is unguarded due to diminished mental status.

Treatment

Treatment requires little thought and much action. Ideally, the patient should receive preoxygenation and ventilation with bag-mask and 100% O_2. *Endotracheal intubation must be accomplished immediately!* These patients do not need sedation or paralysis; if they did, they would conform to the description of the crashing patient. Rapid orotracheal intubation in recumbency is the technique of choice. All other choices are more time-consuming, and in this patient *there is no time*. Blind nasotracheal intubation is not appropriate as there is not enough airflow to guide tube directioning and one cannot be guaranteed success since the procedure is performed blindly. A Sellick manuever is absolutely essential: any aspiration in this patient would be fatal. Once intubated, several rapid and forceful ventilations with the bag should be performed, expanding collapsed alveoli and loosening secretions, followed by vigorous suctioning. This cycle should be repeated several times in the first few minutes after intubation and before the endotracheal tube is connected to the ventilator. Sedation with or without paralysis should not be necessary in the immediate postintubation period because the patient is too weak and lethargic to fight the ventilator, but it may become necessary as the patient revives.

If several attempts at orotracheal intubation fail, the alternatives mentioned above for the crashing patient must then be entertained. Those requiring the least time and equipment (e.g., tactile intubation) are obviously the most appropriate under these extreme circumstances. One must carefully monitor ABGs following institution of mechanical ventilation; the objective should be normalization of the pH, not PCO_2. Overventilation to normalize the PCO_2 in any patient with chronic ventilatory failure will result in alkalosis and risks serious dysrhythmias.

Pharmacologic therapy must not be neglected once the patient is being ventilated. In-line nebulized β-agonists and anticholinergics should be administered. Terbutaline can be given subcutaneously. Intravenous corticosteroids should be administered.

These patients have acute cor pulmonale and may have concomitant left ventricular failure. They are subject to a wide variety of both ventricular and atrial ectopic rhythms. Pharmacologic therapy for these rhythms should be undertaken only if serious hypotension or malignant ventricular rhythms are not rapidly reversed by mechanical ventilation and proper oxygenation.

PREHOSPITAL CONSIDERATIONS

Education of prehospital personnel must emphasize the clinical characteristics of the stable, crashing, and crashed patient with COPD so that appropriate decisions pertaining to airway support may be made. Important historical data to be obtained by emergency medical personnel include chronic medications, use of home O_2, and the need for previous intubation and mechanical ventilation. Unfortunately, therapeutic prehospital options are limited. The stable patient with COPD should be treated with 1 to 2 Liters of O_2 by nasal cannula or 24% to 28% O_2 by Venturi mask. Cardiac monitoring is necessary. Subcutaneous terbutaline may be administered at the scene or en route to the hospital. Some emergency medical systems can provide delivery of nebulized bronchodilators en route and if available, their use is encouraged. Prehospital use of metered-dose inhaler bronchodilators should be considered if nebulized agents are not available. Although aminophylline has long been a standard bronchodilator administered in the field, time should not be wasted on the scene attempting to achieve intravenous access, preparing medication, and attempting to achieve a controlled infusion as more effective and rapidly acting bronchodilators (i.e. β2-agonists) are available. Immediate and rapid transport to the ED where multiagent therapy is available is of greatest benefit to these patients.

The crashing patient presents a dilemma. Patients with COPD in respiratory distress who remain awake and alert should be treated at the scene and en route with O_2, subcutaneous terbutaline, and inhaled bronchodilators (if available) and transported rapidly to the ED. The decision to intubate should be made in conjunction with medical control. Potential indications for intubation include progressive somnolence, hypotension, and prolonged transport times. Should intubation be necessary but unsuccessful, repeated attempts should not be made; rather bag-valve-mask ventilation with 100% O_2 should be instituted along with rapid transport to the ED.

The crashed patient requires immediate endotracheal intubation. If endotracheal intubation cannot be accomplished, support with 100% O_2 and bag-valve-mask ventilation should be instituted. If possible, intravenous fluid should be administered en route to treat hypotension. Rapid transport to the ED is mandatory.

REFERENCES

1. Snider GL, Kleinerman J, Thurlbeck WM, et al: The definition of emphysema: Report of a National Heart, Lung, and Blood Institute, Division of Lung Diseases workshop. *Am Rev Respir Dis* 1985; 132:182–185.
2. Schmidt GA, Hall JB: Acute on chronic respiratory failure. *JAMA* 1989; 261:3444–3453.
3. Hall J, Keamy MF: Artificial airways in the critically ill patient. *Pulmonary Crit Care Update* 1986; 2:2–8.
4. Weinberger SE, Schwartzstein RM, Weiss JW: Hypercapnia. *N Engl J Med* 1989; 321:1223–1231.
5. Sharp JT, Drutz WS, Moisan T, et al: Postural relief of dyspnea in severe chronic obstructive pulmonary disease. *Am Rev Respir Dis* 1980; 122:201–211.
6. Browning IB, D'Alonzo GE, Tobin MJ: Importance of respiratory rate as an indicator of respiratory dysfunction in patients with cystic fibrosis. *Chest* 1990; 97:1317–1321.
7. Gravelyn TR, Weg JR: Respiratory rate as an indicator of acute respiratory dysfunction. *JAMA* 1980; 284:1123–1125.
8. Tobin MJ, Perez W, Guenther SM, et al: Does rib cage–abdominal paradox signify respiratory muscle fatigue? *J Appl Physiol* 1987; 63:851–860.
9. Roussos C, Fixley M, Gross D, et al: Fatigue of inspiratory muscles and their synergistic behaviour. *J Appl Physiol* 1979; 46:897–904.
10. Cohen CA, Zagelbaum G, Gross D, et al: Clinical manifestations of inspiratory muscle fatigue. *Am J Med* 1982; 73:308–316.
11. Nowak RM, Tomlanovich MC, Sarker DD, et al: Arterial blood gases and pulmonary function testing in acute bronchial asthma; predicting patient outcomes. *JAMA* 1983; 249:2043–2046.
12. Tobin MJ: Respiratory monitoring. *JAMA* 1990; 264:244–251.
13. Bone RC, Pierce AK, Johnson RL: Controlled oxygen administration in acute respiratory failure in chronic obstructive pulmonary disease. *Am J Med* 1978; 65:896–902.
14. Francis PB: Acute respiratory failure in obstructive lung disease. *Med Clin North Am* 1983; 67:657–668.

15. Aubier M, Murciano D, Fournier M, et al: Effects of the administration of O_2 on ventilation and blood gases in patients with chronic obstructive pulmonary disease during acute respiratory failure. *Am Rev Respir Dis* 1980; 122:747–754.
16. Aubier M, Murciano D, Fournier M, et al: Central respiratory drive in acute respiratory failure of patients with chronic obstructive pulmonary disease. *Am Rev Respir Dis* 1980; 122:191–199.
17. Sassoon CS, Hassel KT, Mahutte CK: Hyperoxic-induced hypercapnia in stable chronic obstructive pulmonary disease. *Am Rev Respir Dis* 1987; 135:907–911.
18. Hudson LD, Monti CM: Rationale and use of corticosteroids in chronic obstructive pulmonary disease. *Med Clin North Am* 1990; 74:661–690.
19. Meduri GU, Conoscenti CC, Menashe P, et al: Non-invasive face mask ventilation in patients with acute respiratory failure. *Chest* 1990; 95:865–870.
20. Brochard L, Isabey D, Piquet J, et al: Reversal of acute exacerbations of chronic obstructive lung disease by inspiratory assistance with a face mask. *N Engl J Med* 1990; 323:1523–1530.
21. Menzies R, Gibbons W, Goldberg P: Determinants of weaning and survival among patients with COPD who require mechanical ventilation for acute respiratory failure. *Chest* 1989; 95; 398–405.
22. Fontanarosa PB, Goldman GE, Polsky SS, et al: Sitting oral-tracheal intubation. *Ann Emerg Med* 1988; 17:336–338.

30

White-out Lung

Jon Jui, M.D.

Robert H. Dailey, M.D.

The assessment and management of a patient with acute respiratory failure presenting with a "white-out" lung (WOL) presents a major challenge to the emergency physician. These patients are often "crashing" or "crashed" and require acute intervention, often before an adequate history or complete physical examination can be performed. The unifying concept of this chapter is the presence of the white-out lung, i.e., lung opacification upon radiography.

Multiple etiologies have been associated with WOL. The most common causes are listed in Table 30–1. Some may be subacute or even chronic, but all either displace, compress, infiltrate, or obliterate pulmonary parenchyma. For practical purposes our discussion is focused primarily on the adult respiratory distress syndrome (ARDS).

ARDS is an acute, severe disorder characterized by diffuse pulmonary infiltrates on chest radiography (Fig 30–1), hypoxemia resistant to oxygen therapy, normal left atrial pressures, and stiff, poorly compliant lungs. (Table 30–2 lists the diagnostic criteria for the diagnosis of ARDS.) The common underlying pathophysiology is an abnormal permeability of the air-blood barrier (the alveolar-capillary membrane). Water rich in plasma constituents escapes the intravascular space into the interstitial space; this fluid then crosses the alveolar epithelium into the alveolar space. Massive shunting also occurs.

The four major causes of lung injury are: (1) direct injury (e.g., toxin inhalation, aspiration of gastric contents), (2) neutrophil-mediated injury (e.g., oxygen free radicals, proteases, platelet activity factor, activated complement, tumor necrosis factor, etc.), (3) arachidonic acid metabolite injury (e.g., prostaglandins, thromboxanes, and leukotrienes), and (4) coagulation product injury (e.g., fibrin degradation products secondary to disseminated intravascular coagulation) (DIC).[1]

ARDS may be thought of as occurring in four stages. This characterization is somewhat artificial owing to the enormous individual variation in clinical expression of this syndrome. *Acute injury* is the first stage. During this phase there may be no symptoms specifically related to the lungs or ARDS. Results of chest auscultation and the chest film are normal unless the primary injury is to the lungs. The *latent period* immediately follows acute injury and lasts about 6 to 48 hours. The only clinical sign may be hyperventilation. The chest film may show fine reticular markings consistent with interstitial fluid. The third stage is *respiratory failure*. These patients require respiratory support (intubation and mechanical ventilation). The *final* or *terminal* stage is that of severe and usually irreversible pulmonary pathologic changes that are incompatible with life.[2]

CLINICAL EVALUATION OF THE PATIENT WITH WHITE-OUT LUNG

These patients are so clearly sick that their evaluation is nearly self-evident. All four vital signs must be taken initially! Particular care must be taken to obtain the patient's temperature; even though the patient is sitting, a core body temperature measurement (rectal, tympanic membrane) is preferable, since mouth breathing will give a falsely low reading. The clinical status of these patients is inherently unstable, so vital signs should be repeated frequently;

TABLE 30–1.

Causes of White-out Lung

1. Adult respiratory distress syndrome (ARDS)
2. Cardiac pulmonary edema
3. Subacute or chronic pulmonary infiltration or fibrosis of diverse cause
4. Massive pleural effusions
5. Tumor masses
6. Acute intrapulmonary hemorrhage
7. Massive atelectasis
8. Miscellaneous others

TABLE 30–2.

Diagnostic Criteria for Adult Respiratory Distress Syndrome* (ARDS)

Clinical
    Acute onset of respiratory distress in a patient with a predisposing condition
Radiographic
    Diffuse infiltrates on chest film
Physiologic
    PaO_2 <50 mm Hg with an FiO_2 >60%
    Total respiratory compliance <50 mL/cm H_2O
    Normal left atrial pressure (PCWP ≤12 mm Hg)

*PaO_2 = arterial oxygen partial pressure; FiO_2 = fractional concentration of oxygen in inspired gas; PCWP = pulmonary capillary wedge pressure.

an automatic pulse and blood pressure–taking device (Dynamap) is an excellent aid. Slowing of the respiratory and pulse rates may indicate either improvement or deterioration. It is ominous if associated with exhaustion, profuse diaphoresis, or clouding of consciousness; these are the classic signs of acute ventilatory failure. The temperature should be repeated if normal initially; fever or hypothermia are such important signs of sepsis that one cannot afford to miss them. The presence or absence of rales and wheezes is helpful diagnostically; if intense wheezing is present, bronchodilators offer a much-needed therapeutic weapon.

Ancillary studies include a complete blood count

(CBC), arterial blood gas (ABG) analysis, pulse oximetry, sputum Gram's stain and culture, chest radiograph, three sets of blood cultures, and an electrocardiogram (ECG). Pulse oximetry is particularly useful in WOL: hypoxemia is usually severe, and therefore the steep slope of the oxygen-hemoglobin dissociation curve pertains, so that O_2 saturation changes significantly with only small changes in arterial oxygen partial pressure (PaO_2). ABGs are necessary to monitor the adequacy of alveolar ventilation (through assessment of the carbon dioxide tension

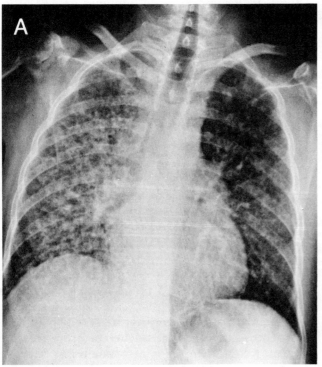
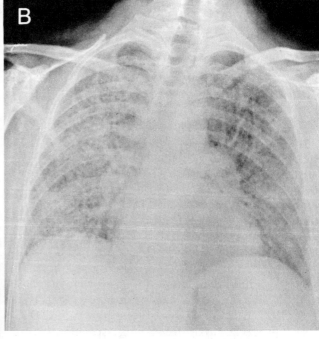

FIG 30–1.
Pneumocystis carinii pneumonia in a hemophiliac patient with AIDS shows progression to involve all parts of both lungs. **A** and **B,** the two views were obtained 5 days apart. (From Armstrong P, Dee P: Infections of the lungs and pleura, in Armstrong P, Wilson AG, Dee P (eds): *Imaging of Diseases of the Chest.* St Louis, Mosby–Year Book, Inc, 1990, p 237. Used by permission.)

[PaCO$_2$]). Although standard posteroanterior (PA) and lateral chest films are desirable, the patient's condition often necessitates a portable film. Every attempt should be made to obtain a sputum specimen. If the specimen is grossly purulent, or upon Gram's stain has many white blood cells (WBCs) and few epithelial cells, the significance of bacteria seen is much enhanced. Blood cultures are mandatory in all cases of WOL to rule out a primary or associated septic process. Gram's stains and cultures of urine, skin lesions, or other possible foci of infection should also be performed as clinically appropriate. A diligent search must be made for occult abscesses, especially within the abdomen.

DIFFERENTIAL DIAGNOSIS

After the above evaluation has been initiated, and once oxygen therapy has been administered (see below), an orderly differential diagnosis should be pursued (see Table 30–1 and Fig 30–2). Usually it

is clear by even a portable chest film whether some process other than ARDS is producing WOL e.g., massive pleural effusions, chronic infiltrative disease, large tumor masses, etc. Once these abnormalities have been ruled out, one must exclude left ventricular failure as either a primary or contributing abnormality. This is often impossible upon initial emergency department (ED) evaluation, and it may require assessment of pulmonary capillary wedge pressure by means of a pulmonary artery catheter. If there is any reasonable suspicion of left ventricular failure, specific therapy should be instituted since the benefits of such therapy outweigh the risks.

Next the multiple agents causing ARDS must be weighed and sifted (Table 30–3). They are often classified by the manner in which they act: (1) those acting primarily on the airway, (2) those acting directly upon the pulmonary vasculature, and (3) those acting directly upon the lung (Table 30–4). Some are self-evident, such as near-drowning, inhalation injury, and high-altitude pulmonary edema. But, more commonly, the cause will not be immedi-

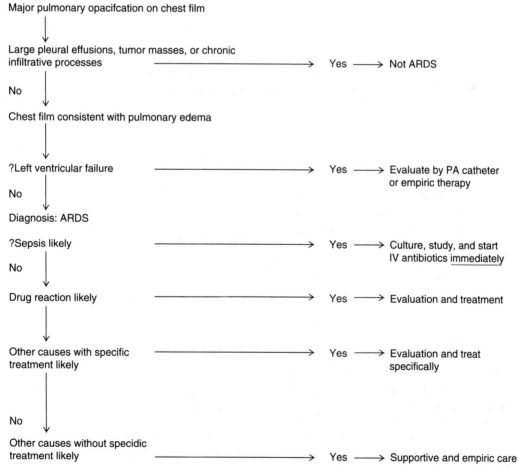

FIG 30–2.
Clinical algorithm for assessment of white-out lung.

TABLE 30–3.

Causes of Adult Respiratory Distress Syndrome (ARDS) in the Emergency Department (ED)*

Airway source
  †Aspiration of gastric contents
  †Near-drowning
  †Diffuse infectious pneumonia
  Smoke inhalation injury
  Irritant gas inhalation
  O_2 toxicity
Vascular route
  †Sepsis
  †Trauma
  †Drug overdose (e.g., aspirin, opiates)
  †Head injury
  Fat embolism
  Pancreatitis
  †Shock
  Toxic shock syndrome
  Surface burns
  †Drug idiosyncratic reaction
  Thrombotic thrombocytopenia
  Leukemia
  Venous air embolism
  Amniotic fluid embolism
  Uremia
  Diabetic ketoacidosis
  †Disseminated intravascular coagulation
  High-altitude pulmonary edema
Direct or physical injury
  †Lung contusion
  Radiation
  Hanging

*Adapted from Tobin MJ: *Essentials of Critical Care Medicine.* New York, Churchill Livingston Inc, 1989, p 172.
†Conditions most common in the ED.

ately apparent. Pneumonia is probably the most common cause of WOL, both in the nonimmunocompromised patient (NICP) and the immunocompromised patient (ICP).[3, 4] Often the clinical picture is confusing—dominated by acute respiratory failure and septic shock instead of cough, fever, and modest pulmonary infiltration. Fever may be absent or missed (the temperature is frequently not taken because of severe respiratory distress). There may be leukopenia instead of leukocytosis. The differential count must be carefully examined for immature granulocytes, toxic granulation, and Döhle's bodies. Unfortunately, neither the absolute WBC or differential count reliably differentiates between viral and bacterial pneumonia, nor do other clinical features. One must be alert today for the possibility of underlying human immunodeficiency virus (HIV) infection or other immunocompromising conditions! Antibiotics must be initiated intravenously (IV) in the emergency department (ED) as soon as blood and sputum (if available) cultures have been obtained!

Pulmonary aspiration of gastric contents is also a very common cause of ARDS. Unfortunately, it is rarely directly observed, and there is no specific diagnostic test. Diagnosis rests upon a high index of suspicion in the susceptible patient (obtundation, poor protective airway reflexes, factors promoting emesis or regurgitation, etc.; see Chapter 2). The clinical picture of sudden dyspnea, tachypnea, shock, and lower lobe infiltrations in the above setting is highly suggestive.

Drugs can produce a wide variety of pulmonary insults (see Table 30–4). Three syndromes are associated with pulmonary opacification. (1) *Drug-induced pneumonitis* presents with insidious onset of nonproductive cough, dyspnea, and fever without chills. The chest film shows a gradual increase of alveolar-interstitial markings, but pleural effusions are rare. (2) *Hypersensitivity* to particular drugs may present with a subacute onset of dyspnea, nonproductive cough, chills, myalgias, and headache. The chest film reveals variable infiltrates and sometimes pleural effusions. Fever, skin rash, and eosinophilia are often present. (3) *Drug-induced pulmonary edema* is an acute and fulminating process, and not associated with the other findings of hypersensitivity reactions. It is most often associated with aspirin or opiate overdoses, and is commonly seen in the practice of emergency medicine[5] (Fig 30–3). Many severe illnesses of diverse etiology can cause ARDS: pancreatitis, dia-

TABLE 30–4.

Agents That Cause Pulmonary Disease

Amiodarone
Amphotericin
Nitrofurantoin
†Heroin
†Methadone
†Propoxyphene
†Aspirin
*Terbutaline
 Gold salts
 Penicillamine
 Hydrochlorothiazide
*Dilantin
*Carbamazepine
 Tocainide
*Lidocaine
*Haloperidol
 Chlordiazepoxide
 Ethchlorvynol
 Imipramine
*Penicillin
 Cancer chemotherapeutic agents
 Paraquat

*Most common.
†Most common causes of emergency department acute pulmonary edema.

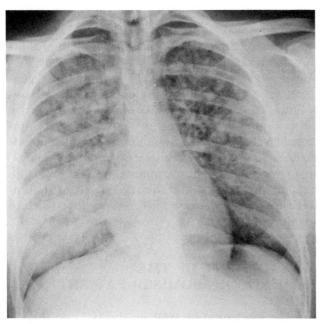

FIG 30–3.
Pulmonary edema due to acute severe laryngospasm following general anesthesia for a meniscectomy. (From Armstrong P: Pulmonary vascular diseases and pulmonary edema, in Armstrong P, Wilson AG, Dee P (eds): *Imaging of Diseases of the Chest.* St Louis, Mosby–Year Book, Inc, 1990, p 395. Used by permission.)

betic ketoacidosis (DKA), uremia, shock, drug overdoses, skin burns, fat embolism, sepsis, and especially any process associated with DIC.

If the ARDS picture cannot be otherwise explained, one must simply search for clues consistent with some of the less common (or even obscure!) causes listed in Table 30–3.

GENERAL TREATMENT CONSIDERATIONS

Unfortunately, there are few specific treatment modalities for WOL. Of course, massive pleural effusions can be drained by thoracentesis, sepsis treated with antibiotics, and opiate or aspirin overdose managed with particular treatment modalities. But treatment is largely supportive and empiric. If no other clear cause for ARDS is apparent, it is wise to assume a drug reaction until proved otherwise, and discontinue previous medications where practicable. Intravenous fluids may be either a curse or a blessing; hypovolemia exacerbates all conditions associated with ARDS, but hypervolemia increases fluid transudation into the pulmonary parenchyma. Central venous pressure (CVP) catheterization may be useful in this circumstance, but a pulmonary ar-

tery catheter is definitive. Considerable controversy exists regarding the use of colloids vs. crystalloids. Since neither has been shown to be superior, cost favors the use of crystalloid.

Diuretics are useful in patients with cardiac failure or gross volume overload, but they cannot otherwise mobilize fluid from the damaged lung. If shock is not corrected by normalization of intravascular volume, pressors such as dopamine should be instituted.

A potential new strategy for improving ventilation in ARDS is inhalation of exogenous surfactant. Although the loss of surfactant is the crucial factor in respiratory distress syndrome of the newborn, it may play an important role in ARDS as well. Currently, pilot clinical trials in adult patients are under way.[6]

Another treatment area involves efforts to control systemic inflammation and thereby reduce the severity or occurrence of ARDS. A number of anti-inflammatory agents have been tried, including corticosteroids, prostaglandin E_1 inhibitors, cyclooxygenase inhibitors, and pentoxifylline. To date, none of these inhibitors have shown a therapeutic benefit compared to conventional supportive therapy. The utility of corticosteroid use in ARDS has been the subject of particular controversy. Sibbald et al.[7] documented a reduction of alveolar-capillary permeability using radiolabeled albumin in 14 of 19 patients with ARDS. Two large, randomized clinical trials have been performed to investigate the utility of steroids in septic shock. Both studies entered patients within 2 hours of shock onset, analyzed only patients with positive blood cultures, and compared the results of early methylprednisolone treatment (30 mg/kg every 6 hours for 24 hours) to placebo. Neither study found that methylprednisolone prevented the development of ARDS or improved the outcome of ARDS.[8, 9] Weigelt et al.[10] evaluated the effect of early methylprednisolone therapy in patients at risk for the development of ARDS. These investigators found that the use of corticosteroids was associated with a significant degree of pulmonary function deterioration as well as a higher incidence of infectious complications.

Prostaglandin E_1 has anti-inflammatory properties and is a potent vasodilator. In a large multicentered study, Bone and colleagues[11] found no improvement in survival between the prostaglandin-treated group and controls, despite significant improvements in cardiac output and O_2 delivery in the prostaglandin-treated group.

The use of specific antibodies against endotoxin

in the setting of sepsis in both animal as well as human studies shows great promise. Two controlled clinical trials have documented the efficacy of monoclonal antibodies against endotoxin in reducing mortality in sepsis and septic shock due to gram-negative bacteria.[12, 13] Commercially available agents have recently been approved for use in the United States. Other measures specific to the particular diagnosis must be considered, e.g., for DIC.

Finally, the emergency physician should admit all WOL patients and consult with a pulmonary or other intensive care specialist as soon as WOL is identified.

OXYGEN THERAPY

Supplemental O_2 is the mainstay of treatment in WOL since all of these patients are, by definition, hypoxemic. Yet even as one administers O_2, one should be thinking physiologically one step further: to O_2-carrying capacity. Thus one must correct the severe anemia early. A rough target hematocrit of 30% is probably appropriate.

Oxygen saturation should be determined before O_2 supplementation is begun. Then a nasal cannula with flows of 5 to 8 L/min should be employed. This provides inspired O_2 concentrations in the range of 35%. If ABGs or pulse oximetry still reveals unsatisfactory O_2 saturations (less than 90%–95%), a nonrebreathing mask should be used. It can achieve inspired oxygen concentrations of 60% to 85% if the mask is tightly fitted. If O_2 saturation is still inadequate, intubation and mechanical ventilation must be undertaken. A volume-cycled ventilator should be used with large tidal volumes (10–15 mL/kg). Initially, 100% O_2 should be given, but rapidly reduced to mitigate O_2 toxicity as gauged by the patient's O_2 saturation. Positive end-expiratory pressure (PEEP) is recommended, since opening closed alveoli improves gas exchange. Lower O_2 concentrations can then be used. High levels of PEEP, however, decrease cardiac output and promote lung leak. The best course is probably to start at low levels (about 5 mL/kg) and then go higher, if necessary, as determined by unsatisfactory oxygenation.[14]

If satisfactory oxygenation cannot be maintained even with high O_2 concentrations and the highest tolerable levels of PEEP, high-frequency and inverse-ratio ventilation might be considered in the intensive care unit (ICU) setting. Advocates of high-frequency ventilation (HFV) suggest that some of the injury seen in ARDS may be secondary to baro-

trauma. HFV involves low tidal volumes with resulting low peak inspiratory pressures and less barotrauma compared to conventional mechanical therapy. However, HFV has not improved survival.[15–17] All else failing, extracorporeal membrane oxygenation (ECMO) may be considered. Zapol and colleagues[18] published the results of a large prospective study comparing ECMO with treatment by conventional mechanical ventilation. Results revealed no differences in survival between the two groups. Availability, cost, the patient's acquiescence to heroic life support procedures, and the reversibility of the underlying cause of ARDS must be considered before ECMO is instituted.

MANAGEMENT OF THE IMMUNOCOMPROMISED PATIENT

The evaluation of WOL in the ICP is a unique and difficult diagnostic and therapeutic challenge to the emergency physician. There are relative degrees of immunocompromise, ranging in severity and significance from chronic alcoholism to acquired immunodeficiency syndrome (AIDS).

The determination of a patient's HIV seropositivity is often impossible in the emergency care setting. One scenario that haunts physicians today is that of the "ordinary community-acquired pneumonia" that transpires subsequently to be an opportunistic infection in the HIV-positive patient. Another nightmare scenario is the patient discharged from the ED with trivial respiratory complaints who returns with WOL 24 hours later. These are two of the ED "faces of AIDS." Thus the index of suspicion for AIDS today must be extremely high!

In the ICP, WOL results from a combination of the following processes: (1) extension of the basic underlying disease process involving the lungs, (2) opportunistic infection, (3) pulmonary reaction to drugs, or (4) a new unrelated disease process. The common underlying pathophysiologic defect in these patients is an impairment of three categories of host defenses: (1) impaired antibody formation (B lymphocyte–mediated), (2) impaired cell-mediated immunity (T lymphocyte–mediated), and (3) granulocytopenia or impaired granulocytic function.

Some causes of pulmonary opacification in AIDS patients, both common and uncommon, and infectious and noninfectious, are listed in Table 30–5. "Normal" bacterial pathogens are not listed, but—interestingly—account for the majority of infections (particularly *Haemophilus influenzae* and *Streptococcus*

TABLE 30–5.

Pulmonary Complications of HIV Infection

Opportunistic infections diagnostic of AIDS
  Pneumocystis carinii pneumonia
  Pulmonary toxoplasmosis
  Extraintestinal strongyloidiasis
  Bronchopulmonary candidiasis
  Pulmonary cryptococcosis
  Disseminated histoplasmosis
  Cytomegalovirus pneumonia
  Herpes simplex pneumonia
HIV-related pulmonary infections
  Tuberculosis
  Nocardiosis
Presumed HIV-related pulmonary disorders
  Lymphoid interstitial pneumonitis
AIDS-related pulmonary neoplasia
  Kaposi's sarcoma
  Non-Hodgkin's lymphoma

pneumoniae).[19, 20] Of opportunistic infections, *Pneumocystis carinii* pneumonia (PCP) is the most common.[21] It occurs in approximately 75% of AIDS patients. As one might expect, the incidence of both multilobar pneumonia and bacteremia exceeds that in NICPs.

If pneumonia is a real possibility, a number of clinical associations may assist the emergency physician in diagnosis. Pneumonitis in the ICP with diarrhea can be seen in patients with legionella, herpes simplex, *Strongyloides, Cryptosporidium,* or cytomegalovirus (CMV). The skin is an important source of clues, and lesions presenting in the patient with sepsis or pneumonia should be biopsied or cultured, or both. Another clue is the degree of hypoxemia found in the ICP. Severe hypoxemia is commonly found in bacterial infections (excluding mycobacteria and *Nocardia*), viruses, and PCP. Patients with mycobacteria, *Nocardia,* and fungi usually demonstrate less severe hypoxemia.

Chest radiograph abnormalities can be of great assistance. The rate of progression of pulmonary infiltrates caused by particular infectious agents is shown in Table 30–6. The type of radiologic infiltrate (consolidated, interstitial, nodular), in concert with the rate of progression, can likewise be diagnostically helpful (Table 30–7). Tables 30–8 and 30–9 list causes and degrees of pleural effusion and cavitary pulmonary lesions in the ICP.

The *management of ICPs* requires rapid diagnosis and effective treatment. Special goals in these patients are: (1) avoidance of unecessary toxic drugs, (2) decreasing the risks of superinfection, and (3) minimizing the chances of inappropriate or inadequate therapy.

Certain points in the history and physical examination should lead one to suspect an opportunistic infection in the ICP: male homosexuality or IV drug abuse; recent weight loss; diarrhea; chronic fever, malaise, fatigue, and weakness; generalized lymphadenopathy; oral thrush; appearance of chronic illness; unusual pulmonary infiltration or opacification; dyspnea or hypoxemia out of proportion to radiographic findings, etc.

When WOL is found in the known or suspected HIV seropositive patient, PCP and other opportunistic infections must head the differential diagnosis. The sputum examination is very helpful in distinguishing between ordinary and opportunistic pneumonias: Polsky et al.[20] reported a positive sputum culture in 11 of 16 AIDS patients with bacterial pneumonia. With PCP the WBC count is rarely elevated; most patients have the lymphopenia and neutropenia characteristic of late-stage HIV infection.[21–24] CD4 counts are usually below 200/mm^3.[22]

TABLE 30–6.

Rate of Progression of Infectious Pulmonary Infiltrates on Chest Radiograph and Potential Underlying Organisms

Acute	Subacute	Chronic
Streptococcus pneumoniae	*Pneumocystis carinii*	Mycobacteria
Staphylococcus aureus	*Aspergillus*	*Coccidioides immitis*
Haemophilus influenzae	Zygomycetes	*Histoplasma capsulatum*
Pseudomonas aeruginosa	*Cryptococcus neoformans*	*Blastomyces dermatitidis*
	Herpes simplex	*Strongyloides stercoralis*
	Varicella-zoster	
	Nocardia	
	Mycoplasma	
	Cytomegalovirus	
	Influenza virus	
	Legionella	
	Mycobacteria	

TABLE 30–7.

Differential Diagnosis of Fever and Pulmonary Infiltrates in an Immunocompromised Patient: Radiographic Abnormality vs. Rate of Progression of Symptoms

Chest Radiographic Abnormality	Etiology According to Rate of Progression of Illness	
	Acute	Subacute-Chronic
Consolidation	Bacterial	Fungal
	Thromboembolic	Nocardial
	Hemorrhage	Tuberculous
	Pulmonary edema	Tumor (viral, pneumocystic, radiation, drug-induced)
Interstitial infiltrate	Leukoagglutinin reaction	Viral
	Pulmonary edema	Pneumocystic
		Radiation
		Drug-induced,
		Fungal, tuberculous, nocardial, tumor
Nodular infiltrate	Bacterial	Tumor
	Pulmonary edema	Fungal
		Nocardial
		Tuberculous

More than 95% of patients with PCP have an elevated serum lactic dehydrogenase (LDH) as contrasted with only 20% with other pulmonary conditions.[25] The chest film is abnormal in 90% of PCP patients.[21] The most common finding is a diffuse increase in interstitial and alveolar markings[26, 27] (Fig 30–4). Consideration of specialized studies by pulmonary or infectious disease consultants should follow: carbon monoxide diffusion capacity and gallium lung scanning (gallium scanning has a 95% sensitivity in PCP); inducing sputum with 3% to 5% saline aerosol (80%–92% sensitivity); fiberoptic bronchoscopy with washings, special cultures, and possibly transbronchial biopsy (87% sensitivity) and bronchoalveolar lavage (86% sensitivity); and transthoracic percutaneous needle aspiration.[21]

Once studied (or even before, if circumstances dictate), treatment (often empiric) is begun. *Antibiot-*

TABLE 30–8.

Causes of Pleural Effusion in the Immunocompromised Patient

Relatively common
  Congestive heart failure
  Pulmonary embolus or infarction
  Bacterial pneumonia, including legionella
Uncommon
  Drug therapy
  Nocardia
  Graft-versus-host disease
Rare
  Pneumocystis carinii pneumonia
  Cytomegalovirus
  Herpesvirus
  Invasive fungal disease

ics should ideally be started in the ED on all ICPs with pulmonary infiltrates believed to be due to an infectious agent!

An ideal chemotherapeutic regimen must be broad-spectrum, achieve high bactericidal concentrations, be nontoxic, and be simple to administer. Both gram-positive and gram-negative bacteria or combinations have frequently been isolated from febrile neutropenic patients. Currently, combined therapy with a β-lactam and an aminoglycoside are recommended. If a high incidence of staphylococci occurs in a given area, the inclusion of a specific antistaphylococcal agent should be added. The appropriate antistaphylococcal antibiotic would be nafcillin or vancomycin, respectively, depending upon whether the organism is anticipated to be methicillin-sensitive or not. The feasibility of monotherapy with such agents as imipenem or ceftazidime in these settings is currently being explored. If PCP is likely, trimethoprim-sulfamethoxazole is the antibiotic of choice (20 mg/kg/day of trimethoprim and 100 mg/

TABLE 30–9.

Conditions and Organisms Associated With Cavitary Pulmonary Lesions in the Immunocompromised Patient

Staphylococcus aureus
Nocardia
Cryptococcus
Aspergillus
Anaerobic bacteria
Tuberculosis
Lymphoma
Wegener's granulomatosis
Pulmonary infarction

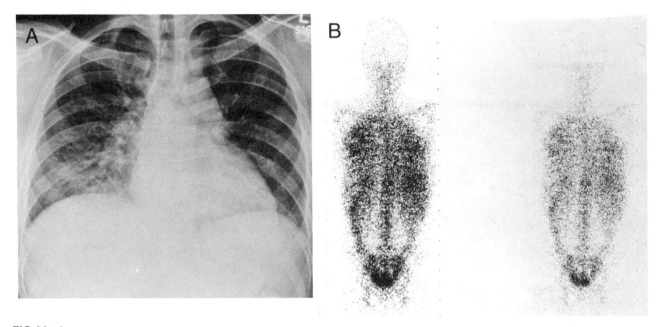

FIG 30–4.
Pneumocystis carinii pneumonia in a man with AIDS. **A,** the chest radiograph showed early diffuse pulmonary infiltration. **B,** the gallium scan shows markedly increased uptake in lungs. (From Armstrong P, Dee P: Infections of the lungs and pleura, in Armstrong P, Wilson AG, Dee P (eds): *Imaging of Diseases of the Chest.* St Louis, Mosby–Year Book, Inc, 1990, p 236. Used by permission.)

kg/day of sulfamethoxazole, IV in four divided doses). The addition of erythromycin (500 mg every 6 hours, IV) is also recommended to cover Legionella, Mycoplasma, and Chlamydia species. Two recent studies have shown that corticosteroids (methylprednisolone 40 mg IV every 6 hours for 7 days) reduces the likelihood of respiratory failure and death in HIV-infected patients with PCP infection.[28, 29]

Scenario 1: The Stable Patient

White-out lung patients usually present as a surprise to the ED; i.e., they have often been quite well without cardiac or pulmonary disease. And, in most instances, the illness has begun and evolved rapidly, usually over a day or two, sometimes even over hours. There is usually a paucity of other clinical findings. Rales or wheezing is almost invariably present, but these findings are outweighed by, and seem not impressive enough to explain, the dyspnea and tachypnea observed. If previously healthy, patients can muster a marked respiratory effort, and may not sweat despite their labored breathing. Use of accessory muscles and retractions are common. At first blush they may be mistakenly diagnosed as hyperventilation syndrome, especially if cyanosis has been corrected by O_2 therapy begun by prehospital care personnel. Another common incorrect first diagnosis is hyperventilation to compensate for a se-

vere metabolic acidosis. However, the true nature of this patient's problem is revealed by a chest film and pulse oximetry (or ABG analysis). The stable patient's radiograph may initially have only modest or beginning WOL, but the findings are generalized. Even if minimal, such radiographic abnormalities are associated with disproportionately significant hypoxemia (60%–80% saturation), often prompting disbelief and repetition of the ABG sampling. The physician's surprise is a measure of the even more marked hypoxemia to come, as the clinical picture frequently worsens. Though hypoxemia is marked, ventilation is quite adequate in the stable patient; the PCO_2 is usually in the range of 20 to 30 mm Hg.

Once WOL is recognized, and while a diagnostic search is underway, O_2 therapy is begun: 5 to 8 L/min by nasal cannula (see above under Oxygen Therapy). If O_2 saturation does not immediately rise above 90%, a nonrebreather mask should be applied. That failing in turn, one needs to prepare for intubation and mechanical ventilation. There is a very important point to be made here: this patient, though stable now, is likely to deteriorate very quickly and to suffer progressive hypoxemia that cannot be adequately treated by just increasing inspired O_2 concentration. One should not wait for the usual indications for intubation: respiratory failure, exhaustion, and altered mental status! One need only be sure that the O_2 saturation is progressively falling despite delivery of O_2 by nonrebreather mask.

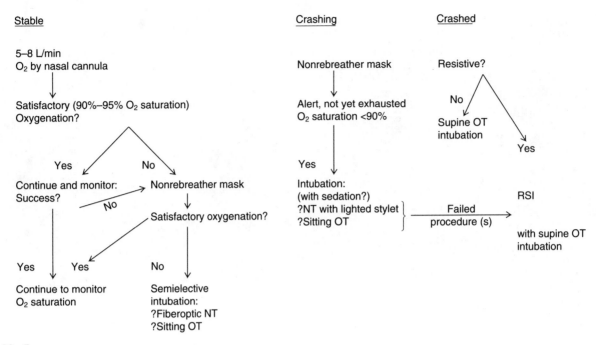

FIG 30–5.
An algorithm for airway management of white-out lung. NT = nasotracheal; OT = orotracheal; RSI = rapid-sequence intubation.

If the tempo of the deterioration is over hours instead of minutes, intubation may be performed semielectively over a fiberoptic endoscope. This is a particularly attractive option since diagnostic sampling of bronchial secretions can be done concomitantly. And the patient enjoys the benefit of a procedure well explained and performed under controlled circumstances.

If, however, the patient is crashing, different methods must be used.

Scenario 2: The Crashing Patient

These patients are alarming. Though alert and orientated, they are clearly in extremis. They are extremely dyspneic, tachypneic (respiratory rate 35–40 breaths/min), and tachycardic (pulse >120 beats/min). Respirations are extremely labored, with full use of accessory muscles and retractions. There is sweating. The chest film shows significant multiple infiltrations or even near-opacification. The O_2 saturation, even with increased fractional concentration of oxygen in inspired gas (FiO_2) provided is frighteningly low. If, with the use of the nonrebreather mask, the O_2 is less than 90%, and if other of the above clinical features obtain, intubation is now necessary. Again, one must not procrastinate!

The procedure of choice is either blind nasotracheal or sitting orotracheal intubation. The choice depends largely upon the past procedural experience of the physician. If nasotracheal intubation is elected, a lighted stylet should be used. Nasotracheal

intubation may precipitate disastrous immediate epistaxis, especially if the nasal passage has not been adequately cocainized. And if the tube is left in long-term, the high incidence of sinusitis must be considered. These disadvantages must be weighed against the advantages of comfort and oral alimentation.

If the patient is apprehensive but alert and orientated, and still has an acceptable PCO_2 (<40 mm Hg), some gentle sedation with an ultra-short-acting sedative (e.g., IV hexobarbital) may make intubation more merciful without risk of significant hypoventilation.

If sitting intubation fails, or acute complications (such as epistaxis) occur, or the patient's oxygenation deteriorates hyperacutely, a crashed scenario has ensued.

Scenario 3: The Crashed Patient

These patients have clearly ineffective respirations, have alterations in mental status that range from disorientation and combativeness to coma, and can be expected to have O_2 saturations less than 70% to 80% despite FiO_2 values 60% to above 70%. As with crashed patients of other clinical cause, they are defined by the need to be intubated immediately.

The procedure of choice depends largely on the patient's mental status. If the patient is comatose, he or she will generally not be resistive, and supine orotracheal intubation without sedation or paralysis can usually be performed without undue difficulty. Care must be taken immediately afterward to return the patient to a sitting position to assure optimal ventilation (unless the patient is in shock). However, if the patient resists intubation, rapid-sequence intubation with short-term sedation and paralysis will be necessary. The need for longer-term paralysis will, of course, depend on the patient's ability to cooperate with the ventilator. (See Oxygen Therapy above for the particulars of ventilator usage and settings.)

An algorithm for airway management in white-out lung is presented in Figure 30–5.

The clinical need for "emergent intubation" raises the major ethical issue of whether to institute assisted ventilation in AIDS patients developing respiratory failure. Although early investigations found a very high mortality rate in intubated AIDS patients, more recent experience suggests that 20% to 30% of these patients survive.[30, 31] Prolonged survival of the AIDS patient after hospitalization is accomplished with such advances as inhaled pentamidine prophylaxis and oral zidovudine. Therefore many leading investigators now recommend that assisted ventilation should generally be provided for patients with respiratory failure due to first-episode PCP who are in relatively good general condition and who desire intensive therapy.

REFERENCES

1. Hatherill JR, Raffin TA: Diagnosis and management of the adult respiratory distress syndrome. *Compr Ther* 1989; 15:21–27.
2. Royal JA, Levin DL: Adult respiratory distress syndrome in pediatric patients: 1. Clinical aspects, pathophysiology, pathology, and mechanisms of lung injury. *J Pediatr* 1988; 112:169–180.
3. Kirsch CM, Sanders A: Aspiration pneumonia. *Otolaryngol Clin North Am* 1988; 21:677–689.
4. Snow RM, Miller WC, Rice DL, et al: Respiratory failure in cancer patients. *JAMA* 1979; 241:2039–2042.
5. Cooper JAD Jr., White DA, Matthay RA: State of the art: Drug-induced pulmonary disease. *Am Rev Respir Dis* 1986; 133:321–340; 488–505.
6. Richman PS, Spragg RG, Merritt TA, et al: Administration of porcine-lung surfactant to humans with ARDS: Initial experience (abstract). *Am Rev Respir Dis* 1987; 135(suppl):A5.
7. Sibbald WJ, Anderson RR, Reid B, et al: Alveolar-capillary permeability in human septic ARDS: Effect of high-dose corticosteroid therapy. *Chest* 1981; 79:133–142.
8. Bone RC, Fisher JR JC, Clemmer TP, et al: Early methylprednisolone treatment for septic syndrome and the adult respiratory distress syndrome. *Chest* 1987; 92:1032–1036.
9. Benard GR, Luce JM, Sprung CL, et al: High-dose corticosteroids in patients with the adult respiratory distress syndrome. *N Engl J Med* 1987; 317:1565–1570.
10. Weigelt JA, Norcross JF, Borman KR, et al: Early steroid therapy for respiratory failure. *Arch Surg* 1985; 120:536–540.
11. Bone RC, Slotman G, Maunder, et al: Randomized double-blind multicenter study of prostaglandin E1 in patients with the adult respiratory distress syndrome. *Chest* 1989; 96:114–119.
12. Ziegler EJ, Fisher CJ Jr, Sprung CL, et al: Treatment of gram-negative bacteremia and septic shock with HA-1 A human monoclonal antibody against endotoxin. *N Engl J Med* 1991; 324:429–436.
13. Ziegler EJ, McCutchan JA, Fierer J, et al: Treatment of gram negative bacteremia and shock with human antiserum to mutant *Escherichia coli*. *N Engl J Med* 1982; 307:1225–1230.
14. Petty TL: The use, abuse, and mystique of positive end expiratory pressure. *Am Rev Respir Dis* 1988; 138:475–478.
15. Carlon GC, Howland WS, Ray C, et al: High-frequency jet ventilation: A prospective randomized evaluation. *Chest* 1983; 84:551–558.
16. Schuster DP, Klain M, Snyder JV: Comparison of high frequency jet ventilation to conventional ventilation during severe acute respiratory failure in humans. *Crit Care Med* 1982; 10:625–630.
17. Wattwil LM, Sjostrand UH, Borg UR: Comparative studies of IPPV and HFPPV with PEEP in critical care patients. *Crit Care Med* 1983; 11:30–37.
18. Zapol WM, Snider MT, Hll DJ, et al: Extracorporeal membrane oxygenation in severe acute respiratory failure: A randomized prospective study. *JAMA* 1976; 242:2193–2196.
19. Witt DJ, Craven DE, McCabe WR: Bacterial infections in adult patients with the acquired immune deficiency syndrome (AIDS) and AIDS-related complex. *Am J Med* 1987; 82:900–906.
20. Polsky B, Gold JW, Whimbey E, et al: Bacterial pneumonia in patients with the acquired immunodeficiency syndrome. *Ann Intern Med* 1986; 104:38–41.
21. Kovacs JA: Diagnosis, treatment, and prevention of *Pneumocystis carinii* pneumonia in HIV-infected patients. *AIDS Updates* 1989; 2 (March/April):1–12.
22. Murray JF, Mills J: Pulmonary infectious complications of human immunodeficiency virus infection. Part I. *Am Rev Respir Dis* 1990; 141:1356–1372.
23. Walzer PD: Diagnosis of *Pneumocystis carinii* pneumonia. *J Infect Dis* 1988; 157:629–632.
24. Hopewell PC: *Pneumocystis carinii* pneumonia: Diagnosis. *J Infect Dis* 1988; 157:1115–1119.
25. Medina I, Mills J, Wofsy C: Serum lactate dehydrogenase levels in *Pneumocystis carinii* pneumonia in AIDS: Possible indicator and predictor of disease, in Pro-

ceedings of the Third International Conference on AIDS, Washington, DC, June 1–5, 1987; vol 3, p 109.

26. Cohen BA, Pomeranz S, Rabinowitz JG, et al: Pulmonary complications of AIDS: Radiologic features. *AJR* 1984; 143:115–122.

27. Goodman PC, Gamsu G: Pulmonary radiographic findings in the acquired immunodeficiency syndrome. *Postgrad Radiol* 1987; 7:3–15.

28. Gagnon S, Boota AM, Fishi MA, et al: Corticosteroids as adjunctive therapy for severe *Pneumocystis carinii* pneumonia in the acquired immunodeficiency syndrome—A double-blind placebo-controlled trial. *N Engl J Med* 1990; 323:1444–1447.

29. Bozzette SA, Sattler FR, Chiu J, et al: A controlled trial of early adjunctive treatment with corticosteroids for *Pneumocystis carinii* pneumonia in the acquired immunodeficiency syndrome. *N Engl J Med* 1990; 323:1451–1457.

30. el-Sadr W, Simberkoff MS: Survival and prognostic factors in severe *Pneumocystis carinii* pneumonia require mechanical ventilation. *Am Rev Respir Dis* 1988; 137:1264–1267.

31. Efferen LS, Nadarajah D, Palat DS: Survival following mechanical ventilation for *Pneumocystis carinii* pneumonia in patients with acquired immunodeficiency syndrome: A different perspective. *Am J Med* 1989; 87:401–404.

32. Zaman MK, White DA: Serum lactate dehydrogenase levels and *Pneumocystis carinii* pneumonia. *Am Rev Respir Dis* 1988; 137:796–800.

31

Overdoses

Roy Magnusson, M.D.

Toxicologic emergencies are a daily event in most busy emergency departments (EDs). Respiratory complications are not only the most common complication in acute poisonings, they are also the most common cause of death.[1-5] Therefore, effective management of the airway and aggressive ventilatory support are critical aspects in the care of seriously poisoned patients. Unfortunately, overdose significantly complicates several aspects of airway management. "Difficult intubations," which occur in 10% to 15% of overdose patients, are associated with a significant increase in mortality.[5] Although drugs and poisons vary considerably in their toxic effects, there are key aspects of supportive care that are common to all poisonings. To emphasize the three pillars of airway management in the poisoned patient, the fundamentals of airway management in this setting are reviewed using three commonly encountered clinical scenarios. An algorithm for airway management of overdose (OD) is presented in Figure 31–1.

Scenario 1: The Alert Patient With Intact Gag Reflex

When patients present with a normal mental status, an intact gag reflex, and without respiratory distress, airway management is routine. However, a variety of special circumstances may complicate airway management even in the alert poisoned patient. The risk of respiratory complication in the alert patient is determined by three key factors: (1) the specific properties of the toxin ingested, (2) the potential for a change in mental status, and (3) the necessity for gastric decontamination.

Certain toxins carry the risk of airflow compromise due to specific direct effects on the airway. Corrosive agents (e.g., acids and alkali) burn the oropharyngeal mucosa and serious airway obstruction may occur due to edema. Cholinergic agents (e.g., organophosphates) cause excessive bronchial secretions.[6] Several toxins have the ability to produce seizures or coma shortly after ingestion. General categories of such drugs include sedative-hypnotics, narcotics, antidepressants, industrial poisons, and insecticides (Tables 31–1 and 31–2). Tricyclic antidepressants, aminophylline, cocaine, amphetamines, and hypoglycemic agent ingestions are the most commonly seen ODs in the ED setting. Patients who present with a normal level of consciousness initially may still be at risk of airflow compromise if the toxin ingested has the potential of causing rapid diminution in mental status.

Several toxins increase the likelihood of aspiration by causing emesis (e.g., aspirin, acetaminophen, iron, and ipecac).[2] Volitile substances with low viscosity (e.g., hydrocarbons) are easily aspirated either during the initial ingestion or upon regurgitation.[6, 7] The severity of pulmonary damage is proportional to the irritant qualities of the ingested toxin. Procedures to decontaminate the gastrointestinal tract increase the risk of aspiration since the patient's ability to protect the airway is compromised during emesis or gastric lavage.[8]

Oxygenation and ventilation may be impaired by exposure to a number of toxins. Pulmonary edema associated with salicylate toxicity is an example of *direct* pulmonary toxicity.[6, 9, 10] Other drugs causing adult respiratory distress syndrome (ARDS) include heroin, barbiturates, colchicine, methadone, tricyclic antidepressants, ethchlorvynol, and propoxyphene.[3, 11-17] Aspiration of gastric contents contributes to hypoxia and respiratory acidosis. Patients with witnessed aspiration develop ARDS 30% and 36% of the time.[18, 19] Paraquat ingestion causes death by acute pulmonary edema and hemorrhage. In patients who survive the initial pulmonary crisis, severe delayed pulmonary fibrosis and death due to respiratory failure occur.[20-22] Many inhaled substances (e.g., ammonia, chlorine, phosgene) cause di-

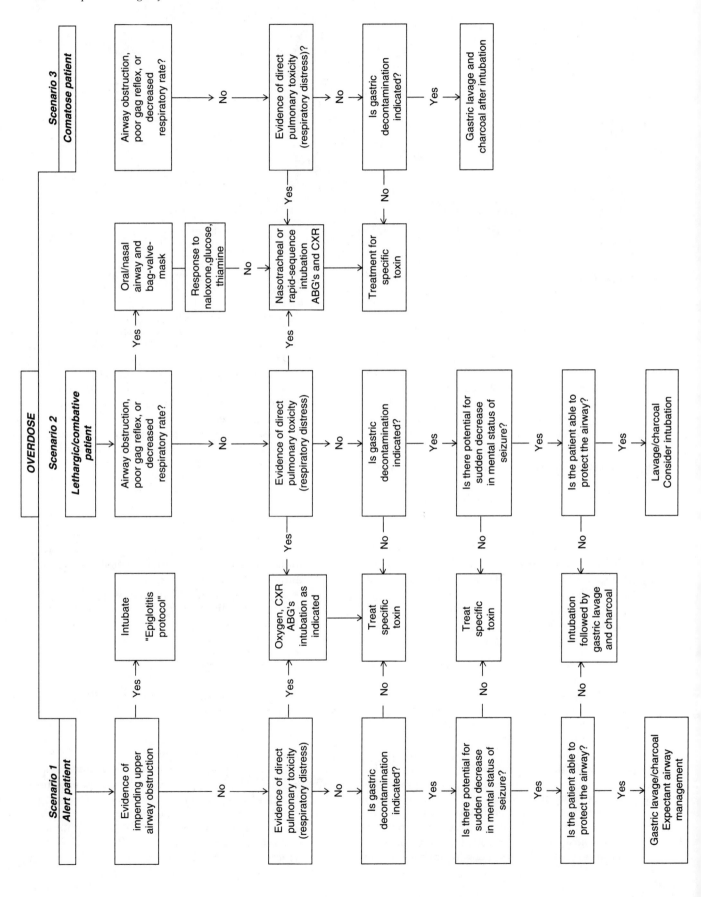

TABLE 31–1.

Toxins Producing Coma

Narcotics
Sedative hypnotics (benzodiazepines, others)
Barbituates
Cyanide
Hydrogen sulfide
Carbon monoxide
Nicotinic acid
Phencyclidine (PCP)
Glutethimide
Alcohols
  Methanol
  Ethylene glycol
  Ethanol
  Isopropanol
Anticonvulsants
  Phenytoin
  Valproic acid
  Others
Monoamine oxidase inhibitors
Cyclic antidepressants
Antihistamines
Bromides
Tranquilizers

TABLE 31–2.

Toxins Producing Seizures

Anticholinergic agents
  Organophosphates
  Physostigmine
Antihistamines
Antidepressants
Antipsychotics
β-Blockers
Camphor
Chlorambucil
Cocaine, lidocaine (local anesthetics)
Cycloserine
Cyclosporin A
Ergonovine
Folic acid
Hypoglycemic agents
Isoniazid
Methylxanthines (theophylline)
Metronidazole
Nalidixic acid
Narcotics
Phencyclidine (PCP)
Sympathomimetics (amphetamines, ephedrine, terbutaline)
Phenytoin

rect bronchial or pulmonary injury resulting in increased secretions, bronchial edema, and small airway hyperreactivity.[23–26]

Airway Management

In the alert patient, airflow obstruction is unusual. Thermal and chemical burns are an exception. The management of oropharyngeal burns is described in Chapter 26. Positioning and suctioning may be necessary in patients with excessive secretions or vomitus in the airway.

If there is evidence of aspiration, the airway is cleared by suctioning to avoid aspiration of additional materials. Arterial blood gas (ABG) measurements and a chest x-ray film (CXR) are helpful in assessing oxygenation, ventilation, and the extent of injury. Oxygen concentration should be increased as needed to maintain an arterial oxygen partial pressure (PaO_2) of 60 mm Hg or greater. Infiltrates on CXR may take hours to develop but, when present, represent significant aspiration requiring further evaluation (ABGs) and treatment. Positioning the patient in order to facilitate airway clearing is important. Alert patients will protect their own airway by sitting up and forward. Do not force patients into a supine position. If a recumbent position is necessary, the left lateral decubitus position is preferable to theoretically keep toxins from moving through the pylorus. If hypoxia (PaO_2 <60 mm Hg) persists despite 100% oxygen therapy, intubation and positive end-expiratory pressure (PEEP) are indicated. Intubation is also indicated when hypoventilation results in acidosis (pH <7.35).

Gastrointestinal Decontamination

When the three pillars of airway management are not initially compromised, the emergency physician must next answer three key questions. First, should the stomach be emptied? Second, what is the potential for a significant decrease in mental status or seizures during emesis or gastric lavage? Third, what is the safest and most effective method of decontamination given the patient's history and condition?

Although gastric decontamination is a standard recommendation for many ingestions, there are situations in which it is contraindicated. Attempts at removing caustic or volatile substances may precipitate additional burn or aspiration. Many substances are

FIG 31–1.
Algorithm for airway management of overdose. *ABGs* = arterial blood gases; *CXR* = chest x-ray film.

so quickly absorbed that emesis or lavage would not be expected to be of benefit beyond a certain time period (e.g., alcohols) *Gastric decontamination should be reserved for those situations where safe removal of a significant amount of a very toxic substance can be expected.* If decontamination is indicated, it must be done in such a way so as to not compromise airway patency, cause aspiration, or impair oxygenation and ventilation. Until recently, ipecac-induced emesis has been standard therapy in alert patients. Ipecac therapy results in emesis within 15 minutes in 60% of patients and within 30 minutes in 90%. Drug recovery of 20% to 40% can be expected if given in the first hour; recovery is minimal after this time period.[27–29] Ipecac is contraindicated if corrosive or volatile substances have been ingested since the risk of additional burn or aspiration is increased.[30] One of the most dangerous experiences in emergency medicine is to administer ipecac to an alert patient only to have that patient become more obtunded or seize just as vomiting begins. It is standard practice to avoid ipecac when toxins known to produce rapid onset of coma or seizures have been ingested (see Tables 31–1 and 31–2). In these patients, gastric lavage is the preferred method of stomach emptying.[30]

Drug recovery with gastric lavage is slightly better than with ipecac and ranges from 30% to 50% when performed immediately post ingestion.[27–29] Recovery percentages decrease rapidly as the time from ingestion to lavage increases. Obtunded patients lavaged within 1 hour of ingestion have better outcomes when compared to patients treated with nasogastric (NG) suction and activated charcoal alone.[31] This benefit, however, disappears at 1 hour post ingestion.[31] In the alert patient with an intact gag reflex, lavage can be performed without intubation. If there is any question about the patient's ability to protect the airway, intubation with a cuffed tube should precede the procedure (see Scenario 2). Alert patients are placed in the left lateral decubitus position in 15 degrees of Trendelenburg's position. A large-bore (36–40F) lavage tube is recommended. Using a bite-block, the tube is gently passed into the mouth as the patient swallows. Patients find this to be a very difficult process and will need to be restrained. Gagging and emesis frequently occur. Therefore, it is imperative that suction and intubation equipment be immediately available and that the process be closely supervised by the emergency physician. Gastric tube placement is checked by both aspirating gastric contents from the tube and by instilling air while auscultating the epigastric area. The

stomach is drained and then aliquots of 200 to 300 mL of normal saline are flushed in and out until the lavage return is clear. Sixty to 90 g of charcoal with sorbitol (1 g/kg in children) is then instilled into the stomach just prior to tube removal.

Oral administration of activated charcoal is now being considered as an alternative to ipecac-induced emesis or lavage in the alert patient: activated charcoal is more comfortable, safer, and may be more effective.[28, 31–33] Charcoal has the added benefit of decreasing the half-life of several drugs even after they have been absorbed.[34] The use of charcoal does have disadvantages. It has been our experience that it is difficult to get patients, especially children, to drink charcoal preparations; and several toxins including heavy metals, iron, lithium, alcohols, and hydrocarbons are not bound by charcoal.[31] Also, charcoal obscures endoscopic examination in patients with caustic esophageal burns and should not be used with acid or alkaline ingestions.[30] Finally, although considered very safe, serious complications of charcoal aspiration have recently been reported including acute airway obstruction, bronchospasm, pneumonia, and fatal bronchiolitis obliterans.[35–37] These are isolated case reports, however, and activated charcoal is used without significant complication in thousands of patients every year.[38] Nevertheless, should aspiration of charcoal occur, aggressive tracheal and upper airway suctioning is required.

Scenario 2: The Stuporous or Agitated Patient

In patients who are uncooperative due to lethargy, confusion, or agitation, airway management is extremely challenging. All of the hazards mentioned for the alert patient exist for the obtunded patient and are magnified by the impaired mental status. In addition, agitation makes theraputic intervention much more difficult. As the level of consciousness decreases, facial and laryngeal muscles relax. If relaxation is profound the tongue may fall posteriorly and obstruct the airway. Gag and cough reflexes diminish along with mental status, leaving the airway less well protected. If emesis occurs in this setting, there is a high risk of aspiration. Respiratory acidosis develops as respiratory drive is impaired to the point of inadequate ventilation. This is particularly important when the toxin ingested is known to produce a metabolic acidosis since the patient's ability to compensate by hyperventilation is diminished. Finally, impaired lung defenses have been demonstrated in patients with altered levels of consciousness, hypoxia, or acidosis. These conditions predispose patients to pneumonia.[6, 39–41]

Management

Assessment of airflow is accomplished by observing chest wall movements for adequate rate and depth of breathing, feeling for airflow over the airway, and listening for upper airway noise (e.g., snoring, stridor). Airway obstruction due to muscle laxity can be initially relieved by jaw thrust or placement of an oral or nasopharyngeal airway. Also, the airway should be cleared of secretions or vomitus with suctioning. Supplemental oxygen (4–6 L by nasal prongs) should be started. If airflow is shallow or absent despite manuvers to open the airway, an oropharyngeal airway should be placed and ventilation assisted with a bag-valve-mask until intubation can be performed. Cricoid pressure applied during assisted ventilation may prevent gastric distention and subsequent regurgitation. Once adequate ventilation and oxygenation is provided, reversible causes of altered mental status such as narcotic OD and hypoglycemia should be treated immediately with a protocol consisting of naloxone 2 mg intravenously (IV) and either 25 g of glucose in 50% D/W or rapid glucose determination (Dextrostix). Thiamine 100 mg IV is given prior to glucose administration in the alcoholic or malnourished patient.

Scenario 2 patients presenting without a clear indication for immediate intubation are often the most challenging to manage. The level of consciousness may range from lethargy to mania. To complicate decisions, the mental status of many patients will wax and wane. The toxins ingested, the potential for emesis, the risk of gastric decontamination procedures, the potential for changes in the level of consciousness, and the ability to monitor these patients must all be considered when evaluating the need for intubation. When in doubt, intubation should precede gastric lavage and instillation of activated charcoal.

Intubating the Combative Overdose Patient

Because combative patients are so difficult to manage, no attempt should be made to intubate without being fully prepared. There needs to be enough manpower to restrain the patient. Medications for sedation or paralysis should be immediately available. Intravenous access should be established. Because of the risk of emesis, suctioning equipment must be available and ready. The laryngoscope, endotracheal tube, and various blades must be tested and functional.

The patient is oxygenated and hyperventilated with 100% oxygen. There are two basic methods available to the emergency physician to intubate these patients: blind nasotracheal intubation and rapid-sequence intubation. Rapid-sequence intubation will be discussed in detail since it has been shown to be superior to blind nasotracheal intubation in this setting.[42]

Although sedation may potentiate the effects of ingested drugs, it may be necessary in agitated patients. A short-acting barbituate, e.g., methohexital (Brevital); a benzodiazepine, e.g., midazolam (Versed); or a narcotic, e.g., fentanyl (Sublimaze) can be titrated IV to sedate the patient during the procedure. Oral or nasotracheal intubation can then be attempted primarily, but if not immediately successful, rapid-sequence intubation should be undertaken.

Succinylcholine is the paralyzing agent of choice for intubation because of its rapid onset (<1 minute) and short duration of action (5–10 minutes). A dose of 1 to 2 mg/kg IV is recommended. Succinylcholine should be used with caution in certain circumstances, however. This drug may aggravate the cholinergic side effects of bradycardia, salivation, and bronchorrhea in cholinergic poisonings. In addition, the effects of succinylcholine may be significantly prolonged in patients with poisonings due to organophosphates and cocaine since these toxins reduce plasma cholinesterase activity, the enzyme which metabolizes succinylcholine. Colistin, lithium, and quinine have also been reported to potentiate the neuromuscular block produced by succinylcholine.[34] Following paralysis, oral intubation as described in Chapter 6 is then performed.

With the airway secure and protected from aspiration, close clinical observation, ABG measurements, and CXR are necessary to determine the need for mechanical ventilation and admission.

Scenario 3: The Comatose Patient

Coma profoundly affects all three pillars of airway management. In some ways, these patients are more easily managed because the indications for intubation are clear and present. On the other hand, the emergency physician must act quickly and definitively under these circumstances. All of the previously mentioned threats to airflow and causes of aspiration exist in these patients. The risk of aspiration is extremely high.

Several threats to adequate oxygenation and ventilation need to be considered in the comatose patient. Firstly, drugs that cause deep central nervous system (CNS) depression, such as narcotics, barbiturates, or tricyclic antidepressants, depress central respiratory drive, producing hypoxia and ventilatory acidosis. Secondly, exposure to carbon monoxide, cyanide, and nitrates or nitrites decreases the oxygen-carrying capacity of hemoglobin, resulting in lactic acidosis which is compounded by circulatory collapse. Thirdly, many toxins (e.g., methanol, ethylene glycol, salicylates) produce severe metabolic acidosis. Since respiratory compensation for severe metabolic acidosis is very important in this setting, even mild sedative-induced hypoventilation is dangerous.

Management

All comatose overdosed patients that do not respond immediately to IV glucose or naloxone must be intubated. Orotracheal or nasotracheal intubation both have their advocates and are generally appropriate (see Chapters 6 and 9, including discussion of indications and contraindications). Naturally, if the patient is apneic or otherwise in extremis, orotracheal intubation is the clearly preferred mode. If the patient is able to successfully resist intubation, and ventilation does not need to be supported immediately, one may wait a short while, observing the patient carefully, to reassess the need for intubation. (Indeed, the patient may gradually wake up.) However, should continued stimulation be necessary for adequate ventilation, endotracheal intubation should proceed.

If the patient requires restraint for intubation, sedation and, that failing, paralysis should precede intubation, as in Scenario 2.

PEDIATRIC CONSIDERATIONS

Airway management of poisoned children is very similar to adult management with a few special considerations. First, the efficacy of gastric lavage is unproven: nasogastric tubes larger than 28F cannot be used and smaller tubes are not as effective.[34] Simple aspiration of gastric contents and instillation of activated charcoal may be the best we can offer this group of patients. Second, the endotracheal tubes used in small children are not cuffed. Protection from aspiration therefore should not be assumed simply because the patent is intubated. Special considerations in pediatric airway techniques are discussed in Chapter 7.

PREHOSPITAL MANAGEMENT

Airway management in the prehospital setting presents additional challenges. Limited equipment, adverse conditions, and the need for transport complicate an already difficult procedure. Gastric decontamination should be avoided in the prehospital setting in which transport times are less than 30 minutes. Ipecac or charcoal could be considered in patients with a recent ingestion and prolonged transport time (>30 minutes). This should be done only after consultation with the on-line physician-advisor.

REFERENCES

1. Jacobsen D, Frederichsen PS, Knutsen KM, et al: Clinical course in acute self-poisonings: A prospective study of 1125 consecutive hospitalized adults. *Hum Toxicol* 1984; 3:107–116.
2. Bouknight RR, Alguire PC, Lofgren RP, et al: Self poisoning: Outcome and complications in the community hospital. *J Fam Pract* 1986; 23:223–225.
3. Goodman JM, Bischel MD, Wagers PW, et al: Barbiturate intoxication. Morbidity and mortality. *West J Med* 1976; 124:179.
4. Neilsen M, Henry J: Respiratory complications (ABC of poisoning). *Br Med J* 1984; 289:614–618.
5. Jay SJ, Johanson WG, Pierce AK: Respiratory complications of overdose with sedative drugs. *Am Rev Respir Dis* 1975; 112:591–598.
6. Taveira da Silva AM: Principles of respiratory therapy, in Goldfrank (ed): *Toxicologic Emergencies.* ed 3. Norwalk, Conn, Appleton-Century-Crofts, 1986, pp 00.
7. Eade NR, Taussig LM, Marks MI: Hydrocarbon pneumonitis. *Pediatrics* 1974; 54:351.
8. Silberman H, Davis SM, Lee A: Activated charcoal aspiration. *N C Med J* 1990; 51:79–80.
9. Bowers RE, Brigham KL, Owen PJ: Salicylate pulmonary edema: The mechanism in sheep and review of the clinical literature. *Am Rev Respir Dis* 1977; 115:261.
10. Thomas C, Gullmer HG: Adult respiratory distress syndrome in salicylate intoxication. *Lancet* 1979; 1:1294.
11. Silber R, Clerkin EP: Pulmonary edema in acute heroin poisoning. *Am J Med* 1959; 27:187.
12. Steinberg AD, Karliner J: The clinical spectrum of heroin pulmonary edema. *Arch Intern Med* 1968; 122:122.
13. Hill RN, Spragg RC, Wedel MK, et al: Adult respiratory distress syndrome associated with colchicine intoxication. *Ann Intern Med* 1975; 83:523.
14. Balk R, Bone RC: The adult respiratory distress syndrome. *Med Clin North Am* 1983; 67:685–700.

15. Glauser FL, Smith WR, Caldwell A, et al: Ethchlovynol (Placidyl) induced pulmonary edema. *Ann Intern Med* 1976; 84:46.
16. Presant S, Knought L, Klassen G: Methadone induced pulmonary edema. *Can Med Assoc J* 1975; 113:966.
17. Varnell RM, Godwin JD, Richardson ML, et al: Adult respiratory distress syndrome from overdose of tricyclic antidepressants. *Radiology* 1989; 170:667–670.
18. Fowler AA, Hamman RF, Good JT, et al: ARDS: risk with common predispositions. *Ann Intern Med* 1983; 98:593–597.
19. Pepe PE, Potkin RT, Reus DH, et al: Clinical predictors of ARDS. *Am J Surg* 1982; 144:124–128.
20. Fairshter RD, Wilson AF: Paraquat poisoning. *Am J Med* 1975; 59:751.
21. Raffin TA, Robin ED, Pickersgill J, et al: Paraquat ingestion and pulmonary injury. *West J Med* 1978; 128:26.
22. Smith P, Heath D: Paraquat lung: A reappraisal. *Thorax* 1974; 29:643.
23. Caplin M: Ammonia-gas poisoning: Forty seven cases in a London shelter. *Lancet* 1941; 2:95.
24. Levy DM, Divertie MB, Litzow TJ, et al: Ammonia burns of the face and respiratory tract. *JAMA* 1964; 190:873–876.
25. Flury KE, Dines DE, Rodarte JR, et al: Airway obstruction due to inhalation of ammonia. *Mayo Clin Proc* 1983; 58:389–393.
26. Reisz GR, Gammon RS: Toxic pneumonitis from mixing household cleaners. *Chest* 1986; 89:49–52.
27. Auerbach P, Osterloh J, Braun O, et al: Efficacy of gastric emptying: Gastric lavage vs emesis induced with Ipecac. *Ann Emerg Med* 1986; 15:692–698.
28. Curtis R, Barone J, Giacona N: Efficacy of ipecac and activated charcoal/cathartic. *Arch Intern Med* 1984; 144:48–52.
29. Tandberg D, Diven B, McLeod J: Ipecac induced emesis vs. gastric lavage. *Am J Emerg Med* 1986; 4:205–208.
30. Rumack BH: *POSINDEX Information System*. Denver, Micromedex Inc, 1990.
31. Kulig K, Bar-Or D, Cantrill S, et al: Management of acutely poisoned patients without gastric emptying. *Ann Emerg Med* 1985; 14:562–567.
32. Neuvonen P, Vartiainen M, Tokola O: Comparison of activated charcoal and ipecac in prevention of drug absorption. *Eur J Clin Pharmacol* 1983; 24:557–562.
33. Tenenbein M, Cohen S, Sitar D: Efficacy of ipecac induced emesis, orogastric lavage and activated charcoal for acute drug overdose. *Ann Emerg Med* 1987; 16:838–841.
34. Ellenhorn MJ, Barceloux DG (eds): *Medical Toxicology*, ed 1, New York, Elsevier Co, 1988.
35. Elliott CG, Colby TV, Hicks HG: Bronchiolitis obliterans after aspiration of activated charcoal. *Chest* 1989; 96:672–674.
36. Menzies DG, Busuttil A, Prescott LF: Fatal pulmonary aspiration of oral activated charcoal. *Br Med J* 1988; 207:450–451.
37. Pollack MM, Dunbar BS, Holbrook PR, et al: Aspiration of activated charcoal and gastric contents. *Ann Emerg Med* 1981; 10:528–529.
38. Litovitz TL, Schmitz BF, Holm KC: Annual report of the American Association of Poison Control Centers national data collection system. *Am J Emerg Med* 1989; 7:495–545.
39. Brayton RG, Stokes PE, Schwartz MS, et al: Effect of alcohol and various diseases on leukocyte mobilization, phagocytosis and intracellular bacterial killing. *N Engl J Med* 1970; 282:123.
40. Green GM: The Amberson lecture: In defense of the lung. *Am Rev Respir Dis* 1970; 102:691.
41. Newhouse M, Sanchis J, Bienenstock J: Lung defense mechanisms. *N Engl J Med* 1976; 295:990.
42. Dronen SC, Merigian KS, Hedges JR, et al: A comparison of blind nasotracheal and succinylcholine-assisted intubation in the poisoned patient. *Ann Emerg Med* 1987; 16:650–652.

32

Cardiac Pulmonary Edema

Kevin Hutton, M.D.

Peter Rosen, M.D.

Pulmonary edema is a common and critical problem in the practice of emergency medicine. Whatever its etiology, pulmonary edema can produce severe hypoxia. A difficult question is when to actively manage the airway. Although laboratory values are of little immediate value to this decision, they may be helpful over time as they reflect a response (or lack thereof) to therapy.

In this chapter, we discuss the issues of when and how to decide upon active airway management. We then present cases to illustrate the problems that need to be solved. The three scenarios to be discussed are (1) simple pulmonary edema (the stable patient), (2) pulmonary edema secondary to pump failure (the crashing patient), and (3) pulmonary edema complicated by renal failure (the crashed patient).

PATHOPHYSIOLOGY

The pathophysiologic mechanisms of pulmonary edema are not completely understood, but it is believed that changes in either the intravascular hydrostatic pressures, the plasma oncotic pressures, or the integrity of the pulmonary microvascular membrane are required for pulmonary edema to develop. The hypoxia of pulmonary edema develops from varying combinations of ventilation-perfusion mismatching, intrapulmonary shunting, bronchospasm, decreased lung compliance, and in some cases permanent parenchymal damage. To differentiate the pathophysiology, authors have categorized pulmonary edema into either permeability (membrane diffusion) edema or hemodynamic (cardiac pump failure)

edema.[1, 2] The focus of this chapter is on hemodynamic edema. Membrane diffusion edema is discussed in Chapter 30.

Hemodynamic pulmonary edema begins with progressive infiltration of edema fluid into the interstitial space and results in positional edema symptoms. The presence of orthopnea, paroxysmal nocturnal dyspnea, and cough is strongly suggestive of early interstitial hemodynamic pulmonary edema, but is usually elicited in the patient's history since upright positioning during transport to the hospital often may reverse the infiltration of edema fluid and thus the patient's symptoms. Recognition in this phase is important, however, as it will prompt interventions (rarely intubation) that will prevent interstitial hydrostatic pressure from exceeding alveolar pressure. If this early phase goes unrecognized, edema fluid will then move into the alveolar space. This later stage, termed *alveolar* or *flocculent pulmonary edema,* is much more serious, and often requires active airway management.[2]

Pulmonary edema of cardiac (pump) origin occurs in two major varieties: high-resistance pump overload, otherwise known as "simple" pulmonary edema, and muscle destruction pump failure, usually accompanying a large anterior wall myocardial infarction. The distinction between the two is that in high-resistance pulmonary edema, the problem originates outside the heart in the hypertensive (extrinsic) overload of the heart's musculature, whereas pump failure edema is intrinsic to the cardiac musculature.[2] While the final common pathway in both is hypoxia and inadequate tissue perfusion, the difference in mechanism is critical and leads to major differences in appropriate therapeutic strategies.

Pathophysiology of Simple (High-Resistance) Pulmonary Edema

In this form of pulmonary edema, the heart is overworked by the increased afterload created by systemic arterial hypertension. The cardiac output is inadequate, pulmonary hypertension ensues, edema fluid develops, and the right heart becomes overworked causing venous preload to increase.[1, 2] Progressive hypoxia occurs that will in turn have a negative effect on pump function, thus producing a cyclic worsening of the clinical picture. This type of edema requires therapies to unload the pump and reduce its workload allowing it to pump more effectively. Active airway control may be required to reverse the hypoxic stress on the myocardium while unloading therapies are allowed time to work.[3-5]

Pathophysiology of Pump Failure Pulmonary Edema

Pump failure edema requires therapies that will fix the pump directly.[3-5] Thus reperfusion with thrombolytic therapy, percutaneous angioplasty, or coronary artery bypass surgery will be needed to improve myocardial muscle function. As the myocardium receives more oxygen, the dyskinesia and ineffective cardiac output should improve and reverse the pump failure. If more than 50% of the left ventricle has been destroyed by ischemia, the pump failure will usually not be reversible without a new pump (cardiac transplantation).[2] Combined with myocardial muscle injury or death, there is often concomitant valve disease from arteriosclerotic cardiovascular disease or rheumatic valve disease that can affect the acuity with which pulmonary edema develops. In some of these pump failure patients, coronary artery reperfusion alone will be inadequate therapy, and the patient will also require valve replacement to overcome the pump failure.

Airway strategy for both forms of pulmonary edema is dependent upon improvement of oxygen delivery to the heart to bolster function while other therapies improve perfusion. But even in simple high-resistance pulmonary edema, oxygen delivery needs to be direct and active airway management may be required. In pump failure, the relief of the work of breathing may provide time to restore the myocardial perfusion. In most of these cases direct airway management is required.

Initially, patients in pulmonary edema compensate for the developing hypoxia by increasing the depth and rate of respiration and by using accessory muscles to overcome failing lung compliance. These mechanisms increase negative intrathoracic pressures, but eventually diaphragmatic and other respiratory muscles fatigue, secretions accumulate, compliance falls further, hypoxia worsens, and cardiac arrest occurs. Whatever the cause, there is established a vicious cycle of failing ventilation, increasing hypoxia, diminishing cardiac output, more hypoxia, more accumulation of secretions, and thus more failure of ventilation.[3-5]

Clinical Presentation of Simple Pulmonary Edema

The patient with simple pulmonary edema presents with hypertension (both by history and at the time of presentation), a gradual onset of dyspnea that worsens (usually in the middle of the night), tachycardia, and perhaps bubbling rales.[3-5] The patient may have coughing and bronchospasm that dominate the picture, but inspiration equals expiration and the cough is usually nonproductive. The jugular veins are distended, and there is often an S3 gallop. The upright chest film may reveal cephalization of the vasculature and perhaps Kerley's A, B, or C lines in early interstitial edema, and will progress to the classic "butterfly-shaped infiltrate" in alveolar edema.[6] These patients, while having laboratory evidence of hypoxia and a frightening clinical appearance, are not usually hypercarbic. The presence of hypercarbia in these patients, however, correlates with a worse outcome.[7] These patients most often respond to unloading therapies, and do not usually require intubation. For them, the indication for intubation is failure to respond to appropriate therapy.[3-5]

Clinical Presentation of Pump Failure Pulmonary Edema

The patient in pump failure edema presents in shock from inadequate perfusion. The blood pressure is low, heart sounds are faint, there is jugular venous distention, but the characteristic gallop rhythm may be obscured by rales and wheezes. Ischemic chest pain may dominate the clinical picture if myocardial infarction is the cause.[2] If these patients cannot be reperfused quickly and effectively, they will likely die. These patients require aggressive airway management.

When cardiac pulmonary edema is caused by congenital heart disease, or by valvular heart disease, the patient often presents in the same fashion as the patient with simple pulmonary edema. These patients present acutely with signs of an overloaded heart, and usually respond to direct cardiac unloading therapies. Their airways need to be actively managed only when they fail to respond to these therapies.

When pulmonary edema is caused by acute fluid overload, as in the patient with renal failure, the problem presents as acute volume overload as opposed to pump disease itself. These patients present with a history of progressive dyspnea and are often in severe ventilatory failure. These patients often require urgent dialysis to unload the heart, but will also require urgent airway management prior to dialysis.

Mechanical compression of the heart caused by tamponade or tension pneumothorax presents with shock but without pulmonary edema; it is best treated by relieving the mechanical compression. Simultaneous active airway management is often necessary to protect the patient while definitive therapeutic surgical procedures are being performed.

ASSESSMENT AND MONITORING

Rapid assessment of the patient in pulmonary edema must address the following points:

1. The patient's ability to protect the airway
2. Level of ventilatory fatigue present
3. Level of ventilatory compensation present
4. Level of hypoxia present
5. The measure needed to reverse the process

In fulminant pulmonary edema this assessment can often be accomplished by observation alone, but in the subacute presentation, assessment is often more difficult.

The patient's ability to protect the airway from aspiration can be ascertained by assessing cough and gag reflexes, and determining how well the edema-associated secretions are being handled. Patients in mild to moderate pulmonary edema may be able to protect their airway without much difficulty. In more severe cases, the patient will appear to be drowning in the secretions and require immediate intubation. Aspiration of gastric fluid is a concomitant serious problem that may need to be prevented by early intubation with cricoid pressure.[8, 9]

The amount of ventilatory fatigue present and the amount of ventilatory compensation remaining is determined primarily by bedside examination. A brief history is helpful and key points to elicit include the duration of symptoms; presence of orthopnea; presence of paroxysmal nocturnal dyspnea; presence of cough; a past medical history of hypertension, heart, or renal disease; and response to therapy at home. Important points on physical examination to look for include the degree of accessory muscle use, presence of retractions, presence of abdominal breathing, and airway patency. Trends in respiratory rate, pulse, and mental status can also be helpful as a progressive decrease in respiratory rate or pulse after tachypnea, or a decreased mental status are highly predictive of the need for intubation. The ability of the patient to count numbers without taking a breath or the number of words a patient can vocalize between breaths are also useful clinical methods for assessing and monitoring the level of ventilatory distress and for predicting when intubation is imminent.

Laboratory values and pulse oximetry have little utility in the fulminant presentation, but in the mild to moderate presentation can be a valuable means of assessing the level of ventilatory compromise. Factoring these data into the clinical picture allows the patient's level of fatigue to be accurately estimated and allows for a gestalt prediction of how much continued hypoxia the patient can tolerate.

Clinical determination of the level of hypoxia without laboratory data can be difficult. Cyanosis is one indication of severe hypoxia, but is not present if oxygen therapy is being provided. Severely anemic patients in pulmonary edema may not have enough desaturated hemoglobin to be clinically cyanotic. Pulse oximetry is a very useful tool for assessing hypoxia, if one remembers that the oxygen saturation curve is sigmoidal and that small changes in saturation from 95% to 90% represent large changes in partial pressure of oxygen (PO_2). Pulse oximetry does not monitor hypercarbia, and desaturation is often a late indicator of the need for intubation. Arterial blood gas (ABG) analysis is the most accurate means of determining the level of hypoxia, but this determination is more useful in the patient who is not responding to therapy. In general, a patient with a PO_2 less than 50 mm Hg, a partial pressure of carbon dioxide (PCO_2) greater than 50 mm Hg, or a saturation of arterial blood with oxygen (SaO_2) less than 90% is severely compromised and in need of intubation. In the decompensated severe pulmonary edema patient, ABG analysis is reserved for postintubation management.

The critical decision to be made from the initial assessment is whether to initiate therapy to break the cycle or to proceed directly to intubation. The results of ABG analysis, peak expiratory flow, spirometry, and chest radiographic studies should be utilized in the assessment of the stable patient. In the unstable, failing patient, however, immediate control of the airway is the priority. In this setting the emergency physician must act on only the initial bedside clinical assessment of the patient.[8, 9] Again, close observation of the patient's level of fatigue, the level of change in mental status, the trends in vital signs, as well as the vocal counting of numbers and words between breaths are the best predictors of the need for immediate intubation.

An algorithm for airway management of pulmonary edema is presented in Figure 32–1.

TREATMENT

Therapy for pulmonary edema must be individualized, but the overall goals are similar in every case, no matter the cause: integrity of airflow, improved oxygenation and ventilation, and protection of the airway from aspiration (the three pillars of airway management). Current therapy includes supplemental oxygen, vasodilatation with nitrates, diuretics, and morphine.[10–12] The calcium channel blocker nifedipine is an excellent afterload reducer in the hypertensive pulmonary edema patient. Naloxone is indicated in opiate-induced pulmonary edema.[3] Additional beneficial treatments in the acute setting are continuous positive airway pressure

(CPAP), or in the intubated patient, positive end-expiratory pressure (PEEP).[13, 14] CPAP is particularly useful when a patient requests not to be intubated and requires only temporary support to reverse the disease process.[14] Bronchodilatation is often needed since bronchospasm can and often does accompany any cause of pulmonary edema. Phlebotomy has been recommended in the past, but presents logistic problems in practice. The volume of blood necessary to reduce intravascular volume significantly is time-consuming to remove and may result in detrimental anemia. Currently hemodialysis is the preferred method of fluid removal. Rotating tourniquets have been recommended in the past, but have proved to be ineffective and possibly detrimental.[15, 16]

INTUBATION

Once the decision to intubate has been made, the patient should be preoxygenated using a nonrebreathing face mask. Spontaneous methods of preoxygenation minimize the gastric insufflation of air seen with assisted methods.[8, 9, 17] Bag-valve preoxygenation devices should always be used in conjunction with cricoid pressure to control gastric dilatation and minimize the risk of aspiration when spontaneous methods fail or are inappropriate.[8, 9, 17] During preoxygenation, intubation and suction equipment should be prepared and tested, intubation drugs and cricothyrotomy equipment should be

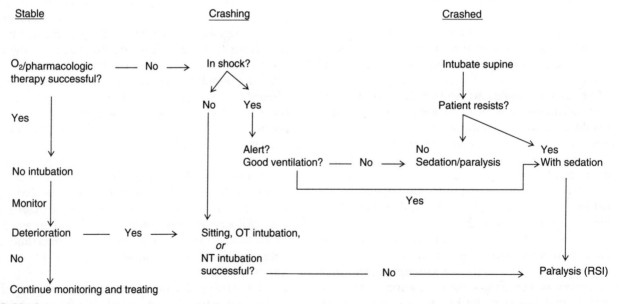

FIG 32–1.
Algorithm for airway management in pulmonary edema. *OT* = orotracheal; *NT* = nasotracheal; *RSI* = rapid-sequence induction.

brought to the bedside, and the operator should mentally rehearse the airway management plan as well as alternative plans to be used if the initial plan fails. Aggressive medical therapy should be instituted simultaneously, but should not delay intubation. To limit complications, intubation must be done as a deliberate, well-planned, and well-executed procedure.

Methods of intubation should be individualized to the patient's condition and to the cause of the pulmonary edema. Nasotracheal intubation should be used for patients who are breathing spontaneously, but intubation by this method becomes more difficult as the depth of respiration diminishes. Nasotracheal intubation is generally not utilized in patients who are apneic; recently, however, a method of blind nasotracheal intubation in the apneic patient using a flexible lighted stylet has been described.[18] Liberal use of lidocaine jelly along with phenylephrine, dilatation of the nostril, sedation, and proper technique are the keys to successful intubation by this method.[8, 9, 17] Orotracheal intubation in the supine position for the patient in hemodynamic pulmonary edema may not be tolerated easily, but this does not preclude supine oral intubation, even in the fulminant presentation. In these patients it may be necessary to use a rapid-sequence induction technique prior to intubation. Sedation must be done cautiously in these patients since it may precipitate cardiac arrest by exacerbating hypoxia. Oral intubation is often preferable to nasal intubation because it allows use of a larger tube that facilitates better suctioning and secretion control. In the combative, hypoxic patient, paralysis is often also required, though these patients are severely fatigued and may tolerate intubation without drugs. Appropriate sedation is desirable since paralytic agents have no effect on consciousness.

Recently, an alternative method of oral intubation with the patient in the seated position has been described.[19] This technique is performed with the operator standing behind and leaning over the patient. It would appear that this method will be useful in this setting, perhaps as the initial procedure of choice.

Continuous cricoid pressure should be applied in all cases to minimize the risk of aspiration, to help in vocal cord visualization, and as a tactile method of endotracheal tube placement verification. Preoxygenation before, and continuous oxygen saturation monitoring during, intubation are prudent. Suction should be used as needed. Once the endotracheal tube is passed through the cords, the cuff is inflated, and 100% oxygen is again applied. The endotracheal tube position must then be verified by multiple clinical methods. Auscultation is unreliable as the sole method of endotracheal tube confirmation because breath sounds may be diminished by the poor compliance and edema fluid. Additional verification methods and a portable chest film should be used for confirmation.[20] If intubation attempts via nasal or oral routes are unsuccessful, the emergency physician must be prepared psychologically as well as technically to perform a surgical airway.[8, 9, 17] Arterial blood gas analysis, radiograph studies, and suctioning of the lower respiratory tract should be done once the tube position is verified.

PEDIATRIC CONSIDERATIONS

Diagnosis and management of pulmonary edema in the pediatric population can be a unique challenge to the emergency physician. It is often complicated by difficulties in clinical assessment. Subtle historical and physical examination findings are usually present, e.g., the heart sounds may be difficult to hear when a normal heart rate is 120 to 140 beats per minute.[21] The relatively infrequent occurrence of pulmonary edema in the pediatric population also make it an entity that is often overlooked in the differential diagnosis of pediatric respiratory disorders. When it does occur, however, it can be classified into similar pathophysiologic categories as for the adult and treated in a similar fashion. True fluid overload pulmonary edema is likely to be iatrogenic in the pediatric patient, but can occur with associated cardiac or renal disease. Congenital heart disease, which occurs in 8 in 1,000 babies, is the most common cause of pediatric pulmonary edema.[22]

Technical constraints in the child, such as differences in anatomy, intubation technique, medication dosages, and methods of oxygen delivery, are important and need to be noted. In general, pediatric intubation up to age 10 years is best accomplished via the oral route using a straight laryngoscope blade. After age 10 a curved blade is more useful.[8, 9, 17] Premedication with atropine and appropriate sedation are also wise. Positive pressure ventilation is useful, but the potential for barotrauma should be monitored closely.[15] Pulse oximetry is prudent though the oximeter may not sense well with extremely fast heart rates, hypotension, or when hypothermia occurs concurrently.

PREHOSPITAL CONSIDERATIONS

The treatment of pulmonary edema in the prehospital environment is dependent upon the skill and judgment of the prehospital care providers. Information such as the patient's location, the distance to the hospital, the technician's level of training and experience, the operational protocols, and the destination policies of the emergency medical services must be factored into treatment decisions. A system with basic emergency medical technicians (EMTs) may best serve the patient by providing oxygen therapy, proper positioning, and rapid transport, whereas advanced life support systems can provide oxygen therapy, cardiac monitoring, nitrates, morphine, nebulized β-adrenergic agonists, and intravenous furosemide. The technician should determine the duration of the symptoms, the patient's ability to speak, the use of accessory muscles, and the level of consciousness. Active airway intervention should be performed on most patients who have changes in mental status or who are unable to utter more than three or four words between breaths. Assisted ventilation can be performed by basic EMTs, and intubation can be performed in paramedical systems. Most advanced life support (ALS) systems are limited to oral tracheal intubation in the supine position, but a few prehospital systems allow awake nasotracheal intubation by paramedical workers. Supine positioning may not be tolerated by some patients and sedation with diazepam may be useful if operating protocols permit its use. A reasonable attempt at intubation should be performed, but excessive delays in transport and iatrogenic complications should be avoided.

The chief difficulty in the field is correct diagnosis. Since acute superimposed on chronic respiratory failure is easy to confuse with pulmonary edema of cardiac origin, many patients in pulmonary edema receive the wrong diagnosis of asthma or COPD. Conversely, many emphysematous patients are misdiagnosed as having pulmonary edema. The paramedic and, in turn, the medical command should not focus upon wheezing, but rather place it in the context of the overall findings. An octagenarian who presents with wheezing is unlikely to be having an acute first episode of asthma. Conversely, a patient who has been on home oxygen, steroids, theophylline, and nebulizers is unlikely to be having acute pulmonary edema. Age, history, and the physical examination findings are all critical to accurate assessment, but when in doubt it is better to opt for supplemental oxygen and rapid transportation to the emergency department rather than try to sort things out in the field. When the clinical picture is confused, and the patient is not in severe distress, withholding potentially harmful treatments such as morphine may be prudent. If the patient is wheezing, nebulizer treatment will be helpful regardless of the cause of the respiratory disease. Even in respiratory failure, oxygen in high volumes is safe so long as the patient can be stimulated and one is prepared to intubate if necessary. Most patients take time to get into trouble, and in most instances can be gotten out of trouble in a measured rather than a precipitous fashion.

The following case scenarios illustrate the appropriate "three-pillar" management of patients presenting with varying types and degrees of hypoxia from pulmonary edema.

Scenario 1: The Stable Patient

This patient has interstitial or early alveolar pulmonary edema; is hypertensive; and will usually present in the middle of the night with a history of paroxysmal nocturnal dyspnea, orthopnea, and dry hacking cough. The patient will be alert, and respirations will be labored but strong. The airway is patent and protected. This patient can generally speak in phrases or short sentences. The patient is anxious but otherwise normal in mentation.

Other clinical findings, such as ABG values and chest films are highly variable and correlate poorly with bedside clinical appearance. These patients are usually only mildly hypoxic (initial pulse oximeter saturations are usually above 90%), but are seldom severely hypercarbic. They usually respond well to intravenous (IV) furosemide, sublingual nitroglycerin, oral or sublingual nifedipine, morphine IV, and continuous oxygen unless cardiogenic shock or renal failure is coincident.

Oxygen therepy consists routinely of 3 to 4 L/min of oxygen administered by nasal cannula. In most cases this will bring oxygen saturation to levels well above 90%. If, however, it does not, one is entering the domain of the "crashing" patient (see below).

Scenario 2: The Crashing Patient

The crashing patient is severely dyspneic and tachypneic, has labored breathing, is diaphoretic from the work of breathing and increased sympathetic outflow, has prominent use of accessory muscles and retractions, can utter only one to three words in succession, and may have frothy avleolor fluid at the lips. *Additionally, and most significantly, observable respiratory exhaustion and beginning lethargy hail the termination of this phase; these are the classic indicators of acute and rapidly progressive ventilatory failure.*

If the patient presents initially with this appearance, one may be able, by virtue of aggressive IV drug administration, to save the day without intubation. The decision not to intubate under these circumstances requires very sophisticated and refined clinical judgment. If one miscalculates, the patient progresses to further hypoxia, hypercarbia, metabolic and ventilatory acidoses, and cardiopulmonary arrest. The patient is then seldom resuscitable. On the other hand, if immediate intubation is attempted in such patients, it may not only be unnecessary but one may confidently anticipate that it will be difficult, time-consuming, and, just possibly, unsuccessful! This "damned-if-you-do, damned-if-you-don't" situation is simply part of any life-threatening emergency condition. A cool head, steady hands, and measured clinical judgment are necessary. The worst possible error here is to wait for the patient to become moribund or to arrest before intubating: better to intubate the difficult patient than the dead patient!

If the initially stable patient deteriorates to a crashing configuration despite all possible IV medications and oxygen therapy, then intubation should be carried out at the earliest possible moment. Procrastination at this juncture is inexcusable! The cycle of respiratory failure aggravating myocardial function and metabolic status aggravating, in turn, respiratory failure is not reversible without external ventilatory support. The clinical direction is inexorably downward, and interventions short of intubation and mechanical intervention have failed.

Nasotracheal intubation is generally the technique of choice if the patient is reasonably cooperative and can wait the 3 to 5 minutes necessary for local anesthesia of the nose and pharynx. One must also keep in mind that this blind technique has a failure rate of 10% to 20% (use of the lighted stylet is highly advisable to decrease this failure rate). Can the patient tolerate several passes with the tube? The trauma of the procedure? Epistaxis? The time lost if the procedure does not go smoothly? If this elegant technique goes smoothly, it is highly gratifying to both patient and physician: the tube is comfortable, stable, and allows alimentation.

If nasotracheal intubation is not elected for any of the above reasons, sitting orotracheal intubation may be a very suitable alternative. All emergency physicians are familiar with the basic technique of oral intubation, and sitting intubation is little different. Unfortunately, few physicians have attempted this procedure, so there is no body of clinical experience. Theoretically, it should share the high success rate and low complication rate of supine orotracheal intubation.

If the above methods are not appropriate or are unsuccessful, crash supine orotracheal intubation must be performed. If the patient effectively resists the procedure, sedation or paralysis, or both, will be necessary. If such is the case, one must be careful to administer sufficient doses of sedating and paralyzing drugs *the first time*. There is not enough time for a stepwise approach!

Scenario 3: The Crashed Patient

The crashed patient is defined by the need for immediate intubation; gross hypoxia, hypercarbia, and acidosis. If the patient has not already aspirated, there is a grave risk of doing so. The patient is about to die. The clinical status runs the short gamut from (a) the lower end of the crashing scenario to (b) apnea or near-apnea with palpable pulses, to (c) full cardiopulmonary arrest. Bradycardia and bradypnea are the rule, as is hypotension. The crashed patient has major alterations in consciousness; at best he or she is lethargic and disorientated; at worst, comatose. The patient is unable to cooperate, and may be frankly combative, often resisting procedures such as venous access and intubation.

Immediate intubation is, of course, mandatory. Preventilation with bag-mask and 100% oxygen should be attempted for only as long as it takes to assemble the intubation equipment. Supine orotracheal intubation is the fastest and surest method to establish a protected airway and initiate ventilatory support. If the patient is unable to resist intubation, of course, no sedation-paralysis is needed. If combative behavior prevents initial attempts, rapid-sequence measures should follow without hesitation. Hand-compressed, bag ventilation with 100% oxygen should follow, and ventilator support as soon thereafter as possible (see Appendix for settings). One then must not forget to return the patient to a sitting position (if not in shock).

Several complicating factors have their own special management considerations that must not be lost sight of in the rush to treat the airway. If the patient is in renal failure, dialysis will likely be necessary to relieve the pulmonary edema; therefore those arrangements should be made at the moment renal failure is identified. If the pulmonary edema is associated with acute myocardial infarction, one needs to consider immediate thrombolytic therapy and cardiology consultation. Finally, in the event of cardiogenic shock, intubation should be undertaken relatively early, and pressors administered.

REFERENCES

1. Haupt MT, Carlson RW: Permeability pulmonary edema and the adult respiratory distress syndrome, in Tintanalli JE, Krome RL, Ruiz E (eds): *Emergency Medicine: A Comprehensive Study Guide*, ed 2. New York, McGraw-Hill Book Co, 1988.

2. Stirling EL: Congestive heart failure, in Rosen P, Baker FJ, Barkin RM, et al (eds): *Emergency Medicine Concepts and Clinical Practice* ed 2. St Louis, Mosby–Year Book, Inc, 1988, pp 1291–1301.

3. Bernard GR, Brigham KL: Pulmonary edema: Pathophysiologic mechanisms and new approaches to therapy. *Chest* 1986: 4:493–594.

4. Guntupalli KK: Acute pulmonary edema. *Cardiol Clin* 1984; 2:183–199.

5. Goldberger JJ, Peled HB, Stroh JA, et al: Prognostic factors in acute pulmonary edema. *Arch Intern Med* 1986; 147:489–493.

6. Robin ED, Cross CE, Zelis R: Pulmonary edema, parts 1 and 2. *N Engl J Med* 1973; 288:239, 292.

7. Aberman A, Fulop M: The metabolic and respiratory acidosis of acute pulmonary edema. *Ann Intern Med* 1972; 76:173.

8. Jordan RC: Airway management. *Emerg Med Clin North Am* 1988; 6:671–686.

9. Kastendieck J: Airway management, in Rosen P, Baker FJ, Barker RM, et al (eds): *Emergency Medicine Concepts and Clinical Practice*, ed 2. St Louis, Mosby–Year Book, Inc, 1988, pp 41–68.

10. Vismara LA, Leaman DM, Zelis R: The effects of morphine on venous tone in patients with acute pulmonary edema. *Circulation* 1976; 2:335–337.

11. Bussman WD, Schupp D: Effects of sublingual nitroglycerin in emergency treatment of severe pulmonary edema. *Am J Cardiol* 1978; 5:931–936.

12. Frazier HS, Yager H: The clinical use of diuretics, part 2. *N Engl J Med* 1973; 288:455–457.

13. Pepe PE, Hudson LD, Carrico CJ: Early application of positive end-expiratory pressure in patients at risk for the adult respiratory distress syndrome. *N Engl J Med* 1984; 5:281–286.

14. Covelli HD, Weled BJ, Beekman JF: Efficacy of continuous positive airway pressure administered by face mask. *Chest* 1982; 2:147–149.

15. Roth A, Hochenberg M, Keren G, et al: Are rotating tourniquets useful for left ventricular preload reduction in patients with acute myocardial infarction and heart failure? *Ann Emerg Med* 1987; 7:764–767.

16. Bertel O, Steiner A: Rotating tourniquets do not work in acute congestive heart failure and pulmonary edema (letter). *Lancet* 1980; 5:762.

17. Hochbaum SR: Emergency airway management. *Emerg Med Clin North Am* 1986; 3:411–425.

18. Verdile VP, Chiang JL, Bedger R, et al: Nasotracheal intubation using a flexible lighted stylet. *Ann Emerg Med* 1990; 5:506–510.

19. Fontanarosa PB, Goldman GE, Polsky SS: Sitting oral-tracheal intubation. *Ann Emerg Med* 1988; 4:336–338.

20. Cheny FW, Posner K, Caplan RA, et al: Standards of care and anesthesia liability. *JAMA* 1989; 261:1599–1603.

21. Fleischer G, Ludwig S: Pulmonary emergencies, in *Pediatric Emergency Medicine*, ed 2. Baltimore, Williams & Wilkins Co, 1988, pp 675–676.

22. Brookfield EG: Guest presentation. Childhood cardiac emergencies, part 1. *PREM Educ Rev* February 1991, pp 15–17.

33

Grand Mal Seizures

Robert H. Dailey, M.D.

Major motor seizures are morbid events. The estimated death rate for sudden unexplained seizures is 1 in 500 to 1,000 epileptic patients per year.[1] There are many possible causes of death, but since death is almost always medically unobserved, precise causation is hard to determine. Some deaths may be related to the underlying disease process that caused the seizure, e.g., meningitis, brain tumor, subdural hematoma, etc. Many deaths have been shown at post mortem to be due to acute pulmonary edema. In one study, 42 of 52 patients had significant pulmonary edema.[1] In another study involving young adults, 8 of 8 patients had pulmonary edema. In most cases, however, pulmonary edema is probably only one of a number of contributing events. Multiple metabolic and other derangements occur during and following seizures: marked adrenergic discharge, decreased cardiac output, hyperthermia, upper airway obstruction secondary to secretions and tongue laxity, severe hypoxia, lactic and ventilatory acidoses, associated toxic overdoses (especially cocaine), and head trauma sustained during the seizure. This chapter concerns itself primarily with the problems related specifically to airway and breathing; these are discussed further in the scenarios below.

A seizure begins with a momentary aura, followed immediately by loss of consciousness, tonic rigidity of all muscles for less than 1 minute, then rhythmic clonic muscular jerking for 1 or more minutes. In the immediate postictal phase all skeletal muscles are flaccid, and the urinary sphincter frequently relaxes (the anal sphincter less frequently). The duration of postictal lethargy and confusion depends on the duration, intensity, and number of immediately antecedent seizures: it is usually minutes, only rarely hours, and tends to be constant in a given patient. Rarely a seizure is not self-limited and either recurs during the postictal period or becomes continuous. These situations define status epilepticus, the most malignant of our scenarios. Status epilepticus carries a mortality rate of 10% to 50%.[3] Therefore special attention is given in this chapter to this scenario.

The scenarios for discussion are (1) the presumed isolated seizure, (2) the postictal state, and (3) status epilepticus. An algorithm for airway management of these patients is presented in Figure 33–1.

SCENARIOS

The Presumed Isolated Seizure Scenario

When faced with an actively seizing patient, it is usually clear to an emergency medical technician (EMT) or bystander whether the seizure is isolated or part of status epilepticus. If isolated, only supportive measures are indicated, since one anticipates that the seizure will terminate spontaneously in less than a minute or two. Even so, limited active treatment is necessary.

There are a number of threats to airflow. Firstly, the teeth are clenched and the lips pursed, limiting air intake through the mouth. Indeed, if there is any significant degree of concomitant nasal obstruction, air intake may be critically impaired. Secondly, oropharyngeal blood may be present from tongue chewing. Such bleeding is usually minimal since the tip or lateral borders of the tongue are generally only contused. However, rarely the tongue may be severely lacerated; this occurs if the tongue was protruded when the head struck the ground at the onset of the seizure. Such a laceration can produce brisk, even tumultuous, bleeding if the lingual artery

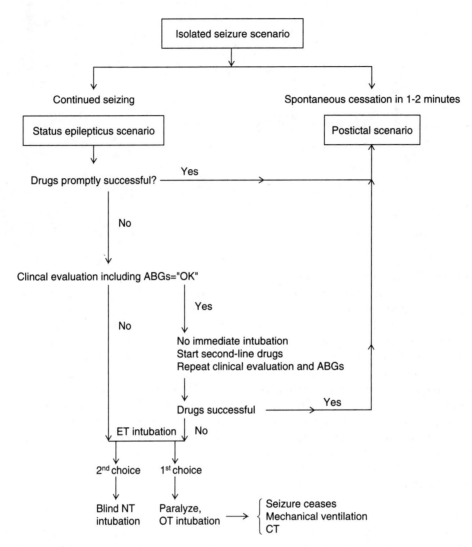

FIG 33–1.
Algorithm for airway management in grand mal seizures. *ABGs* = arterial blood gases; *ET* = endotracheal; *NT* = nasotracheal; *OT* = oro-tracheal; *CT* = computed tomography.

has been lacerated. Thirdly, saliva adds its measure of obstruction, since the seizing patient cannot swallow it. Fourthly, if the patient is supine, the tongue obstructs the posterior oropharynx.

Aspiration is probably not a major accompaniment of active seizing. It is not described in two large series discussing status epilepticus.[4, 5] This might be surprising if one did not consider the physiology: the actively seizing patient simply cannot neurologically produce the complex coordinated act of retching. Although regurgitation of stomach contents can occur, it is apparently rare. The volume of blood-tinged saliva usually present is small and not acidic, so it poses relatively little threat as an aspirate. Rarely, a tooth or fragment thereof may be loosed into the airway by a seizure; this threat should at least be considered and sought.

One would expect ventilation and oxygenation to be impaired during a single motor seizure, since both the diaphragm and accessory respiratory muscles are contracting spasmodically and rapidly. Are such "panting" respirations ineffectual? One study examined arterial blood gases (ABGs) in eight patients 0 to 4 minutes following a single seizure.[6] The mean partial pressure of carbon dioxide (PCO_2) was 45 mm Hg (range: 31–65 mm Hg). This is a slender database, but suggests that a severe and prolonged seizure can produce significant hypoventilation. In this study individual partial pressure of oxygen values (PO_2) were not reported (nor their range) and there was no information regarding oxygen administration; these omissions make it impossible to assess the presence of hypoxemia in this study. However, in those instances in which upper airway obstruction

(UAO) and hypoventilation coexist, hypoxemia is indeed likely to be present. Certainly, digital oximetry is warranted to quickly assess the matter.

Management

Airway treatment for the presumed isolated seizure is simple and supportive. Since the teeth are clenched, oral secretions are usually not accessible to suctioning. Nonetheless, external oral suctioning might be worthwhile, and sometimes tonsillar or catheter suctioning of the oropharynx is possible despite teeth clenching. The risk of epistaxis from nasopharyngeal suctioning may outweigh its possible benefit. Turning the seizing patient on his side (yes, it is possible) and administering a jaw thrust usually suffices to overcome tongue obstruction. Should a dental screw or some other such device be used to open the mouth to decrease airway obstruction and allow tonsillar suction to be used? Certainly a theoretical case can be made for such a maneuver, but I believe that (1) it is technically difficult to perform in the rigid and jerking patient, and (2) by the time one completes this action, the seizure has terminated anyway. The insertion of a nasopharyngeal trumpet should be considered; it can improve nasal patency, overcome tongue obstruction, and even provide a safe portal for nasopharyngeal suctioning. If properly lubricated and gently inserted, the risks of epistaxis are minimal. It can also provide ongoing airway protection in the postictal period.

To best prevent aspiration from regurgitation, the torso should probably be slightly elevated, though this is unproven (see Chapter 2). Suctioning of blood and saliva has been mentioned above. A dental and oropharyngeal examination to exclude dental fragments should accompany the search for a chewed or lacerated tongue in the immediate postictal period. In the rare event of voluminous tongue bleeding, immediate suturing is necessary. This can be done without medication if the patient is comatose postictally, but more often local (and possibly parenteral) analgesia would be needed.

Ventilation and oxygenation are relatively easily attended to. Should one assist ventilation with nasopharyngeal airway and bag-valve-mask? If the seizure is of short duration it is probably neither practicable nor necessary. However, if the seizure is prolonged, it may be advisable, although it may be difficult to achieve a good face-to-mask seal secondary to sweat and froth; also, it may be hard to ventilate adequately in the face of spasmodic respiratory movements. Unquestionably, however, supplemental O_2 should be given: it cannot hurt, may help, and is easy to administer by nasal cannula or mask. If severe hypoxemia is demonstrated by oximetry, a nonrebreathing mask should be used.

The Postictal Scenario

Upon cessation of the last clonic jerks of a seizure, the patient takes several gasping respirations, then appears to hyperventilate, presumably in response to ventilatory and lactic acidoses. Voluntary and reflex muscle activity rapidly returns and the level of consciousness improves. Lactic acidosis clears in about 1 hour if liver function is intact.[6] Fever secondary to muscle hyperactivity is present in almost half of patients, is probably proportional to the severity and duration of the seizure, and may last up to 2 days.[7]

Management

If the patient returns to consciousness in a matter of minutes, the airway precautions taken in the first scenario (active seizing) will well satisfy our three pillars of airway management. However, in those instances in which postictal lethargy persists for many minutes or hours, greater vigilance is necessary: regular checks for oral bleeding and secretions, assessments of vital signs and mental status, and assurance of airway patency. The patient should be kept on his or her side (best supported front and back with pillows), with side rails up and the nasopharyngeal airway in place.

The risk of vomiting and aspiration should be small unless (1) the mental status remains depressed, and (2) there is some underlying cause for emesis. Fortunately, this combination of events is rare.

Although hyperpnea and tachypnea are commonly observed in the immediate postictal period, the expected alveolar hyperventilation has not been confirmed in the one study that examined it. Orringer et al.[6] found a mean PCO_2 of 39 mm Hg 15 minutes postictally in their eight patients, but at least one patient's PCO_2 was above 50 mm Hg during the entire hour of study.[6] Whether this patient had a concomitant ventilatory problem is unknown. However, it seems unlikely that hypoventilation should extend so late into the postictal period, and it would not square with the hyperpnea and tachypnea commonly seen. Though hypoxemia was not documented by Orringer et al., supplemental O_2 could not help but improve the metabolic milieu for the recovering brain.

One must be alert to one special circumstance in the postictal patient. A particular series of changing breathing patterns developing in the first 15 to 20 minutes of observation suggests acute increased intracranial pressure (ICP) with brainstem compression affecting central nervous system (CNS) respiratory control. One should look for the temporal sequence of, first, marked central hyperventilation, then Cheyne-Stokes respirations, then ataxic (irregular) breathing, and finally *apnea*. These abnormal respiratory patterns mandate intervention (intubation) before apnea occurs (especially since apnea in the nonintubated patient reliably happens in the computed tomography [CT] suite). If nasotracheal intubation is performed, the patient should be premedicated with intravenous (IV) lidocaine and a rapid-acting barbiturate to mitigate increased ICP (see Chapter 24). Otherwise, the patient can be paralyzed and intubated orotracheally (see Status Epilepticus below). A "stat" CT must be performed to rule out treatable causes of increased ICP. Also, the patient must be hyperventilated, to diminish brain volume (see Chapter 24).

Status Epilepticus Scenario

For our purposes, *status epilepticus* may be defined as continuous major motor seizure activity or as discrete seizures occurring within minutes of one another. This condition entrains major problems with airway and breathing.

All of the factors (described above) causing airway obstruction during a single seizure are, of course, operative in status epilepticus: decreased airflow through the mouth, blood and saliva in the oropharynx, and obstructing tongue. However, as opposed to the situation of a single seizure, in status epilepticus these factors persist and so are far more threatening. As during single seizures, aspiration should not pose a major problem in status epilepticus.

Although the data of Orringer et al. for ventilation and oxygenation in single seizures were largely inconclusive, Aminoff and Simon provide us with a clearer picture in status epilepticus.[4] ABG samples were obtained in 70 patients in status epilepticus. Thirty (43%) were hypoventilating, and the PCO_2 of almost half of those 30 patients exceeded 60 mm Hg! PO_2 data were not provided, but hypoxemia should be assumed.

Management

In considering airway control in status epilepticus one needs to take a broader look at the threats to the brain. It has been demonstrated that the metabolic abnormalities consequent to major motor activity are more devastating to the brain than the uncon-

trolled electrical discharges of the seizure.[8] Thus, for metabolic as well as airflow and ventilation considerations, the major skeletal muscle contractions must be promptly terminated. It is difficult to say with precision how quickly status epilepticus must be controlled, but a sensible clinical approach can be outlined (see Fig 33–1). First, all the measures for airway management of the presumed single seizure are instituted. Then the routine initial IV medications (thiamine, glucose, lorazepam [Ativan], or diazepam [Valium]) are administered; they will control the seizure activity very promptly in the majority of cases, and we revert then to our postictal scenario. However, if these drugs are *not* immediately successful, major additional measures become necessary.

Phenytoin (Dilantin) and phenobarbital are begun, but these will take some 20 to 30 minutes to become fully effective. It is then crucial to assess the clinical, metabolic, and ventilation-oxygenation status of the patient, i.e., check for hypotension, high fever, and dysrhythmias, and obtain ABG samples. *Any of these clinical situations or the alarming combination of lactic acidosis, hypoxemia, hypoventilation, and ventilatory acidosis mandates immediate endotracheal (ET) intubation and active ventilation and oxygenation.* In effect, this means rapid-sequence orotracheal (OT) intubation with succinylcholine followed by pancuronium (Pavulon) paralysis. Special care to secure a biteblock is necessary, because as paralysis wears off and seizures return, one may be witness to the excruciating spectacle of an ET tube being at once occluded and rendered unremovable by firmly clenched teeth! Blind or lighted nasotracheal (NT) intubation can be entertained. However, the guiding airstream is either impaired or absent; the danger from epistaxis is augmented by the impossibility of adequate oropharyngeal suctioning; and NT intubation is subject to some measure of increased ICP—an added insult to an already injured brain. Also, paralysis and OT intubation confer other advantages: the motor activity of the seizure is completely terminated; one can immediately ensure adequate mechanical ventilation and oxygenation; one can, if necessary, hyperventilate the patient to produce brain shrinkage and so decrease ICP; and the patient is rendered motionless for CT scanning. It is probably advisable to allow the pancuronium to wear off (about 45 minutes) after the CT scan so that one can assess mental status and seizure activity, both of which, of course, will be masked by paralysis. Also, by this time the phenobarbital and phenytoin regimen may have terminated the brain discharges, and one does not wish a patient to return to consciousness while paralyzed. If the patient is seen to be still seizing, pancuronium can be readministered, etc.

What is done with the patient who continues to seize after drug therapy, but who has acceptable clinical signs and ABG values? This patient is probably safe to support without intubation until such time as secondary drugs (phenobarbital, phenytoin, ?lidocaine, ?valproic acid, ?paraldehyde, etc.) have failed or in whom repeat clinical signs and ABG values have deteriorated. But intubation must be performed eventually for airway protection, as in all cases of prolonged unconsciousness.

GRAND MAL SEIZURES: PEDIATRIC PERSPECTIVE*

The presentation of major motor seizures in children is similar to that in adults. The exception to this lies primarily with the neonate, who produces significantly different manifestations than those seen in an adult or older child. Because the neonate's subcortical structures are more mature than the cortex, the neonate's seizures are manifested more by respiratory abnormalities, chewing, ocular signs, tone changes, and focal motor twitching.

For the isolated seizure in a child, little more than supportive care is indicated. Most often the isolated seizure is secondary to a febrile illness and lasts only a few minutes. The patient requires a workup for infection or metabolic disorders; however, if this workup is negative, the seizure often goes untreated.

Airway management for the isolated seizure in a child is similar to that for the isolated seizure in the adult, with the exception that nasopharyngeal airways in the child must be used with caution because of abundant adenoidal tissue and the possibility of airway trauma. Oxygen is always indicated, if available. Positive pressure ventilation during the seizure is difficult at best, and in the young child often leads to gastric distention.

The postictal state should be relatively uneventful after an isolated seizure. If the seizure is prolonged and treated with antiepileptic agents, the postictal state often is modified by neurologic depression secondary to drug therapy. Frequently the use of phenobarbital in combination with a benzodiazepine may lead to significant depression of consciousness and respiratory compromise.

Since the child's history may be uncertain because of events transpiring during unsupervised

---

play, a high index of suspicion of an underlying head injury should be maintained in all cases. In addition, nonaccidental trauma should always be suspected and would not be confirmed on routine history taking.

If the patient's neurologic status deteriorates or tracheal intubation is required to secure the airway and provide ventilation and oxygenation, the patient is given an anesthetizing dose of a barbituate or benzodiazepine and a muscle relaxant, to facilitate placement of the ET tube. The barbiturate of choice usually is sodium pentothal, and the muscle relaxant of choice usually is succinylcholine, to provide immediate airway access with a rapid-sequence technique. As soon as the airway is secured, further sedation or paralysis, or both, are provided so that a CT scan can be immediately obtained. As with nasopharyngeal airways, noted above, NT intubation is contraindicated.

Status epilepticus requires immediate pharmacologic therapy. As with adults, the first-line therapy is a benzodiazepine, such as diazepam or lorazepam (Ativan). Once the seizures have stopped, it is essential that a loading dose of an appropriate longer-acting antiepileptic drug be given. The most frequently used drugs for this purpose are phenobarbital and phenytoin. Because the combined use of diazepam and phenobarbital causes synergistic respiratory depression, the use of lorazepam plus phenytoin in the immediate postseizure period is gaining popularity. Phenytoin, in combination with the benzodiazepine, will produce less immediate respiratory depression and also will allow for better assessment of the postictal state.

If initial attempts at pharmacologic therapy are unsuccessful in stopping status epilepticus, tracheal intubation often is pursued, even in the presence of adequate ventilation and oxygenation, for airway protection and for facilitation of much higher doses of drug therapy. Intravenous bolus injection of barbiturates and other respiratory depressants to near-toxic levels often may be required and necessitates prophylactic airway management.

REFERENCES

1. Leestma JE, Walczak T, Hughes JR, et al: A prospective study on sudden unexpected death in epilepsy. *Ann Neurol* 1989; 26:195–203.
2. Terrence CS, Ral GR, Perrper GA: Neurogenic pulmonary edema in unexpected and unexplained death of epileptic patients. *Ann Neurol* 1981; 9:458.

---

*This section was prepared by William W. Feaster, M.D.

3. Simon RP: Physiologic consequences of status epilepticus. *Epilepsia* 1985; 26(suppl 1):58.

4. Aminoff MJ, Simon RP: Status epilepticus: Causes, clinical features and consequences in 98 patients. *Am J Med* 1980; 69:657–666.

5. Janz D: Status epilepticus and frontal lobe lesions. *J Neurol Sci* 1964; 1:446–457.

6. Orringer CE, Eustace JC, Wunsch CD, et al: Natural history of lactic acidosis after grand mal seizures. *N Engl J Med* 1977; 297:796–799.

7. Wachtel TJ, Steele GH, Day JA: Natural history of fever following seizure. *Arch Intern Med* 1987; 147:1153–1155.

8. Meldrum BS, Vigouroux RA, Brierley JB: Systemic factors and epileptic brain damage. *Arch Neurol* 1973; 29:82–87.

34

Croup and Epiglottitis

Jonathan T. Clarke, M.D.

William W. Feaster, M.D.

There is a small margin for error in the management of pediatric airway emergencies. Croup and epiglottitis are the most common causes of acute upper airway obstruction in children. These two diseases can be differentiated by their history of onset, physical examination, and radiographic appearance. Both, however, may lead to a rapid deterioration of the airway and respiratory failure or arrest.

CROUP
(LARYNGOTRACHEOBRONCHITIS)

This disease impacts on the pediatric airway primarily because of the anatomic differences of the subglottic region in children. The pediatric airway is characterized by delicate mucosa with loose submucosal tissue which tends to accumulate edema fluid freely, and by floppy and compliant laryngeal tissues which tend to collapse with turbulent flow and exaggerated negative intrapleural pressure.[1] Moreover, for at least the first 6 years of life, the narrowest part of the tracheal airway in children is the cricoid ring, a circular cartilage just below the thyroid cartilage. The cricoid cartilage encircles the airway and creates a fixed narrowing. When the mucosal and submucosal tissues are injured or inflamed, swelling occurs, with further narrowing of the airway. The child presents with upper airway obstructive symptoms which may include stridor, retractions, tachypnea, and tachycardia.

Croup typically presents between the ages of 3 months and 3 years, but is most life-threatening in the first 2 years of life, when the airway is the most vulnerable. Croup begins most commonly with the symptoms of an upper respiratory infection, with coryza, cough, and fever, consistent with its usual viral etiology. The cough, which initially may have an associated wheeze or bronchitic component, assumes primarily a barking quality. As airway inflammation gives way to airway narrowing, stridor becomes the predominant symptom, first only during crying, then with every breath. An anteroposterior (AP) neck film shows the classic "steeple" sign, indicating a narrowed subglottic region (Fig 34–1). Infrequently, croup in children can progress to profound respiratory failure and even cardiac arrest.

EPIGLOTTITIS

Unlike croup, which is primarily a viral disease of young children, epiglottitis has a bacterial etiology and can be seen in adults as well as in children. The peak incidence of epiglottitis is between the ages of 2 and 7 years, but it has been reported in patients ranging in age from 7 months to 90 years.[2] Epiglottitis is a rapidly progressive illness characterized by high fever, sore throat, and hoarseness, progressing to stridor, drooling, and air hunger. The child characteristically will have a postural preference: sitting, leaning forward, with the head in the sniffing position, and the mouth open. The diagnosis is based on the clinical presentation and the lateral neck film, rather than an airway examination. The lateral neck film shows the "thumb sign" of a swollen epiglottis, with indistinct aryepiglottic folds corresponding to severe inflammation and swelling of all the supraglottic structures (Fig 34–2). The most important characteristic not to forget: epiglottitis can rapidly

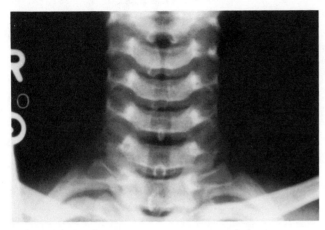

FIG 34–1.
Classis "steeple" sign indicates a narrowed subglottic region.

and unpredictably progress to complete airway obstruction.[3–5] Airway protection with an endotracheal tube is paramount.

BACTERIAL TRACHEITIS

Bacterial tracheitis has features of both croup and epiglottitis: there is often a prodrome of mild upper respiratory symptoms, followed by rapidly progressive stridor, high fever and toxic symptoms, and a barky cough.[6] The age of the child ranges from infancy to early adolescence. Examination of the trachea reveals a red, swollen mucosa covered with thick, copious pus. The AP and lateral neck films can look just like croup, but the purulent debris can give a shaggy tracheal wall border and even be confused with a foreign body. Intubation is re-

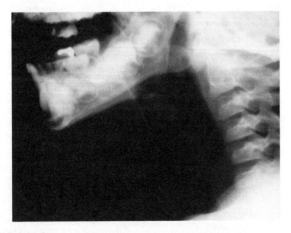

FIG 34–2.
"Thumb sign" of a swollen epiglottis shows severe inflammation and swelling of all supraglottic structures.

quired to maintain a patent airway much more frequently than is required with croup.[7]

DIFFERENTIAL DIAGNOSIS

Since therapeutic interventions differ for croup and for epiglottitis, it is important to make an accurate diagnosis. A history of a gradual-onset viral-like illness with low-grade fever, cough, and hoarse voice favors the diagnosis of croup. Epiglottitis is characterized by abrupt onset of toxic symptoms of high fever (>39° C), lethargy, irritability, sore throat, and muffled voice.

If the diagnosis is unclear in a child with only mild or moderate respiratory distress, AP and lateral neck films can be helpful.[4] However, in a child with significant respiratory distress from impending upper airway obstruction, it is unnecessary and potentially dangerous to stress the child and to take the time to get radiographs.[8]

Croup and epiglottitis can be confused with other, less common, infectious causes of upper airway obstruction. Bacterial tracheitis should be considered in the child who has a croupy cough and hoarse voice but also has high fever, toxicity, and worsening stridor that may not respond to racemic epinephrine aerosols. Infections in the pharynx, such as tonsillitis or peritonsillar abscess in the older child or retropharyngeal abscess in the younger child (infancy to 3 years), also can cause progressive upper airway obstruction.

Foreign body aspiration and lower airway disease can also produce symptoms of upper airway obstruction. Classically, children with foreign body aspiration are 6 months to 4 years old and have a history of a sudden choking episode, followed by coughing or respiratory distress. However, in at least a third of cases, there is no such history.[1] There can be a silent period followed by a gradual progression of respiratory symptoms mimicking epiglottitis, croup, or asthma, depending on the location and type of foreign body. Children with lower airway disease, such as bronchiolitis and asthma, who are in severe respiratory distress, sometimes can be challenging in the differentiation from children with croup.

Scenario 1: Croup With Mild Respiratory Compromise

With a mild narrowing of the subglottic airway, airflow is preserved but symptoms of a croupy cough and mild stridor dominate. Agitation increases stridor, so therapeutic interventions should be minimal or atraumatic.

The child is alert and has good airway reflexes. Skin color is pink in room air. The breath sounds are normal with good aeration, and the child has only mild retractions, if any. Stridor is heard only on inspiration and not at all when the child falls asleep. Cool mist therapy reduces the cough and stridor associated with croup. Invasive tests, such as arterial blood gas (ABG) determinations, are not needed. In fact, any unnecessary maneuvers, such as trying to put an oxygen mask on a young child, are counterproductive because they induce agitation and worsen stridor. Mist can be delivered in a hood or tent, or simply blown by the face with corrugated tubing.

Management

Most of these children can be managed with only routine supportive therapy (mist, decongestants, fever control) and parent education. If the symptoms progress, with harsh breath sounds, increased retractions, and worsening stridor, see the next scenario.

Scenario 2: Croup With Moderate Respiratory Distress

As subglottic narrowing worsens, airflow becomes compromised, leading to stridor at rest, sometimes on both inspiration and exhalation. On chest examination there are retractions, tachypnea, and poor air entry. Oxygenation can become an issue. The least traumatic method of monitoring is with the pulse oximeter. Supplementing mist with oxygen is certainly indicated. Racemic epinephrine aerosols may be used to constrict the blood vessels to the subglottic area and reduce the narrowing and edema formation. If racemic epinephrine is used, the disease is severe enough to warrant close observation in the emergency department or hospital ward for a minimum of 6 hours, because the duration of effect of racemic epinephrine varies from a few minutes to several hours, and after the effect wears off, the child can deteriorate quite rapidly. Racemic epinephrine aerosols should improve the symptoms of croup at least transiently. If they do not improve the symptoms significantly, consider other diagnoses, such as bacterial tracheitis.

Management

Racemic epinephrine is the front-line therapy for croup. Children with significant respiratory distress often require frequent treatments, as often as

every hour, or even continuous therapy. These children require intensive care unit (ICU) observation and monitoring. Also, it would be difficult to argue against the use of steroids with this type of patient. Steroid therapy with this disease has been controversial. There is no evidence that steroids are helpful in viral croup, but in severe cases a short course of high-dose steroids appears to be safe and is often used.[3, 9, 10]

Children with moderate respiratory distress need an intravenous line to provide hydration and, if necessary, to provide access for medications to facilitate intubation. If the child is unstable, oral feeding is stopped to assure an empty stomach in case intubation is subsequently required. If the child is stable, clear liquids are acceptable.

Supplemental oxygen is delivered with mist in all cases. Hiding an unstable child in a frosted mist tent may be unwise. All patients' oxygenation should be monitored with a pulse oximeter. Ventilation is assessed subjectively by following air entry and respiratory rate. Airway reflexes remain intact unless severe obtundation from carbon dioxide retention is present. If the clinical findings progress to more severe stridor and ventilatory insufficiency, demonstrated by decreased aeration, CO_2 retention, and cyanosis, see the next scenario.

Scenario 3: Croup With Severe Respiratory Distress

As the subglottic airway becomes critically narrowed, stridor is severe on inspiration and expiration, or it can even be diminished as air entry becomes markedly decreased. Retractions are severe with use of accessory muscles. Skin color is dusky or cyanotic. Fatigue or CO_2 retention can cause the child to fall asleep. In the case of CO_2 retention, air movement on examination is severely compromised and hypoxemia may be present.

If the child does not immediately improve with a racemic epinephrine aerosol, intubation in order to bypass airway obstruction is required. Such an intubation may be extremely difficult and should be performed by an anesthesiologist, if possible, with a surgeon at hand to provide a surgical airway if needed.

The supraglottic anatomy is normal in croup and visualization of the cords is not affected. The difficulty is in passing the tube below the vocal cords through a narrow subglottic region. If clinically and radiologically the diagnosis is clearly croup, anesthesia with thiopental (Pentothal) and succinylcholine in the emergency department will facilitate intubation. Prior to laryngoscopy, positive pressure ventilation with oxygen and racemic epinephrine, with a bag-valve-mask apparatus, often will prevent cardiac arrest from hypoxia during the intubation attempt. Several sizes of lubricated endotracheal tubes with stylets in place should be available for intubation, and a tube that is 1 mm inside diameter (ID) smaller than usual for the child's age should be used initially.

Management

If intubation attempts fail, a needle cricothyroidotomy with a 16-gauge intravenous over-the-needle catheter should be performed immediately. A 3.0-mm endotracheal tube connector will attach directly to the catheter to allow insufflation with high-pressure oxygen. Alternatively, a 3-mL syringe can be attached to the catheter, the plunger removed from the syringe, and an 8.0-mm endotracheal tube connector attached to the barrel of the syringe. Needle cricothyroidotomy is only a temporizing procedure. Secure airway control must be achieved as rapidly as possible with an endotracheal tube or formal tracheostomy.

Scenario 1: Epiglottitis With Mild to Moderate Respiratory Distress

Epiglottitis actually is "panglottitis" or supraglottitis, because the inflammation involves all of the supraglottic structures and the epiglottis is not always the most inflamed. The classic symptoms are the four D's: dysphagia, dysphonia, drooling, and inspiratory respiratory distress.[10] As soon as the diagnosis of epiglottitis is considered, the anesthesiologist, appropriate surgeon, and the operating room (OR) must be notified immediately. Do not wait until the diagnosis is confirmed. Remember that epiglottitis can rapidly and unpredictably progress to respiratory failure, so, until the airway is secured, the child must be constantly attended by a physician skilled in intubation.[11]

Routine treatment in some emergency departments includes ABG assessment for every patient with respiratory symptoms. Children with upper airway obstruction who are otherwise healthy actually do a good job of maintaining adequate tidal volumes for a while, until they fatigue and "crash"; thus, ABG values are unreliable predictors of severity or progression of upper airway obstruction. Furthermore, any invasive testing is contraindicated in these children until the airway is secure, because it can precipitate acute deterioration. The child should be minimally stimulated and allowed to assume a position of comfort (often sitting, leaning forward). Supplemental oxygen should be provided if the child accepts it.

Management

In many cases the diagnosis is clear from the clinical presentation, and no other tests are needed.[3, 5, 9, 10] If the diagnosis is not certain and the child is stable, a lateral neck film can be helpful. Oropharyngeal examination for visualization of the epiglottis should be performed only if the radiograph is equivocal and if emergency airway equipment is immediately available.

As soon as the diagnosis is made, the child should immediately be accompanied to the OR by the anesthesiologist, and a mask induction with halothane and oxygen begun. Children with suspected epiglottitis should not be managed conservatively. Attempting to treat a child with epiglottitis with just antibiotics and observation runs a significant risk of death or hypoxic brain damage.[10, 12] Except in the very mildest cases, the child will benefit from emergency endotracheal intubation in the OR by an anesthesiologist, with a surgeon skilled in endoscopy and tracheostomy standing by. In contrast, other invasive procedures, such as blood tests, should be delayed until after the airway is secured. The most important characteristic not to forget: epiglottitis can rapidly and unpredictably progress to complete airway obstruction.[3-5]

Scenario 2: Epiglottitis in Extremis

If a child develops complete airway obstruction, the priority is established by the standard ABCs of advanced cardiac life support (ACLS): clear the airway, and ventilate with oxygen with positive pressure, with bag-valve-mask apparatus. Protection of the airway from aspiration of gastric contents is not as high a priority as establishing an airway. Cricoid pressure can be employed, but care must be taken not to obstruct the airway. In the child with epiglottitis, even with apparent complete obstruction, gentle assisted positive pressure ventilation is often surprisingly easy. The inflamed supraglottic structures fall over the airway, obstructing it with a negative-pressure spontaneous breath. Positive pressure often can push air past the supraglottic obstruction. Sedation may be required, but laryngoscopy is performed without muscle relaxants, in case visualization of the larynx is totally obscured by the abnormality present. In this case, air moving through an obscured opening may create bubbling with secretions, which helps locate the laryngeal orifice. If the child is not breathing spontaneously, a squeeze on the chest will often produce enough air bubbles to show where to put the endotracheal tube. The child is intubated orally with a lubricated tube with a stylet, using with the initial pass a tube 1 mm ID smaller than

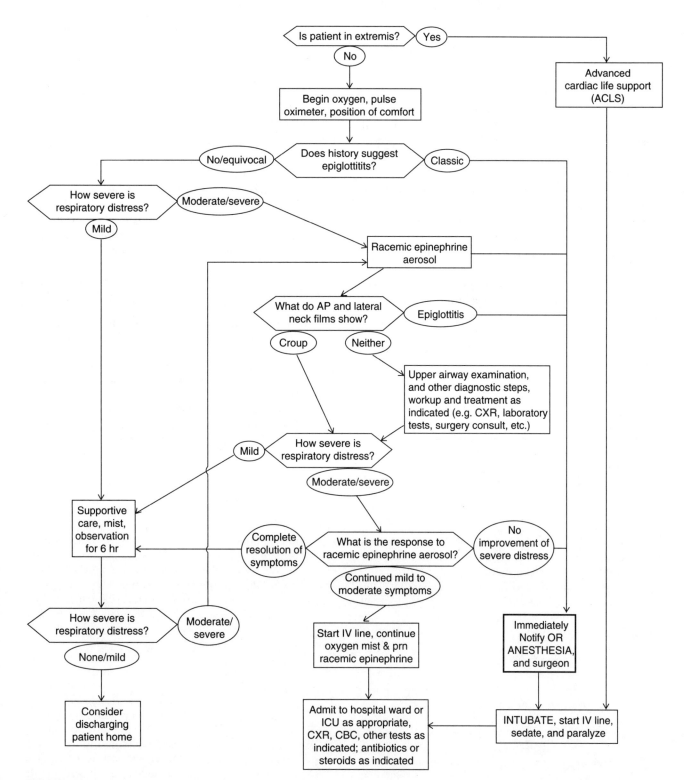

FIG 34–3.
Algorithm for airway management of the child with croup or epiglottitis.

normal for the child's age. If intubation attempts
fail, a needle cricothyroidotomy should be performed immediately, to temporize until the airway is
secured, as described above in the croup with severe
distress scenario.

Management

After the airway is established, a muscle relaxant
is given, the tube secured, and proper tube placement confirmed on the chest film. A nasogastric tube
is placed and the stomach emptied. Cultures of the
epiglottis and blood are sent, and antibiotics are
started. Cefuroxime or cefotaxime are recommended because they cover the most common causative organism, *Haemophilus influenzae* type B.

The child is taken to the ICU for ventilation and
monitoring. Paralysis and sedation are continued for
1 to 2 days. After repeat laryngoscopy to assure reduction of erythema and swelling, sedation is
stopped and the child is extubated.

An algorithm for airway management of the
child with croup or epiglottitis is presented in Figure
34–3.

REFERENCES

1. Downes JJ, Godinez RI: Acute upper-airway obstruction in the child, in Hershes S (ed): *ASA Refresher
Courses in Anesthesiology,* vol 8. Philadelphia, JB Lippincott Co, 1980, pp 29–48.

2. Singer JI, McCabe JB: Epiglottitis at the extremes of
age. *Am J Emerg Med* 1988; 6:228.
3. Kilham H, Gillis J, Benjamin B: Severe upper airway
obstruction. *Pediatr Clin North Am* 1987; 34:1.
4. Deeb ZE: Approach to supraglottitis. *Emerg Med Clin
North Am* 1987; 5:353.
5. Kronick JB, Kissoon N, Frewen TC: Guidelines for
stabilizing the condition of the critically ill child before transfer to a tertiary care facility. *Can Med Assoc
J* 1988; 139:213.
6. McNamara RM, Altreuter RW, Malone DR: Bacterial
tracheitis: A resurfacing airway emergency. *Am J
Emerg Med* 1987; 5:224.
7. Zalzal GH: Stridor and airway compromise. *Pediatr
Clin North Am* 1989; 36:1389.
8. Cote CJ, Todres ID: The pediatric airway, in Ryan
JF, et al (eds): *A Practice of Anesthesia for Infants and
Children.* Orlando, Fla, Grune & Stratton Inc, 1986,
pp 35–57.
9. Davis HW, Gartner JC, Galvis AG, et al: Acute upper
airway obstruction: Croup and epiglottitis. *Pediatr
Clin North Am* 1981; 28:859.
10. Diaz JH: Croup and epiglottitis in children: The anesthesiologist as diagnostician. *Anesth Analg* 1985;
64:621.
11. Kimmons HC, Peterson BM: Management of acute
epiglottitis in pediatric patients. *Crit Care Med* 1986;
14:278.
12. Vernon DD, Sarnaik AP: Acute epiglottitis in children: A conservative approach to diagnosis and management. *Crit Care Med* 1986; 14:23.

Appendix

Ventilator Settings

Herbert Rogove, D.O.

TERMINAL SHOCK AND CARDIOPULMONARY ARREST

Rationale

The resuscitation of the postcardiac arrest and shock patient should include respiratory support to ensure adequate oxygenation and ventilation for the low flow state. Attention should also be directed toward minimizing the work of breathing and consequently oxygen utilization to ensure optimal support of cardiac function.

Settings

Mode: Patients seem to tolerate the assist-control mode of ventilation or even an SIMV mode as long as the required minute ventilation is delivered.
Tidal volume: 12–15 mL/kg.
Ventilatory rate: Adjusted to maintain arterial $PaCO_2$ and pH within a normal range. An initial rate of 12 breaths per minute is acceptable.
FiO_2: Start at 100% and ultimately wean to 50% as soon as the patient's hemodynamics and gas exchange are stabilized.
Other: PEEP should be added if hypoxemia persists despite 100% FiO_2.

FACIAL AND NECK TRAUMA

Rationale

Protection of the airway is the main concern and greatest threat to patient survival. Associated bleeding and edema may cause asphyxia, induce cardiac arrest, or result in aspiration.

Settings

Mode: Patients may be ventilated either in the assist-control or SIMV mode depending upon how effortless the patient's work of breathing appears.
Tidal volume: 12–15 mL/kg.
Ventilatory rate: Should be adjusted so that the arterial pH and $PaCO_2$ are compatible.
FiO_2: Start at 100% FiO_2 and titrate to 50% or less to maintain an $SaO_2 \geq 90\%$.

HEAD INJURY AND PRESUMED INCREASE IN ICP

Rationale

The clinician should provide for adequate oxygen exchange in a severely injured and hypoxic brain. Hyperventilation will help to control cerebral blood flow and elevation of ICP.

Settings

Mode: Patients should initially be placed in the assist-control mode of ventilation.
Tidal volume: Start at 12 mL/kg in an attempt to minimize an increase in transpulmonary and ultimately intracranial pressures. The tidal volume can be maximized at 15 mL/kg, but the potential exists for increasing ICP.
Ventilatory rate: Should be titrated at a level to maintain $PaCO_2$ at 25–30 mm Hg. Starting at a rate of 12 breaths per minute is a reasonable initial setting.
FiO_2: Should be maintained initially at 100% and then titrated to maintain a PaO_2 >100 mm Hg. This will optimize the chance of providing adequate oxygenation in a state of injured and edematous cerebral tissue.
Other: Sedation and paralysis may be indicated if the patient is agitated, but only after an examination by the appropriate neurosurgeon or neurologist.

CHEST INJURY

Rationale

Patients with blunt chest injuries usually have associated rib fractures and often a lung contusion. It is the underlying lung contusion rather than a flail chest that often creates difficulty with oxygenation. Also, pain may cause splinting-induced hypoventilation.

Settings

Mode: Some patients, particularly younger ones, can be successfully managed by using face CPAP. If intubation is required, placing the patient on assist-control mode and sedating will often improve oxygenation and chest wall stabilization.

Tidal volume: 12–15 mL/kg should suffice.

Ventilatory rate: 10–12 breaths per minute to initiate ventilator support is appropriate. Subsequent arterial blood gases can be utilized for further adjustment.

FiO_2: If the initial blood gases are not available, begin at 100% FiO_2 and titrate to 50% as the patient stabilizes.

Other: CPAP or PEEP should be instituted at 5 cm H_2O until a satisfactory SaO_2 is attained (usually ≥90%). Levels can be increased by 2–5 cm H_2O.

AIRWAY BURNS: CHEMICAL AND THERMAL

Rationale

The patient's upper airway should be directly visualized to evaluate the extent of injury. Utilizing a bronchoscope may enable the clinician to pass an endotracheal tube over the bronchoscope quickly and easily. A major goal is to maintain airway control.

Settings

Mode: The patient, if awake and of reasonable prior health, can be placed immediately on SIMV both as a mode of ventilation and means to wean when appropriate.

Tidal volume: 12–15 mL/kg.

Ventilatory rate: If the patient has only the burn as the major problem and looks as though he or she will wean easily, an SIMV rate of 6 breaths per minute may be all that is needed. If, however, the patient has preexisting lung disease, other system problems, or is malnourished, then a less stressful rate of 12 breaths per minute can be initiated. Subsequent arterial blood gases will help to make additional changes.

FiO_2: If hypoxemia is a major problem, then starting at an FiO_2 of 100% is acceptable. For those patients who are not hypoxemic and require airway management primarily for protection, an FiO_2 starting at 50% will be sufficient.

Other: If aspiration begins to cause hypoxemia, PEEP should be added. It is important to understand that prophylactic PEEP does *not* prevent acute lung injury.

ATRAUMATIC ACUTE UPPER AIRWAY OBSTRUCTION

Rationale

Acute upper airway obstruction may occur secondary to anatomic swelling from causes such as anaphylaxis, drug reaction, or infections. Aspiration of a foreign body may also occlude major airways and will therefore require immediate removal.

Settings

Mode: For patients who are not intubated, if the airway is anatomically narrowed by swelling, the use of a mixture of helium (70%) and oxygen (30%) may help to initially provide for adequate oxygenation until a decision to intubate is made. Intubated patients may be best served by either SIMV or assist-control mode.

Tidal volume: 12–15 mL/kg.

Ventilatory rate: Depending upon the severity of the respiratory failure, the patient can be started at a rate of 6–12 breaths per minute on SIMV. Arterial blood gases and clinical examination will help to arrive at the best rate.

FiO_2: Only if oxygenation becomes a problem should an FiO_2 higher than 50% be utilized. Most patients do well with 50% or less.

ASTHMA

Rationale

Patients who develop status asthmaticus unresponsive to bronchodilators and steroids are at risk for acute respiratory failure and may require emergent intubation. Severe bronchospasm occurs, and the tracheobronchial tree is filled with inspissated secretions which prevent adequate ventilation.

Settings

Mode: Patients should be immediately sedated and placed on assist-control mode. If, despite sedation, agitation continues, then start the patient on a paralyzing agent along with sedation.

Tidal volume: 12–15 mL/kg.

Ventilatory rate: A rate starting at 12 breaths per minute is titrated until the respiratory acidemia is corrected and the $PaCO_2$ begins to decline.

FiO_2: Starting at 100% FiO_2 and titrating to 50% or less is a reasonable goal once adequate ventilation is attained.

Other: Ensure adequate humidification in consultation with the respiratory therapist.

COPD

Rationale

Acute respiratory failure in a patient with COPD is frequently due to either infection or cor pulmonale. Looking for a cause is extremely important so that the appropriate therapeutic modalities (i.e., antibiotics or inotropic support) can be started immediately.

Settings

Mode: Place the patient on either SIMV or assist-control mode to support ventilation.

Tidal volume: 12–15 mL/kg.

Ventilatory rate: Should adjust the rate to normalize pH. Remember that *overcorrecting* the $PaCO_2$ to normal in a patient who usually retains $PaCO_2$ may cause significant acid-base alterations.

FiO_2: The occasional patient with advanced disease usually tolerates an SaO_2 even slightly lower than 90%; however, during the acute event, a level of 90% or greater is safe.

Other: PEEP should be avoided unless the patient has an acute lung injury with bilateral infiltrates or refractory hypoxemia.

WHITE-OUT LUNG

Rationale

Acute lung injury from multiple causes results in a noncompliant or stiff lung. Aggressive measures to minimize fluid overload and support the patient's hemodynamics are mandatory. Patients may progress quickly from an early state of a normal PaO_2 and $PaCO_2$ to severe hypoxemia and hypercapnia. Intrapulmonary shunting is a major defect.

Settings

Mode: Depending upon the patient's underlying condition, the patient may tolerate CPAP or SIMV as an initial mode of therapy. Assist-control may be needed if either of the previous modes fail.

Tidal volume: An initial setting of 12 mL/kg if significant levels (>10 cm H_2O) of PEEP are used. The rationale is to keep the peak airway pressures as low as possible and thereby avoid barotrauma.

Ventilatory frequency: A rate should be set at 10–12 breaths per minute with adjustments based upon blood gas measurement of pH and $PaCO_2$.

FiO_2: Start at 100% FiO_2 in all patients and decrease to 50% or less as the patient responds to therapy.

Other: PEEP is one of the mainstays of treatment. Start at 5 cm H_2O and increase by 2–5 cm H_2O. Hemodynamic monitoring may be required if high levels of PEEP are employed.

OVERDOSES

Rationale

Oversedation from drug overdose may cause respiratory depression and inability to clear secretions. Loss of airway security and the potential for aspiration are high.

Settings

Mode: If a patient is having difficulty initiating spontaneous respirations, a reasonable level of SIMV or assist-control mode will support the patient until he or she is awake. Arterial blood gases will help to guide therapy.

Tidal volume: 12–15 mL/kg.

Ventilatory rate: 12 breaths per minute can be adjusted according to subsequent arterial blood gases. In cases of tricyclic overdose, the rate should be adjusted to keep the pH at 7.50 or greater.

FiO_2: Start at 100% and begin to decrease to 50% according to the patient's tolerance. Utilization of pulse oximetry may be helpful.

Other: If the patient aspirates, has diffuse bilateral infiltrates, and is beginning to require an increase in FiO_2, consider starting 5 cm H_2O of PEEP.

CARDIAC PULMONARY EDEMA

Rationale

The hypoxemia of cardiogenic pulmonary edema is the result of ventilation-perfusion mismatching and a small increase in intrapulmonary right-to-left shunting. Because of the accumulation of interstitial edema, the lungs become less compliant and therefore hypoxemia is accompanied by an increased work of breathing (tachypnea and abnormal ventilatory pattern).

Settings

Mode: The patient may be placed in the SIMV mode. If the patient is extremely dyspneic and cannot decrease the work of breathing by an adequate SIMV, then switching to an assist-control mode may afford ventilatory relief.

Tidal volume: 12–15 mL/kg.

Ventilatory rate: Should be started at about 12 breaths per minute and titrated upward by clinical response (decrease in tachypnea) and arterial blood gases (avoid hyperventilation and associated alkalosis).

FiO_2: Begin at 100% and titrate to 50% to maintain SaO_2 >90%.

Other: PEEP may be added to attain a 50% FiO_2. This modality mainly benefits the cardiac patient because it may decrease left ventricular afterload.

GRAND MAL SEIZURES

Rationale

The seizure itself may result in loss of respiratory mechanics due to tonic contractions and also alteration of respiratory pattern such as apnea and Cheyne-Stokes respiration. Sympathetic discharge during seizures may manifest as an increase in secretions. Loss of airway protection may predispose to aspiration.

Settings

Mode: Patients may be placed in either the SIMV or assist-control mode.
Tidal volume: 12–15 mL/kg.
Ventilatory rate: Should initially be set at 12 breaths per minute and adjusted to patient response evaluated by respiratory rate, pattern of ventilatory ease, and arterial blood gases.
FiO_2: Should start at 100% and titrate to 50% or less as soon as the patient's SaO_2 stabilizes at >90%.

Index